T AND B LYMPHOCYTES:
RECOGNITION AND FUNCTION

Academic Press Rapid Manuscript Reproduction

Proceedings of the 1979 ICN–UCLA Symposia on
Molecular and Cellular Biology held in Keystone,
Colorado, March 25–30, 1979

ICN–UCLA Symposia on Molecular and Cellular Biology
Volume XVI, 1979

T AND B LYMPHOCYTES: RECOGNITION AND FUNCTION

edited by

FRITZ H. BACH
Immunology Research Center
University of Wisconsin
Madison, Wisconsin

BENJAMIN BONAVIDA
Department of Microbiology and Immunology
University of California, Los Angeles
Los Angeles, California

ELLEN S. VITETTA
Department of Microbiology
University of Texas Southwestern Medical School
Dallas, Texas

C. FRED FOX
Department of Microbiology and Molecular Biology
University of California, Los Angeles
Los Angeles, California

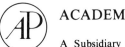

ACADEMIC PRESS   1979

A Subsidiary of Harcourt Brace Jovanovich, Publishers

New York   London   Toronto   Sydney   San Francisco

ACADEMIC PRESS, INC.
111 Fifth Avenue, New York, New York 10003

United Kingdom Edition published by
ACADEMIC PRESS, INC. (LONDON) LTD.
24/28 Oval Road, London NW1 7DX

ISBN 0-12-069850-1

PRINTED IN THE UNITED STATES OF AMERICA

79 80 81 82   9 8 7 6 5 4 3 2 1

CONTENTS

C. T- AND B-CELL MARKERS AND DIFFERENTIATIONS

II. TRIGGERING AND TOLERANCE VIA RECEPTOR INTERACTIONS

A. EARLY EVENTS IN LYMPHOCYTE ACTIVATION

B. ROLE OF SURFACE IMMUNOGLOBULIN AND OF ANTIGEN
      RECEPTORS WITH B-CELL TRIGGERING AND TOLERANCE

C. ROLE OF ANTIGEN BINDING CELLS IN THE IMMUNE RESPONSE

CONTRIBUTORS

Numbers in parentheses refer to chapter numbers

ACTON, RONALD T. (52), Department of Microbiology, University of Alabama, Birmingham, Alabama 35294

ADORINI. LUCIANO (21, 44), Department of Microbiology, University of California, Los Angeles, California 90024

AHMANN, GERALD B. (35), National Cancer Institute, Bethesda, Maryland 20205

AHMED, AFTAB (12, 13), Naval Medical Research Institute, Bethesda, Maryland 20014

ALTER, BARBARA J. (56), Immunobiology Research Center, University of Wisconsin, Madison, Wisconsin 53706

AMOS, D. BERNARD (66), Duke University Medical Center, Durham, North Carolina 27710

ANDERSSON R. (47), Department of Immunology, Uppsala University Biomedical Center, Uppsala, S-751 23, Sweden

ASHMAN, ROBERT F. (20, 22), Department of Microbiology and Immunology, University of California, Los Angeles, California 90024

ASOFSKY, RICHARD (11), National Institutes of Health, Bethesda, Maryland 20205

BACH, BRUCE ALLEN (38), Department of Pathology, Harvard Medical School, Boston, Massachusetts 02115

BACH, FRITZ H. (5, 10, 56), Immunobiology Research Center, University of Wisconsin, Madison, Wisconsin 53706

BAKER, P. E. (68), Hematology Research Laboratory, Dartmouth Medical School, Hanover, New Hampshire 03755

BALDWIN, R. W. (64), Cancer Research Campaign Laboratories, University of Nottingham, England

BENACERRAF, BARUJ (38), Department of Pathology, Harvard Medical School, Boston, Massachusetts

BENJAMIN, CHRISTOPHER D. (44), Department of Microbiology, University of California, Los Angeles, California 90024

BENJAMIN, DAVID (58), Department of Biology, City of Hope National Medical Center, Duarte, California 91010

BINZ, H. (47), Institute of Medical Mikrobiologie, University of Zurich, Zurich, Switzerland

BLACK, PAUL L. (51), Department of Microbiology, University of Texas Health Science Center, Dallas, Texas 75235

BONA, COSTANTIN (45, 46), Laboratory of Immunology, National Institutes of Health, Bethesda, Maryland 20014

BONAVIDA, BENJAMIN (49, 60), Department of Microbiology and Immunology, University of California, Los Angeles, California 90024

BRENAN, MARY (58), Transplantation Biology Unit, Clinical Research Center, Watford Road, Harrow, Middlesex HA1 3UJ, England

BRENNAN, CAROLE(16), National Institutes of Health, Bethesda, Maryland 20014

BROWN, ALAN R. (38), Department of Pathology, Brandeis University, Waltham, Massachusetts 02154

BURAKOFF, S. (65), Department of Pathology, Harvard Medical School, Boston, Massachusetts 02115

BYERS, V. S. (64), Department of Dermatology, University of California, School of Medicine, San Francisco, California 94143

CAPRA, J. DONALD (4, 6), Department of Microbiology, University of Texas, Southwestern Medical School, Dallas, Texas 75235

CECKA, J. MICHAEL (37), Department of Zoology, University College, London WC1, England

CHAN, CHRISTINA (43), Laboratory of Immunology, National Institutes of Health, Bethesda, Maryland 20205

CHEN, C. (28), National Institutes of Health, Bethesda, Maryland 20014

CHRISTADOSS, PREMKUMAR (26), Department of Immunology, Mayo Clinic, Rochester, Minnesota 55901

CLARKE, JESSICA ANNE (21), Department of Microbiology, University of California, Los Angeles, California 90024

CLEMENT, LORAN (43), Laboratory of Immunology, National Institutes of Health, Bethesda, Maryland 20205

COLLAVO, DINO (71), Genetics Unit, Institute of Pathological Anatomy, University of Padua, Padua, Switzerland

COOK, RICHARD G. (4), Department of Microbiology, University of Texas, Southwestern Medical School, Dallas, Texas 75235

COSENZA, HUMBERTO (37), Basel Institute for Immunology, Basel, Switzerland

COUDERC, JACQUES (21), Department of Microbiology, University of California, Los Angeles, California 90024

CRUMPTON, MICHAEL J. (1), National Institute for Medical Research, Mill Hill, London NW7 1AA, United Kingdom

CUNNINGHAM, ALASTAIR J. (27), Ontario Cancer Institute, University of Toronto, Toronto, Ontario, Canada M4X 1K9

DAVID, CHELLA S. (26, 37), Department of Immunology, Mayo Clinic, Rochester, Minnesota 55901

DENNERT, GUNTHER (69), Department of Cancer Biology, The Salk Institute for Biological Studies, San Diego, California 92112

DIENER, ERWIN (23, 41), Department of Immunology, University of Alberta, Edmonton, Alberta, Canada T6G 1H7

DOCKRELL, HAZEL (18), Department of Immunology, Middlesex Hospital Medical School, London, England

DOHERTY, PETER C. (55), The Wistar Institute, Philadelphia, Pennsylvania 19104

DUTTON, R. W. (34), Department of Biology, University of California, at San Diego, La Jolla, California 92093

EL-GAMIL, MONA (2), Immunology Branch, National Cancer Institute, Bethesda, Maryland 20205

ENGERS, HOWARD (71), Department of Immunology, Swiss Institute for Experimental Cancer Research, CH-1066 Epalinges Lausanne, Switzerland

ERB, PETER (37), Institute of Medical Microbiology, University of Basel, Basel, Switzerland

FATHMAN, C. G. (61), Department of Immunology, Mayo Clinic, Rochester, Minnesota 55901

FELDMANN, MARC (37), Department of Zoology, University College, London WC1, England

FESTENSTEIN, HILLIARD (63), Department of Immunology, London Hospital Medical College, London E1 2AD, England

FINBERG, R. (65), Department of Pathology, Harvard Medical School, Boston, Massachusetts 02115

FISCHER LINDAHL, KIRSTEN (63), Basel Institute for Immunology, Grenzacherstrasse 487, CH-4058 Basel, Switzerland

FLIEGER, N. (54), Irvington House Institute, New York University Medical Center, New York, New York 10016

FORMAN, J. (51), Department of Microbiology, University of Texas, Health Science Center, Dallas, Texas 75235

FRISCHKNECHT, H. (47), Institute of Medical Microbiologie, University of Zurich, Zurich, Switzerland

GERSHON, R. K. (62), Section of Comparative Medicine, Yale University School of Medicine, New Haven, Connecticut 06510

GILLIS, STEVEN (68), Hematology Research Laboratory, Dartmouth Medical School, Hanover, New Hampshire 03755

GIORGI, JANIS V. (72), Immunobiology Laboratories, University of New Mexico, Albuquerque, New Mexico 87131

GIVOL, DAVID (50), Department of Chemical Immunology, Weizmann Institute, Rehovot, Israel

GOLUB, SID (63), Department of Bacteriology, University of California, Los Angeles, California 90024

GOODMAN, JOEL W. (48), Department of Microbiology and Immunology, University of California, San Francisco, California 94143

GRANGER, G. A. (49), Department of Microbiology and Immunology, University of California, Los Angeles, California 90024

GREENE, MARK IRWIN (38), Department of Pathology, Harvard Medical School, Boston, Massachusetts 02115

GRONOWICZ, EVA (19), Immunology Division, Stanford University, Stanford, California

HAAS, WERNER (71), Basel Institute of Immunology, Basel, Switzerland

HARVEY, M. A. (44), Department of Microbiology, University of California, Los Angeles, California 90024

HATHCOCK, KAREN S. (35), National Cancer Institute, Bethesda, Maryland 20205

HAYAKAWA, KYOKO (32, 40), Department of Immunology, University of Tokyo, Tokyo, Japan

HAYES, COLLEEN E. (10), Immunobiology Research Center, University of Wisconsin, Madison, Wisconsin 53706

HENGARTNER, H. (61), Department of Immunology, Mayo Clinic, Rochester, Minnesota 55901

HENGARTNER HANS (71), Basel Institute of Immunology, Basel, Switzerland

HENKART, PIERRE (67), Immunology Branch National Institutes of Health, Bethesda, Maryland 20205

HOWIE, SARAH (37), Basel Institute for Immunology, Basel, Switzerland

HENLEY, SUSANNE L. (52), Department of Microbiology, University of Alabama, Birmingham, Alabama 35294

HISERODT, JOHN C. (49), Department of Microbiology and Immunology, University of California, Los Angeles, California 90024

HODES, RICHARD J. (35), National Cancer Institute, Bethesda, Maryland 20205

HORNBECK, PETER V. (48), Department of Microbiology and Immunology, University of California, San Francisco, California 94143

JAMES, ROGER (37), Department of Zoology, University College, London WC1, England

JANEWAY, CHARLES A. (18, 36, 62), Department of Pathology, Yale University School of Medicine, New Haven, Connecticut 06510

JOHNSTONE, ALAN P. (1), National Institute for Medical Research, Mill Hill, London NW7 1AA, England

JONES, BARRY (18), Department of Pathology, Yale University, New Haven, Connecticut 06510

JOHSSON, B. (47), Department of Immunology, Uppsala University Biomedical Center, Uppsala, S-751 23, Sweden

KANELLOPOULOS-LANGEVIN, COLETTE (11), Laboratory of Microbiological Immunity, National Institutes of Health, Bethesda, Maryland 20205

KANG, C.-Y. (51), Department of Microbiology, University of Texas Health Science Center, Dallas, Texas 75235

KANOWITH-KLEIN, SUSAN (20), Department of Microbiology and Immunology, University of California, Los Angeles, California 90024

KAPPLER, JOHN W. (39), Department of Microbiology, University of Rochester, Rochester, New York 14642

KATZ, DAVID H. (33), Scripps Clinic and Research Foundation, La Jolla, California 92037

KELLER, DANIEL M. (39), Department of Microbiology, University of Rochester, Rochester, New York 14642

KESSLER, STEVEN (12), Naval Medical Research Institute, Bethesda, Maryland 20014

KIM, K. JIN (11), National Institutes of Health, Bethesda, Maryland 20205

KISZKISS, PATRICIA (2), Immunology Branch, National Cancer Institute, Bethesda, Maryland 20205

KOHLER, H. (8), La Ribida University of Chicago Institute, Chicago, Illinois 60649

KONTIAINEN, SIRKKA (37), Department of Bacteriology and Immunology, University of Helsinki, Helsinki, Finland

LAMBERT, EDWARD H. (26), Department of Immunology, Mayo Clinic, Rochester, Minnesota 55901

LASAROW, ELISABETH H. (27), Department of Microbiology and Immunology, University of California, Los Angeles, California 90024

LENNON, VANDA A. (26), Department of Immunology, Mayo Clinic, Rochester, Minnesota 55901

LEWIS, GEORGE K. (48), Department of Microbiology and Immunology, University of California, San Francisco, California 94143

LILLY, FRANK (57), Department of Genetics, Albert Einstein College of Medicine, Bronx, New York 10461

LIPSKY, PETER E. (30), Department of Internal Medicine, University of Texas Health Science Center, Dallas, Texas 75235

LUCAS, DAVID (19), Department of Microbiology, University of Arizona, Tucson, Arizona 85724

LUNNEY, JOAN K. (2), National Cancer Institute, Building 10, Room 4B17, Bethesda, Maryland 20205

MACY, ERIC M. (17), Department of Microbiology and Immunology, University of California, Los Angeles, California 90024

MAKELA, OLLI (16), National Institutes of Health, Bethesda, Maryland 20014

MANN, DEAN L. (2, 3), National Cancer Institute, Bethesda, Maryland 20205

MARCHALONIS, JOHN J. (50), Cancer Biology Program, Frederick Cancer Research Center, Frederick, Maryland 21701

MARGOLIASH, E. (28), National Institutes of Health, Bethesda, Maryland 20014

MARRACK, PHILIPPA (39), Department of Microbiology, University of Rochester, Rochester, New York 14642

MATSUNAGA, TAKESHI (58), Department of Biology, City of Hope, National Medical Center, Duarte, California 91010

MAURER, P. H. (28), National Institutes of Health, Bethesda, Maryland 20014

MAURER, PAUL (37), Department of Biochemistry, Jefferson Medical College, Philadelphia, Pennsylvania 19107

McCONNEL, HARDEN M. (67), Department of Chemistry, Stanford University, Stanford, California 94305

McDEVITT, H. O. (54), Irvington House Institute, New York University Medical Center, New York, New York 10016

McKEAN, DAVID J. (7), Department of Immunology, Mayo Clinic, Rochester, Minnesota 55901

McKENZIE, IAN F. C. (37, 71), Department of Medicine, Austin Hospital, Melbourne, Australia

MELCHERS, FRITZ (19), Institute for Immunology, Basel, Switzerland

MERRILL, JEAN E. (20), Department of Virology, Karolinska Institute, Stockholm, Sweden

MERRYMAN, C. F. (28), National Institutes of Health, Bethesda, Maryland 20014

MERUELO, DANIEL (54), Irvington House Institute, New York University Medical Center, New York, New York 10016

MESCHER, MATTHEW F. (65), Department of Pathology, Harvard Medical School, Boston, Massachusetts 02115

MILLER, ALEXANDER (21, 22, 44), Department of Microbiology, University of California, Los Angeles, California 90024

MITCHISON, N. A. (31), University College, Department of Tumor Biology, London WC1 6BT, England

MOCHIZUKI, DIANE (14), Department of Microbiology, University of California, Irvine, California 92717

MOLLER, GORAN (19), Immunobiology, Karolinska Institute, Stockholm, Sweden

MOND, JAMES J. (16), National Institutes of Health, Bethesda, Maryland 20014

NABHOLZ, MARKUS (71), Swiss Institute for Experimental Cancer Research, CH-1066 Epalinges Lausanne, Switzerland

NADLER, PAUL I. (35), National Cancer Institute, Bethesda, Maryland 20205

NAKOINZ, ILONA (15), Sloan-Kettering Institute, Rye, New York 10580

NATHENSON, STANLEY G. (6), Albert Einstein College of Medicine, Bronx, New York 10461

NISONOFF, ALFRED (38), Department of Pathology, Brandeis University, Waltham, Massachusetts 02154

NONAKA, M. (40), Department of Immunology, University of Tokyo, Hongo, Tokyo, Japan

NORTH, MARCEL (71), Genetics Unit, Swiss Institute for Experimental Cancer Research, CH-1066 Epalinges Lausanne, Switzerland

OI, VERNON T. (73), Department of Genetics, Stanford University School, Stanford, California 94305

OKUMURA, KO (32, 40), Department of Immunology, University of Tokyo, Hongo, Tokyo, Japan

O'TOOLE, MARGOT (29), Department of Pathology, Tufts University School of Medicine, Boston, Massachusetts 02111

OWENS, MICHAEL J. (1), National Institute for Medical Research, Mill Hill, London NW7 1AA, England

OZATO, KEIKO (2), National Cancer Institute, Bethesda, Maryland 20205

PAIGE, CHRISTOPHER J. (15), Sloan-Kettering Institute, Rye, New York 10580

PANFILI, P. R. (34), Department of Biology, University of California at San Diego, La Jolla, California 92093

PARISH, CHRIS (37), Department of Microbiology, John Curtin School of Medical Research, Canberra, Australia

PARKS, D. ELLIOT (24), Department of Immunopathology, Scripps Clinic and Research Foundation, La Jolla, California 92037

PAUL, W. E. (16), National Institutes of Health, Bethesda, Maryland 20014

PLATA, FERNANDO (57), Department of Genetics, Albert Einstein College of Medicine, Bronx, New York 105461

POTTER, MICHAEL (7), National Cancer Institute, Bethesda, Maryland 20014

RALPH, PETER (15), Sloan-Kettering Institute, Rye, New York 10580

REES, ANNE (37), Department of Zoology, University College, London WC1, England

SACHS, DAVID H. (2, 11, 59), Immunology Branch, National Cancer Institute, Bethesda, Maryland 20205

SAITO, T. (70), Laboratory for Immunology, Chiba University, Chiba, Japan

SCHER, IRWIN (12), Naval Medical Research Institute, Bethesda, Maryland 20014

SCHWARTZ, ANTHONY (62), Section of Comparative Medicine, Yale University School of Medicine, New Haven, Connecticut 06510

SCHWARTZ, RONALD (28), National Institute of Allergy and Infectious Diseases, National Institutes of Health, Bethesda, Maryland 20014

SERCARZ, ELI E. (21, 44), Department of Microbiology, University of California, Los Angeles, California 90024

SHEARER, GENE (60), Immunology Branch, National Cancer Institute, Bethesda, Maryland 20205

SHEN, F. W. (47), Sloan–Kettering Cancer Center, New York, New York 10021

SHERMAN, LINDA(65), Department of Cellular and Developmental Immunology, Scripps Clinic and Research Foundation, La Jolla, California 92037

SHEVACH, ETHAN M. (43), Laboratory of Immunology, National Institutes of Health, Bethesda, Maryland 20205

SHINOHARA, NOBUKATA, (2, 59), National Cancer Institute, Bethesda, Maryland 20205

SHIOZAWA, CHIAKI (391), Department of Immunology, University of Alberta, Edmonton, Alberta, Canada T6G 1H7

SIEGELMAN, MARK H. (4), Department of Microbiology, University of Texas Southwestern Medical School, Dallas, Texas 75235

SIMPSON, ELIZABETH (58, 73), Transplantation Biology Unit, Clinical Research Center, Watform Road, Harrow, Middlesex HA1 3UJ, England

SINGER, ALFRED(35), National Cancer Institute, Bethesda, Maryland 20205

SINGH, BHAGIRATH (23, 41), University of Alberta, Medical Science Building, Edmonton, Alberta, Canada T6G 2H7

SLAVIN, SHIMON (25), Department of Medicine, Hadassah Hebrew University School of Medicine, Jerusalem, Israel

SMITH, D. (54), Irvington House Institute, New York University Medical Center, New York, New York 10016

SMITH, K. A. (68), Hematology Research Laboratory, Dartmouth Medical School, Hanover, New Hampshire 03755

SOLINGER, A. M. (28), National Institutes of Health, Bethesda, Maryland 20014

SONIK, SIKANDER (41), Department of Immunology, University of Alberta, Edmonton, Alberta, Canada T6G 2H7

STEIN, KATHRYN E. (16), Laboratory of Immunology, National Institutes of Health, Bethesda, Maryland 20014

STEVENS, RONALD H. (17), Department of Microbiology and Immunology, University of California, Los Angeles, California 90024

STIMPFLING, J. H. (28), National Institutes of Health, Bethesda, Maryland 20014

STROBER, SAMUEL (13, 25), Stanford University School of Medicine, Stanford, California 94305

STUTMAN, OSIAS (9), Sloan–Kettering Institute for Cancer Research, New York, New York 10021

SWAIN, SUSAN L. (34), Department of Biology, University of California, San Diego, La Jolla, California 92093

SWIERKOSZ, JAMES E. (39), Department of Microbiology, University of Rochester School of Medicine and Dentistry, Rochester, New York 14642

SY, MAN-SUN (38), Department of Pathology, Harvard Medical School, Boston, Massachusetts 02115

TADA, TOMIO (32, 40, 70), Department of Immunology, University of Tokyo, Tokyo, Japan

TAKEI, I. (70), Laboratory for Immunology, Chiba University, Chiba City, Chiba, Japan

TANIGUCHI, MASARU (32, 70), Laboratory for Immunology, Chiba University, Chiba City, Chiba, Japan 280

THOMAN, MARILYN (14), Department of Immunopathology, Scripps Clinic and Research Foundation, La Jolla, California 92037

THOMAS, DAVID W. (43), Department of Pathology, The Jewish Hospital of St. Louis, St. Louis, Missouri 63110

TODD, IAN (37), Department of Zoology, University College, London WC1, England

TORANO, ALFREDO (37), Department of Zoology, University College, London WC1, England

UHR, JONATHAN W. (4, 51), Department of Microbiology, University of Texas Southwestern Medical School, Dallas, Texas 75235

ULTEE, M. E. (28), National Institutes of Health, Bethesda, Maryland 20014

VITETTA, ELLEN S. (4, 20, 51), Department of Microbiology, University of Texas Southwestern Medical School, Dallas, Texas 75235

VON BOEHMER, HARALD (71), Basel Institute of Immunology, Basel, Switzerland

WAGNER, H. (42), Institut für Medical Mikrobiologie, D-65 Mainz, West Germany

WARNER, NOEL L. (72), Immunobiology Laboratory, University of New Mexico, Albuquerque, New Mexico 87131

WATERFIELD, J. DOUGLAS (69), Department of Cancer Biology, Salk Institute for Biological Studies, San Diego, California 19211

WATERS, C. A. (23), University of Alberta, Edmonton, Alberta, Canada T6G 2H7

WATSON, ANDREW (5), Immunobiology Research Center, University of Wisconsin, Madison, Wisconsin 63706

WATSON, JAMES (14), Department of Microbiology, University of California, Irvine, California 92717

WEIGLE, WILLIAM O. (24, 27), Department of Immunopathology, Scripps Clinic and Research Foundation, La Jolla, California 92037

WEISSMAN, IRVING L. (55), Department of Pathology, Stanford University School of Medicine, Palo Alto, California 94305

WHISNANT, CAROL C. (66), Duke University Medical Center, Durham, North Carolina 27710

WIGZELL, H. (47), Department of Immunology, Uppsala University Biomedical Center, Uppsala S-751 23, Sweden

WILLIAMSON, A. R. (8), Department of Biochemistry, University of Glasgow, Glasgow G12 8QQ, Scotland

WILSON, DARCY (50), Department of Pathology, University of Pennsylvania School of Medicine, Philadelphia, Pennsylvania 19104

WINGER, LARRY (37), Department of Zoology, University College, London WC1, England

WISE, KIM S. (52), Department of Microbiology, University of Alabama, Birmingham, Alabama 35294

WOODY, J. N. (37), Immunology–Oncology Division, Georgetown University Medical School, Washington DC 20007

WORTIS, HENRY H. (29, 36), Department of Pathology, Tufts University School of Medicine, Boston, Massachusetts 02111

YAMAMOTO, HIROSHI (33), Institute for Cancer Research, Osaka University Medical School, Fukushima-ku, Osaka 553, Japan

YANO, A. (28), National Institutes of Health, Bethesda, Maryland 20014

ZARLING, DAVID A. (5), Immunobiology Research Center, University of Wisconsin, Madison, Wisconsin 53706

ZINKERNAGEL, ROLF M. (53), Department of Immunopathology, Scripps Clinic and Research Foundation, La Jolla, California 92037

PREFACE

The major raison d'être for the organization of this conference was to attempt to organize symposia and workshops that would deal with at least some of the areas of immunobiology in which progress at the molecular level was either already being made or in which systems seemed ripe for investigations at this level. Although description at any level is phenomenological, it seems clear that molecular definition of component parts of complex reactions would, in many cases, serve to clarify what at the moment are some of the most difficult areas to interpret. It seems to us that the active participation and contributions of our many colleagues who attended the meeting, in both the plenary sessions and the workshops, assured whatever success this meeting had in achieving this end. Certainly several areas of active investigation were presented and discussed in which our understanding is progressing at the molecular level. In addition, and perhaps more exciting (as the future always seems to be), model systems were presented that offer great promise for the "molecularization" of investigations in certain areas of immunobiology.

Central to many questions is, of course, our understanding of the cell membrane. This has been an area in which enormous progress has been made from some perspective and yet in which the enormity of problems, technical and conceptual, that remain seems almost overwhelming. The ability to study surface molecules following labeling and immunoprecipitation with respect to their primary sequence, degree of glycosylation, and their tertiary or quaternery structure is most encouraging and important. Techniques developed for determining whether membrane glycoproteins are "transmembrane" or not are paving the way for a presumed eventual understanding of the role of these molecules in cell activation and regulation. Thus, at the conference there was extensive presentation and discussion of the parameters just discussed with regard to the varied products of the major histocompatibility complex as well as other receptors on cells of the immune system. In addition, perhaps very importantly, attention is being turned to the changes in patterns of glycosylation as a cell is virally infected or differentiates.

One of the next orders of complexity deals with interactions between different molecules in the membrane of the same cell or between a molecule(s) in the membrane of one cell interacting with a molecule(s) in the membrane of, or secreted by, a second cell; this is an area around which several critical questions currently facing the immunobiologist revolve. Directly relating to this question are problems of associative recognition—the recognition by T-lymphocytes of a foreign determinant in association with a "self" major histocompatibility complex encoded molecule. Techniques such as capping have provided valuable information with regard to possible molecular associations but have left most investigators concerned about possible artifacts such as the "serological rake" effect of including in a "cap" molecules that are caught up in the antigen–antibody network that forms during capping. At least two approaches were discussed at the conference that would cause one to be optimistic that answers may soon be forthcoming at the molecular level regarding such molecular associations. First, the use of artificial membranes (lipid vesicles) for the incorporation of antigens such as those encoded by the major histocompatibility complex or such antigens plus virally determined molecules has already permitted certain conclusions regarding the molecular requirements for recognition by T-lymphocytes at both the afferent and efferent level. Second, chemical crosslinking of cell surface components with a variety of different crosslinking reagents should, conceptually, allow one to map "nearest-neighbors" of any molecule on the cell surface against which a serological reagent exists. One could even dream that with a technology such as this, receptors of one cell could be studied with regard to the molecules that they recognize on the surface of a second cell. Here too, however, formidable technological problems are apparent, which dictate a major effort for continued improvement in our ability to handle the membrane molecules without losing their antigenic (functional) properties and yet allowing their study following cleavage of the crosslinking reagent.

The molecular nature of a T-cell receptor is the other side of the coin that addresses the question of the target(s) recognized by T-lymphocytes. Several laboratories discussed data dealing with this problem and attempting to resolve the issue of the apparent differential recognition by T-and B-cells while both use the same V_H genes. One of the most exciting approaches to this area, which has been discussed for several years, is to use the antiidiotypic antibody that recognizes shared determinants on the immunoglobulin directed at a given antigen and the T-cells responsive to that antigen. The recent realization that antiidiotypic sera directed at T-cells responding to allogeneic major histocompatibility complex encoded antigens contain separate antiidiotypic antibody populations reactive with the T_h and the T_c cells, responding to the different antigens of that haplotype, suggest that this approach will truly help dissect the problem of the T-cell receptor even with respect to the functionally disparate subclasses of T-lymphocytes.

Antiidiotypic sera, together with the activity of "regulator" T-cells, were discussed, once again, in some detail with regard to their role in networks of regulation of the immune response. Parallel advances in our understanding of subclasses of T-lymphocytes with the increasing information on the effect of antiidiotype sera can be expected to provide major advances in our understanding. Whether the degree of complexity that lies ahead as one considers the possible combinations and permutations of all these factors will allow eventual intelligent and predictive manipulation of the immune response has no answer at present; any guess in this regard will no doubt depend on the personal philosophy of the person making the estimate.

"Factors" that influence the immune response have been among the most ill-defined areas of study in this broad field until quite recently. Not only were data presented at this meeting that provided information regarding at least several of the factors at the molecular level, but also the existence of hybridomas producing antigen-specific factors provides a tool that should allow exacting molecular characterization and testing of these factors.

Although perhaps a little further molecular dissection, the increasing knowledge regarding functionally diverse subpopulations of T-lymphocytes, and the availability of sera directed at differentiation antigens on these cells will allow further dissection of this very complex cellular system. Two findings, intimately interrelated, that perhaps offer an area of great hope for progress involve T-cell growth factor (TCGF) and cloning of T-lymphocytes. It has been known for approximately three years that supernatants of mitogen-activated mixed leukocyte cultures allow bulk culture of either nonstimulated or alloantigen activated T-lymphocytes. Such cells, or those obtained by multiple restimulation with antigen, maintain functional specificity. At least in mouse, there are several published reports demonstrating that T_c derived in this manner can be cloned (although only a few of these reports have demonstrated subcloning). In addition, T-lymphocytes that are probably not T_c have been cloned and used for immunogenetic definition of major histocompatibility complex encoded antigens. Work was presented at this meeting demonstrating that human T-lymphocytes can also be cloned and both noncytotoxic proliferating T-lymphocytes and T_c can be so obtained. These technologies will add greatly to the information being gained through the use of T-lymphocyte tumors. Although much less emphasized, continuing studies were presented regarding heterogenity of B-lymphocytes as well as macrophages, describing to the latter cell type differential function depending on Ia antigen expression or nonexpression.

No attempt has been made in this preface to present, even in outline form, a complete review of topics discussed during the course of the meeting. One feels guilty not to mention in more detail areas such as cell interactions, genetic control of immune response to syngeneic tumors or in autoimmunity, or genetic control of the increasingly investigated Iat antigens. We hope that the reader will find in these pages the same stimulation that we found. We express our gratitude, once again, to the participants as well as the staff that were instrumental in any success that the meeting enjoyed.

We wish to acknowledge the ongoing support that the Life Sciences Division of ICN Pharmaceuticals, Inc., donates to this series and to the National Institutes of Health for Contract No. 263-79-C-0222. This generous award from NIH was jointly sponsored by The Fogarty International Center, National Cancer Institute, National Institute of Allergy and Infectious Diseases, National Institute on Aging and Bureau of Biologics, and the Food and Drug Administration.

ROLE OF THE STRUCTURE OF THE PLASMA MEMBRANE'S CYTOPLASMIC FACE IN LYMPHOCYTE FUNCTION

Michael J. Crumpton, Alan P. Johnstone
and Michael J. Owen

National Institute for Medical Research,
Mill Hill, London NW7 1AA, U.K.

ABSTRACT   Compelling arguments suggest that the cytoplasmic face of the lymphocyte surface membrane plays
important roles in controlling lymphocyte behaviour, most
probably via the regulation of signal transduction. Various
approaches to designating the structure of the inner membrane
surface have been established. First, sealed inside-out
plasma membrane vesicles were separated by coupling dextran
T10 density gradient centrifugation with fractionation on
Con A-Sepharose. Second, antisera against inside-out pig
lymphocyte plasma membrane vesicles recognise a major plasma
membrane polypeptide that is most probably albumin. The
significance of this observation as well as the origin and
location of the albumin is discussed. Third, a lipophilic,
photoactivatable label for polypeptides has been evaluated.
Evidence is presented that labeling is restricted to the non-
polar portions of membrane proteins that are in contact with
lipid. In this case the reagent can be used to distinguish
integral from peripheral membrane proteins.

INTRODUCTION

The lymphocyte surface mediates antigen (mitogen)
recognition and regulates the immediate biochemical consequences of antigen recognition that are ultimately expressed
as cell growth, division and differentiation (1). It also
mediates recognition and interaction with other cells. In
the latter respect, the major histocompatibility antigens are
especially important. Thus, the classical major transplantation antigens (H-2D and H-2K antigens in mice, and HLA-A, B
and C antigens in humans) play important roles in the interaction of T-cytotoxic (killer) cells with target cells,
whereas Ia antigens (HLA-DRw antigens in humans) mediate
interaction between immunocompetent cells (e.g. helper,
suppressor and activated macrophages) (2).
Regulation of lymphocyte behaviour by the surface structure includes two important stages, namely recognition and
signal transduction. The initial regulatory event is the
interaction of an extracellular ligand with a specific
receptor. The ligand may be antigen (mitogen), a processed
form of antigen such as a soluble factor, or the surface of

an accessory cell. Ligand-receptor interaction generates a
signal that is transmitted across the surface membrane into
the cell interior. The nature of the signal(s) and the
mechanism of its transmission have not been defined, although
it has been argued that it corresponds to an influx of Ca^{2+}
(1). The latter arguments are not, however, compelling due
to various reasons especially the failure of some workers to
measure influx (3).

The orientation of receptors in the membrane and the
nature of the association of intracellular contractile
elements with the membrane are of especial importance in view
of their potential contribution to signal transduction. Thus,
a priori reasoning suggests that transmembrane polypeptides
are of particular significance since they may function both
as receptors and as direct transmission channels connecting
the extra- and intra-cellular compartments. Similarly if,
as has been suggested, patching and capping play important
roles in modulating recognition of antigen (4,5), then knowledge of the molecular basis of redistribution is essential
to the comprehension of the regulation of lymphocyte behaviour. Although the molecular basis of redistribution has yet
to be established, according to a consensus of opinion it is
mediated by contractile elements within the cell (6). In
this respect the close association of the cytoskeleton with
the inner face of the plasma membrane is especially pertinent.
A transmembrane orientation may also be important since it
would provide a direct means for interactions with contractile
proteins at the inner membrane surface to be expressed as
changes in the cell surface structure. One possible model is
based upon the premises that each transmembrane protein
possesses a low affinity binding site for actin and that
cross-linkage of a particular surface antigen stabilises its
association with actin through the increase in affinity
resulting from multivalent interaction (7). Alternative, but
less satisfying, explanations are that actin is associated
with a transmembrane polypeptide ('protein X' or 'peg
protein') which binds any aggregated surface receptor (6,8).

If the above suppositions are correct then delineation of
how the lymphocyte surface structure regulates lymphocyte
behaviour depends upon knowledge of various aspects especially
the orientation of surface receptors, the structure of the
inner membrane surface, the mode of attachment of membrane
proteins with the lipid bilayer (whether peripheral or integral) and the nature of the putative association between
transmembrane and contractile proteins. This chapter is
concerned with the establishment of experimental approaches
to the resolution of these questions especially the structure
of the plasma membrane's cytoplasmic face.

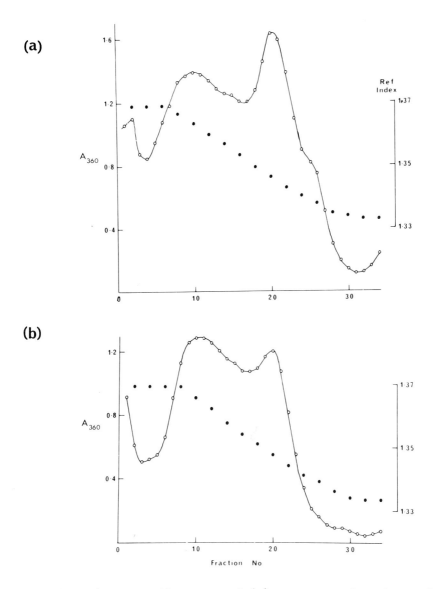

FIGURE 1. Centrifugation of (a) microsome fraction and (b) plasma membrane fraction recovered from a sucrose gradient on continuous gradients of dextran T10 (average molecular weight, 10000). The microsome and plasma membrane fractions were isolated from pig mesenteric lymph node as previously described (10). The distribution of membrane was monitored by turbidity (O, A_{360}) and of dextran by refractive index (●).

SEALED INSIDE-OUT MEMBRANE VESICLES

Previous studies of the orientation of lymphocyte cell
surface antigens and of the structure of the inner membrane

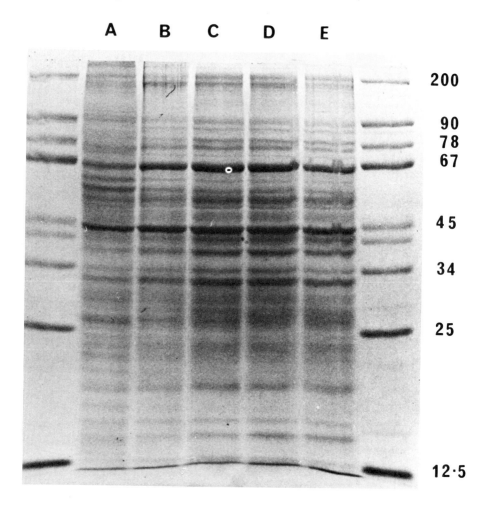

FIGURE 2.   Polyacrylamide gel electrophoresis in sodium
dodecylsulfate of (A) pellet from dextran gradient (Fig. 1),
(B) unsealed membrane vesicles (Fig. 1), (C) sealed membrane
vesicles (Fig. 1), (D) fraction of sealed vesicles not bound
(unretarded) by Con A-Sepharose, (E) fraction of sealed
vesicles bound by Con A-Sepharose (retarded) and subsequently
eluted by agitation in the presence of α methyl mannoside.
The unlabeled tracks represent standard proteins. Polypeptides were revealed by staining with Coomassie blue.

surface were based upon the availability of inside-out plasma
membrane vesicles (9). These studies were restricted by a
number of problems including the low and variable yield of
sealed membrane vesicles. As a result, alternative, more
reproducible methods were sought for preparing such vesicles.
    Previously lymphocyte plasma membrane was isolated from
the microsome fraction by centrifuging on a discontinuous
sucrose gradient (10) prior to the separation of the sealed
vesicles on a dextran T10 gradient (9). Under the latter
conditions, vesicles that are impermeable to dextran (i.e.
sealed) collect within the gradient at a density of about
1.03g/ml, whereas vesicles that are permeable to dextran (i.e.
unsealed) have a higher density (11). It seemed possible
that the prior contact with sucrose influenced the extent of
sealing of the vesicles as defined by exclusion of dextran
T10. Figure 1 compares the behaviour of the microsome
fraction when centrifuged on a continuous gradient of dextran
T10 with that of the plasma membrane fraction recovered from
a sucrose gradient. It is apparent that the size of the peak
corresponding to the sealed vesicles (dextran density 1.03
g/ml) relative to that of the unsealed vesicles (dextran
density 1.11g/ml) is much larger for the microsome compared

TABLE I

PERMEABILITY OF PIG LYMPHOCYTE PLASMA MEMBRANE
FRACTIONS TO ^{14}C-INULIN RELATIVE TO ^{3}H$_2$O[a]

Sample	Ratio (c.p.m.) ^{14}C-inulin to ^{3}H$_2$O[b]
Control (no membrane)	1.01
Unsealed membrane vesicles	1.04; 1.01[c]
Sealed membrane vesicles	0.82; 0.83[c]

[a]Membrane that had been incubated with ^{14}C-inulin
and ^{3}H$_2$O was separated by centrifuging through a sucrose
cushion. The tube was frozen, the bottom portion was cut off
and counted.
    [b]The ratio of ^{14}C-inulin to ^{3}H$_2$O was ascribed a
value of 1.
    [c]Two separate experiments.

with the plasma membrane fraction. Positive evidence was
obtained that both the sealed and unsealed peaks of the
microsome fraction represented plasma membrane by recentri-
fuging them on continuous sucrose gradients; under these
conditions they located at closely similar sucrose densities
(1.14 and 1.13g/ml respectively). Also, as shown in Figure

2, the sealed and unsealed membrane peaks (tracks C and B respectively) possessed very similar polypeptide chain compositions as revealed by polyacrylamide gel electrophoresis in sodium dodecylsulfate.

Although the above results are consistent with the microsome fraction containing plasma membrane vesicles that are sealed to dextran T10, this interpretation relies heavily upon indirect arguments (11). Direct evidence was sought in support of the 1.03g/ml dextran density fraction being sealed. Table I shows that this fraction was significantly less permeable to ^{14}C-labeled inulin of 5000 molecular weight than $^{3}H_2O$. In contrast, the putative unsealed vesicles were equally permeable to inulin and water.

The sealed membrane vesicles were next fractionated on a column of Con A-Sepharose. As described previously (12), about 50% of the added membrane (estimated as protein) passed straight through the column (i.e. was unretarded). In contrast, essentially no membrane was bound if the competing sugar (α methyl mannoside) was added to the membrane prior to its addition to the column. It has been argued previously that right-side-out membrane vesicles are bound by Con A via their exposed carbohydrate, whereas inside-out vesicles have no exposed carbohydrate and thus are not bound. Evidence in support of this view includes the different labeling patterns produced by lactoperoxidase catalysed iodination of the Con A-unretarded fraction and whole lymphocytes (9), the properties of antisera raised against the Con A unretarded fraction (9,12) and the marked similarity in polypeptide compositions of the Con A-unretarded and the Con A-bound fractions (Fig. 2, tracks D and E respectively). Alternative explanations of the fractionation on Con A-Sepharose that do not include a difference in membrane orientation are, however, possible. In particular, it has been suggested that both the bound and unretarded fractions have a right-side-out orientation but that they differ in the complement of their glycoproteins, especially one of high affinity of about 55000 molecular weight (13). This explanation appears, however, unlikely to be correct in the present case since the Con A-unretarded and retarded fractions showed no apparent differences in their Con A-binding proteins including the 55000 molecular weight region (Figure 3).

STRUCTURE OF THE INNER MEMBRANE SURFACE

The structure of the inner surface of lymphocyte plasma membrane has been probed using antisera raised in rabbits against the Con-A unretarded fraction of pig lymphocyte

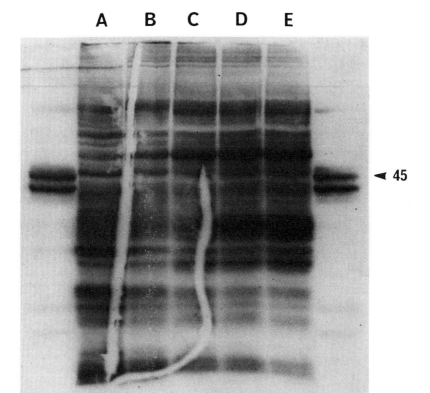

FIGURE 3. Autoradiograph of the polyacrylamide gel shown in Figure 2 that had been stained with ^{125}I-labeled Con A as described by Robinson et al. (14).

plasma membrane. Evidence was obtained that such antisera contain antibodies against actin and several non-glycosylated proteins including one of about 68000 molecular weight (15). The latter polypeptide is a major component of pig lymphocyte plasma membrane as judged from the intensity of Coomassie blue staining (Figure 2). The results of various experiments including peptide fingerprint analysis and immunological reactivity indicate that it is similar if not identical with pig serum albumin (16). This conclusion is supported by the results presented in Figure 4 which shows that the 68000

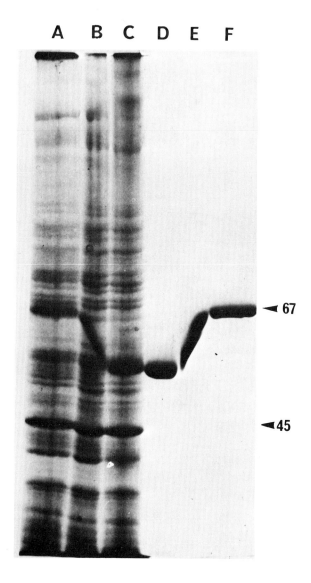

FIGURE 4. Polyacrylamide gel electrophoresis in sodium dodecylsulfate of pig lymphocyte plasma membrane (tracks A, B and C) and of pig serum albumin (tracks D, E and F). Samples in tracks A and F were reduced with dithiothreitol prior to adding to the gel. All other samples were not reduced.

TABLE II

BINDING OF ^{125}I-LABELED PIG ALBUMIN TO
LYMPHOCYTE PLASMA MEMBRANE

Sample	Radioactivity added (c.p.m.)	Radioactivity recovered (c.p.m.)[c]	Binding (%)
Lymphocytes [a]	141000	520	0.37
Lymphocyte plasma membrane [b]	697000	930	0.13

[a] Pig lymphocytes incubated with ^{125}I-labeled albumin prior to cell disruption and separation of the plasma membrane fraction.

[b] Purified lymphocyte plasma membrane was incubated with ^{125}I-labeled albumin and then washed three times by sedimentation.

[c] Radioactivity associated with the recovered plasma membrane.

molecular weight reduced polypeptide behaves as a 55000 molecular weight polypeptide when not reduced and that this unique behaviour is shared by an authentic sample of albumin.

Albumin associated with purified plasma membrane may, theoretically, have been adsorbed from the serum either prior to or during cell breakage. Alternatively, it may have been synthesised by the cells. The results shown in Table II argue strongly against the former possibility and further suggest that the albumin is firmly attached to the plasma membrane (i.e. does not exchange with soluble albumin). On the other hand, no direct evidence was obtained for pig lymphocytes synthesising albumin by immunoprecipitation with anti-(albumin) serum of Nonidet P40 lysates of cells that had been incubated for 6 hr with ^{35}S-methionine.

The presence in the anti-(inside-out vesicle) serum of antibodies against albumin suggests that albumin is associated with the inner membrane surface. This suggestion is also consistent with the failure of anti-(albumin) serum to stain pig lymphocytes as judged by immunofluorescence and the failure to detect ^{125}I-labeled albumin after lactoperoxidase catalysed iodination of viable cells. Further work is necessary in order to evaluate the significance of these observations. In particular, it is important to determine whether albumin is a common constituent of the purified plasma membrane fractions isolated from different lymphocyte sub-populations and from different species.

DESIGNATION OF PERIPHERAL versus
INTEGRAL MEMBRANE PROTEINS

Hexanoyl diiodo-N-(4-azido-2-nitrophenyl)-tyramine containing ^{125}I has been evaluated as a lipophilic photoactivatable reagent for labeling membrane proteins (17). The
following data indicate that labeling was most probably restricted to the non-polar portion of the polypeptide chains
inserted in the lipid bilayer. First, the reagent has a
partition coefficient for octanol and water of about 10^6.
Second, under the conditions used for labeling of lymphocyte
plasma membrane (50μCi of the azide in 10μl of methanol
illuminated with light of less than 430nm for 20 min at 20°C
with 1mg of membrane protein in 1.0ml of 10mM tris HCl
buffer, pH 7.4), greater than 98% of the added radioactivity
was associated with the plasma membrane. Third, pronase
digestion of ^{125}I-nitrene-labeled lymphocyte plasma membrane
(0.1% by weight of pronase for 15 min at 37°C) caused no
significant loss of protein-bound radioactivity (less than 1%).
In contrast, under the same conditions about 70% of the radioactivity incorporated into the proteins of lymphocyte plasma
membrane by lactoperoxidase-catalysed iodination was released.
Fourth, polypeptides that are extrinsic to the lipid bilayer
of lymphocyte plasma membrane contain little if any radioactivity. Thus, immunoprecipitin analysis of ^{125}I-nitrene-
labeled lymphocyte plasma membrane revealed no detectable
radioactivity in the β_2-microglobulin component of the human
major transplantation antigens (HLA-A and B antigens),
whereas the 43000 molecular weight polypeptide, which has a
transmembrane orientation (9), was strongly labeled.

Although the above interpretations are not definitive, the
results argue strongly in support of the reagent providing a
valuable probe for distinguishing integral from peripheral
membrane proteins. The reagent has not yet been applied to
studies of the inner membrane surface, but questions concerning the labeling (or not) of B lymphocyte membrane-bound
immunoglobulin have yielded interesting results. Thus,
Figure 5 shows that the reagent labeled the μ chain but not
the L chain of the immunoglobulin associated with the purified
plasma membrane of human B lymphoblastoid BRI 8 cells. Identical results were obtained with the plasma membrane fractions
of Daudi cells (a Burkitt's lymphoma) and mouse spleen except
that with mouse spleen both the μ and δ chains were labeled.
These results suggest that B-lymphocyte surface immunoglobulins resemble other cell surface glycoproteins in being
attached to the membrane via a hydrophobic sequence. If the
results are assessed in conjunction with the recent report

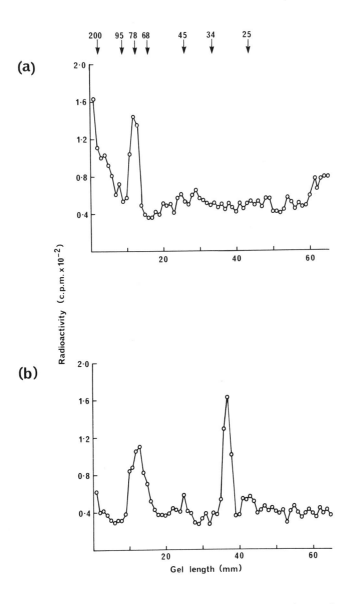

FIGURE 5. Polyacrylamide gel electrophoresis in sodium dodecylsulfate of the immunoprecipitates obtained by reacting the deoxycholate-solubilised plasma membrane of human BRI 8 cells with a rabbit anti-(human immunoglobulin) serum. The plasma membrane had been radioiodinated prior to solubilisation by either (a) the lipophilic nitrene or (b) lacto-peroxidase-catalysed iodination. The gels were dried and divided into 1mm slices prior to counting.

that the μ chain of the membrane-bound immunoglobulin of Daudi
cells has a different C-terminal sequence than that of the
secreted μ chain (18), then they further indicate that the
non-polar region is most probably located at the C-terminus.

DISCUSSION

Compelling arguments can be invoked in support of the
cytoplasmic face of the lymphocyte surface membrane playing
important roles in the regulation of lymphocyte behaviour
particularly in relation to signal transduction and to the
redistribution of cell surface components induced by interaction with multivalent ligands. By analogy with the erythrocyte membrane (19) the inner surface of lymphocyte plasma
membrane should comprise the 'tails' of cell surface transmembrane glycoproteins, peripheral non-glycosylated proteins
especially actin and other contractile proteins, as well as
(possibly) integral proteins which dip into but do not span
the lipid bilayer, (i.e. are not expressed on the cell surface). The nature of the proteins on the inner membrane
surface and of their interactions with one another have,
however, yet to be defined. One promising approach to this
definition is to analyse inside-out membrane vesicles whose
surface has been labeled vectorially using a non-penetrating
reagent. Fractionation of lymphocyte plasma membrane preparations on dextran T10-density gradients, as recommended by
Steck (11), and on columns of Con A-Sepharose (12) has been
used to prepare such vesicles that are sealed to lactoperoxidase, but the yield was low and not very reproducible
(9). The present results suggest that prior separation of
the plasma membrane fraction on sucrose gradients (10) has a
detrimental affect upon the proportion of sealed vesicles as
well as on their degree of sealing. When this step was
replaced by centrifuging on a dextran T10 density gradient,
the membrane vesicles collecting at a dextran density of
1.03g/ml were isolated in high yield (Figure 1). Positive
evidence for sealing was obtained by showing that these
vesicles were less permeable to inulin of 5000 molecular
weight than vesicles collecting at a dextran density of 1.11
g/ml (Table I). When the membrane of dextran density 1.03
g/ml was subsequently fractionated on Con A-Sepharose about
50% failed to bind. This lack of binding has been equated
with an inside-out orientation. Although this interpretation
is supported by various persuasive arguments (9,12,15), these
arguments are by no means unequivocal. Further evidence in
support of the former interpretation was obtained in the
present study by showing that the bound and unbound membrane
fractions possessed the same complement of Con A-binding
proteins (Figure 3).

Antisera prepared against the inside-out membrane vesicles should provide a valuable probe for dissecting the structure of the plasma membrane's cytoplasmic face. Such antisera contain antibodies against several non-glycosylated membrane proteins, as judged by their lack of binding to lentil lectin, including actin (15). Evidence has now been obtained, in the case of pig mesenteric lymph node lymphocyte plasma membrane, that one of the antibodies recognises albumin and that purified pig lymphocyte plasma membrane contains albumin as a major component (16) (see also Figures 1 and 4). Although these two observations suggest that albumin is present on the inner surface of the plasma membrane, this interpretation is premature and must await the resolution of the important question as to whether the albumin is synthesised by pig lymphocytes or is acquired passively from the serum. In this context, the recent report that rabbit lymphocytes, particularly B-cells, synthesise albumin is especially interesting (20).

In the case of the erythrocyte, the peripheral membrane proteins are primarily located on and mainly comprise the inner surface (19). If this situation is common to all cell types, then methods of distinguishing peripheral from integral membrane proteins will be especially valuable for studies of the composition of the membrane's cytoplasmic face. Hexanoyl-diiodo-N-(4-azido-2-nitrophenyl)-tyramine appears likely to satisfy the requirement for a probe for integral proteins, as judged by its affinity for lipid bilayers and by its capacity to label known integral polypeptides but not peripheral polypeptides. The observation that this reagent labeled the μ and δ chains of membrane-bound immunoglobulin is particularly interesting since it implies strongly that B-cell surface immunoglobulins (IgMs and IgD) are attached to the membrane via a non-polar segment.

REFERENCES

1. Crumpton, M.J., Allan, D., Auger, J., Green, N.M., and Maino, V.C. (1975). Phil. Trans. Roy. Soc. 272, 173.
2. Katz, D.H., and Benacerraf, B. (eds.). (1976). "The Role of the Products of the Histocompatibility Gene Complex in Immune Responses". Academic Press, New York.
3. Hesketh, T.R., Smith, G.A., Houslay, M.D., Warren, G.B., and Metcalfe, J.C. (1977). Nature, 267, 490.
4. Edelman, G.M. (1976). Science, 192, 218.
5. Schreiner, G.F., and Unanue, E.R. (1976). Adv. Immunol. 24, 38.
6. de Petris, S. (1977). In "Dynamic Aspects of Cell Surface Organization" (G. Poste and G.L. Nicolson, eds.), pp.643-

728. Elsevier/North Holland Biomedical Press, Amsterdam.

7. Karash, F. (1976). Contemp. Top. Mol. Immunol. 5, 217.

8. Bourguignon, L.Y.W., and Singer, S.J. (1977). Proc. Nat. Acad. Sci. 74, 5031.

9. Walsh, F.S., Barber, B.H., and Crumpton, M.J. (1978). In "Cell Membrane Receptors for Drugs and Hormones: a Multidisciplinary Approach" (L. Bolis and R.W. Staub, (eds.), pp. 9-22. Raven Press, New York.

10. Crumpton, M.J., and Snary, D. (1974). Contemp. Top. Mol. Immunol. 3, 27.

11. Steck, T.L. (1974). J. Cell Biol. 62, 1.

12. Walsh, F.S., Barber, B.H., and Crumpton, M.J. (1976). Biochem. 15, 3557.

13. Resch, K., Loracher, A., Mahler, B., Stoeck, M., and Rode, H.N. (1978). Biochim. Biophys. Acta, 511, 176.

14. Robinson, P.J., Bull, F.G., Anderton, B.H. and Roitt, I.M. (1975). FEBS Lett. 58, 330.

15. Walsh, F.S., Barber, B.H., and Crumpton, M.J. (1977). Biochem. Soc. Trans. 5, 1134.

16. Owen, M.J., Barber, B.H., Faulkes, R.A., and Crumpton, M.J. (1978). Biochem. Soc. Trans. 6, 920.

17. Hebden, G.M., Knott, J.C.A., and Green, N.M., unpublished observations.

18. Williams, P.B., and Grey, H.M. (1978). Fed. Proc. 37, 1838.

19. Steck, T.L., and Hainfeld, J.F. (1977). In "International Cell Biology 1976-1977" (B.R. Brinkley and K.P. Porter, eds.), pp. 6-14. Rockefeller University Press, New York.

20. Teodorescu, M., Debates, M.J., and Dray, S. (1977). In "Regulatory Mechanisms in Lymphocyte Activation" (D.O. Lucas, ed.), pp. 450-452. Academic Press, New York.

Ia ANTIGEN CROSSREACTIONS BETWEEN SPECIES

D. H. Sachs, M. El-Gamil, P. Kiszkiss, J. K. Lunney,
D. L. Mann, K. Ozato, and N. Shinohara

Immunology Branch, National Cancer Institute,
National Institutes of Health, Bethesda, MD 20205

ABSTRACT   Significant crossreactions have been observed between mouse Ia^k alloantigens and Ia antigens of several other species. Crossreactions with products of the mouse I-A locus were not always seen and were distinct for different species. However, crossreactions with products of the I-E/C loci were observed on all species tested and appeared to be with determinants common to all of these species. The mouse strains producing these crossreacting anti-I-E/C^k antibodies were of the H-2^b and H-2^s haplotypes, and for neither of these haplotypes have we been able to demonstrate I-E/C products by the use of appropriate allo- or xenoantisera. It thus appears that the I-A crossreactions may represent true crossreactions between alleles of polymorphic systems, while the I-E/C crossreactions may result from detection of determinants common to the I-E/C analog of all species which are for some reason not expressed in certain mouse strains. These findings may thus have both practical and theoretical implications.

INTRODUCTION

The detection of serological crossreactions between the products of the H-2K and H-2D regions of the mouse major histocompatibility complex provided the first clue that these two regions may have been derived from common primordial genes (1). This hypothesis has now been substantiated in a number of laboratories by the demonstration of marked sequence homologies between molecules encoded by the H-2K and H-2D regions (2-6). Thus serological crossreactions can provide a useful probe for studying the evolutionary relationships between genes determining polymorphic antigenic systems. It has therefore been for both theoretical as well as obvious practical reasons that we have pursued the crossreactivity patterns of mouse anti-Ia alloantisera with lymphocytes of other species.

15

ISBN 0-12-069850-1

The first such crossreaction we have studied was observed by chance during the testing of a Bl0.D2 anti-Bl0.BR antiserum on rat spleen cells. This antiserum, which was intended as a negative control, produced a cytotoxicity pattern on rat splenic target cells similar to what one might expect for anti-Ia antiserum killing. An examination of the same cross-reaction in the combination Bl0.D2 anti-rat tested on Bl0.BR spleen cells showed a similar cytotoxicity pattern. This latter antiserum was then examined on a panel of recombinant H-2 haplotypes and the genes responsible for this Ia-like activity were mapped to the I-A subregion (7). By a variety of criteria, including immunoprecipitation analyses and tissue distribution studies, this crossreaction was shown to be characteristic of classical B cell Ia alloantigens.

We have subsequently extended these studies to the examination of mouse alloantisera crossreactions with several other species, including pig (8) and human (9). In addition, we have attempted to use antisera raised in other species to define possible new alloantigenic specificities in the mouse. Our results indicate that crossreactions between species can be observed for Ia antigens determined both by the I-A subregion and the I-E/C subregions. However, there seem to be major differences in the basis of the crossreactions observed with Ia antigens determined by these two subregions, and these differences may have implications for the basis of polymorphism of the Ia antigens.

METHODS

Animals. Mice were either purchased from The Jackson Laboratory, Bar Harbor, Maine, or were raised in our own mouse colonies. Rats were purchased from Microbiological Associates, Bethesda, Maryland. Swine were from our partially inbred herd of miniature swine housed at the NIH Animal Center, Poolesville, Maryland.

Serology. Methods for production of alloantisera and xenoantisera against lymphoid cells have been previously described (10). A goat antiserum to mouse Ia antigens was prepared by immunizing a goat with a purified cell-free product from a mouse B cell tumor cell line, which will be described in detail elsewhere (Sachs, Kiszkiss, and Kim, manuscript in preparation). The goat was boosted 3 times with this purified Ia antigen preparation in complete Freund's adjuvant, and the serum was absorbed extensively with insolubilized fetal calf serum and mouse globulins, after which its reactivity was exclusively with mouse Ia antigens by immunoprecipitation criteria.

Lymphoid populations from mouse and rat spleens were prepared as previously described (11). Peripheral blood lymphocytes of swine and human donors were prepared by Ficol Hypaque
separation (12), and in the case of human lymphoid cells,
rosetting with sheep red cells was performed by published
methods (13). The JY human B cell line was carried in long-
term tissue culture (14).

Complement-mediated cytotoxicity assays and absorptions
of cytotoxicity were performed by previously described methods
(11), as was staining for surface immunoglobulin (10).

Isolation and Characterization of Labeled Cell-Surface
Antigens. Lymphoid glycoproteins were labeled with ^{3}H-leucine,
solubilized in NP-40 and purified by lentil lectin chromatography. Indirect immunoprecipitation was carried out using
S. aureus Cowan I strain fixed bacteria as the precipitating
agent and immune complexes were eluted in SDS and mercaptoethanol and were analyzed by electrophoresis on 10% SDS polyacrylamide gels (PAGE). All of these methods have been
described previously (7).

RESULTS

In our original studies of the crossreaction between
mouse alloantisera and rat Ia antigens, the reactivity on rat
lymphocytes was observed using an antiserum produced in the
strain combination H-2^d anti-H-2^k (7). In subsequent analyses
and screening assays of mouse alloantisera with lymphoid cells
from other species, we have consistently found that antisera
directed to products of the I genes have contained cross-
species reactive anti-Ia antibodies, while such activity in
antisera directed to other I region alleles has generally been
weak or absent (8,9,15). One of the most potent antisera
examined in this regard has been the A.TH anti-A.TL antiserum
(I^s anti-I^k). By cytotoxic analysis, this antiserum was positive with lymphoid cells of all rats, hamsters, swine, and
human beings tested, while the reciprocal antiserum, A.TL anti-
A.TH, was uniformly negative (8,9, and unpublished
observations).

The levels of cytotoxicity produced by this antiserum
were furthermore consistent with the percentage of B cells in
fractionated populations of lymphoid target cells from these
other species. For example, when human peripheral blood
lymphocytes were examined, only approximately 5-10% positivity
by cytotoxicity was observed before fractionation. However,
after sheep red cell rosetting had been performed, the non-
rosetting cells showed approximately 35% cytotoxicity with
this antiserum. As can be seen in Fig. 1, this cytotoxicity
correlated well with the Ig staining of each of the fraction-

ated populations. In addition, a human B cell line (JY)
showed approximately 80% positivity with this antiserum.
        When immunoprecipitation experiments were performed on
^{3}H-leucine labeled lymphocytes from these different species,
and the precipitated antigens were examined on PAGE analysis,
peaks consistent with Ia antigens were observed in every case
(Fig. 2).
        As shown in Table I, the availability of the B10.HTT ani-
mal, in the H-2 haplotype of which a recombination between the
I-J and I-E subregions has been demonstrated, has made possible the production of antisera directed to products of different subregions coding for Ia antigens in the same combination
as the polyvalent antiserum A.TH anti-A.TL (i.e., Ia^s anti-
Ia^k). Since the predominant reaction of the B10.D2 anti-
B10.BR antiserum with rat Ia antigens had been previously
demonstrated to involve a specificity determined by the I-A
subregion, it was anticipated that the majority of these

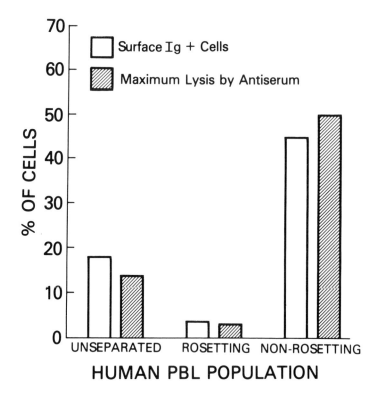

FIGURE 1. Comparison of surface Ig staining and cytotoxicity by A.TH anti-A.TL antiserum on subpopulations of
human peripheral blood lymphocytes separated by SRBC rosetting.

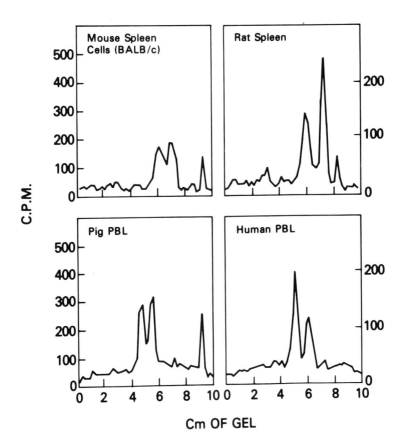

FIGURE 2. Immunoprecipitation analysis of A.TH anti-A.TL antiserum on ³H-leucine labeled antigen preparations of different species. In each analysis alloantisera with known specificity for Ia antigens of the species being tested were also employed, and in every case the Ia peaks were in identical position to those seen in these figures. This figure is a composite from several independent experiments using slightly different electrophoretic techniques, so that relative positions of peaks do not necessarily reflect molecular weight differences.

interspecies crossreactions would likewise be with determinants encoded by this subregion. However, the reactivities with subregion specific antisera produced in the combination Ia^s anti-Ia^k were found to be predominantly with determinants encoded by the I-E/C subregions. As can be seen in Figure 3, the anti-I-ABJ^k antiserum showed significant reactivity only

TABLE I

PRODUCTION OF SUBREGION SPECIFIC ANTISERA

Strain	Haplotype	Origin of Regions							
		K	A	B	J	E	D	S	D
A.TL	t1	s	k	k	k	k	k	k	d
A.TH	t2	s	s	s	s	s	s	s	d
B10.HTT	t3	s	s	s	s	k	k	k	d
A.SW, B10.S	s	s	s	s	s	s	s	s	s

As seen from the haplotypes of origin, (A.SWxB10.HTT) anti-A.TL$_k$ can detect ABJ^k, and (A.THxB10.S) anti-B10.HTT can detect EC^k, both of which are included in A.TH anti-A.TL.

with rat lymphocytes. Human nonrosetted lymphocytes showed slight reactivity (0-15% above complement controls in 6 experiments), and this antiserum was totally unreactive with pig peripheral blood lymphocytes (PBL). On the other hand, as shown in Figure 4, the anti-I-E/C^k antiserum was significantly reactive with lymphoid cells of all species tested.

It thus appears that the predominant crossreactive specificities recognized by mouse alloantisera on pig, human, and even rat lymphoid cells are between Ia antigens of these other species and mouse Ia determinants of the I-E/C subregions. Cross absorption studies were performed in order to determine whether these crossreactions were with the same or different determinants on the different species tested. Absorption of the A.TH anti-A.TL antiserum with lymphocytes of rats and pigs and with JY tumor cells was capable of clearing reactivity with rat, pig, and human cells, respectively. The absorbed antisera did not show any appreciable reduction in cytotoxic activity against mouse lymphoid cells, indicating that in addition to the crossreactive antibodies, there were also alloantibodies present which did not crossreact with the other species. This was true of the subregion specific antisera as well, although in the case of the anti-I-E/C^k antiserum, absorption to completion with either rat or human cells diminished the reactivity on mouse lymphocytes to an extent much greater than did comparable absorptions of the A.TH anti-A.TL antiserum or of the anti-I-ABJ^k antiserum. This decrease in reactivity was greater than could be explained by dilutional artifacts alone.

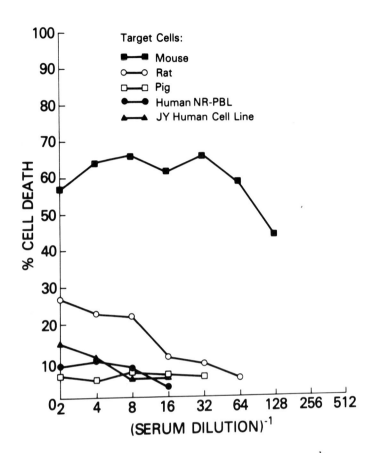

FIGURE 3. Cytotoxicity patterns of anti-ABJ^k subregion specific antiserum on lymphocytes of other species. The serum (A.SWxB10.HTT) anti-A.TL was tested on lymphoid cells from each of the species shown.

Absorption of the anti-I-ABJ^k antiserum with human cells decreased reactivity on rat lymphocytes, but did not eliminate it, presumably indicating species differences in the cross-reactive determinants detected by the anti-I-ABJ^k antiserum. On the contrary, absorption of the anti-I-E/C^k antiserum with lymphocytes of any of the crossreactive species cleared reactivity to all of the other crossreactive species, presumably indicating that the reactivity was with a determinant shared extensively between species. It is important to note, however, that in these absorption studies the absorbed antiserum is inevitably diluted (1:2 to 1:8) because of the large volume of lymphoid cells needed to clear the reactivity. Thus, low

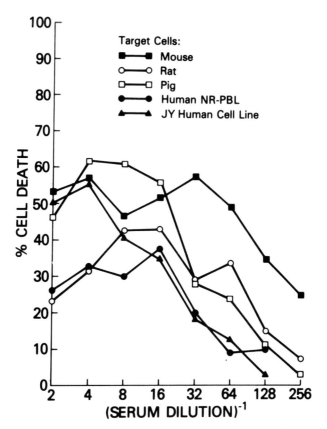

FIGURE 4. Cytotoxicity patterns of anti-E/C^k subregion
specific antiserum on lymphocytes of other species. The serum
(A.THxB10.S) anti-B10.HTT was tested on lymphoid cells from
each of the species shown.

levels of reactivity to determinants not shared by all species
could conceivably be overlooked.
    Considering the predominant reactivity of anti-I-E/C^k
antisera with all other species tested, including rat, one
might ask why our original study showed the predominant crossreactive Ia determinant to be encoded by the I-A subregion (7).
It seemed to us that a likely explanation might be that the
serum used in those studies was produced in the combination
H-2^d anti-H-2^k, both of which haplotypes express I-E/C antigens, and share a predominant Ia specificity determined by the
I-E/C subregion, Ia.7. Conceivably, then, the predominant
crossreactive determinants detected on other species would be

shared by animals of the $\underline{H-2}^d$ and $\underline{H-2}^k$ haplotypes, thereby
precluding production of antibodies to such determinants.
Such an explanation would imply, however, something very
peculiar about the $\underline{I-E/C}$ subregions of strains of mice producing this crossreactive antiserum. Such strains would presumably be lacking in a determinant which is shared not only
by $\underline{H-2}^k$ and $\underline{H-2}^d$ mice, but by all other species tested. One
possible explanation for this unusual situation might be that
such strains are lacking either in the genes or in the expression of the genes determining I-E/C antigens, and thereby are
capable of producing antibodies to common determinants of the
products of these subregions as well as to possible alloantigens determined by these subregions. Consistent with this
hypothesis has been the observation that B10 anti-B10.D2 and
B10 anti-B10.A antisera ($\underline{H-2}^b$ anti-$\underline{H-2}^d$ and $\underline{H-2}^b$ anti-$\underline{H-2}^a$,
respectively) also showed I-E/C crossreactions with rat Ia
antigens (data not shown).

Failure to detect any alloantigens determined by the
$\underline{I-E/C}$ subregions of $\underline{H-2}^b$ and $\underline{H-2}^s$ is also consistent with such
an hypothesis. As shown in Table II, attempts to produce anti-
sera in combinations which should potentially detect these
products have been unsuccessful, as have absorptions of potent
polyvalent anti-Ia antisera with cells from appropriate recombinant $\underline{H-2}$ haplotypes. Since such an hypothesis would have
important implications relative to the evolution of these
antigens, we have produced and examined two highly crossreactive xenoantisera in an attempt to detect $\underline{I-E/C}$ subregion
products of the $\underline{H-2}^b$ and $\underline{H-2}^s$ haplotypes. So far our data,
which are as yet complete only with the $\underline{H-2}^b$ haplotype, have
failed to demonstrate any I-E/C^b product. The first antiserum
tested was a hyperimmunized rat anti-C57BL/10 xenoantiserum.
This antiserum precipitated molecules with appropriate molecular weight for Ia antigens from lymphocyte antigen preparations of all mouse strains tested, including B10 and B10.A.
As seen in Figure 5, pretreatment of a B10 antigen preparation
with an anti-I-A^b antiserum did not leave any residual Ia
antigens which could be precipitated by this xenoantiserum.
In addition, when a similar experiment was performed on a
B10.A lymphocyte antigen preparation, preprecipitation of the
I-A components left Ia antigens precipitable by an anti-I-E/C^k
reagent, but no such molecules could be precipitated by the
rat anti-B10 antiserum. This result implies that no antibodies were produced in the rat reactive with mouse specific
determinants on an E/C type molecule.

The second xenoantiserum tested was a goat antiserum produced against Ia antigens purified from a B cell tumor supernatant. It was shown by sequential precipitation analysis
that this antiserum reacted with both I-A and I-E/C products
of both the $\underline{H-2}^a$ and $\underline{H-2}^d$ haplotypes (data not shown). In

TABLE II

FAILURE TO DETECT I-E/C ALLOANTIGENS IN H-2[b] AND H-2[s] HAPLOTYPES

Strain	Haplotype	Presumed Haplotype Origin							
		K	A	B	J	E	C	S	D
B10·A	a	k	k	k	k	k	d	d	d
B10	b	b	b	b	b	b	b	b	b
B10·A (2R)	h2	k	k	k	k	k	d	d	b
B10·A (4R)	h4	k	k	b	b	b	b	b	b
A·TL	t1	s	k	k	k	k	k	k	d
A·TH	t2	s	s	s	s	s	s	s	d
B10·HTT	t3	s	s	s	s	k	k	k	d

Serum Tested	Initial Titer[-1]	Absorbing Cells	Target Cells	Presumed Specificity	Titer[-1]
B10 α B10·A	64	B10·A (4R)	B10·A (2R)	I–BJEC[a]	8
B10·A α B10	64	B10·A (2R)	B10·A (4R)	I–BJEC[b]	<2
A·TH α A·TL	1024	B10·A (4R)	B10·A	I–BJEC[k]	320
A·TL α A·TH	1024	B10·HTT	B10·S	I–E/C[s]	<2

fact, it removed all Ia antigens from solubilized lymphoid cells of these haplotypes, leaving no Ia molecules detectable even by potent polyvalent Ia alloantisera. When this xenoantiserum was tested on a B10 antigen preparation, it likewise cleared all Ia activity from the preparation. However, in sequential precipitation analyses, when the I-A[b] molecules had been removed, this xenoantiserum failed to precipitate any other Ia-like molecules. Thus, our results with both of these xenoantisera have failed to reveal any evidence for expression of an E/C product by the H-2[b] haplotype.

DISCUSSION

Crossreactions between murine Ia antigens and Ia-like antigens of other species have now been observed for Ia determinants encoded by both the I-A and I-E/C subregions. In both cases the antigens were detected by alloantisera, presumably implying that the antigenic determinants are "alloantigens" in

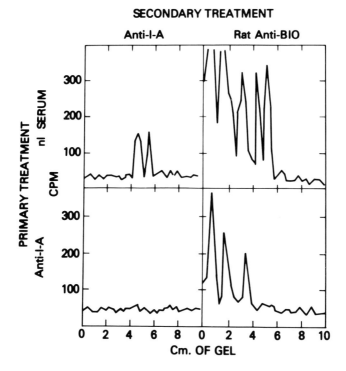

FIGURE 5. Co-precipitation analysis using ^{3}H-leucine
labeled B10 antigen. Aliquots of antigen were pretreated with
the serum shown on the left (normal serum or anti-Ia.8 antiserum) and supernatants after precipitation with Staph. Cowan
I were subdivided and treated again with the antisera shown at
the top (anti-Ia.8 or xenogeneic rat anti-B10). The peaks
corresponding to Ia antigens (4 to 6 cm of gel) were removed
by the pretreatment with the I-A specific alloantiserum regardless of which antiserum was used for secondary treatment,
indicating the absence of any additional Ia products detectable by the xenoantiserum.

the mouse species. However, on more detailed analysis, the
basis of these crossreactions appears to be different for the
two subregions examined.

Crossreactivity with I-A antigens was seen predominantly
in the rat. Reactivity with pig was totally negative, and
reactivity with human lymphocytes was very weak. In addition,
by crossabsorption studies, the crossreactive determinants
detected on rat lymphocytes appeared not to be the same as
those detected on human lymphocytes. Absorption with neither

human nor rat lymphocytes was capable of removing reactivity
toward mouse lymphocytes. The crossreactions observed with
I-A^k antigens thus appear to be with different determinants
for different species. As we have previously suggested, the
predominance of crossreactivity with products of the H-2^k
haplotype may signify that the I-A^k alleles are closer than
other alleles to the primordial I-A gene product (7,9). The
differences in crossreactive determinants shared may reflect
different pathways of divergence from this common ancestor.

On the other hand, the crossreactions of anti-I-E/C^k
reagents appear to be common to all other species tested
within the limits of our assays. There are additional mouse
antigens determined by the E/C subregions, since anti-I-E/C^k
antisera are not cleared of reactivity with mouse lymphocytes
by absorption with other species. However, such absorptions
do markedly diminish titers of anti-I-E/C reactivity, beyond
what would be expected on the basis of dilution, and beyond
what is observed for similar absorptions of anti-I-ABJ^k
reagents. It would thus appear that the interspecies crossreactions with I-E/C^k are with determinants which are more
similar between species than are the determinants crossreactive with I-A^k. This is consistent with the relative levels
of polymorphism detected within the mouse species by alloantisera, since the vast majority of Ia specificities have been
mapped to the I-A subregion, and only a very few to the I-E/C
subregions (16).

A possible interpretation of these data is that the major
I-E/C "alloantigen" is really not an alloantigen in the usual
sense, but is rather the result of reactivity against a common determinant of the I-E/C product which is missing in
certain H-2 haplotypes, notably H-2^b and H-2^s. Our serologic
data using alloantisera and our immunoprecipitation studies
using potent crossreactive xenoantisera are both consistent
with this hypothesis, and will be presented in detail elsewhere (Ozato, El-Gamil, Lunney, and Sachs, manuscript in preparation). However, our studies with xenoantisera indicate
that if an E/C product is produced by the H-2^b haplotype, it
is of such weak antigenicity as not to be detected by the rat,
and has no shared determinants with the E/C product of other
mouse haplotypes which can be detected by a goat antibody
broadly crossreactive with other E/C molecules. It thus seems
possible that H-2^b and H-2^s do not express the antigenic
determinants of E/C products at all. These strains therefore
produce antibodies against determinants of the E/C^k product
which crossreact broadly with mouse strains expressing E/C
products and with the other species tested. The basis of this
failure to express E/C antigens is unclear, but could involve

deletion of a structural gene or of a gene regulating expression of either the E/C product or of an antigenic moiety associated with that product (eg., a carbohydrate determinant).

Immunochemical analyses of human Ia alloantigens have so far characterized only one Ia product (17), although there is serologic evidence for more than one such product (18). By the limited sequence analyses so far available, the human Ia heavy chain appears to be most homologous with the heavy chain of the I-E/C product, and shows no apparent homology with the heavy chain of the I-A product (19). Although most of these studies have been performed using xenoantisera, the same products are apparently detectable with human B cell alloantisera (17). It is thus possible that in man the analog of the I-E/C subregion may be the more polymorphic antigenic system. The fact that the predominant reactivity of crossreactive alloantisera tested on human lymphocytes appears to be with the I-E/C product and that there is sequence homology between the heavy chains of the human Ia alloantigen and the mouse E/C antigens may indicate that the crossreactive determinants are determined by the Ia heavy chain. However, much more extensive sequence information would be necessary to substantiate such an hypothesis.

These results appear to us to have both practical and theoretical implications. From a practical viewpoint, the potent reactivity of certain mouse alloantisera with Ia antigens of other species may provide useful anti-Ia reagents in situations in which genetic or ethical considerations do not permit the production of such antisera by direct immunization. Such reagents could be used for studies requiring anti-Ia reactivity in which polymorphism of the determinant recognized is not a necessary feature. For example, such reagents might be used to block Ia-dependent cellular interactions or to purify Ia antigens or factors bearing Ia determinants.

From a theortical viewpoint, the observation of these interspecies crossreactions probably indicates the conservation of the relevant genetic information during evolution. Such conservation is most readily explained on the basis of functional properties of the gene products. Although the function of these products is still only a matter of speculation, it is difficult to conceive of the generation of such an extensive polymorphism if that polymorphism itself were not of some selective advantage in terms of function. As such, it is perhaps surprising that the $H-2^b$ and $H-2^s$ haplotypes do not appear to express the I-E/C subregions at all. Perhaps the low level of alloantigenic polymorphism of these subregions relative to the I-A subregion may indicate that, at least in the mouse, the function of the I-A subregion is of much greater importance than that of the I-E/C. This might then explain the ability of certain mouse strains to survive (at least in a laboratory situation) without the expression of E/C antigens. In man the predominant polymorphism so far observed at the alloantigenic level appears to be with the analog of the E/C subregion. One might predict that extensive polymorphism of at least one Ia locus will be found in every species, and that in different species different I region analogs may be more or less polymorphic. Such expansion and contraction of genetic diversity would have certain similarities to the postulated evolution of multigene families (22), although there is no compelling reason as yet to suppose that the extensive polymorphism of Ia loci implies multiple copies of the relevant genes.

ACKNOWLEDGMENT

The authors express their thanks to Mrs. Judith Jaworek for expert secretarial assistance.

REFERENCES

1. Shreffler, D. C., David, C. S., Passmore, H. C., and Klein, J. (1971). Transplant. Proc. 3, 176.
2. Henning, R., Milner, R. J., Reske, K., Cunningham, B. A., and Edelman, G. M. (1976). Proc. Nat. Acad. Sci. USA 73, 118.
3. Silver, J., and Hood, L. (1976). Proc. Nat. Acad. Sci. USA 73, 599.
4. Ewenstein, B. M., Freed, J. H., Mole, L. E., and Nathenson, S. G. (1976). Proc. Nat. Acad. Sci. USA 73, 915.
5. Capra, J. D., Vitetta, E. S., Klapper, D. G., Uhr, J. W., and Klein, J. (1976). Proc. Nat. Acad. Sci. USA 73, 3661.
6. Coligan, J. E., Kindt, T. J., Ewenstein, B. M., Uehara, H., Nisizawa, T., and Nathenson, S. G. (1978). Proc. Nat. Acad. Sci. USA 75, 3390.
7. Sachs, D. H., Humphrey, G. W., and Lunney, J. K. (1977). J. Exp. Med. 146, 381.
8. Lunney, J. K., and Sachs, D. H. (1979). J. Immunol. 122, 623.
9. Lunney, J. K., Mann, D. L., and Sachs, D. H. (submitted)
10. Sachs, D. H., and Cone, J. L. (1973). J. Exp. Med. 138, 1289.
11. Sachs, D. H., Winn, H. J., and Russell, P. S. (1971). J. Immunol. 107, 481.
12. Boyum, A. (1968). Scand. J. Clin. Invest. 21, 97.
13. Jondal, M., Holm, G., and Wigzell, H. (1972). J. Exp. Med. 136, 207.
14. Romano, P. J., and Mann, D. L. (1976). Tissue Antigens 8, 9.
15. Shinohara, N., Lunney, J. K., and Sachs, D. H. (1978). J. Immunol. 121, 637.

16. David, C. S. (1976). Transplant. Rev. 30, 299.
17. Snary, D., Barnstable, C., Bodmer, W. F., Goodfellow, P., and Crumpton, M. J. (1977). Cold Spring Harbor Symp. 41, 379.
18. Mann, D. L., Kauffman, J., Robb, R., and Strominger, J. Transplant. Proc. (in press).
19. Springer, T. A., Kaufman, J. F., Terhorst, C., and Strominger, J. L. (1977). Nature 268, 213.
20. Silver, J., Russell, W. A., Reis, B. L., and Frelinger, J. A. (1977). Proc. Nat. Acad. Sci. USA 74, 5131.
21. McMillan, M., Cecka, J. M., Murphy, D. B., McDevitt, H. O., and Hood, L. (1977). Proc. Nat. Acad. Sci. USA 74, 5135.
22. Hood, L., Campbell, J. H., and Elgin, S. C. R. (1975). Annual Rev. Genet. 9, 305.

EVIDENCE THAT MORE THAN ONE GENE LOCUS CONTROLS
EXPRESSION OF HUMAN B-CELL ALLOANTIGENS

Dean L. Mann

Immunology Branch, National Cancer Institute,
National Institutes of Health, Bethesda, Maryland   20205

ABSTRACT   Human B-cell alloantigens (DRw) are thought
to be the serologic correlate of the Dw antigens
defined in MLR. The latter are under genetic control
of the MHC with a number of alleles at a single locus.
In family studies where inheritance of DRw antigens
was determined, it was observed on several occasions
that "DRw" specificities were found to be inherited
with the same HLA haplotype. In sequential immunoprecipitation studies of soluble B-cell alloantigens,
3 molecular components having the electrophoretic
characteristics of human "Ia-like" antigen were found.
The results indicate that 2 loci control the expression of human B-cell alloantigens.

INTRODUCTION

Genes in the human MHC control the expression of
antigens expressed preferentially on peripheral blood B
cells (1, 2, 3) and monocytes and to a lesser extent
(quantitatively) on T cells (4). These antigens are
detected serologically in complement-dependent cytotoxicity tests with the isolated B cells or monocytes.
In earlier studies, these serologically detected antigens
were found to correlate in reaction patterns with the Dw
antigens defined by mixed lymphocyte reactions (MLR) (5).
These latter antigens (Dw) are controlled by genes of
the MHC that are generally considered to be products of
alleles at a single locus (6). Whether or not the Dw and
DRw antigens are structural equivalents remains an open
question.
     Studies of DRw antigens clearly demonstrate control
by genes of the MHC. Observations made in B cell typing
patients with sicca syndrome and systemic lupus erythematosus suggested the possibility that more than one locus
controlled the expression of these antigens (7, 8).
Analysis of family studies where more than 1 member had

31

ISBN 0-12-069850-1

either of the above 2 diseases indicated that a single
haplotype controlled the expression of 2 distinct B-cell
alloantigens. The results of studies of one representative
family will be shown in this report.

Multiple gene control of B-cell alloantigens was further
indicated in sequential immunoprecipitation analysis of soluble B-cell membrane antigens. These results will also be
summarized.

METHODS AND MATERIAL

The preparation of peripheral blood lymphocytes,
isolation of B lymphocytes, serologic reagents used and
the methods of typing are detailed elsewhere (9).

Immunoprecipitation studies were performed on solubilized membrane antigens labeled with ^{3}H-leucine, from the
lymphoblastoid B-cell line J.Y. having the HLA type A2,
B7, DRw4,6. All antirsera used in this analysis were Ia737
(anti-DRw4,4x7), Ia715 (anti-DRw2,6), Ial72 (anti-DRw3,5,6)
and a heteroantiserum prepared by the immunization of a
rabbit with an isolated membrane antigen having a molecular
weight of 23,000 and 30,000 daltons. The latter antiserum
reacts in cytotoxicity assays with monocytes and B lymphocytes only. The details of the immunoprecipitation technique and analysis are reported elsewhere (10).

RESULTS

The results of the analysis of B-cell typing of a
family with several members having the diagnosis of systemic
lupus erythematosus (SLE) is shown in Table 1.

We previously reported the increased frequency of the
DRw2 and/or DRw3 antigens in patients with SLE. In
addition, the antiserum Ia715 reacted with B cells from 75%
of the individuals in the disease population studied compared
to 14% of a normal control population. The latter antiserum
reacts in a normal population showing a significant correlation with DRw2 and 6 antigens. Serum Ia715 reacts
with cells from the mother and 3 offspring following the
maternal B haplotype which appears to be controlling the
DRw3 antigen. The results suggest that in addition to the
2 DRw specificities a third B-cell alloantigen is genetically controlled by the MHC.

Immunoprecipitation analysis of P-40 solubilized
membrane antigens from a B lymphoid cell line was carried
out in an attempt to determine the number of antigen bearing

TABLE 1
B-CELL ALLOANTIGEN TYPING, FAMILY STUDY

Parents			Offspring		
	Haplotype	HLA Antigens		Haplotype	
Mother	A.	A2, B51, DRw7	1.	B.	A1, B8, DRw3, Ia715
	B.	A1, B8, DRw3, Ia715[a]		D.	A29, B12, DRw4
			2.	B.	A1, B8, DRw3, Ia715
Father	C.	A3, B35, DRw6		D.	A29, B12, DRw4
	D.	A29, B12, DRw4	3.	A.	A28, B51, DRw7
				C.	A3, B35, DRw6
			4.	B.	A1, B8, DRw3, Ia715
				C.	A3, B35, DRw6

[a]Sera Ia715 reactions appear to detect an additional
B-cell antigen.

molecules. It has previously been determined that the
human DRw antigens are analogous to the murine Ia antigens
in that precipitation with anti-DRw sera results in the
isolation of 2 molecules with approximate molecular weights
of 29,000 and 34,000 daltons when solubilized with deter-
gents and 23,000-30,000 daltons when solubilized with papain
(10). The results of sequential precipitation with the above
mentioned antisera as measured by migration characteristic
in 10% polyacrylamide gels in SDS and under reducing
conditions are summarized in Table 2.

In Table 2 a positive sign indicates the precipitation
of components with approximate molecular weights of 29,000-
34,000 daltons. A negative sign indicates no radioactive
peaks on the gels. The reproduction of the electrophoretic
profiles observed in these analyses is reported elsewhere
(11). The significant observation in this analysis is the
result of the precipitation with Ia715 and Ia172. These
antisera detect a common specificity, DRw6. Serum Ia172,
however, precipitates an antigenic moiety in addition to
that precipitated by Ia715. This conclusion is based on
the observation that when first clearing for the DRw6
antigen with the serum Ia715 an additional 29,000-34,000
molecular component is precipitated by the Ia172 serum.

TABLE 2
SUMMARY OF RESULTS OF SEQUENTIAL PRECIPITATION
OF SOLUBILIZED "DRw" ANTIGEN ANTISERA USED IN
2nd PRECIPITATION AND DRw ANTIGENS DETECTED

1st precipitat- ing antisera	NHS	Ia715 DRW2,6	Ia737 DRw4	Ia172 DRw3,5,6	Rabbit[a] anti 23-30
NHS	−	+	+	+	+
Ia715	−	−	+	+	+
Ia737	−	+	−	+	+
Ia172	−	−	+	−	+
anti 23-30	−	−	−	−	−

[a]Antisera prepared against papain solubilized B-cell
antigen and absorbed with packed pooled platelets.

In the reciprocal sequence Ia172 clears for the DRw6 specificity as evidenced by the absence of radioactive peaks in
subsequent precipitation attempts with Ia715. Thus, serum
Ia172 appears to contain 2 antibodies, 1 directed against
the DRw6 specificity and a second against an additional
B-cell alloantigen. The results of these experiments
demonstrate that at least 3 Ia-like antigenic moieties can
be isolated from a single cell source, thus 3 gene products.

DISCUSSION

The conclusion drawn from the above studies is that
more than 1 gene locus controls the expression of the
human B-cell antigens. In a recent report Tosi and
associates (12) described their findings which are similar
to those described in the latter portion of this paper. In
addition to the precipitation of 2 DRw antigens with
appropriate alloantisera, another B-cell alloantigen could
be isolated. Their approach attempted to quantitate the
amount of alloantigen precipitated compared to the total
amount of antigen as identified by a heteroantiserum. Their
results suggest a fourth antigen which may be the product of
the allele at the second locus.
The definitive serologic description of multiple loci
awaits the identification of a recombinant event in the
genetic region controlling B-cell alloantigen expression.
If one is to identify such recombinants the approach to
serologic analysis of these alloantigens must be different
from that currently employed by most investigators. This

approach has heretofore related all serologic reactions to
their Dw association. Our studies and those of Gibofsky et
al. (13) on disease association with the MHC have clearly
demonstrated that a single or several antisera may react
with a much higher frequency in the disease population compared to the frequency of reactions of sera identifying DRw
specificities in that same population or a normal population. Using the sera which identify D-cell alloantigens
other than DRw specificities will result in a clearer understanding of the genetic control of human Ia-like antigens.

ACKNOWLEDGMENTS

     I wish to acknowledge the contribution of the following
associates to the contents of this manuscript: Drs. A.H.
Johnson, H. Moutsopoulus, T. Chused, J. Reinertson, and
J. Klippel.

REFERENCES

1.   Mann, D.L., Abelson, L., Harris, S., and Amos, D.B.
     (1976). Nature 259, 143.
2.   Mann, D.L., Abelson, L., Henkart, P., Harris, S., and
     Amos, D.B. (1975). Proc. Natl. Acad. Sci. USA 75, 5103.
3.   Barnstable, C.J., Jones, E.A., Bodmer, W.F., Bodmer,
     J.G., Arce-Gomez, B., Snarg, D., and Crumpton, M.J.
     (1976). Cold Spring Harbor Symp. Quart. Biol. 41, 443.
4.   Mann, D.L., and Sharrow, S.O. Manuscript in preparation.
5.   Van Rood, J.J., van Leeuwen, A., Keuning, J.J., and
     Blusse van oud Alblos, A. (1975). Tissue Antigens 5, 73.
6.   Amos, D.B., and Bach, F.H. (1968). J. Exp. Med. 128, 623.
7.   Moutsopoulos, A.M., Chused, T.M., Johnson, A.H., Knudsen,
     B., and Mann, D.L. (1978). Science 199, 1441.
8.   Reinertsen, J., Klippel, J., Johnson, A.M., Steinberg,
     A., Decker, J., and Mann, D.L. (1978). N. Engl. J. Med.
     299, 515.
9.   Nelson, D.L., Strober, W., Abelson, L., Bundy, B., and
     Mann, D.L. (1977). J. Immunol. 118, 943.
10. Nilsson, S., Schwartz, B.D., Waxdal, M., Green, I.,
     Cullen, S., and Mann, D.L. (1977). J. Immunol. 118,
     1271.
11. Mann, D.L., Kauffman, J., Orr, H., Robb, I., and
     Strominger, J. (1979). Transpl. Proc. In press.
12. Tosi, R., Tanigaki, N., Centis, D., Farrara, G.B., and
     Pressman, D. (1978). J. Exp. Med. 148, 1592.
13. Gibofsky, A., Winchester, R.J., Patarroyo, M., Fortino,
     M., and Kunkel, H.G. (1978). J. Exp. Med. 148, 1728.

STRUCTURAL ANALYSIS OF THE I-A AND I-E/C ALLOANTIGENS[1]

Richard G. Cook, Ellen S. Vitetta, Mark H. Siegelman,
Jonathan W. Uhr, and J. Donald Capra

Department of Microbiology, University of Texas Southwestern Medical School, Dallas, Texas 75235

ABSTRACT The I-A and I-E/C alloantigens isolated from
radiolabeled murine splenocytes were examined for structural variation by NH_2-terminal sequence analysis and
comparative tryptic peptide mapping. For the I-A
antigens (k and b haplotypes), allelic variation was
demonstrated in the α subunits by peptide mapping and in
the β subunits by peptide mapping and sequence analysis.
Comparative peptide analysis of the α and β subunits from
appropriate recombinants indicated that both subunits are
encoded in the I-A subregion. Allelic differences were
also shown for the E/C alloantigens by NH_2-terminal
sequence analysis (β chains) and by tryptic peptide comparisons (α and β chains). Further analysis of several
intra-I-region recombinants revealed that the E/C α chain
was encoded by the E/C subregion, while the β chain was
encoded by the I-A or B subregions.

INTRODUCTION

The murine Ia alloantigens are cell surface glycoproteins
encoded by the I-region of the H-2 complex (1, 2). Their relationship to the various immune responses controlled by the
I-region has become increasingly evident through numerous
studies showing inhibition of function by anti-Ia alloantisera
(3, 4). This suggests that the Ia antigens may function as
receptor molecules which mediate interactions among cells or
between cells and antigens.

Two I-subregions, A and E/C[2], encode products which can
be detected by biochemical techniques. These molecules are
found predominantly on B lymphocytes (2, 5) and are co-
expressed on the same cell as demonstrated by both functional

[1]This work was supported in part by generous grants from
the National Institutes of Health, American Cancer Society,
and National Science Foundation.
[2]Due to our present uncertainty as to whether Ia specificity 7 is encoded by the I-E or I-C subregions, the
designation E/C will be utilized.

(6) and biochemical techniques (7). Both the A and E/C alloantigens consist of two subunits, α and β, with apparent mw
of 31-34,000 and 26-29,000 daltons, respectively. In an
effort to gain insight into the extent and nature of structural variation which exists in these putative receptor
molecules, our laboratories over the past two years have
studied the A and E/C antigens at the primary structural level. This article will describe recent structural data on
these molecules and present a tentative model for the genetic
organization of the genes encoding Ia antigens.

METHODS

Splenocytes from various congenic strains were either
radiolabeled for 6-8 hr with ^{3}H- or ^{14}C-amino acids (8-10) or
surface labeled with ^{125}I by the lactoperoxidase catalyzed
iodination technique (11). Cells were lysed with detergent
(NP40) and the internally labeled lysates were chromatographed on lentil lectin-sepharose to enrich for glycoproteins
(12). The lectin adherent glycoprotein pools were cleared of
Ig and non-specific material with rabbit anti-mouse Ig and
Staphylococcus aureus (S. aureus), and then the I-A and/or
I-E/C alloantigens were immunoprecipitated with appropriate
alloantisera and S. aureus. The Ia α and β subunits were resolved by sodium dodecyl sulfate polyacrylamide gel electrophoresis (SDS-PAGE) (12).
Isolated α and β subunits were examined for structural
variation by two techniques — NH$_2$-terminal sequence analysis
(9, 13, 14) and comparative tryptic peptide mapping using
cation exchange chromatography (10). For comparative peptide
analysis, double label (^{3}H and ^{14}C) techniques were utilized.

RESULTS

Structural Characterization of the I-A Alloantigens. We
have examined the A^k, A^b, and A^d alloantigens for electrophoretic variation by SDS-PAGE using sensitive double label
(^{3}H and ^{14}C) techniques (12). Under reducing conditions, the
α and β subunit apparent mw for all three of these products
are 34,000 and 26,000 daltons, respectively. In the absence
of reducing agent, approximately 80% of the A alloantigens
exist as disulfide bonded α-β dimers (mw 65,000) in detergent
lysates. However, the disulfide bonding of the α and β chains
is apparently an artifact of the detergent lysis procedure,
since lysis in the presence of alkylating agents eliminates
the formation of the α-β dimers.
NH$_2$-terminal sequence data on the A^k and A^b antigens is
shown in Table I (14). The α subunits of the k and b alleles
appear identical, although only six assignments have been

made in the first 20 residues. The other positions are apparently occupied by those amino acids (gly, glu, gln, asp, asn) which are poorly incorporated by normal splenocytes. In

TABLE I
PARTIAL NH$_2$-TERMINAL AMINO ACID SEQUENCES OF I-A ALLOANTIGENS[a]

	1	2	3	4	5	6	7	8	9	10	11	12	13	14	15	16	17	18	19	20
A_α^b				ILE		ALA			VAL			TYR				VAL	TYR			
A_α^k				ILE		ALA			VAL			TYR				VAL	TYR			
A_β^b				SER		ARG	HIS	PHE	VAL	TYR		PHE	—	—	—		TYR	PHE		
A_β^k				SER		ARG	HIS	PHE	VAL	—		PHE	PRO	PRO	PHE		TYR	PHE		

[a]Dashes at positions 9, 12, 13, and 14 of the β polypeptides indicate sequence differences between A^k and A^b. These haplotype associated differences are also enclosed in a box.

contrast, the β subunits from these two haplotypes show significant structural variation — positions 9, 12, 13, and 14 are different in the k and b β chains. This suggests that β subunit of the A alloantigen is encoded within the major histocompatibility complex (MHC).

Evidence that the α chain is also MHC encoded has come from comparative peptide mapping studies. As shown in Fig. 1, extensive allelic (k vs b haplotypes) variation was detected in the α and β subunits by this technique. These allelic α and β subunits show only 50-60% coincident elution of tryptic peptides; this probably corresponds to about an 80-90% homology at the amino acid sequence level. A similar degree of structural variation has also been shown in preliminary experiments comparing the A^k with the A^d and A^r subunits (not shown).

While both the α and β subunits of the A alloantigen show allelic variation, it was possible that one subunit was encoded by the A subregion and the other by some other H-2 locus, as has been shown for the E/C alloantigen (see following section). To ascertain whether both subunits were controlled by the A subregion, the α and β chains of B10.A were compared with those of the recombinants B10.A(4R) and A.TL; all three strains are k haplotype in A, but B10.A(4R) is b to the right of A and A.TL is s to the left of A:

		I				
	K	A	B	J	E	C
B10.A	k	k	k	k	k	d
B10.A(4R)	k	k	b	b	b	b
A.TL	s	k	k	k	k	k

By tryptic peptide mapping, the α and β subunits of B10.A
were identical to those of B10.A(4R) and A.TL (not shown).
Thus, it appears that <u>both</u> the α and β chains of the A alloantigens are encoded by the <u>A</u> subregion.

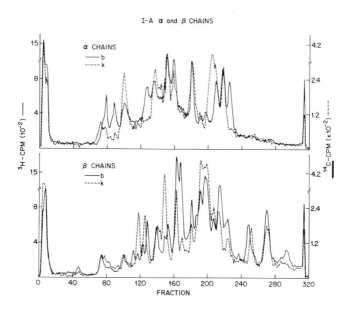

Fig. 1. Ion exchange chromatrography of tryptic digests
of the α (upper panel) and β (lower panel) subunits of the A^k
and A^b alloantigens. ^{3}H-labeled A^b α and β subunits are
compared with ^{14}C-labeled A^k α and β subunits.

<u>Structural Characterization of the I-E/C Alloantigens</u>.
Four alleles of the <u>E/C</u> subregion product have been analyzed
by SDS-PAGE (12). Under reducing conditions, the α and β subunits of <u>k</u> and <u>r</u> haplotypes have apparent mw of 34,000 and
28,000 daltons, while the subunit mw of the <u>p</u> and <u>d</u> products
are 31,000 and 29,000 daltons. The cause of this <u>apparent</u> mw
variation in allelic products is not known, but may result
from a) variation in the degree of glycosylation, b) the size
of the polypeptide chain, or c) differences in conformation of
the polypeptides. Unlike the I-A alloantigens, the E/C α and
β subunits do not tend to form disulfide bonded α-β dimers
during detergent lysis (12, 15).
    The subunits of <u>k</u> and <u>r</u> haplotype have been analyzed for
NH$_2$-terminal sequence (Table II) (14). There were no differences in the α chains, although three positions assigned for <u>k</u>
were not identified for <u>r</u> due to insufficient incorporation of
those amino acids. Allelic variation in sequence was found in

TABLE II
PARTIAL NH$_2$-TERMINAL AMINO ACID SEQUENCES OF I-E/C ALLOANTIGENS[a]

	1	2	3	4	5	6	7	8	9	10	11	12	13	14	15	16	17	18	19	20	21	22
E/C$_\alpha^k$	ILE	LYS			HIS	THR	ILE	ILE		ALA		PHE	TYR	LEU	LEU	PRO			ARG			PHE
E/C$_\alpha^r$	ILE	LYS			HIS	*	ILE	ILE		*		PHE	TYR	LEU	LEU	*			ARG			PHE
E/C$_\beta^k$	VAL	ARG		SER	ARG	PRO		PHE	LEU		TYR	—	LYS	SER				PHE	TYR			
E/C$_\beta^r$	VAL	ARG		SER	ARG	PRO		PHE	LEU		TYR	SER	THR	SER				PHE	TYR			

[a]The asterisks at positions 6, 10, and 16 of the E/C$^r_\alpha$ polypeptide indicate that THR, ALA, and PRO were not tested. The dash at position 12 of the E/C$^k_\beta$ polypeptide indicates that SER is not present. Haplotype associated differences between the β polypeptides of E/C^k and E/C^r are enclosed in a box.

the β subunits at positions 12 and 13. The E/C^d β chain, which was examined by McMillan et al. (16) and Allison et al. (17) differs from both k and r, having a val at position 12. Thus, like the A subregion alloantigens, NH$_2$-terminal sequence variation between E/C allelic products can only be detected in the β subunits.

The E/C alloantigens of k, r, p, and d haplotypes have also been examined structurally by comparative mapping of tryptic peptides (10). A summary of these results is shown in Table III. A small degree of variation (∿10%) was detected in the α chains. In contrast, the E/C β chain comparisons showed significant allelic variation — 48%, 48%, and 69% coincident elution of d, p, and r tryptic peptides when compared to k.

TABLE III
TRYPTIC PEPTIDE COMPARISONS OF E/C α AND β POLYPEPTIDES

E/C Subregion Haplotype	No. of Tryptic Peptides	No. of Shared Peptides	Percent Coincidence[a]
k	14	13	84
p	17		
k	14	13	93
d	14		
k	14	14	97
r	15		
k	14	7	48
p	15		
k	14	7	48
d	15		
d	14	9	69
r	12		

[a]Percent coincidence determined by the following formula:

$$\frac{\text{No. of shared peptides}}{\text{Average no. of peptides}} \times 100.$$

These results, in conjunction with the NH$_2$-terminal sequence data, indicate that the E/C β chains, and probably the E/C α chains, are encoded within the MHC.

Using the technique of 2-dimensional (2-D) gel analysis, Jones et al.(18) have shown that the E/C alloantigens are controlled by two different I-region loci — one in A and the other in E/C. In an effort to confirm and extend these observations to the more conventional α-β subunit nomenclature, and also to determine the possible nature of the electrophoretic variations observed by 2-D gels, we have compared the E/C α and β subunits from appropriate I-region recombinants by peptide mapping (19). A summary of these studies is shown in Table IV; all strains were k/d haplotype in E/C, but varied in A (k, b, or s). The E/C α chains from B10.A, B10.A(3R), B10.A(5R), and B10.HTT showed coelution of all tryptic peptides. However, there were notable differences among the β subunits; Fig. 2 shows that there are distinct tryptic peptide differences between the β subunits of B10.A and 3R or 5R (differences denoted by arrows). The bottom panel is a control showing the reproducibility of the system. The differences between 5R and B10.A indicate that the β chain is encoded to the left of I-J. A comparison of the β subunits from B10.A and B10.AQR revealed no peptide differences (not shown); this maps the E/C β chain structural gene to the right of H-2K and into I-A or B. In other experiments, we found that the β chains of 3R and 5R are identical (both are b in I-A,B); also, the E/C β subunit from B10.HTT is distinct from the β chains of both B10.A and 3R (or 5R). Thus, the E/C β subunit is encoded in the I-A or B subregion, while the E/C α chain by definition must be encoded in the E/C subregion. This implies that allospecificities mapped to the E/C subregion are controlled by the α subunit.

TABLE IV
SUMMARY OF PEPTIDE MAPPING DATA ON THE E/C ANTIGENS FROM RECOMBINANT STRAINS[a]

Strains	K	A	B	J	E	C	S	G	D	α	β
				I							
B10.A	k	k	k	k	k	d	d	d	d	100	100
B10.AQR	q	k	k	k	k	d	d	d	d	ND	100
B10.A(5R)	b	b	b	k	k	d	d	d	d	100	60
B10.A(3R)	b	b	b	b	k	d	d	d	d	100	60
B10.HTT	s	s	s	s	k	k	k	k	d	100	56

(% of Coelution of Tryptic Peptides with B10.A E/C Subunits shown in α and β columns; H-2 Haplotypes shown in K–D columns)

[a]The arrows indicate that the β chain must be encoded to the right or left of that locus.

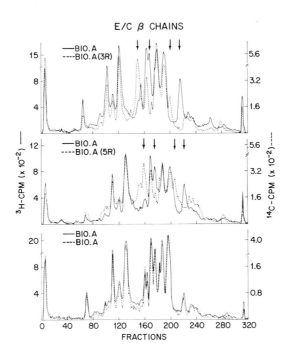

Fig. 2.   Ion exchange chromatography of tryptic digests of E/C β polypeptides. ³H-labeled E/Cᵏ β chains from B10.A are compared with ¹⁴C-labeled E/Cᵏ β chains from B10.A(3R) (panel A), B10.A(5R) (panel B) and B10.A (panel C). Major peptide differences are denoted by arrows.

CONCLUSIONS

1. Primary structural differences exist between the A and E/C alloantigens. Although both the A and E/C antigens consist of two polypeptide chains, α and β, they can be differentiated by their apparent subunit mw, and by their capacities to form disulfide bonded α-β dimers during detergent lysis. By NH_2-terminal sequence analysis and tryptic peptide mapping analysis there is no apparent homology between the A and E/C α chains, or β chains.

2. Allelic variation is detected in the α and β subunits of both the A and E/C antigens. There are multiple amino acid sequence differences between allelic β chains of the A and E/C molecules; thus far no allelic variation in the α subunits has been detected by sequence analysis. Comparative tryptic peptide analysis has demonstrated marked allelic variation

(∿40-50%) in the A α, A β, and E/C β chains and detectable
(∿10%) variation in the E/C α allelic products. Since congenic mouse strains, which theoretically differ only at the
MHC, have been utilized, the allelic variation observed indicates that all four subunits (A α and β, E/C α and β) are
encoded within the MHC.

  3. The I region encodes the α and β subunits of both the
A and E/C alloantigens. By comparative tryptic peptide
analysis of the A and E/C molecules from appropriate intra-
H-2 recombinants, it was shown that both the α and β subunits
of the A alloantigen are encoded in the I-A subregion, while
the E/C α and β subregions are encoded by the E/C and A, B
subregions, respectively. Fig. 3 presents our current interpretation of the genetic organization and expression of the A
and E/C alloantigens. To our knowledge, there is no biological precedent for a two chained molecule, not synthesized as a
polyprotein, which contains subunits encoded by linked genes;
to date there is no evidence for or against the synthesis of
the Ia antigens as polyproteins which are then cleaved to
yield α and β subunits. Finally, although there is presently
no obvious explanation for why linked genes should encode the

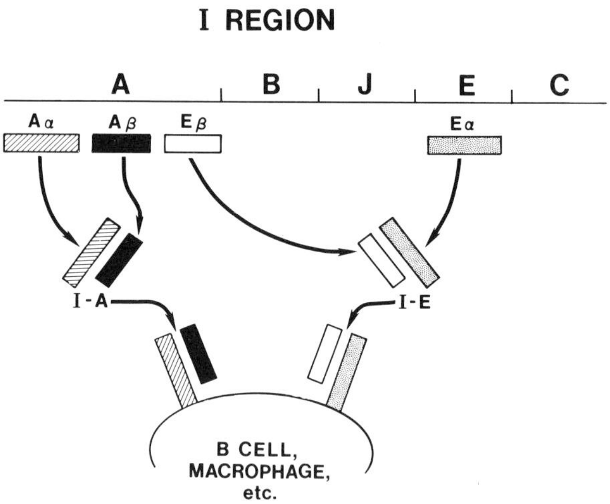

Fig. 3.   Interpretive model of the genetic organization
and expression of the A and E/C alloantigens. The order of
the A α, A β, and E β "genes" in the A subregion is not known;
also, our results have not eliminated the B subregion as the
locus which encodes E β. For simplicity, E is used instead
of E/C.

Ia α and β subunits, the two gene (<u>A</u> and <u>E/C</u>) control of the E/C antigens does offer a possible molecular mechanism for the observed gene complementation requirement (20) for responsiveness to certain antigens.

ACKNOWLEDGEMENTS

We wish to thank S. Kourvelas, M. Bagby, P. Liu, Y.-M. Tseng, S. Lin, B. Himmel, Y. Chinn, T. Wallis, B. Tierney, D. Atherton, and P. Frank for excellent technical assistance during various phases of this work, and J. Hahn for careful and patient preparation of this manuscript.

REFERENCES

1. Klein, J. (1975). "Biology of the Mouse Histocompatibility -2 Complex" Springer-Verlag, New York.
2. Cullen, S.E., Freed, J.H., and Nathenson, S.G. (1976). Transplant. Rev. 20, 236.
3. Schwartz, R.H., David, C.S., Sachs, D.H., and Paul, W.E. (1976). J. Immunol. 117, 531.
4. Frelinger, J.A., Neiderhuber, J.E., and Shreffler, D.C. (1975). Science 188, 268.
5. Vitetta, E.S., and Capra, J.D. (1978). Adv. Immunol. 26, 148.
6. Frelinger, J.A., Hibbler, F.J., and Hill, S.W. (1978). J. Immunol. 121, 2376.
7. Vitetta, E.S., and Cook, R.G. (1979) J. Immunol., in press.
8. Vitetta, E.S., Capra, J.D., Klapper, D.G., Klein, J., and Uhr, J.W. (1976). Proc. Natl. Acad. Sci. USA 73, 905.
9. Cook, R.G., Vitetta, E.S., Uhr, J.W., Klein, J., Wilde, C.E., and Capra, J.D. (1978). J. Immunol. 121, 1015.
10. Cook, R.G., Vitetta, E.S., Uhr, J.W., and Capra, J.D. (1979). J. Mol. Immunol., in press.
11. Vitetta, E.S., Baur, S., and Uhr, J.W. (1971). J. Exp. Med. 134, 242.
12. Cook, R.G., Uhr, J.W., Capra, J.D., and Vitetta, E.S. (1978). J. Immunol. 121, 2205.
13. Cook, R.G., Vitetta, E.S., Capra, J.D., and Uhr, J.W. (1977). Immunogenetics 5, 437.
14. Cook, R.G., Siegelman, M.S., Capra, J.D., Uhr, J.W., and Vitetta, E.S. (1979). J. Immunol., in press.
15. Schwartz, B.D., and Cullen, S.E. (1978). Springer Seminars in Immunopathology 1, 85.
16. McMillan, M., Cecka, J.M, Murphy, D.B., McDevitt, H.O., and Hood, L. (1978). Immunogenetics 6, 137.

17. Allison, J.P., Walker, L.E., Russell, W.A., Pellegrino, M.A., Ferrone, S., Reisfeld, R.A., Frelinger, J.A., and Silver, J. (1978). Proc. Natl. Acad. Sci. USA 75, 3953.
18. Jones, P.P., Murphy, D.B., and McDevitt, H.O. (1978). J. Exp. Med. 148, 925.
19. Cook, R.G., Vitetta, E.S., Uhr, J.W., and Capra, J.D. (1979). J. Exp. Med., in press.
20. Benacerraf, B., and Dorf, M.E. (1976). Cold Spring Harbor Symp. Quant. Biol. 41, 465.

H-2^b STRUCTURE ON MOUSE LEUKEMIA CELLS[1]

David A. Zarling,[2,3] Andrew Watson,[3]
and Fritz H. Bach[3,4]

Immunobiology Research Center
University of Wisconsin, Madison, 53706

ABSTRACT Mouse major histocompatibility (H-2^b) antigens
on RBL-5A leukemia cells can be chemically cross-linked
to form several different H-2^b containing polypeptide
products. These products include apparent dimers
comprised of one H-2^b heavy (46,000 daltons) and one
light (12,000 daltons) chain, intrachain cross-linked
H-2^b heavy chain monomers, and several other species of
higher molecular weight H-2^b polypeptide complexes.

INTRODUCTION

H-2 antigens are cell surface glycoproteins composed of
two different chains with apparent molecular weights (M_r) of
46,000 (heavy chain) and 12,000 daltons (β_2-microglobulin,
light chain) (for review see 1,2). Detergent solubilized
H-2 molecules bear alloantigenic determinants and carbohydrate
moieties solely on the heavy chain; non-covalently bonded
light chains are unglycosylated and devoid of alloantigenic
sites. When H-2 molecules are detergent extracted without
prior alkylation of the cells, at least one disulfide bond
is formed between two heavy chains. When cells are pretreated
with an alkylating agent such as iodoacetamide, disulfide
bonds between heavy chains are not formed in detergent
extracts. Thus, the majority of H-2 heavy chains do not
appear to exist as disulfide bonded dimers on the cell
surface (1,2,3). However, it is not known whether H-2
antigens naturally exist as non-covalently associated dimers
or multimers in the cell membrane. H-2 antigens are involved
in cell-cell interactions and are specifically recognized on
mouse tumor cells as target molecules by allogeneic- or
syngeneic-immune cytotoxic thymus-derived lymphocytes (4-10).

[1] Supported by NIH Grants CA-16836 and CA-9106
[2] Department of Pathology
[3] Immunobiology Research Center
[4] Departments of Medical Genetics and Surgery

We have previously analyzed the structure of Rauscher
murine leukemia virus envelope glycoprotein (R-MLV gp70) on
the surface of R-MLV transformed and virus producing C57BL/6
(H-2^b) mouse leukemia cells (RBL-5A) (11). A 70,000 dalton
protein on the surface of RBL-5A cells which is identifiable
by means of immunoprecipitation with αR-MLV gp70 serum, can
be chemically cross-linked to form dimers and trimers (11).
These dimer and trimer structures may be the 80-100 Å R-MLV
gp70-containing knobs, which have been visualized by electron
microscopy on R-MLV infected cell surfaces (12). R-MLV gp70
may also be associated with polypeptides other than gp70 in
cross-linked high molecular weight complexes (11).
     In studies analoagous to those conducted on R-MLV gp70,
we have used chemical cross-linking to analyze the structure
of H-2^b and its neighboring polypeptide antigens on RBL-5A
cells.

RESULTS

H-2^b Heavy and Light Chains. The structure of H-2^b
antigens on RBL-5A cells was examined (Figure 1). Cells
were ^{125}I-labeled (lactoperoxidase) and extracted (13) with
Nonidet P40, NP-40. Immunoprecipitates were prepared (13)
using specific αH-2^b or αR-MLV gp70 sera (8), and polypeptides
were separated by SDS-PAGE under reducing conditions (8).

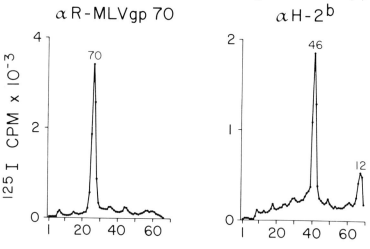

FIGURE 1. Radioiodinated RBL-5A cells were NP-40
extracted and polypeptides immunoprecipitated with αH-2^b
(right) or αR-MLV gp70 serum (left) were separated by
reducing SDS-PAGE (10% acrylamide).

Figure 1 (right) shows αH-2^b serum precipitated polypeptides with apparent M_r of 46,000 and 12,000 daltons (designated as H-2 heavy and light chains, respectively). The αH-2^b serum shown in Figure 1 was harvested 1 week after 6 successive weekly innoculations of young (5 to 6 week old) B10.D2 (H-2^d) mice with C57BL/6 (H-2^b) spleen cells and did not contain αR-MLV gp70 reactivity. R-MLV gp70 (approximately 70,000 daltons) was immunoprecipitated independently of H-2^b heavy and light chains (Figure 1, left). Thus, in RBL-5A extracts no NP-40 detergent stable association of H-2^b and either R-MLV gp70 or other polypeptide antigens was detectable.

H-2^b Cross-Linking. Complexes which might not be detergent stable were sought by chemical cross-linking prior to solubilizing the cells. The rate of cross-linking of H-2^b polypeptides on the surface of RBL-5A cells was measured. Radioiodinated RBL-5A cells were cross-linked at 0°C with 1 mM bis-[2-(succinimidooxycarbonyloxy)ethyl]sulfone (14), (BSOCOES), for 0.17, 0.3, 0.5, 1, 6, 10, or 20 min. Reactions were terminated with arginine. NP-40 extracts were immunoprecipitated with αH-2^b serum and the polypeptides separated by reducing SDS-PAGE. Figure 2 shows the electrophoretic patterns of cross-linked products. At least six species of polypeptides, in addition to H-2^b heavy and light chains were apparent. Polypeptides N, P, Q and HMW were formed first (0.3 min of cross-linking), followed by polypeptides O (0.5 min), and R (6 min). After longer cross-linking (15, 30, 45, 60, or 90 min), peaks N, O, P, Q, R, and HMW were present and persisted for at least 90 min and no additional polypeptides were produced (data not shown).

Figure 3 shows immunoprecipitates from cross-linked RBL-5A polypeptides separated by SDS-PAGE in slab gels (15) and detected by autoradiography (16). Anti-H-2^b serum precipitated 46,000 and 12,000 dalton proteins from non-linked RBL-5A cells (Figure 3, lane 8, 0 min); long x-ray film exposure times revealed trace amounts of a 120,000 dalton component. Polypeptides N (58,000 daltons), O (104,000), P (120,000), Q (doublet; with a mean M_r of 178,000 daltons), several bands at position R (205,000 to 235,000) and HMW ($>$ 350,000) were precipitated from BSOCOES-linked cells (lane 7, 15 min; lane 6, 30 min). For comparison, the extracts were reacted with αR-MLV gp70 serum, which precipitated a 70,000 dalton polypeptide (Figure 3, lane 2, 0 min). Polypeptides A (140,000 daltons) and B (210,000) were present in the BSOCOES-linked extracts (lane 3, 15 min; lane 4, 30 min). No labeled material was precipitated with normal goat (lane 5, 15 min) or mouse serum (not shown). Thus, polypep-

αH-2^b

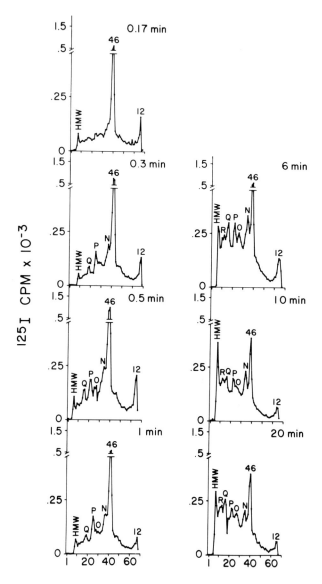

FRACTION NUMBER

FIGURE 2. Radioiodinated cells were BSOCOES-linked for the times shown and αH-2^b precipitated polypeptides were separated by reducing SDS-PAGE (5% acrylamide).

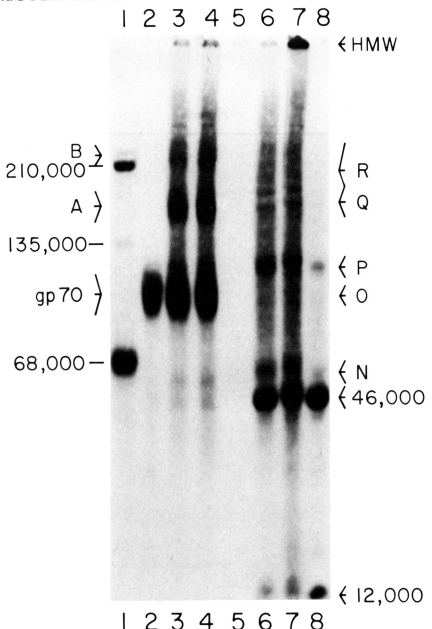

FIGURE 3. Radioiodinated cells were BSOCOES-linked for 0, 15, or 30 min and immunoprecipitated polypeptides were separated by reducing SDS-PAGE (4% acrylamide). Lane 1, M_r markers; 2, 0 min cross-linking, αgp70 serum; 3, 15 min, αgp70; 4, 30 min, αgp70; 5, 15 min, normal serum; 6, 30 min, αH-2^b; 7, 15 min, αH-2^b; 8, 0 min, αH-2^b.

tides A, B, and HMW, in addition to a 70,000 dalton protein
were precipitated with αR-MLV gp70 serum (Figure 3). Polypeptides N, O, P, Q, R, and HMW, in addition to 46,000 and
12,000 dalton polypeptides, were precipitated with αH-2^b
serum (Figures 2 and 3).

   Cleavage of Cross-linked Polypeptides. The compositions
of some cross-linked polypeptides were analyzed. RBL-5A
cells were radioiodinated and BSOCOES-linked for 60 min at
0°C. Polypeptides B, A, and gp70, immunoprecipitated with
αR-MLV gp70 serum, were electrophoresed under reducing
conditions in a first dimension slab gel (4% acrylamide)
with BSOCOES-links intact. The gel lane containing B, A,
and gp70 was removed, treated with base (pH 11.6, 2 hrs,
37°C), and neutralized (pH 7.2). Cleavage products were
analyzed on a second dimension reducing SDS-polyacrylamide
slab gel (4% acrylamide). A and B were cleaved to polypeptides of an approximate M_r of 70,000 daltons (Figure 4).
Under these conditions the cleavages of polypeptides A and B
was nearly complete or complete (Figure 4 and not shown).
Thus, A (140,000 daltons) and B (210,000 daltons) are cross-
linked dimers and trimers of a 70,000 dalton polypeptide
(Figure 4).

   In another experiment, cells were radioiodinated and
BSOCOES-linked for 30 min at 0°C. Reactions were terminated
by incubation with arginine for 20 min at 0°C and the cells
were washed and incubated with 1% iodoacetamide in phosphate
buffered saline for an additional 30 min at 0°C. Extracts
were precipitated with αH-2^b serum and proteins separated by
two-dimensional reducing SDS-PAGE in slab gels as described
above. Figure 5 shows that cross-linked polypeptide N
(58,000 daltons) was partially cleaved to 46,000 and 12,000
dalton products. Therefore, polypeptide N appears to be
composed of dimers consisting of at least one H-2^b heavy
(46,000) and one light chain (12,000). Also shown in Figure
5 is the partial cleavage of a polypeptide of an apparent M_r
of 46,000 daltons from a polypeptide (indicated with a ✶ in
the first dimension) of apparent M_r of 35,000 daltons in the
first dimension SDS-polyacrylamide gel. This ✶ polypeptide,
originally immunoprecipitated with αH-2^b serum, is likely to
be an intrachain BSOCOES-link(s) in an H-2^b heavy chain
monomer. Its faster migration than non-linked (46,000
dalton) heavy chains in the first dimension could be due to
the ✶ polypeptide being less extended in SDS than non-linked
heavy chains. Table 1 summarizes the results of these and
other similar experiments where some of the components of
BSOCOES-linked polypeptides on RBL-5A cells were analyzed.

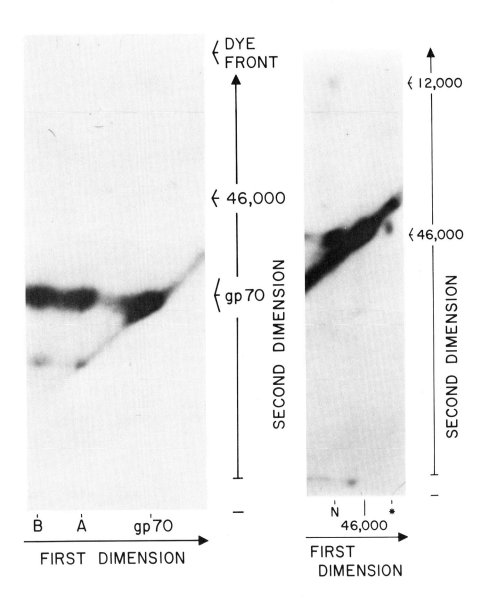

FIGURE 4. Cleavage of BSOCOES-linked polypeptide B (210,000) and A (140,000) to a 70,000 dalton product.

FIGURE 5. Cleavage of N (58,000) to 46,000 and 12,000 dalton products and * (35,000) to a 46,000 dalton product.

TABLE I

COMPOSITIONS OF BSOCOES-LINKED POLYPEPTIDES ON RBL-5A CELLS[a]

BSOCOES-linked polypeptide	Approx. M_r (daltons) with:		Proposed Structure
	Links-intact	Links-removed	
B	210,000	70,000	gp70 trimer
A	140,000	70,000	gp70 dimer
N	58,000	46,000 + 12,000	H-2 heavy and light chain dimer
*	35,000	46,000	H-2 heavy chain monomer (intrachain linked)

[a]Polypeptides B and A were precipitated with αR-MLV gp70 serum. N and * were precipitated with αH-2[b] serum.

These cross-linking experiments show αR-MLV gp70 serum immunoprecipitated dimers and trimers of MLV gp70 and αH-2[b] serum immunoprecipitated apparent dimers, consisting of one H-2[b] heavy and one light chain, and intra-chain cross-linked H-2[b] heavy chain monomers. Several other species of H-2[b] containing BSOCOES cross-linked polypeptides from RBL-5A cell surfaces remain to be analyzed after cleavage of the cross-links (Figures 2 and 3). Preliminary results (not shown) indicate that polypeptides O and P can be partially cleaved to polypeptide products of an apparent M_r of 46,000 daltons. Furthermore, HMW polypeptides immunoprecipitated with αH-2[b] serum, were partially cleaved to polypeptides with apparent molecular weights of 46,000, 12,000, and 70,000 to approximately 130,000 daltons (data not shown). Thus, is it possible that H-2[b] polypeptides may associate with other H-2[b] heavy chains or even other polypeptides than H-2[b].

DISCUSSION

Polypeptide neighbors to H-2[b] antigens on RBL-5A leukemia cells have been measured using chemical cross-linking with BSOCOES, a 13 Å homo-bifunctional reagent reactive with lysine residues (11,14). Without cross-linking, no detergent stable association of H-2[b] with other polypeptides was detected in RBL-5A extracts. Cross-linking reactions were performed with radioiodinated RBL-5A cells at 0°C and polypep-

tides separated by SDS-PAGE under reducing conditions. The
reducing conditions used prevented possible formation of
artifactually-linked complexes due to disulfide exchange
reactions. Following BSOCOES-linking of RBL-5A cells and
immunoprecipitation with αH-2[b] serum, apparent dimers were
formed of one polypeptide with a M_r of 46,000 and one of
12,000 daltons. Apparent intrachain cross-linked 46,000
dalton polypeptide monomers were also observed. The 46,000
and 12,000 dalton polypeptides, initially immunoprecipitated
with αH-2[b] serum, are probably H-2[b] heavy and light chains.
However, peptide mapping and/or immunoprecipitation of these
cleavage products will be required to confirm that these
molecules are heavy and light chains. These cross-linking
results indicate that there may be a native close physical
association between one H-2 heavy and one light chain on the
cell surface. This is in agreement with the findings of
Cunningham et al. (2) and Henning et al. (3) who showed that
papain-treatment of H-2[b] molecules on ^{125}I-labeled cells
generated a large H-2[b] heavy chain fragment non-covalently
associated with an intact light chain. These researchers
have also shown that the majority of H-2[b] heavy chains on
the cell surface are not linked by disulfide bonds and thus
might exist either as one heavy chain or possibly as a
non-covalently associated heavy chain dimer. In preliminary
experiments, they found that disulfide bridge formation
between two H-2[b] heavy chains on the cell surface can be
facilitated by treatment of cells with 0-phenanthroline and
copper sulphate prior to alkylation, conditions which catalyze
disulfide bond formation. Therefore, they suggest that some
H-2[b] molecules could be close enough to one another to exist
as non-covalently bonded heavy chain dimers (2,3). Our
measurements showing the formation of cross-linked, αH-2[b]
immunoprecipitable, polypeptides with molecular weights like
0, P, Q and R are consistent with the possibility that a
significant amount of ^{125}I-labeled H-2[b] molecules on RBL-5A
cell surfaces could be close enough to one another to exist
as either non-covalently bonded heavy chain dimers or possibly
higher multimers. The partial cleavages of 46,000 dalton
polypeptides from cross-linked polypeptides 0 and P is
consistent with the hypothesis that heavy chain dimers may
exist. However, cleavage of 0 and P was not complete, thus
the possibility also exists that these molecules could
contain polypeptides other than H-2 heavy chains. The
composition of the large HMW polypeptides ($\geq$ 350,000 daltons),
immunoprecipitated with αH-2[b] serum, appears to be complex.
These cross-linked HMW polypeptides have not been shown to
contain a single M_r species and will require analysis in
first dimension gels allowing separation of polypeptide

complexes of up to several million daltons. Since HMW polypeptides could be comprised of different M_r species, it is difficult to interpret the partial cleavage of 46,000, 12,000, and 70,000 to 130,000 dalton polypeptides from HMW immunoprecipitated with αH-2^b serum. However, the data obtained so far is consistent with the idea that H-2^b could also be natively associated with polypeptides other than H-2^b on the surface of RBL-5A cells. A similar conclusion has been obtained after analysis of partial cleavage products of BSOCOES-linked HMW polypeptides immunoprecipitated with αR-MLV gp70 serum (11).

In summary, H-2^b antigens on RBL-5A cells can be cross-linked to form apparent dimers comprised of one heavy and one light chain, intra-chain cross-linked heavy chain monomers and several other species of higher molecular weight H-2^b polypeptide complexes.

ACKNOWLEDGEMENTS

We thank R. E. Duke, Department of Biochemistry and Biophysics Laboratory, University of Wisconsin, for suggesting the use of BSOCOES in these studies, providing the reagent, and assisting in the cross-linking experiments.

REFERENCES

1. Uhr, J.W., Vitetta, E.S., Klein, J., Poulik, M.D., Klapper, D.G. and Capra, J.D. (1976). C.S.H. Symp. Quant. Biol. 41, 363.
2. Cunningham, B.A., Henning, R., Milner, R.J., Reske, K., Ziffer, J.A. and Edelman, G.M. (1976). C.S.H. Symp. Quant. Biol. 41, 351.
3. Henning, R., Milner, R.J., Reske, K., Cunningham, B.A. and Edelman, G.M. (1976). Proc. Nat. Acad. Sci. 73, 118.
4. Bach, F.H., Bach, M.L. and Sondel, P.M. (1976). Nature 259, 273.
5. Schrader, J.W., Cunningham, B.A. and Edelman, G.M. (1975). Proc. Nat. Acad. Sci. 72, 5066.
6. Blank, K.J. and Lilly F. (1977). Nature 269, 808.
7. Gomard, E., Duprez, V., Reme, T., Colombani, M.J. and Levy, J.P. (1977). J. Exp. Med. 146, 909.
8. Zarling, D.A., Keshet, I., Watson, A. and Bach, F.H. (1978). Scand. J. Immunol. 8, 497.
9. Watson, A., Zarling, D.A. and Bach, F.H. The availability for recognition of normal H-2 antigens by cytotoxic-T-lymphocytes on a Rauscher virus transformed cell, RBL-5A. Submitted, 1979.

10. Germain, R.N., Dorf, M.E. and Benacerraf, B. (1975). J.
     Exp. Med. 142, 1023.
11. Zarling, D.A., Duke, R.E., Watson, A. and Bach, F.H.
     Mapping of cell surface polypeptide antigens by chemical
     cross-linking with BSOCOES: Rauscher MLV envelope
     glycoprotein neighbors on mouse leukemia cells.
     Submitted, 1979.
12. Demsey, A., Kawka, D. and Stackpole, C.W. (1977) J.
     Virol. 21, 358.
13. Ledbetter, J., Nowinski, R.C. and Emery, S. (1977). J.
     Virol. 22, 65.
14. Tesser, G.I., de Hoog-Declerk, R.A.O.M.M. and Westerhuis,
     L.W. (1975). Hoppe-Seyler's Z. Physiol. Chem. 356,
     1625.
15. Swank, R.T. and Munkres, K.D. (1971). Anal. Biochem.
     39, 462.
16. Laskey, R.A. and Mills, A.D. (1977). FEBS Letters 82,
     314.

WORKSHOP SUMMARY: CHEMISTRY OF MHC PRODUCTS
J. Donald Capra and Stanley G. Nathenson, The
University of Texas Health Science Center at
Dallas, 5323 Harry Hines Blvd., Dallas, Texas
75235 and Albert Einstein College of Medicine,
Bronx, New York 10461

Class I Products

Sequence studies of HLA antigens presented by Orr, Robb,
Bilofsky, Wu, Kabat and Strominger covered their published
as well as recent sequence data on HLA-A and HLA-B heavy
chains. Their progress on this problem has been extremely
impressive with nearly all of the sequence of the HLA-B7
molecule completed. The general features of the HLA heavy
chain glycoproteins were discussed. Two cysteine loops are
present, the first loop beginning at position 101 links to
165. The second loop beginning at 203 links to 258. The
sequences around the second cysteine loop show homology to
the immunoglobulin constant (C_H) domains. HLA-A2 and HLA-B7
antigens show high homology with each other with specific
portions being nearly identical. Areas of particular variability are also noted, for example between position 65 and
80. A hydrophobic region consisting of approximately 20-25
residues was demonstrated near the C-terminus. This is the
postulated membrane spanning region.

Biochemical characterization of major histocompatibility
antigens of the rabbit was presented by Kimball, Coligan and
Kindt. RLA antigens were isolated from radiolabeled
extracts of a rabbit tumor cell line by affinity chromatography with sheep anti-rabbit β_2-microglobulin. The 43,000
dalton glycoprotein was characterized by a variety of physical-chemical techniques. N-terminal amino acid sequence
analysis was performed on the first 35 residues. A 91%
homology existed between RLA and HLA-A2 and H-2K^b. No
evidence of multiple products was noted.

Radio sequence analysis of the H-2K^b MHC product of EL-4
was reported by Coligan, Kindt, Ewenstein, Uehara, Martinko
and Nathenson. Data was presented on the nearly completed
sequence (the first 280 residues) of the EL-4 H-2K^b glycoprotein. Cyanogen bromide cleavage yields 5 major products
which comprise the antigenic fragment released by papain
cleavage. The Ib CNBr product which was still too large
to sequence from the N-terminal was further cleaved by the
enzyme Thrombin into 3 pieces and these were sequenced separately. The overall characteristics of the molecule were
noted to be similar to that of the HLA heavy chain glycoproteins. In contrast, however, carbohydrate was found on

two sites at positions 86 and 176, whereas in the HLA glyco-
proteins carbohydrate has only been reported at position 86.
Although regions of clustered variability between H-2 and
HLA-A2 were noted, the overall sequence homology was 70-80%.

Sequence analysis of the H-2D^d glycoprotein was reported by
Nairn, Coligan, Kindt and Nathenson. Using the same techniques as reported by Coligan, et al. 70 residues have been
sequenced for the H-2D^d glycoprotein. Of importance were the
following findings: the absence of methionine at position 52
and substitution at position 98 of methionine for an isoleucine carried in the K^b glycoprotein. Eleven out of 70 positions were different.

Partial N-terminal amino acid sequences of mouse transplantation antigens were presented by Maizels, Frelinger and Hood.
Analysis of the partial sequence of the N-terminal of four
different H-2 antigens showed that no K-ness or D-ness was
distinguishable by sequencing or by serological or functional
assays. Some H-2 N-termini appeared to be more homologous to
HLA than to the other H-2 antigens.

Studies on the K^b locus mutants was presented by Nathenson,
Ewenstein, Uehara and Yamaga. Twelve MHC mutants of the
H-2K^b gene have been described. Through the use of peptide
mapping techniques of the CNBr fragments of the K^b glycoprotein the peptide differences between a mutant glycoprotein
and parent glycoprotein could be analyzed. In the bm 3 mutant two peptide changes were found, each due to single amino
acid alteration. In the bm 1 mutant a single amino acid
change was noted. Since these changes appear to be the only
ones found between the mutant and parent glycoprotein, the
authors tentatively concluded that the biological recognition
occurring in allogeneic recognition between parent and mutant
was due to the small alterations in the MHC primary structure.
Single point mutations could be the mechanism by which polymorphism is introduced into the H-2 K and D glycoprotein system.

Structural studies on H-2K antigens isolated from murine thymoma was presented by Hunter, Mole, Paslay and Bennett. Using
extracts from the AKR-derived thymoma, BW5147, the H-2K^k
alloantigen has been isolated. Sequence studies have been
initiated on this glycoprotein. An additional glycoprotein
of approximately 70,000 may also be present in the BW5147
cell line, either carrying H-2K^k determinants or associated
during immunoprecipitation, or other isolation procedures.

Two studies on the H-2L molecule were presented. Sears,

Wilson, Polizzi and Nathenson reported on peptide mapping of
H-2.4 (H-2D^d) and H-2.28 (H-2L^d) which indicated a sharing
of many of the major peptides. The small number of differences suggested that the H-2 antigens were not more homologous to each other than to any other H-2 antigens.

H-2L analysis was also described by Rose, Hansen, Sachs and
Cullen who utilized a slightly different antiserum (BALB/c
H-2D^b mutant anti-BALB/c antiserum) and showed that the L^d
molecule and L^q molecule were 65% homologous whereas the L^q
and D^q molecule showed 81% homology. It is noted that the
K^k and K^r are the only other allelic products with such great
homology as shown between the L^q and D^q. These studies
together with those of Sears establish that the L molecule
is separable but highly homologous to the D molecule.

Class II Products
    Biochemical analyses of the I region gene products has been
done primarily by two-dimensional gel electrophoresis (2-D
gels) and peptide mapping as amino acid sequence analysis of
these gene products is much less advanced than for the K and
D gene products. Jones, Murphy and McDevitt have utilized
2-D gels to extend their observations concerning two-gene
complementation for the expression of the I-E/C gene product.
Their major new observation is that surface expression of the
beta chain in two haplotypes (b and s) can be obtained if
the alpha chain in the E subregion is derived from the k, d,
p or r haplotype in either recombinant strains or in F1
heterozygotes. These data were interpreted to indicate that
the alpha chain is needed in order to get expression of the
beta chain in the E subregion. Cook, Siegelman, Vitetta,
Capra and Uhr have demonstrated that both chains of the A
subregion are encoded within the A subregion and by a sensitive peptide mapping procedure have extended the Jones'
observation in the E subregion concerning two-gene complementation that the structural gene for the beta chain was
actually encoded in the A subregion.

Whether those haplotypes which do not express an E region
gene product detected by specificity 7 antisera do, indeed,
contain such a gene product on the cell surface was the subject of considerable controversy. Jones and her colleagues
have been unable to demonstrate such molecules by looking
at whole cell lysates in 2-D gels. However, Lafuse, Neely,
McKean and David presented evidence that with xenoantisera
such gene products can be demonstrated.

Dancey, Cullen and Schwartz demonstrated that both chains in

the E subregion were spatially close together on the cell
surface despite their non-covalent linkage. After treating
cells with chemical cross-linkers, both chains could be isolated and they were found to be cross-linked.

Two papers dealt with cross-reactions between mouse and
human Ia antigens. Lunney, Mann and Sachs demonstrated a
DR-like molecule in man by alloantisera directed against the
E subregion of the mouse. Delovitch had similar results.

Both Lampson and Levy and Mann separately presented evidence
for the existence of more than one locus controlling the
expression of human B-cell alloantigens. Lampson's data was
based on the production of a "hybridoma" antibody which precipitated a molecule from human lymphoblastoid cell lines
with a slightly different molecular weight than that obtained
with several other hybridoma antibodies. In addition, this
molecule could be precipitated even after clearing with antisera directed against the more well known human B-cell alloantigens. In family studies, he concluded that multiple
genes control the expression of B-cell alloantigens.

In the closing moments of the workshop, Phillips, Streilein
and Duncan presented evidence that Syrian hamsters contained
I region gene products.

Class III Products

   Carroll and Capra presented evidence that the structural
gene for the murine Ss protein (C4) was encoded within the S
region of the murine major histocompatibility complex. Using
a direct precipitation technique and a peptide analysis procedure, they were able to demonstrate a structural variation in
the beta chain of this three-chain molecule.

In summary, the major issues discussed at the workshop concerned homologies between MHC gene products and other molecules. Tentatively, it appears that the K and D gene products in the mouse and the HLA-A and -B gene products in man
show modest homology with immunoglobulin, and high degrees
of homology with each other. The I region gene products
demonstrate no significant homology to other molecules, however, the murine E/C gene products are homologous to the
human DR antigens. It appears that all four chains of the
characterized murine I region molecule (I-A and I-E/C) are
encoded within the MHC. Finally, there is now documented
structural polymorphism of the class III antigens and the
human I region is now being subdivided as has the mouse.

GENETIC MECHANISMS OF ANTIBODY DIVERSITY
IN BALB/c KAPPA VARIABLE REGIONS[1]

D. J. McKean and M. Potter

Mayo Medical School, Mayo Clinic, Rochester, MN 55901
and
National Cancer Institute, National Institutes of Health,
Bethesda, MD 20014

ABSTRACT   Amino acid sequences of 14 BALB/c Vκ-21 kappa
variable regions (Vκ) are compared in order to elucidate
the genetic mechanisms of antibody diversity. These Vκ
sequences can be designated into at least six distinct
subgroups which are each thought to be encoded by
different germ line genes. Data is presented which
suggests that Vκ genes can independently assort with
different Joining segment (Jκ) genes during differentiation to produce complete kappa variable regions.
Although antibody diversity is probably generated by
both somatic mutation and by association of different
Vκ and Jκ segments, evidence is presented which suggests
that the majority of the functional Vκ diversity is
encoded within the germ line.

INTRODUCTION

The genetic basis of antibody diversity has been one of
the most intriguing questions of modern molecular biology.
Over the past 15 years there has been much debate about how
an individual could produce the large number of different
immunoglobulin (Ig) molecules which are found in serum.
Ig heavy and light chains are composed of variable and
constant regions which are each encoded by separate genes (1).
X-ray crystallography of Ig molecules have shown that the
variable regions are comprised of framework segments which
determine the conformation of the variable domain and com-
plementarity-determining regions (CDR) which form the antigen
binding site (2,3). In order to explain the genetic origin of
Ig variable region diversity three basic theories have been
proposed. The somatic mutation theory contends that variable
region diversity is generated by random mutation or hyper-
mutation during ontogeny from a relatively few germ line

[1]This work was supported by NIH grant AI 15414

genes (4). The germ line theory contends that each variable
region polypeptide is encoded by a different germ line gene
(5). The minigene theory contends that variable region
diversity is generated during ontogeny by rearrangement of
genes which encode segments of the variable region (6).

In recent years studies to define the genetic basis of
antibody diversity have focused on the Ig protein and gene
structures from inbred strains of mice (BALB/c, NZB). These
strains are highly inbred (thereby minimizing any genetic
polymorphisms) and can readily be induced to produce plasmacytomas.

Lambda light chains comprise a small fraction (~5%) of
the mouse light chains in serum. Amino acid sequence studies
of mouse λ variable regions (Vλ) have shown that Vλ has a
very limited amount of structural diversity (7). Nucleic
acid hybridization and gene-sequencing studies have suggested
that Vλ variability is generated somatically by mutation of a
single germ line gene (8,9,10).

Mouse κ light chains, which comprise approximately 95%
of serum light chains, have extensive variable region (Vκ)
diversity (11). When 80 available Vκ amino terminal sequences
are compared, 34 different groups (based on sequences which
differ by three or fewer residues) can be designated (11).
Available sequence data from complete Vκ regions has shown
that such differences within the Vκ amino terminus are predictive of extensive sequence differences throughout the
variable region (12). These extensive differences between
groups have been interpreted to indicate that different groups
are encoded by distinct germ line Vκ genes (12). We will
present data in this paper which indicates that at least some
of these groups are in fact comprised of a number of Vκ
sequences which are encoded by six or more germ line genes.

RESULTS AND DISCUSSION

For the past several years we have directed our efforts
to analyzing the extent and pattern of diversity within a
single BALB/c Vκ group: Vκ-21. After several Vκ-21 K chains
were identified in a random screening of Vκ amino acid
sequences, heterologous antisera were prepared which would
identify Vκ-21 K chains as free Bence Jones proteins or in
intact Ig molecules (13). Two serologically distinct sets
of Vκ-21 K chains were identified with these antisera. These
two serologically defined Vκ-21 sets probably represent evolutionarily divergent subgroups of Vκ-21 K chains with significant structural differences.

Vκ-21 specific antisera have been used by us and Julius
et al. (14) to screen BALB/c myeloma tumors in order to

identify VK-21 myelomas for sequence analysis. These VK-21
myelomas should represent an unbiased sampling of the VK-21
serogroups in the myeloma pool because they have been identified by their similar serological determinants
and not selected for similar hapten binding reactivities.
Julius et al. (14) have also shown that VK-21 light chains
represent a significant fraction of VK chains (7-10%) in
normal serum. Thus, VK-21 light chains are expressed in a
relatively high proportion of both myeloma proteins and
normal serum Igs. The VK-21 K chains have probably been maintained in Mus musculus because they contribute to antibodies
that react with antigens common in the mouse environment.
Studies are underway to identify the contribution of VK-21
light chains in normal antibody responses to defined antigens.

   VK-21 Diversity. Table 1 shows the sequences of fourteen BALB/c VK-21 variable regions. These fourteen sequences
are classified on the basis of their amino terminal sequence
homology into a single group (VK-21). They can, however, be
subdivided into at least six distinct subgroups on the basis
of common sets of amino acids that are shared throughout their
V regions (21 A,B,C,) or on the basis of homology with NZB
VK-21 sequences (21 D,E,F) (15). These six subgroups differ
from each other by 6 to 22 (out of 99) amino acids throughout
the V region segment (residues 1 to 95). Residues 96 (or 95)
to 107 are considered as part of the joining (JK) segment
which has been shown to be under the control of a separate
DNA gene segment (16) and will be considered later.
   The sequences within subgroups share common amino acids
throughout their V segments and these shared residues are
different for different subgroups. It is unlikely that
sequences in different subgroups could have been randomly
generated in somatic cells from a common germ line structural
gene (parallel mutation). Thus, these six subgroups are most
likely encoded by at least six germ line genes. A recent
hybridization study using VK-21 DNA probes concluded that
there were from four to six germ line genes encoding VK-21
regions (17). Based on the trend of newly found VK-21
sequences to either be designated into new or existing subgroups, we believe the actual number of BALB/c VK-21 genes to
be 10-12. The determination of the exact number of genes
encoding VK-21 polypeptides will have to await analysis by
direct gene sequencing.
   The substitutions which are observed between residues
1 to 95 within subgroups are very limited in number. Out of
the 9 VK-21 region segments where most or all of the sequence
is complete, 3 VK regions differ by 2 residues from the most
commonly occurring subgroup (prototype) sequence and 5 have

TABLE 1

BALB/C Vκ-21 SUBGROUPS

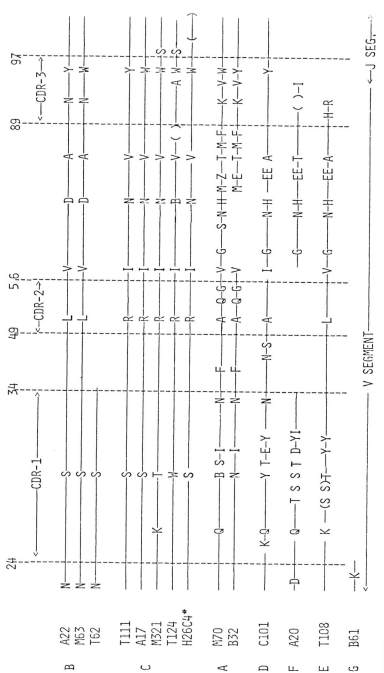

*H26C4 BALB/C HYBRIDOMA WAS THE GENEROUS GIFT OF DR. W. GERHARD IN COLLABORATION WITH DR. M. CANCRO

no sequence differences. The intrasubgroup substitutions
are all found within the first CDR (positions 27,27d,28) or
the third CDR (position 94) and consist of both conservative
(glu-gln, thr-ser) and nonconservative (lys-glu, trp-ser)
differences. When compared to the prototype sequence these
substitutions can all be produced by single base substitutions
at the DNA level. The presence of single base substitutions
occurring in complementarity determining regions within the
Vκ-21 subgroups resembles the pattern of variation described
in Vλ (18).

    Diversity of the J Segment. The part of the V region
between residues 96 (or 97) and 107 has been referred to as
the joining (Jκ) segment (16). The DNA which encodes the
Jκ segment has been shown from both Vκ and Vλ gene sequencing
studies to be separated from the DNA segment which encodes
the V region residues 1 to 95 (or 96) by noncoding DNA. The
actual end of the V segment (residues 95 or 96) and beginning
of the J segment (residues 96 or 97) is uncertain because of
the triplet codon redundancy at the DNA which encodes the
end of V and the beginning of J (18).

    Position 96 in the BALB/c Vκ-21 sequences is comprised
of either trp or tyr residues and both alternatives are found
within each of the Vκ-21 A, B and C subgroups. The trp-tyr
alternative is even more unusual in that it requires a two
base substitution. It, therefore, is likely that the codon
encoding position 96 is the first coding residue of the Jκ
segment. Seidman et al. have recently presented evidence
from DNA sequencing experiments of MOPC 41 (Vκ-9) that position 96 is indeed encoded by the Jκ gene (18).

    There are three different Jκ segments associated with
the variable regions in the Vκ-21C subgroup. These same Jκ
segments are found in other Vκ-21 subgroups and in other non
Vκ-21 variable regions. This suggests that Jκ segments can
independently associate with different V region genes. Since
residues 96 and 97 are located in the third CDR, the association of different Jκ regions containing substitutions at
residues 96 or 97 could potentially alter antigen binding.
Thus, the association of different Jκ segments with different
Vκ regions could generate antibody diversity.

    Although DNA sequencing studies have not defined the
total number of different Jκ genes, eight different Jκ segments have been identified in BALB/c mice and eight in NZB
mice for a total of ten different J segments in the two
strains (Table 2).

TABLE 2
J SEGMENTS IN BALB/c AND NZB Vκ-21

96											107	BALB/c (22,23)	NZB (15)
W	T	F	G	G	G	T	K	L	E	I	K	+	+
Y												+	+
W				S								+	+
R												+	+
L			A						L			+	+
P												+	+
F			S									−	+
W							D					−	+
I			S									+	−
I			A						L			+	−

In the three dimensional model of M603 (2) the majority of the J segment lies clearly outside of the third CDR. Substitutions in these framework parts of the J segments should have little effect on antigen binding. Half of the substitutions observed in the J segments occur in the framework part of the polypeptide. These framework substitutions do not appear to cause significant structural changes in the Ig computer-simulated three dimensional models (based on M603 three dimensional structure). Although variability in the amino terminus of the Jκ segments may be maintained in the genome of the mouse to generate antibody diversity, a relatively large proportion of the Jκ segment diversity may be due to gene duplication and genetic drift.

The BALB/c Vκ-21 sequences presented in this paper suggest that Vκ groups are encoded by at least six germ line genes. Nucleic acid hybridization (17) and Southern blot analysis of Vκ-21 (19) and Vκ-13 (20) light chain variable region groups have also indicated that there are from 6-10 genes per group. Based on the available myeloma amino terminal Vκ sequence data, a total of 34 Vκ groups have been identified (11,21). A statistical analysis of these data has suggested that there may be on the order of 50 Vκ groups in the BALB/c genome (7). Although this calculation is based on the myeloma Vκ pool, there is evidence that the number of Vκ-21 sequences in the myeloma pool is representative of that found in normal serum (14). Although there will probably be a considerable range in the number of germ line genes encoding each of the 50 groups, if each group is encoded by an average of 10 germ line genes, then there would be 500 germ line genes encoding Vκ. As previously described, Vκ diversity might be increased by random association of Vκ with Jκ during lymphocyte differentiation. Although this association could

increase Vκ diversity by another factor of 10, Vκ-Jκ association will probably play a minor diversity generating role.
These data predict that a large proportion of Vκ diversity is
encoded in the germ line.

The existence of multiple Vκ-21 variable regions with
subgroup specific residues scattered throughout both the CDR
and framework regions argues strongly against a minigene
theory of antibody diversity. The minigene theory would predict that CDR would be interchanged between subgroups (or
groups). Instead, the CDR and framework regions are coordi-
nately expressed.

How much does somatic mutation generate antibody diversity? One cannot determine from these Vκ sequences if intrasubgroup substitutions are encoded in the germ line or are
generated by somatic mutation. In order for these substitutions to be encoded in the germ line, however, the nucleic
acid hybridization (8) and Southern blot analyses (9,10) will
have had to substantially underestimated the number of genes
encoding different Vκ subgroups. It seems most likely, therefore, that intrasubgroup substitutions are generated somatically.

Although our data are limited, the diversity pattern of
the Vκ-21C subgroup would suggest that somatic diversity may
generate only a minor part of Vκ variability. Three of the
five Vκ-21C sequences are identical (to residue 95) while the
two sequences which are different vary only at two positions.
This variability pattern is similar to that observed in Vλ.
Twelve out of eighteen Vλ sequences are identical while the
remaining six Vλ differ by one to three amino acid substitutions (7). The intrasubgroup diversity of Vκ-21C and Vλ is
very limited when compared to the amount of diversity observed
between Vκ-21 subgroups (6 to 22% different; average: 16%) or
between different Vκ groups (40-50% different).

Vκ-21 Evolution. We would anticipate that the evolutionary processes generating the Vκ-21 variable regions are
representative of Vκ evolution in general.

The overall three dimensional contour of the light (V_L)
and heavy chain (V_H) variable region CDRs which combine to
produce antigen binding sites capable of binding common
environmental pathogens should be conserved in evolution.
Gene duplication and genetic drift should allow these V_L (or
V_H) to diversify by introducing CDR substitutions which produce subtle differences in the three dimensional contour of
the antigen binding site. Thus, the antigen binding sites
which are made by the products of these duplicated V genes
would still fit the overall contour of the pathogen's antigenic determinant. At the same time the subtle CDR differences could enable the combining site to bind antigenic

variants of the pathogen which are similarly generated during evolution. Mutations which produced major modifications of the CDR could have changed the antigen binding site to the degree that it no longer bound the pathogen's antigenic determinant.

The Vκ-21 ancestral gene product could have proved useful by contributing to antibodies which provided protection against a common environmental pathogen. This gene, after undergoing gene duplication and mutation, could have generated the different Vκ-21 subgroups. The overall size and general homology of the CDR in different Vκ-21 subgroups have been maintained. This would, in general, conserve the CDR three dimensional contour. The CDR contact residues, however, have mutated in evolution producing subtle differences in the Vκ CDR structure. Different Vκ-21 subgroups can in fact be characterized by these distinct CDR substitutions. These subtle differences resulting in modifications of the antigen binding site are presumably generated continuously, not only during the evolution of the species, but also during ontogeny by somatic mutation.

The Vκ-21 subgroup can be divided into two evolutionarily related but separate serogroups. Serogroup 1, composed of Vκ-21B and C, probably represents a relatively recent duplication of Vκ-21 genes. The other serogroup is composed of Vκ-21 A, D, E and F. These subgroups are more structurally heterogeneous although they share a number of subgroup specific residues (68,74,76,80) which make them distinct from Vκ-21B and C subgroups.

We will have to wait for DNA sequencing studies of Ig genes to provide us with a more accurate estimate of the number of Vκ genes. We will also need additional protein Vκ sequences to quantitate the effects of somatic mutation on the total amount of antibody diversity exhibited by individual animals. In spite of these inadequacies in our knowledge, we may be well on the way to understanding the basic contributions of each of the different genetic mechanisms to the generation of antibody diversity.

REFERENCES

1. Dreyer, W. J., and Bennett, J. C. (1965). PNAS 54, 864.
2. Segal, D., Padlan, E. A., Cohen, G. H., Rudicoff, S., Potter, M., and Davies, D. R. (1974). PNAS 71, 4298.
3. Poljak, R. J., Amzel, L. M., Chen, B., Phizackerley, R. P. and Saul, F. (1974). PNAS 71, 3440.
4. Cohn, M. (1974). In "Progress in Immunology" (L. Brent and J. Halborow, eds.), 11, 261-284. Elsevier and North-Holland, New York.

5. Weigert, M., Cesari, I. M., Yonkovich, S. J., and Cohn, M. (1970). Nature 228, 1045.
6. Wu, T., and Kabat, E. (1970). J. Exp. Med. 132, 211.
7. Weigert, M., and Ribblet, R. (1976). Cold Sp. Harb. Symp. Quant. Biol. 41, 837-846.
8. Leder, P., Honjo, T., Seidman, J., and Swan, D. (1976). Cold Sp. Harb. Symp. Quant. Biol. 41, 855-862.
9. Tonegawa, S., Hozumi, N., Matthyssens, G., and Schuller, R. (1976). Cold Sp. Harb. Symp. Quant. Biol. 41, 877-889.
10. Benard, O., Hozumi, N., and Tonegawa, S. (1978). Cell 15, 1133.
11. Potter, M. (1977). Adv. Immun. 5, 141.
12. McKean, D. J., Potter, M., and Hood, L. (1973). Biochemistry 12, 260.
13. McKean, D. J., Bell, M., and Potter, M. (1978). PNAS 75, 3913.
14. Julius, M., McKean, D. J., Potter, M., and Weigert, M. In preparation.
15. Weigert, M., Gatmaitan, L., Loh, E., Schilling, J., and Hood, L. (1978). Nature 276, 785.
16. Brack, C., Hirama, M., Lenhard-Schuller, R., and Tonegawa, S. (1978). Cell 15, 1.
17. Valbuena, O., Marcu, K. B., Weigert, M., and Perry, R. P. (1978). Nature 276, 780.
18. Seidman, J., Max, E., and Leder, P. Per Communication.
19. Lenhard-Schuller, R., Hohn, B., Brack, C., Hirama, M., and Tonegawa, S. (1978). PNAS 75, 4709.
20. Seidman, J., Leder, A., Edgell, M. H., Polsky, F., Tilghman, S. M., Tiemeier, D. C., and Leder, P. (1978). PNAS 75, 3881.
21. Potter, M. Unpublished data.
22. Kabat, E. A., Wu, T. T., and Bilofsky, H. (1976). Variable Regions of Immunoglobulin Chains, Medical Computer Systems, Bolt, Beranek and Newman, Cambridge, MA.
23. Rao, D. N., Rudicoff, S., and Potter, M. (1978). Biochemistry 17, 5555.

WORKSHOP SUMMARY: "Origin of Antibody Diversity".
A.R. Williamson, Department of Biochemistry, University of
Glasgow, Glasgow G12 8QQ, Scotland and H. Köhler, La Rabida –
University of Chicago Institute, East 65th Street at Lake
Michigan, Chicago, Illinois 60649.

Introducing the topic of the workshop A.R. Williamson
divided questions concerning the generation of diversity into
two sets: 1) at the genotype level; and 2) at the level of
phenotypic expression. Focussing on the genotypic aspect one
can ask questions dealing with the most recent advances in
studies of the organization of the Ig genes. i) What are the
number of germ line V gene segments and the "joining" (J)
segments? ii) Do J segments add to Ab specificity or do they
increase Ab redundancy? Relating genotype to phenotype one
can ask: i) Is gene counting sufficient for recognizing the
full extent of diversity? ii) How do V gene sets, defined by
DNA hybridization, relate to V region groups and subgroups
defined by amino acid sequences? iii) Since there is control
of gene expression operating in the generation of diversity
and since this expression seems to be under genetic control,
should this mechanism be described as genetic or somatic?

H. Köhler picked up this last point and quoted Jerne
(1970) who made the distinction between the total (genetic)
repertoire and the available (phenotypic) repertoire. Since
there is an obvious relationship between these two one might
ask whether it is still appropriate to continue analyzing the
repertoire at the protein sequence level or the idiotypic or
Ag-specificity level. He emphasized that though the questions
of the generation of diversity (GOD) is now being addressed
with the new methodology of DNA sequencing there remains an
equally important interest in the generation of operational
diversity (GOOD) which is the province of Immunologists
studying the mechanisms involved in controlling immune
responses.

L. Hood summarized the current status in the analysis of
Ig genes referring to published and unpublished data of his
and other laboratories (Leder, Mach, P erry, Tonegawa).
Immunoglobulins V region phenotypes can be categorized as
follows: 1) Groups, based on amino acid sequence identity at
the 20-25 N-terminal residues. 2) Subgroups, based on amino
acid sequence identity, or near identity, of the entire V
regions. The number of subgroups could approximate the
number of germ line genes. V genes have been counted using
the following techniques with the indicated results:

	COT DNA SATURATION	SOUTHERN BLOT	CLONE/SEQUENCING
V_λ	1-3	-	1-3	$2V_\lambda$ (by sequence)
V_κ MOPC149	-	-	∿10	10 minimum
V_κ *	-	-	6-25	-
$V_\kappa 21$ group	1-3	4-6	>10	-

*Range of six V_κ groups

Hood suggested that to fully understand antibody diversity we need to know the relative contributions of: 1) germ line V genes, 2) somatic mutations and 3) combinatorial joining of J-segments with V-segments.

B. Birshtein summarized her studies on the isolation and characterization of heavy variants of the MPC-11 line which secretes an IgG_{2b} myeloma protein. She described several mutants which have deletions and characteristics of the IgG_{2a} subclass. All of these variants however, carry the same idiotype. Most of the deletions have been observed at the domain boundaries but one has a deletion within a domain. Hood asked for some indications on the ordering of C-genes. Birshtein said that the data from MPC11 and P3 (Köln group) are consistent with the model proposed by Honjo; i.e. μ, γ3, γ1, γ2b, γ2a, α, Givol wanted to know if the data are in agreement with class-switches observed during immune responses. Birshtein replied that some variants might reflect normal translocation but differences involving J segments have not yet been seen.

McKean discussed his sequence data on the $V_{\kappa 21}$ subgroup. He pointed out that the diversity generated by combinatorial events between V- and J-segments might not contribute to the antibody specificity since it affects residues mostly outside the third complementarity determining region, CDR, i.e. after position 96. He also presented evidence for two serologically distinct groups of $V_{\kappa 21}$ proteins, both expressed in most strains of mice. He presented an evolutionary scheme for the two serogroups based on different levels of expression in different strains.   P. Gearhart queried whether the size of the J-segment could be determined by amino acid sequence analysis.   Hood argued that J could be defined without DNA sequencing and used the analogy of the original recognition of the V-C joining sequence region.

J. Owen then described the expression of the $V_{\kappa 21}$ subgroup in induced antibodies against influenza virus. These

antibodies were produced by single clones in splenic fragments
or by hybridomas.   Screening of myeloma proteins has not
shown a V$_{\kappa 21}$ protein with antibody activity.   She stated
that the analysis of monoclonal antibodies with known specificity can be useful in analysing the contribution of the light
chain to the antigen specificity using H-L hybridization.
Furthermore one can evaluate the role of IR genes on the
expression of the V$_{\kappa 21}$ subgroup.

P. Gearhart asked whether the sequence diversity seen in
myeloma proteins is similar to that seen in antibodies.   She
analyzed the sequence of several phosphorylcholine (PC) binding hybridomas which were of the non-T15 idiotype.   One
hybridoma had a light chain similar to MOPC603 myeloma (PC
binding); another had a heavy chain similar to MOPC460
myeloma (DNP binding).   These data indicate that the non-T15
anti-PC antibodies belong to different subgroups than those
defined by the major family of PC myeloma proteins.

K. Denis described isolation of hybridoma lines from
neonatal anti-DNP clones.   Since the neonatal repertoire is
more restricted than the adult these hybridomas might provide
information on germ line genes.   Comparing neonatal clonotypes with adult clonotypes at the amino acid-sequence level
could reveal the role of somatic mutation in diversification.
Anti-idiotypic sera have been raised against hybridoma antibodies and can be used to study normal expression.

C. Kolb discussed her finding of the expression of latent
allotypes in SJL mice.   Expression of the Ig-1a allotype was
observed during the course of an anti-allotypic response to
Balb/c allotype.   She concluded that these SJL mice must have
two structural genes for allotypes (Ig-1b and Ig-1a) and that
some control is operating in the expression of these genes.
M. Bosma reported finding latent allotypes in AKR mice. Most
strains have the U10-173 V$_H$ 'allotype' marker while AKR does
not.   However, a nude mutant of AKR expresses the U10-173
marker.   This seems to implicate the thymus in the control of
V$_H$ expression.   B. Ashman suggested measuring expression of
the U10-173 markers in neonatally thymectomize AKR. S. Weiss
discussed the diversity of λ chains in the Bas mutant rabbit
and suggested that in rabbits λ chains may be as diverse as
κ chains.   This would argue for regulation of light chain
expression.

H. Köhler thanked all participants of the workshop and
predicted that in the future much effort will be devoted to
the study of regulatory mechanisms controlling the expression
of V and C genes.

DEVELOPMENT OF T CELLS IN THE MOUSE[1]

Osias Stutman

Memorial Sloan-Kettering Cancer Center
New York, New York 10021

ABSTRACT Although we have gained a substantial amount
of insight into the functional heterogeneity of T cells
and the complex restrictions for appropriate interaction
and regulation of T cell function, the models for T cell
development are still simplistic and cannot accomodate
with ease the functional heterogeneity of the T cell
compartment in the periphery. A model is proposed which
integrates differentiation, selection of repertoire and
specialization of T cells, as a consequence of intra
and extrathymic differentiation of hemopoietic stem
cells which interact with "inducer" cell populations.

INTRODUCTION

Two experimental facts are generally accepted concerning T cell development: 1) T cells are derived from hemopoietic stem cells which are influenced or processed by the
thymus and 2) the thymus is an absolute requirement for the
differentiation of T cells (1-5).
The observation that the immunologically competent cells
in thymectomized mice grafted with a thymus were almost entirely of host origin (6), was interpreted as the consequence
of either the thymus producing humoral factors acting on host
cells (7) or that the host cells were modified into immunological competence by migration through the thymus (1). Both
the humoral thymic factors (8, 9) and the phenomena of thymus traffic and cell processing (1, 5) are well documented
events, although there is still controversy concerning the
multiplicity and nature of the thymic "hormones", their
possible mechanism of action, the type of cells responsive
to those factors, the type of cells that are actually exported by the thymus and the role of intra and extrathymic
steps in T cell development, etc. (5, 8-10). Furthermore,
although "humoral" and "cellular" components appear as part
of the T cell differentiation mechanism, we still ignore the
actual role and magnitude of each of those components in T

[1]The experimental part of this work was supported by USPHS
grants CA-08748, CA-15988 and CA-17818.

cell development and renewal under physiological conditions,
either during ontogeny or in the adult (5, 10).

In the past five years, a substantial amount of information and theory on the complexities of function, interaction and regulation of peripheral T cells, has been incorporated into our immunological knowledge (11, 12). Both the
phenomenon of MHC-restriction of T cell function (13) as well
as the ability to define subsets of T cells with different
functional properties (14), posed problems to the accepted
models of T cell development (3, 4, 15). For example, the
generally accepted model for T cell development is rather
simplistic (3, 4, 15), even considered inadequate by its own
supporters (4, 15), and clearly incapable of accomodating
the facts about heterogeneity of the T cell pool, and how
such heterogeneity is generated (10).

INTRATHYMIC AND POSTTHYMIC MATURATION

The demonstration of a population of immunologically
competent T cells within the thymus (16-18), was rapidly
developed into a model of T cell differentiation, based on
the following sequence of events taking place within the thymus proper: stem cell---> thymocyte---> "mature" thymus lym-
phocyte---> peripheral T lymphocyte (15, 17). Thus, the whole
process of T cell differentiation was made intrathymic, and
the "mature" thymus lymphocyte was equated with the population of cells ready for export (15, 17). However, an alternative hypothesis was available, which proposed that what
the thymus exported after processing was not necessarily an
immunologically competent mature T cell, but rather a "rec-
ognizable" committed precursor without detectable immune
functions, termed "postthymic" (19-21). This postthymic
precursor (PTP) cell was immunologically incompetent but displayed surface antigens of the T lineage (22). Thus, further maturation in the periphery of the thymus-processed PTP
cells, probably under the influence of thymic humoral factors, appears as one major pathway for generation of competent T cells (5, 10, 22). Using PTP cells with defined chromosome markers, we could show directly that the Lyt 123 PTP
cells can give rise both to Lyt 1 and Lyt 23, as well as
Lyt 123 cells (10, 23). Whether this circuit is the only
one for replenishing the T cell pool, still remains to be
defined. Recent evidence has shown that, although the thymus
exports Lyt 123 cells, an important component of Lyt 1 as
well as a small component of Lyt 23 cells was also detected
(24). However, based on our own studies with chromosome
markers in thymectomized hosts, it was apparent that most of
the T cells responding to mitogens or allogeneic cells in
vitro were derived from the injected PTP cells (10, 23).

Thus, this theory proposed an intrathymic step for irreversible commitment of precursors of hemopoietic origin to the T lineage and an extrathymic one of further maturation and expansion of the PTP cells into immunologically competent T cells (19-22). These two steps were also considered as part of the export-import function of the thymus, usually termed thymus traffic (1, 5). And the hemopoietic cells capable of migration to the thymus were loosely termed "prethymic" (19-22), and clearly include the "prothymocyte" population defined by the in vitro induction studies (25) and the repopulation of irradiated thymuses (26).

Figure 1 shows in schematic form a summary of our studies on thymus traffic (5, 10, 27-20). In the first part of the experiments, a "probe" of cells with the T6T6 chromosome marker, derived from hemopoietic tissues is injected into 60-day old neonatally thymectomized syngeneic mice, which also receive a thymus graft. At different times after the procedure, chromosome analysis of the thymus grafts could show that indeed, T6T6 of hemopoietic origin could be detected within the graft. Yolk sac, fetal liver, fetal blood and adult bone marrow shared this capacity to migrate and proliferate in the thymus (27-30). However, in later studies we could show that yolk sac cells require an additional step (i.e. migration to fetal liver) before being able to migrate to thymus, while fetal liver or adult bone marrow do not (30). The next step of the experiments included the transfer of the thymus from the primary animals to a secondary recipient, and in these animals the only source of T6T6 cells was the thymus graft proper, containing the injected hemopoietic cells of embryonic or adult origin. The export function of the thymus was thus measured, or better the "processing" and subsequent export of the cells, and indeed we could demonstrate that progeny of the injected T6T6 cells of embryonic or adult origin could be detected in lymph nodes and thoracic duct and that such cells could react to mitogens such as phytohemagglutinin, concanavalin A and allogeneic cells, but not to bacterial lipopolysaccharides (5, 10, 27-30). Thus, we could provide the formal proof that thymus processing through "traffic" was truly a differentiation pathway for the T lineage. Recent experiments have also confirmed that yolk sac cells can appear within thymus in a model involving orthoptic injection of yolk sac cells into embryos (31).

Although the experimental models which use lethal whole body irradiation have shown that the thymus can be repopulated by allogeneic hemopoietic cells, traffic of hemopoietic cells to the thymus in models that do not use irradiation shows a marked syngeneic preference (5, 10, 32). When allogeneic cells, even matched for the MHC, are used in the mo-

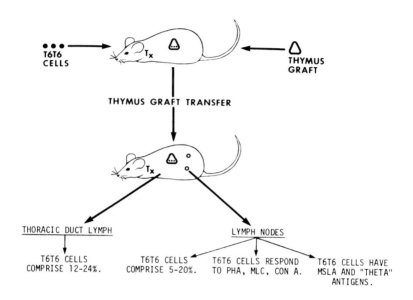

THYMUS GRAFT TRANSFER

THORACIC DUCT LYMPH

T6T6 CELLS
COMPRISE 12-24%.

LYMPH NODES

T6T6 CELLS
COMPRISE 5-20%.

T6T6 CELLS RESPOND
TO PHA, MLC, CON A.

T6T6 CELLS HAVE
MSLA AND "THETA"
ANTIGENS.

Figure 1.   Schematic representation of the two step experimental model to study migration of hemopoietic T6T6 cells
into the thymus and the export to periphery of the thymus-
processed T6T6 cells in the secondary hosts.   The recipients
of thymus grafts were 60-day old neonatally thymectomized
CBA/H mice.   The T6T6 cells were from yolk sac, embryonic
liver, embryonic blood or adult bone marrow.   Thoracic duct
and lymph node cells usually tested 30 days after thymus
graft.

del depicted in Figure 1, the proportion of cells that can
penetrate, remain and divide within the thymus graft is extremely low when compared to a syngeneic probe (5, 10, 32).
In reality, the allogeneic probe, under such experimental conditions, is competing with the host's own hemopoietic cells
which are syngeneic for the thymus graft (10).   In addition,
we could show that syngeneic preference of thymus traffic is
radiosensitive, and can be abolished by 750R of whole body
irradiation (10).   Thus, as it will be further discussed in
the paper, these types of findings agree well with the recently described "instructive" role of the thymic stroma in determining the range of reactivities to modified self (33, 34).
        In addition to its difficulties in explaining T cell
subset diversification, the "classic" T cell developmental

theory [i.e. the whole process being intrathymic and an equation of the mature subpopulation of thymocytes with the fraction that is exported (15, 17)] had one major experimental
result to explain. That was the evidence by Elliott (35, 36),
that the steroid-resistant population in thymus appeared as
a resident population. It was specifically such steroid-
resistant population that was considered the candidate for
export (3, 4, 15, 17). However, there is strong evidence
that such steroid-resistant population is not undergoing re-
placement for relatively long periods of time (36, 37) and
that in a model as the one described in Figure 1, there is
no evidence of any detectable export to the periphery for
7 months or more after thymus grafting (5). Thus, the
steroid-resistant population appears as a resident population
in thymus and does not represent the fraction that is exported (5, 10, 35-37). Whether these types of intrathymic resident populations are regulators of T cell maturation or specificity via selection mechanisms, or play other yet undefined
functions, deserves further study.

Thus, based on the above results, it is possible that
hemopoietic immigrants in the thymus may have three choices:
1) to become part of the pool of cells which will be exported
to the periphery, most probably as PTP cells; b) enter the
pool of thymocytes which are not exported and die within the
thymus and c) become part of the intrathymic pool of mature
T cells, which are not exported (5, 10). Figure 2 shows this
proposed differentiation pathway for the T lineage, including
prethymic, intrathymic and postthymic events. If the possibility of some form of selection taking place in the thymus
(33, 34, 37-39) is considered, the first two, and perhaps all
three choices within thymus would represent a single process
of negative selection, and only the cells with the appropriate repertoire would be allowed to emigrate as PTP cells
(10). Thus, the PTP cells in the periphery, are not only
irreversibly committed for the T lineage, but are also committed for restricted recognition to the MHC determinants displayed in the intrathymic environment (10, 33). However,
further postthymic maturation or refinement of the restricted recognition is associated in the periphery to other
"inducer" cells (see next section) in the lympho-hemopoietic
tissues (10, 33). The differentiated progeny of the PTP cells
in the periphery, will have the repertoire of the PTP cell
but will also differentiate in a new microenvironment and
acquire an additional repertoire for cell-cell interaction
(33).

The availability in the periphery of the PTP compartment
that can be driven into further differentiation by thymic
humoral factors and perhaps by antigen or other yet undefined
influences, has the advantage of presenting an economic way

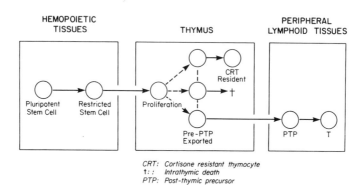

HEMOPOIETIC
TISSUES   THYMUS

PERIPHERAL
LYMPHOID TISSUES

Pluripotent   Restricted   Proliferation
Stem Cell   Stem Cell

CRT
Resident

†

Pre-PTP
Exported   PTP   T

CRT: Cortisone resistant thymocyte
†::   Intrathymic death
PTP: Post-thymic precursor

Figure 2.   Prethymic, intrathymic and postthymic steps
for T cell development.

for maintaining homeostasis of the renewing T cell pool, and
is symmetrical with other models of cell renewal and differentiation on the hemopoietic series. In addition, it permits a further selection of effector cells with the appropriate interaction molecules (10, 33). Whether expansion
of the PTP pool is the only mechanism of T cell renewal in
the periphery is still open to investigation. The model
also agrees with the requirements for MHC regulation of immune reactivity, as well as with the instructional role of
the thymus in determining T cell specificity (33, 34). Thus,
the intrathymic step would permit the development of the
appropriate recognition units for self-MHC and non-self (i.e.
would offer the "restrictive" environment, see 33, 34, 38),
while the postthymic maturation would permit the functional
diversification of T cell subclasses, including the T help
required for modified-self specific cytotoxicity (33) as
well as for other types of cell interactions and functions.
        The demonstration that the thymus exports to periphery
Lyt 123 as well as Lyt 1 cells (24), would suggest that Lyt
subclass diversification may take place already within thymus, an interesting possibility that deserves further study.

As was discussed in previous paragraphs, we still don't know if the Lyt 123 PTP cell represents the only cell-differentiation circuit induced by the thymus. However, the recent evidence that the MHC-restrictive event also takes place within thymus (33, 34) should be considered in relation to the Scollay et al. (24) results. The procedure for demonstration of the export of Lyt cells included intrathymic labelling with fluorescein isothiocyanate (FITC) and subsequent analysis of the peripheral tissues using the fluorescence-activated cell sorter (24). However, one wonders at the validity of the procedure since it has been shown that FITC-conjugated cells can elicit syngeneic cytotoxic T cell responses (40), i.e. can be recognized as "modified self". Even though the Scollay et al. experiments were short term (3 hrs after intrathymic labelling) it is quite possible that intrathymic selective mechanisms may already be operative for or against the FITC-conjugated cortical thymocytes, raising some interesting questions concerning the detected exported T cells, which obviously need further study.

A MODEL FOR FUNCTIONAL T DEVELOPMENT

The basic process of T cell differentiation is probably inseparably related with the process of selection for T cell repertoire as well as specialization into the different functional subsets of T cells (10). We recently proposed that the three integrated events (differentiation, selection and specialization) are the consequence of the appropriate or concordant matching of precursor and "inducer" cell populations, both at intra and postthymic locations, and that the thymic humoral "factors" are a necessary but not sufficient signal for functional differentiation (10). Furthermore, in the absence of "inducer" cells or as a consequence of inappropriate or non-concordant matches, non-functional differentiation, probably doomed to negative selection in vivo, takes place (10). The model also proposes that major histocompatibility (MHC) determinants are important in permitting the appropriate matching, either as the complementary sites allowing effective interactions or as special regions for the anchorage of other cell-interaction moieties (10).

I will not dwell on details of the model, since it was extensively discussed in a previous publication (10), however it is worthwhile indicating that: a) the model fits well with our understanding of thymus traffic and postthymic differentiation; b) it fits well with the intrathymic step of development of MHC-restriction (33, 34) as well as with the postthymic step (33) and even provides for the "restricting cell" required for the ontogeny of T cell precursors (38); c) the model also incorporates selection for appropriate matching

via excess intrathymic cell production (10) and d) explains
the "non-functional" differentiation obtained in vitro when
only thymic humoral factors are used to drive differentiation.
    "Matching" is used as an operational term. We still do
not know if matching is mediated by like-like structures or by
congruent antigen-antibody like interactions. The nature of
the "inducer" cell, both in thymus and periphery is also not
defined (except for the evidence that in the thymus it may be
in the "radioresistant" portion of the thymic stroma, see 33,
34). Characterization of "inducer" cells and determination if
they are the same as the "restrictive" cell, appears as important avenues for exploration. Perhaps the definition of the
mechanics of the interactions between precursor and inducer
cells may serve to clarify the mechanism of restrictive
recognition and the development of the T cell repertoire
(33, 34, 38, 39).

REFERENCES

1. Ford, C.E. (1966). In "The Thymus: Experimental and Clin-
    ical Studies" (G.E.W. Wolstenholme and R. Porter, eds.),
    p. 131. Little, Brown & Co., Boston.
2. Miller, J.F.A.P. and Osoba, D. (1967). Physiological Rev.
    74, 437.
3. Greaves, M.F., Owen, J.J.T. and Raff, M.C. (1974). "T and
    B Lymphocytes: Origins, Properties and Role in Immune Res-
    ponses." American Elsevier Publ., New York.
4. Cantor, H. and Weissman, I.L. (1976). Progr. Allergy 20, 1.
5. Stutman, O. (1977). Contemp. Topics Immunobiol. 7, 1.
6. Dalmasso, A.P., Martinez, C., Sjodin, K. and Good, R.A.
    (1963). J. Exp. Med. 118, 1089.
7. Osoba, D. and Miller, J.F.A.P. (1963). Nature 199, 653.
8. Bach, J.F. and Carnaud, C. (1976). Progr. Allergy 21, 342.
9. Stutman, O. and Good, R.A. (1973). Contemp. Topics Immuno-
    biol. 2, 299.
10. Stutman, O. (1978). Immunological Rev. 42, 138.
11. Sercarz, E.E., Herzenberg, L.A. and Fox, C.F., eds. (1977).
    "The Immune System: Genetics and Regulation." Academic
    Press, New York.
12. "Origins of Lymphocyte Diversity" (1977). Cold Spring
    Harbor Symp. Quant. Biol. 41.
13. Zinkernagel, R.M. and Doherty, P.C. (1977). Contemp.
    Topics Immunobiol. 7, 179.
14. Cantor, H. and Boyse, E.A. (1977). Contemp Topics Immuno-
    biol. 7, 47.
15. Raff, M.C. (1973). Nature 242, 19.
16. Blomgren, H. and Anderson, B. (1969). Exp. Cell Res. 57,
    185.
17. Raff, M.C. (1971). Nature New Biol. 229, 182.

18. Leckband, E. and Boyse, E.A. (1971). Science 172, 1258.
19. Stutman, O., Yunis, E.J. and Good, R.A. (1969). J. Exp. Med. 130, 809.
20. Stutman, O., Yunis, E.J. and Good, R.A. (1970). J. Exp. Med. 132, 583.
21. Stutman, O., Yunis, E.J. and Good, R.A. (1970). J. Exp. Med. 132, 601.
22. Stutman, O. (1975). Ann. N.Y. Acad. Sci. 249, 89.
23. Stutman, O. and Shen, F.W. (1979). Transplant. Proc. 11, 907.
24. Scollay, R., Kochen, M., Butcher, E. and Weissman, I. (1978). Nature 276, 79.
25. Scheid, M.P., Goldstein, G., Hammerling, U., and Boyse, E.A. (1975). Ann. N.Y. Acad. Sci. 249, 531.
26. Basch, R.S. and Kadish, J.L. (1977). J. Exp. Med. 145, 405.
27. Stutman, O. (1970). In "Fifth Leukocyte Culture Conference" (J. Harris, ed.), p. 671. Academic Press, New York.
28. Stutman, O. and Good, R.A. (1971). Transplant. Proc. 3, 923.
29. Stutman, O. (1972). In "Membranes and Viruses in Immunopathology" (S.B. Day and R.A. Good, eds.), p. 437. Academic Press, New York.
30. Stutman, O. (1976). Ann. Immunol. (Inst. Pasteur) 127C, 943.
31. Weissman, I.L., Baird, S., Gardner, R.L., Papaioannou and Easchke, W. (1977). Cold Spring Harbor Symp. Quant. Biol. 41, 9.
32. Stutman, O. and Good, R.A. (1969). Exp. Hematol 19, 12.
33. Zinkernagel, R.M. (1978). Immunological Rev. 42, 224.
34. Bevan, M.J. and Fink, P.J. (1978). Immunological Rev. 42, 3.
35. Elliott, E.V., Wallis, V. and Davies, A.J.S. (1971). Nature New Biol. 234, 77.
36. Elliott, E.V. (1973). Nature New Biol. 242, 150.
37. Jerne, N.K. (1971).Eur. J. Immunol. 1,1.
38. Cohn, M. and Epstein, R. (1978). Cell. Immunol. 39, 125.
39. Langman, R.E. (1978).Rev. Physiol. Biochem. Pharmacol. 81, 1.
40. Starzinski-Powitz, A., Pfizenmaier, K., Rollinghoff, M., and Wagner, H. (1976). Eur. J. Immunol. 6, 799.

T-CELL-SPECIFIC MURINE Ia ANTIGENS: SEROLOGY OF I-J and I-E SUBREGION SPECIFICITIES[1]

Colleen E. Hayes[2] and Fritz H. Bach

From the Immunobiology Research Center and
Departments of Medical Genetics and Surgery
University of Wisconsin
Madison, Wisconsin 53706

ABSTRACT Antibody to I-region-encoded structures
expressed on thymus-derived (T) but not B lymphocytes
has been produced by immunizing recipient mice with
I-region congenic, concanavalin A-stimulated donor
thymocytes. T cell Ia antigens have been mapped to the
I-J and I-E subregions; other subregions are under
investigation. T lymphocytes purified by either of two
methods from peripheral lymphoid organs are lysed by
antiserum and complement. Purified B lymphocytes
are neither directly lysed, nor do they absorb
T-cell-reactive antibody. We conclude that a system of
unique T cell Ia specificities may be observed by
suitably altering conventional immunization protocols
for Ia antiserum production.

INTRODUCTION

The murine major histocompatibility complex (H-2)[1]
I-region was identified as that chromosomal segment wherein
map the genes regulating antibody production to chemically-
defined antigens in inbred mice (1,2). This segment has
since proven to be a cluster of critically important immunoregulatory loci (3-5). Because of their potential relevance
to immunoregulatory mechanisms, identification and structural
analysis of I-region gene products has been the focus of
intensive research.

    I-region congenic mice reciprocally recognize cellular
antigens (Ia antigens) when cross-immunized with lymphoid

[1]This work is supported in part by NIH grants CA 16836,
AI 11576 and AI 15588 and National Foundation-March of Dimes
grants 5-192 and 1-246.
[2]This investigation was carried out in part while
C.E.H. was a fellow of the Helen Hay Whitney Foundation.

tissue (6-10). Ia antigens are presently considered to be
primarily B (immunoglobulin-bearing) cell structures (3-10).
Although thymus-derived (T) cells participate in $\underline{I}$-region-
controlled immunoregulatory phenomena, exquisitely sensitive
techniques are required to detect T cell Ia antigens (11-14).
    Twenty-three Ia specificities are presently recognized.
While some studies suggest that Ia antigens are concordently
expressed by T and B lymphocytes (11,15,16), limited experimental evidence is available regarding the commonality or
uniqueness of B and T cell Ia molecules. Thus, complete
absorption by cortisone-resistant thymocytes of cytotoxic
anti-Ia antibody (11), and presence of Ia specificities 1
through 10 and 22 on lipopolysaccharide-stimulated splenocytes as well as concanavalin A (con A)-stimulated thymocytes
(15,16) suggest coincidence of Ia antigen expression. On
the other hand, functional studies suggest that T cells may
carry $\underline{I}$-region encoded determinants not found on B cells
(17,18).
    Hypothesizing that commonly used immunization protocols
might favor production of B cell Ia antibodies, we have
sought to maximize the immunogenicity of T cell Ia antigens
by immunizing $\underline{I}$-region congenic mice with con A-stimulated
thymocytes. In two strain combinations, (B10 x B10.D2)F_1
anti-B10.A(5R) and (B10.HTT x A.TH)F_1 anti-A.TL, we have
produced cytotoxic antibody against T cell specificities
(19,20). B lymphocytes neither react with, nor absorb T
lymphocyte reactive antibody. On the basis of these experiments, we suggest the existance of a T cell unique, Ia
antigen system to which antisera may be prepared by suitably
altering conventional immunization protocols.

METHODS

    Antiserum production. Con A-stimulation of thymocytes,
immunization, and bleeding schedules have been fully described (19).
    Dye exclusion microcytotoxicity assay. Antibody-
dependent cell lysis was measured as described (19). Rabbit
serum (19) or guinea pig serum (20) served as complement
(C'). Percentage of cells lysed was calculated according to
the formula:

$$\% \text{ cells lysed} = 100 \left[\frac{\% \text{ dead experimental} - \% \text{ dead C' control}}{100\% - \% \text{ dead C' control}} \right]$$

    Cell separation. Macrophages were removed from lymphoid
cell suspensions by adherence to plastic. T cells were
prepared either by nylon wool column passage (21), or by

TABLE I
H-2 HAPLOTYPE OF ORIGIN OF RECOMBINANT STRAINS

Strain	Haplotype	H-2 Region								
				I						
		K	A	B	J	E	C	S	G	D
A.TH	t1	s	s	s	s	s	s	s	s	d
A.TL	t2	s	k	k	k	k	k	k	k	d
B10.HTT	t3	s	s	s	s	k	k	k	k	d
B10.A	a	k	k	k	k	k	d	d	d	d
B10.A(3R)	i3	b	b	b	b	k	d	d	d	d
B10.A(4R)	h4	k	k	b	b	b	b	b	b	b
B10.A(5R)	i5	b	b	b	k	k	d	d	d	d
B10.S(9R)	t4	s	s	?	k	k	d	d	d	d
C57BL/6-H-2^k	k	k	k	k	k	k	k	k	k	k

anti-immunoglobulin plus complement lysis of lymphoid cells.
B cells were obtained by anti-Thy 1.2 plus complement lysis
of spleen cells. Cells were assayed for surface immunoglobulin by immunofluorescence, for Thy 1.2 by dye exclusion microcytotoxicity, and for phagocytic cells by latex ingestion.

RESULTS

Recipient (B10 x B10.D2)F_1 mice produced cytotoxic
antibody against donor B10.A(5R) lymph node cells after the
sixth injection with con A-stimulated B10.A(5R) thymocytes
(19). (Haplotypes of origin of strains used in this study
are given in Table I.) (B10 x B10.D2)F_1 anti-B10.A(5R)
serum could potentially contain antibody to I-J^k and I-E^k-
encoded specificities. Reaction with B10.A($\overline{3R}$) cells, in
the absence of reactivity with C57BL/10 or B10.D2 cells,
demonstrated anti-I-E^k antibody (Table II). I-E^k reactivity
was supported by B10.HTT cell lysis using B10.S-absorbed
serum (Table II). The antiserum contained anti-I-J^k antibody
as well; B10.A(3R) absorbed serum lysed B10.A(5R) lymph node
cells (Fig. 1).

When lymph node, spleen, and thymus cells were examined
for expression of I-J^k and I-E^k antigens, it was clear that
the structures detected were not distributed among lymphoid
cells in the same pattern as are conventional B cell Ia
antigens. Specifically, the antiserum produced against con
A-stimulated thymocytes was most cytotoxic to lymph node
cells (Table I, Fig. 2), whereas anti-B cell Ia sera exhibit
strongest reactivity with splenocytes (3-5). Since splenocytes contain a high percentage of immunoglobulin positive
(B) cells, yet were only weakly reactive, it appears that
the antigens detected are expressed by cells other than B

TABLE II

CELLULAR DISTRIBUTION OF I-J AND I-E ANTIGENS

Antiserum	Test Strain	I-region Detected	Percentage Cells lysed[a]		
			Lymph node	Spleen	Thymus
(B10 x B10.D2)F$_1$ anti-B10.A(5R)[1]	B10.BR	J,E	27±3	5±2	<3
	B10.A(5R)[c]	J	12±3	ND[b]	<3
	B10.A(3R)	E	20±5	ND	<3
	B10.HTT[d]	E	20±5	ND	<3
(B10.HTT x A.TH)F$_1$ anti-A.TL	A.TL	A,B,J	45±6	ND	ND
	B10.A(4R)	A	47±12	ND	ND
	B10.A(5R)	J	25±6	8±3	<3
	B10.S(9R)	J	17±4	ND	ND
	A.TL[e]	J	19±4	ND	ND

a. mean ± S.D.
b. not determined.
c. B10.A(3R)-absorbed serum
d. B10.S-absorbed serum
e. B10.A(4R)-absorbed serum

lymphocytes. Further evidence was obtained by titrating
(B10 x B10.D2)F$_1$ anti-B10.A(5R) serum on nylon wool nonadherent lymphocytes. These cells, which are >90% Thy 1.2
positive, gave strongly positive reactions whether derived
from lymph node or spleen (Fig. 2). It must be noted that
nylon wool column passed cells required a short period of
culture (~6 hr.) to re-express antigens apparently stripped
off by the column. Anti-immunoglobulin plus complement-
treated splenocytes were unreactive (<3% lysis). These
findings suggest that the antigens detected are singularly
expressed on T lymphocytes with respect to these populations.
    In a second system, recipient (B10.HTT x A.TH)F$_1$ mice
produced antibody cytotoxic to peripheral A.TL lymphocytes
when immunized with con A-stimulated A.TL thymocytes (20).
Pooled antiserum obtained after the seventh immunization
lysed A.TL lymph node cells (45 ± 6% lysis, Table II).
Autoantibodies against B10.HTT, A.TH, and (B10.HTT x A.TH)F$_1$
lymph node cells were not detected (< 3% lysis). This
antiserum can potentially contain antibody to cellular
structures whose expression is governed by I-A^k, I-B^k,
and/or I-J^k genes. Serum reactivity with recombinant
B10.A(4R) was observed (Table II). C57BL/10 lymphocytes did
not react. This suggests that antigens mapping in the I-A
region are detected by the antiserum, and/or that a K^k-region
gene product exhibits cross-reactivity. (K^k region crossreactivity is not a likely explanation on the basis of

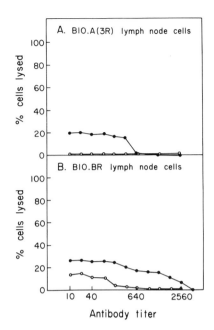

Figure 1.   Cytotoxicity of (B10. x B10.D2)F$_1$ anti-
B10.A(5R) serum on B10.A(3R) and B10.BR lymph node cells.
(●) unabsorbed serum; (o) B10.A(3R)-absorbed serum.

cellular distribution studies, H-2K antigens being ubiquitous
in their distribution). Exhaustive absorption with B10.A(4R)
lymph node cells left serum reactivity on A.TL lymphocytes
which could be due either to an I-B^k or an I-J^k-encoded
antigen (Table II). Antiserum titration on recombinant
B10.A(5R) lymph node cells indicated the presence of anti-
I-J^k antibody, since neither B10.D2 nor C57BL/10 cells
react. The antiserum was analyzed for antibody to I-B^k
region-encoded antigens; exhaustive absorption with B10.A(4R)
then with B10.A(5R) lymph node cells left no reactivity on
B10.A lymph node cells. This suggests that antibody to an
I-B^k gene product was not produced. Since B10.S lymphocytes
were not lysed by B10.A(4R)-absorbed serum, and further,
antibody to I-B^k gene products was not apparent, reactivity
with B10.S(9R) cells must also be due to cytotoxic anti-I-J^k
antibody (Table II). Thus, antibody to I-J^k encoded specificities was observed by titration of B10.A(4R)-absorbed
serum on A.TL cells, and by titration of unabsorbed serum on
B10.A(5R) and B10.S(9R) lymphocytes.
      Previous results (19) as well as functional studies
(18) suggested that I-J antigens are structures unique to T

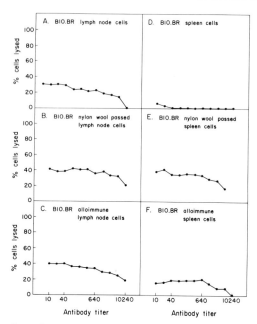

Figure 2.   Cytotoxicity of (B10. x B10.D2)F$_1$ anti-
B10.A(5R) serum on B10.BR lymphocytes.

lymphocytes.   It was of interest, therefore, to assess
whether the I-J^k antigen detected by (B10.HTT x A.TH)F$_1$
anti-A.TL serum exhibited the same restricted cellular
distribution pattern.   B10.A(5R) lymph node cells (25 ± 6%)
were lysed to a far greater extent than spleen cells (8 ±
3%), whereas thymocytes were unreactive (<3%).   When B and T
lymphocytes were separated using either anti-Thy 1.2 (for B)
or anti-immunoglobulin (for T) plus complement, these cell
populations were clearly distinguishable by reactivity with
the antiserum.   B cells were 82 ± 11% Ig positive, 5 ± 4%
phagocytic, and <3% Thy 1.2 positive; T cells were 12 ± 11%
Ig positive, 5 ± 3% phagocytic, and 87 ± 14% Thy 1.2 positive.   As shown in Fig. 3, T cells were lysed (maximal lysis
22 ± 3%; half-maximal lysis at a dilution of 1:320), B cells
were not (<3% lysis).
     Fig. 4 presents the results of absorption studies
carried out to determine whether B cells might express I-J
determinants in densities too low to activate complement, or
alternatively, might be more resistant to complement lysis
than T cells under the conditions employed.   The upper
panels of Fig. 4 confirm the absence of antibodies cytotoxic
to B cells in (B10.HTT x A.TH)F$_1$ anti-A.TL serum.   Moreover,
absorption of antiserum with increasing numbers of B cells

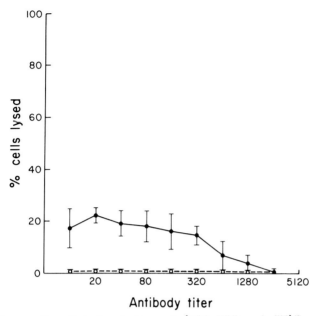

Figure 3.   Cytotoxicity of (B10.HTT x A.TH)F$_1$ anti-A.TL
serum on B10.A(5R) lymphocytes (o) B cells; (●) T cells.

did not diminish residual cytotoxic activity on T lymphocytes
(lower left panel), whereas T cell absorption did (lower
right panel). We conclude from these experiments that B
cells do not express the I-J^k-encoded structures detected by
this antiserum.

DISCUSSION

These experiments illustrate the production of cytotoxic
antibodies to I-region-encoded T cell antigens by immunization of I-region congenic mice with con A-stimulated thymocytes. The fact that this protocol yields high-titered
antibody, whereas conventional immunization protocols do
not, may be explained by one or several considerations.
Both I-J and I-E determinants have been detected on con
A-reactive T cells (16,22). Thus, altered antigen density,
selective expansion of that population which is positive, or
presentation of a weakly immunogenic Ia antigen together
with a strongly immunogenic structure on the thymocyte blast
("hapten-carrier" type effect) may have contributed to
increased T cell Ia antigen immunogenicity.
Compelling evidence is provided by these results that T
cells carry unique I-region associated antigens. Firstly, B

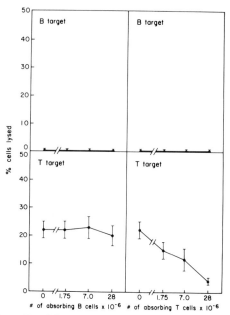

Figure 4.   Residual cytotoxicity of (B10.HTT x A.TH)F$_1$ anti-A.TL serum on B10.A(5R) B or T lymphocytes following absorption with B or T cells.

and T lymphocytes have been separated and antigen expression studied by direct cytotoxicity on purified and characterized cell populations.   T but not B cells are reactive.   Secondly, quantitative absorption analysis indicates that T but not B lymphocytes absorb T cell reactivity.   By these criteria, B cells do not express the I-J and I-E antigens detected by the antisera described herein at all, or do so with much diminshed antigen density.   Being carried by T but not B lymphocytes, these Ia antigens are distinct from "classical" Ia antigens (3-5).

The uniqueness and/or commonality of B and T lymphocyte Ia antigen expression merits detailed consideration.   It is generally agreed that I-region encoded antigens are easily demonstrated on B lymphocytes, but detected with difficulty on T cells (3-5).   Four studies suggest coincident Ia antigen expression by T and B lymphocytes (11,15,16,23).   Unfortunately, studies showing T and B cell reactivity with a multispecific antiserum are difficult to interpret because it is not clear whether the same or distinct antibody populations account for cytotoxic reactivities (11,23).   Similarly, it is difficult to discern duality or singularity of Ia antigen presentation in studies on mitogen-stimulated lymphocytes (15,16). These studies presume first, that mitogen-stimulated cells represent purified cell populations, and second, that mitogen stimulation does not induce the appearance of antigens for which both T and B cells carry structural genes, but whose expression is normally strictly regulated. Both assumptions are difficult to verify. Thus, the question of duplicity in T and B cell Ia antigen expression is unresolved.

Functional studies argue convincingly in favor of unique, I-region encoded T cell structures. Murphy et al determined that an anti-I-J antiserum removed suppressor T cells although it was not detectably cytotoxic to T cells by cell enumeration (18). Activity was absorbed by T but not B lymphocytes (24). Our results substantiate by serology what was shown by functional studies. Further experiments using Ia antisera which are not broadly specific with purified, characterized lymphoid cells will be required to establish whether unique structures are encoded by genes elsewhere in the I-region as well.

The finding that antibodies to I-J and I-E-controlled Ia antigens represented on T cells may be raised by immunizing with con A-induced thymocyte blasts is of significance to both Ia antigen serology and functional studies of T cell subpopulations. Specifically, a group of "Iat" antigens may be detectable by altering conventional immunization protocols in a variety of ways. It will be of great interest to discover whether structure-function relationships exist between serologically-defined Iat structures and functionally distinct T lymphocyte populations.

ACKNOWLEDGMENTS

The authors wish to extend their gratitude to Mr. J.M. Maier, whose excellent technical skill and unusual dedication contributed to the completion of the work, and to Ms. Cindy Smith and Ms. Michelle Howard for their capable assistance in preparing this manuscript.

REFERENCES

1. McDevitt, H.O., Deak, B.D., Shreffler, D.C., Klein, J., Stimpfling, J., and Snell, G.D. (1972). J. Exp. Med. 135, 1259.
2. Benacerraf, B., and McDevitt, H.O. (1972). Science (Wash. D.C.) 175, 273.
3. Shreffler, D.C., and David, C.S. (1975). Adv. Immunol. 20, 125.

4. Katz, D.H., and Benacerraf, B., eds. (1976). "The
    Role of Products of the Histocompatibility Gene Complex
    in Immune Responses," Academic Press, New York.
5. McDevitt, H.O., ed. (1978). "Ir Genes and Ia Antigens."
    Academic Press, New York.
6. David, C.S., Shreffler, D.C., and Frelinger, J.A.
    (1973). Proc. Natl. Acad. Sci. U.S.A. 70, 2509.
7. Hauptfeld, V., Klein, D., and Klein, J. (1973).
    Science (Wash. D.C.) 181, 167.
8. Hämmerling, G.J., Deak, D.B., Mauve, G., Hämmerling,
    U., and McDevitt, H. (1974). Immunogenetics 1, 68.
9. Götze, D., Reisfeld, R.A., and Klein, J. (1973). J.
    Exp. Med. 138, 1003.
10. Sachs, D., and Cone, J.L. (1973). J. Exp. Med. 138,
    1289.
11. Frelinger, J.A., Niederhuber, J.E., David, C.S., and
    Shreffler, D.C. (1974). J. Exp. Med. 140, 1273.
12. Fathman, C.G., Cone, J.L., Sharrow, S.O., Tyrer, H.,
    and Sachs, D. (1975). J. Immunol. 115, 584.
13. Krammer, P.H., Hudson, L., and Sprent, J. (1975). J.
    Exp. Med. 142, 1403.
14. Elkins, W.L., Klinman, N.R., and Mayol, R. (1977). J.
    Immunol. 118, 998.
15. David, C., Meo, T., McCormick, J., and Shreffler, D.C.
    (1976). J. Exp. Med. 143, 218.
16. Shreffler, D.C., David, C.S., Cullen, S.E., Frelinger,
    J.A., and Neiderhuber, J.E. (1976). Cold Spring
    Harbor Symp. Quant. Biol. 41, 477.
17. Lonai, P., and McDevitt, H.O. (1974). J. Exp. Med.
    140, 1317.
18. Murphy, D.B., Herzenberg, L.A., Okumura, K., Herzenberg,
    L.A., and McDevitt, H.O. (1976). J. Exp. Med. 144,
    699.
19. Hayes, C.E., and Bach, F.H. (1978). J. Exp. Med. 148,
    692.
20. Hayes, C.E., and Bach, F.H. (1979). Submitted for
    publication.
21. Julius, M.H., Simpson, E., and Herzenberg, L.A. (1973).
    Eur. J. Immunol. 3, 645.
22. Frelinger, J.A., Niederhuber, J.E., and Shreffler, D.C.
    (1976). J. Exp. Med. 144, 1141.
23. Götze, D. (1975). Immunogenetics 1, 495.
24. Murphy, D.B., Okumura, K., Herzenberg, L.A., Herzenberg,
    L.A., and McDevitt, H.O. (1976). Cold Spring Harbor
    Symp. Quant. Biol. 41, 497.

B CELL LYMPHOMA LINES AS POTENTIAL MODELS FOR THE STUDY OF B CELL SUBPOPULATIONS

Colette Kanellopoulos-Langevin, K. Jin Kim,
David H. Sachs[1] and Richard Asofsky

Laboratory of Microbial Immunity
National Institute of Allergy and Infectious Diseases
National Institutes of Health
Bethesda, Maryland 20205

ABSTRACT   The surface characteristics of a panel of BALB/c lymphomas have been examined. It was found that these in vitro cell lines express different surface immunoglobulin classes and several other B cell markers (Ia and LyM antigens, Fc (IgG) receptors), suggesting that they represent different B cell subpopulations. Three different cell lines were selected for further investigation of the possible relationship between Fc (IgG) receptors and alloantigens on their surface.   Three different patterns of inhibition by the alloantisera tested (anti-Ia, anti-H-2D and anti-LyM) were observed. Preliminary data suggest that these inhibitions are not due only to Fc portions of the alloantibodies. These cell lines may be useful as models of distinct B cell subpopulations.

INTRODUCTION

Several laboratories have described lymphoid tumors from different species which retained specialized, differentiated characteristics such as T or B cell morphology and markers (1-8). Therefore it is possible that these tumors could be useful models for the study of T or B cell populations not readily available from a normal animal.

In our laboratory, we have adapted to tissue culture and characterized five spontaneously derived BALB/c lymphoma lines (K46, L10A, X16C, A20 and M12) and one 1-ethyl-1-nitrosourea induced BALB/c tumor line (BALENLM 17) (9). This report reviews the results obtained with these homogeneous in vitro

[1]Immunology Branch, National Cancer Institute, National Institutes of Health, Bethesda, Maryland 20205.

cell lines, which indicate that they could be useful models
in the study of markers of B cell subpopulations, and their
possible interactions.

MATERIALS AND METHODS

Mice. BALB/cAnN were obtained from the Animal Production Unit at the National Institutes of Health, Bethesda, MD.
Adult mice of both sexes aged 8-16 weeks were used.
    Antisera and tumor cell culture conditions, EA rosetting,
inhibition of EA rosetting and antibody dependent cytotoxicity
techniques have been described in detail elsewhere (9, 10).

Indirect Immunofluorescence Staining and Flow Microfluorometry (FMF) Analysis. Tumor cells were stained by indirect immunofluorescence technique as described before (9).
For the detection of surface IgD, cells were first exposed to
rabbit anti-mouse δ serum (or rabbit anti-KLH serum as a
control) and then mixed with fluorescein-labeled (fl.) goat
anti-rabbit immunoglobulins. Cells were then analysed by
FMF as described by Loken et al. (11).

Cell Surface Iodination and Polyacrylamide Gel Electrophoresis (PAGE) Analysis. K46 cells were labeled with
^{125}Iodine (^{125}I) by the lactoperoxidase-catalyzed procedure
(12). Cells were lysed with Nonidet P40 and cell lysates
were ultracentrifuged at 100,000 g for one hour. Surface-
labeled immunoglobulins (Ig) were precipitated by appropriate
anti-Ig sera and by Cowan I as described (13). Immune precipitates were then subjected to PAGE on 10% slab gels (14).
Autoradiographs of dried gels were developed using high speed
X-ray film.

Mild Reduction and Alkylation of Alloantibodies. 4 ml of
anti-Ia serum (A.TH anti-A.TL) and 4 ml of anti-H-2D serum
(A.SW anti-A.TH) were precipitated with 44% ammonium sulfate.
The precipitates were resuspended in saline and reprecipi-
tated with 33.5% ammonium sulfate. The pellets were dissolved
in 1 ml of Phosphate buffered saline pH 7.2 (PBS) and dialysed
against the same buffer. The protein concentration was then
adjusted to 1 mg per ml and the two Ig enriched preparations
were reduced with dithiothreitol (0.01M) for 30 minutes at
37°C; iodoacetamide (0.03M) was then added and the mixture
incubated at 37°C for an additional 30 minutes. The two
preparations were then dialysed thoroughly against PBS.

Trypsin Treatment of Tumor Cells. Tumor cells were washed three times with Hanks' balanced salt solution (HBSS). 5×10^6 cells were resuspended in 4.5 ml of prewarmed HBSS and 0.5 ml of Trypsin ("10X" Grand Island Biological Co., Grand Island, N.Y.) were added to reach a final concentration of 0.25%. The mixture was incubated for 15 or 30 minutes at 37°C. Five ml of cold PBS + 10% fetal calf serum + 0.1% sodium azide were added to stop the reaction and prevent possible resynthesis of the digested surface proteins.

RESULTS

A summary of the characteristics of the cell lines is presented in Table I. It appeared that all cell lines had several properties of B cells: 1) they had surface immuno-globulins (sIg); 2) they bore receptors for the Fc portion of IgG, but not for the third component of complement; 3) they did not phagocytize latex particles nor give positive staining for esterases; 4) all but one (M12) bore Ia antigens, and 5) all had LyM antigens on their surfaces. In addition, these cell lines had different classes of sIg: four (K46, X16C, L10A and BALENLM 17) had sIgM but no IgG or IgA, the two others (A20 and M12) had no sIgM but gave positive staining with fluoresceinated polyvalent goat anti-mouse immunoglobulin antibodies.

Another class of immunoglobulin has been shown to be present on most normal splenic B cells: IgD. We have recently investigated this question with the tumor lines using in-direct immunofluorescence staining and analysis in PAGE of the immune precipitates from ^{125}I surface labeled cell lysates. A typical experiment on K46 is shown in Fig. 1a, 1b and Fig. 2. It can be seen that a specific staining for IgD was detected by flow microfluorometry and that a specific pre-cipitate containing IgD was obtained from the same cells. The presence of membrane IgD was also demonstrated on L10A, X16C, BALENLM 17, while A20 and M12 had much lower amounts, if any (R. Laskov et al., manuscript in preparation).

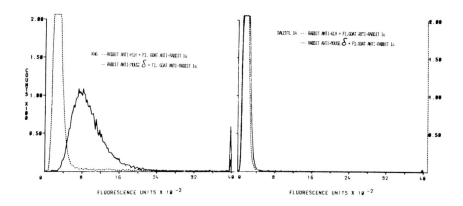

FIGURE 1a.   FMF detection of sIgD on K46 cells.
(left)

FIGURE 1b.   In the same experiment, staining of a T
(right)   lymphoma line BALENTL 14.

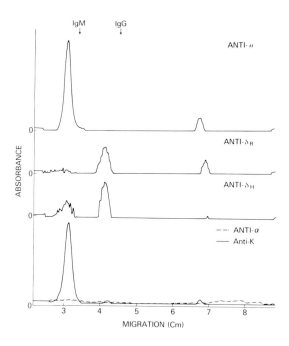

FIGURE 2.   Analysis in PAGE of immune precipitates with
anti μ, δ, α, κ antibodies) from [125]I
surface labeled K46 cells.

TABLE I

SUMMARY OF THE CHARACTERISTICS OF BALB/c LYMPHOMA LINES

Cell Lines	Surface Ig	Ia	LyM 1.2	Fc(IgG) Rec.	C' Rec.	Latex particle uptake	Esterase activity
K46	μ, poly+++	+	+	+	-	-	-
L10A	μ, poly+++	+	+	+	-	-	-
X16C	μ, poly+++	+	+	+	-	-	-
BALENLM 17	μ, poly+++	+	+	+	-	-	-
A20	poly++	+	+	+	-	-	-
M12	poly ±	-	+	+	-	-	-

We also examined normal spleen cells or tumor cells for a possible interaction between Fc (IgG) receptors and surface alloantigens as described previously by Dickler et al. (15-17). The cell lines were each homogeneous as compared to heterogeneous spleen cell populations (15-19). We found that Fc receptors on K46 and X16C, as well as on a normal BALB/c spleen cell population, could be inhibited by alloantisera directed against all cell surface antigens tested (anti-Ia, anti-LyM and anti-H-2D sera). This blocking phenomenon was not modified by addition of sodium azide (0.1%) to the medium or by the EA rosetting technique used in the assay (i.e., sheep red blood cells (SRBC) coated with mouse antibodies or ox red blood cells coated with rabbit antibodies). In contrast, EA rosettes of A20 and M12 were no longer inhibited by anti-H-2D sera in the presence of sodium azide, whereas they were still inhibited by anti-LyM sera in the same conditions. Anti-Ia sera gave no inhibition on M12 (Ia-) but inhibited very effectively A20 cells (Ia+) even in the presence of sodium azide. Therefore, it appeared that the cell lines fell into three different categories whether we looked at their surface phenotypes or at the relationship between their surface markers.

The possible role of Fc portions of alloantibodies in these inhibitions was investigated as follows: Ig fractions from alloantisera were reduced and alkylated under mild conditions so that interchain disulfide bonds would be primarily broken, leaving intact as much as possible their antigen-binding capacity. This treatment has been shown to remove complement binding activity from antibodies (20) and we found that it prevented EA rosette formation when SRBC were sensitized with anti-SRBC antibodies after such treatment, although the hemagglutinating activity was not affected (data not shown). This is in agreement with Michaelsen et al. (21) who found they could still inhibit antibody dependent cell cytotoxicity reactions but not induce them after mild reduction and alkylation of rabbit antibodies. Reduced and alkylated anti-Ia and anti-H-2D antibodies were used to inhibit EA rosetting (Table II). No modification was observed in the inhibition by anti-Ia; but anti-H-2D antibodies were no longer inhibitory on A20 and M12, whereas they still significantly blocked EA rosettes on K46 and the normal BALB/c spleen cell control. FMF analysis of the indirect immunofluorescence staining (using alloantibodies and fluoresceinated goat anti-mouse IgG2 antibodies) showed no difference between the treated and the control preparations, demonstrating that the antigen binding capacity of the treated antibodies was not affected (Fig. 3a,3b).

TABLE II

INHIBITION OF EA (SRBC) ROSETTES BY ANTI-Ia AND
ANTI-H-2D ANTIBODIES AFTER MILD REDUCTION AND ALKYLATION

Cell suspension	%Inhibition by			
	αIa[a]	αIa R.A.[b]	αH-2D	αH-2D R.A.
Normal BALB/c spleen	80	80	87.6	72.8
K46	93	89.6	95.1	58.8
A20	96.8	93.6	43.9	3.1
M12	ND[c]	ND	65.3	3.2

[a] α= anti-

[b] R.A. = reduced and alkylated (see Methods)

[c] ND = Not done

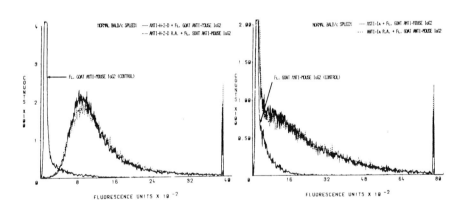

FIGURE 3a.   FMF analysis of indirect immunofl. staining
(left)   with R.A. (---) or non modified (____) anti-
              H-2D antibodies.
FIGURE 3b.   Same experiment with anti-Ia antibodies.
(right)
Cells mixed only with fl. goat anti-mouse IgG2 gave a fluorescent profile - indicated by arrows.

TABLE III

EA (SRBC) ROSETTING ON B CELL LYMPHOMAS AFTER
TRYPSIN TREATMENT

Cell lines	Time of incubation	%EA rosettes $(0.1\% \text{ NaN}_3)^a$	Indirect immuno fl. staining[b] (Ia)
K46	-	85	>90%++++
	15 min.	90	>90%++
	30 min.	88	80%-, 20% ±
A20	-	97	>90%++++
	15 min.	97.5	>90%++
	30 min.	98	>90% ±
M12	-	94	>90%-
	15 min.	97	>90%-
	30 min.	96	>90%-

[a]NaN_3 = sodium azide

[b]numbers indicate percentages of fluorescent positive
cells; number of crosses indicates the brightness of
fluorescence.

Recent findings of two distinct types of Fc receptors on
some macrophage tumor lines (22-26) suggested the possibility
of different Fc receptors on our cell lines explaining the
different inhibition patterns of EA rosetting by alloantisera.
One of the major differences between the two Fc receptors on
macrophage cell lines is their trypsin sensitivity. We thus
subjected our cell lines to trypsin digestion for up to 30
minutes after which we tested them for EA rosetting capacity.
As shown in Table III, no decrease in the percentages of EA
rosettes was observed whereas Ia antigens (assayed by indirect immunofluorescence staining) had been stripped from
the cells in the same time.

DISCUSSION

In the present report, we reviewed the properties and
surface characteristics of a panel of BALB/c lymphomas.
These cell lines presented three different surface phenotypes:
1) four (K46, X16C, L10A, BALENLM 17) are sIg+, sIgM+, sIgG-,
sIgA-, Ia+, Fc(IgG) receptor + and LyM+; 2) one (A20) is sIg+,

sIgM-, sIgG-, sIgA-, Ia+, Fc(IgG) receptor + and LyM+; 3) another one (M12) is sIg+, sIgM-, sIgG-, sIgA-, Ia-, Fc(IgG) receptor + and LyM+. In addition, blocking of EA rosettes by alloantisera was found different among the three categories. These findings support the hypothesis that these cell lines represent normal B cell subpopulations. Another property of the majority of normal splenic B cells is the presence of surface IgD. We found that Ig of this class could be detected on the surface of K46, L10A, X16C and BALENLM 17. Using K46, A20 and M12 we studied the interaction between Fc(IgG) receptors and alloantigens, and investigated the possible role of Fc portions of alloantibodies in the blocking of Fc receptors by alloantisera. The reduction and alkylation experiment we described brings preliminary evidence that the sodium azide resistant inhibitions of EA rosetting might not be due to Fc portions of alloantibodies. Nevertheless, in order to exclude any participation of Fc portions in the phenomenon, and to distinguish between an inhibition by cross-linking of alloantigens and a "ligand-induced alteration" as described by Dickler et al.(17), additional inhibition experiments are needed using Fab fragments of alloantibodies. Different Fc receptors have been described on macrophage cell lines (22-26) and Herpes virus infected cells (27,28). Another aspect of the heterogeneity of our cell lines might reside in different Fc receptors. We tested the trypsin sensitivity of Fc(IgG) receptors on three cell lines and they all appeared trypsin resistant. These preliminary results do not eliminate the possibility of more subtle differences between Fc receptors on the different cell lines.

Not only are these cell lines useful for the description and characterization (and possibly purification) of normal B cell markers but they are also good models to study other B cell properties such as surface molecule interactions, B cell physiology and function. As an illustration of the last point, these tumor lines have been used in various studies such as biosynthesis of membrane associated Ig (29), induction of secretion of IgM after fusion with MPC 11.4T00.1L1 myeloma (30), production of lymphotoxin (31) and antigen presentation (32).

ACKNOWLEDGMENTS

The authors gratefully acknowledge Dr. Irwin Scher and Robert Habbersett for their cooperation in the F.M.F. analysis of SIgD, Susan O. Sharrow for her expert assistance in the F.M.F. analysis of binding of R.A. alloantibodies and Mrs. Olive Childers and Virginia Shaw for skillfully typing this manuscript.

REFERENCES

1. Trainin, Z., and Klopfer, U. (1971). Cancer Res. 31, 1968.
2. Dickler, H. B., Siegal, F. P., Bentwich, Z. H., and Kunkel, H. G. (1973). Clin. Exp. Immunol. 14, 97.
3. Pichler, W. J., Broder, S., Muul, L., Magrath, I., and Waldmann, T. A. (1978). Eur. J. Immunol. 8, 274.
4. Shevach, E. M., Stobo, J. D., and Green, I. (1972). J. Immunol. 108, 1146.
5. Ramasamy, R., and Munro, A. J. (1974). Immunol. 26, 563.
6. Kim, K. J., Weinbaum, F. I., Mathieson, B. J., McKeever, P. E., and Asofsky, R. (1978). J. Immunol. 121, 339.
7. Mathieson, B. J., Campbell, P. S., Potter, M., and Asofsky, R. (1978). J. Exp. Med. 147, 1267.
8. Bergman, Y., and Haimovich, J. (1977). Eur. J. Immunol. 7, 413.
9. Kim, K. J., Kanellopoulos-Langevin, C., Merwin, R. M., Sachs, D. H., and Asofsky, R. (1979). J. Immunol. 122, 549.
10. Kanellopoulos-Langevin, C., Kim, K. J., Sachs, D. H., and Asofsky, R. (1979). (submitted for publication).
11. Loken, M. R., and Herzenberg, L. A. (1975). Ann. N. Y. Acad. Sci. 254, 163.
12. Marchalonis, J. J., Cone, R. E., and Santer, V. (1971). Biochem. J. 124, 921.
13. Cullen, S. E., and Schwartz, B. D. (1976). J. Immunol. 117, 136.
14. Flemming, H., and Haselkorn, R. (1974). Cell. 3, 159.
15. Dickler, H. B., and Sachs, D. H. (1974). J. Exp. Med. 140, 779.
16. Dickler, H. B., Cone, J. L., Kubicek, M. T., and Sachs, D. H. (1975). J. Exp. Med. 142, 796.
17. Dickler, H. B., Kubicek, M. T., Arbeit, R. D., and Sharrow, S. O. (1977). J. Immunol. 119, 348.
18. Krammer, P. H., and Pernis, B. (1976). Scand. J. Immunol. 5, 205.
19. Schirrmacher, V., Halloran, P., and David, C. S. (1975). J. Exp. Med. 141, 1201.
20. Isenman, D. E., Dorrington, K. J., and Painter, R. H. (1975). J. Immunol. 114, 1726.
21. Michaelsen, T. E., Wisloff, F., and Natvig, J. B. (1975). Scand. J. Immunol. 4, 71.
22. Walker, W. S. (1976). J. Immunol. 116, 911.
23. Unkeless, J. C. (1977). J. Exp. Med. 145, 931.
24. Heusser, C. H., Anderson, C. L., and Grey, H. M. (1977). J. Exp. Med. 145, 1316.

25. Anderson, C. L., and Grey, H. M. (1978). J. Immunol. 121, 648.
26. Diamond, B., Bloom, B. R., and Scharff, M. D. (1978). J. Immunol. 121, 1329.
27. Adler, R., Glorioso, J. C., Cossman, J., and Levine, M. (1978). Infec. and Immun. 21, 442.
28. McTaggart, S. P., Burns, W. H., White, D. O., and Jackson, D. C. (1978). J. Immunol. 121, 726.
29. McKeever, P. E., Kim, K. J., Nero, G. B., Laskov, R., Merwin, R. M., Logan, W. J., and Asofsky, R. (1979). J. Immunol. (In press).
30. Laskov, R., Kim, K. J., and Asofsky, R. (1979). PNAS 76, 915.
31. Aksamit, R. R., and Kim, K. J. (1979). J. Immunol. (In press).
32. Schwartz, R. H., Kim, K. J., Asofsky, R., and Paul, W. E. (1979). In "Regulatory Role of Macrophages in Immunity" (A. S. Rosenthal and E. R. Unanue, eds.), Academic Press, New York. (In press).

CHARACTERIZATION OF A NON-H-2 LINKED GENE CLUSTER CODING
FOR THE MURINE B CELL ALLOANTIGENS LYB-2, LYB-4, AND LYB-6[1]

Steven Kessler, Aftab Ahmed, and Irwin Scher

Uniformed Services University of the Health Sciences and
Naval Medical Research Institute, Bethesda, Maryland 20014

ABSTRACT   Lyb-6 is the 45,000 dalton polypeptide, B
lymphocyte surface membrane target of an antiserum
raised in CBA/N mice against CBA/J spleen cells. The
antigen is identified by its mobility (reduced) in
sodium dodecyl sulfate-polyacrylamide gel electrophoresis after immunoprecipitation from radioiodinated
cells of appropriate mouse strains. The B cell localization of this antigen was verified by the inability
of extensive absorptions with cells from nonlymphoid
tissues to remove Lyb-6 reactivity from this serum,
and by the ability to isolate this antigen from B cell
populations but not from B cell-depleted populations.
Because the strain distribution of Lyb-6 (further defined as the 6.1 allele) was strikingly similar to the
published distributions of Lyb-2.1 and Lyb-4.1 (defined
serologically), we performed linkage analyses for these
and other markers in (C57BL/6 x DBA/2)F_1 x C57BL/6 backcross mice. The results indicated conclusively that
Lyb-2, -4, and -6 are products of distinct genes which
are linked to the Mup-1 locus on chromosome 4. The
pattern of recombinations observed establishes the
probable gene order as Lyb-2-Lyb-4-Lyb-6-Mup-1, with
a recombination frequency of 3-5% between the Lyb-2
and Lyb-6 loci.

[1]Supported in part by the Uniformed Services University
of the Health Sciences Research No. CO8310 and in part by the
Naval Medical Research and Development Command Work Unit No.
MO095-PN.001-1030. The opinions and assertions contained
herein are the private ones of the writers and are not to be
construed as official or reflecting the views of the Navy
Department or the naval service at large. The experiments
reported herein were conducted according to the principles
set forth in the "Guide for the Care and Use of Laboratory
Animals," Institute of Laboratory Resources, National Research Council, DHEW, Pub. No. (NIH) 78-23.

INTRODUCTION

The constellation of surface membrane constituents of
mouse B lymphocytes includes a diverse array of serologically, immunochemically, and functionally defined antigens and
receptors. The known murine Lyb antigens which, by definition, are present only on B cells, comprise only a small proportion of these membrane markers. However, this fact belies
their current and potential significance in lymphocyte biology. The importance of these latter antigens is based on two
principles. First, among B lymphocytes there is great functional heterogeneity (1, 2), and several of the Lyb antigens
serve to identify certain B cell subpopulations (3, 4).
Second, as more factors and mediators to which B cells specifically respond are found, and as mechanisms of cellular
interaction in immunity are further unraveled, the search
will intensify to identify the surface membrane structures
which are involved in these interactions. The Lyb antigens
are obvious candidates for such roles.

Although the Lyb antigens are identified with the use of
antisera, this does not imply the existence of a requisite
assay system for their definition. Indeed, it is important
to distinguish between the way in which an antigen is originally defined and other assays which are aimed at further
characterization. While most surface membrane markers, including the antigens Lyb-1 (5), Lyb-2 (6), Lyb-4 (7), and
Lyb-5 (4), have been defined using serological (cytotoxicity)
techniques, conclusions regarding B cell specificity have
also been obtained with combined functional and immunofluorescent techniques (Lyb-3) (3) or functional assays alone
(Lyb-7) (8). In the latter case B cell specificity is
deduced by the inability of other cell types to absorb out
the antiserum activity.

It is possible to intentionally raise antisera against
Lyb antigens that are restricted to subpopulations of B cells.
In all cases where this has been done, use has been made of
the CBA/N mouse system. CBA/N mice have an X chromosome-link-
ed immune defect which is associated with the deficiency of a
mature or late-developing subpopulation of B cells comprising
approximately half the entire B cell population in spleens of
normal adult mice (9). Heterozygous F_1 male mice which carry
the CBA/N X chromosome also exhibit the immune defect. Thus,
by immunizing (CBA/N x BALB/c)F_1 male mice with BALB/c spleen
cells, it is possible to obtain an antiserum which detects a
cell surface component on mature B cells (Lyb-3). Similarly,
an antiserum raised in C57BL/6 mice against DBA/2 splenocytes
and subsequently absorbed extensively with (CBA/N x DBA/2)F_1
male splenocytes and thymocytes also recognizes a marker of a

mature B cell population (Lyb-5). Lyb-7 was discovered as a
second (noncytotoxic) specificity in anti-Lyb-5 serum which is
not genetically linked to Lyb-5, but it is not yet clear
whether the antigen itself, as opposed to its functional properties, is restricted to a B cell subpopulation.

Recently, employing immunochemical approaches, we identified another Lyb antigen which we term Lyb-6 (10, 11).
Anti-Lyb-6 serum is raised in CBA/N mice; however, unlike
Lyb-3 and Lyb-5, the antigen appears to be present on a majority of B cells. Lyb-6 is also the first Lyb antigen whose
biochemical detection, notably, its mobility in sodium dodecyl
sulfate-polyacrylamide gel electrophoresis (SDS-PAGE) has preceded its serological or functional detection. The molecule
precipitated by anti-Lyb-6 serum is a 45,000 dalton polypeptide. This is a property which is shared in common with anti-
Lyb-2 and Lyb-4 sera (12; unpublished observations; and R. E.
Humphreys, personal communication) and is potentially of tre-
mendous significance because of the similarity in size to H-2
antigens (13) and several other H-2 linked alloantigens (14-
16). In addition to data which substantiates the properties
of Lyb-6 stated above, we also present in this report preliminary evidence which indicates that the genes that code for
Lyb-2, Lyb-4, and Lyb-6 are distinct but closely linked, and
that they are unlinked to the genes that code for H-2.

METHODS

Animals. Mice were obtained from The Jackson Laboratory
and from the Small Rodents Laboratory of NIH.

Antisera. Antiserum which defines Lyb-6 by immunoprecipitation was produced by repeated intraperitoneal injections of
adult CBA/N mice with CBA/J spleen cells. Anti-Lyb-2.1 serum
(C3H.I x C57BL/6 anti-I/St ascites tumor I.29) was a generous
gift of Drs. M. Scheid and E.A. Boyse of Memorial Sloan-
Kettering Cancer Center. Anti-Lyb-4.1 serum (C57BL/KsJ anti-
DBA/2N spleen cells) was made as previously described (7).
Anti-H-2.31 serum was produced in B10.A mice immunized against
the BALB/c fibrosarcoma Meth A. Antiserum against H-2 and Ia
antigens of the H-2^k haplotype (C3H.SW anti-C3H) was a gift
of Dr. D. Sachs of NIH.

*Cell-Surface Membrane Radioiodination and Immunoprecip-
itation.* Methods for lactoperoxidase-catalyzed iodination
with ^{125}I and antigen immunoprecipitation with antisera and
protein A-bearing *Staphylococcus aureus* were as detailed
previously (17, 18).

Polyacrylamide Gel Electrophoresis and Fluorography.
Antigens eluted in SDS-urea after immunoprecipitation were
reduced in 5% mercaptoethanol and electrophoresed in a discontinuous SDS buffer system on polyacrylamide gel slabs, as
described elsewhere (19). The gels were processed for fluorography on X-ray film (20), and radioactivity vs. mobility
profiles were produced with a scanning densitometer.

Fluorescence Activated Cell Sorting. Purification of
surface immunoglobulin (Ig) positive and negative fractions
of splenocytes with the fluorescence activated cell sorter
(FACS) has previously been described (4).

RESULTS

Molecular Properties of Lyb-6. DBA/2 splenocytes (Lyb-6
positive) were radioiodinated by the lactoperoxidase method
and portions of the NP-40 detergent lysate were incubated
with CBA/N anti-CBA/J serum or with anti-H-2.31 serum. The
immune complexes were then precipitated with the staphylococ-
cal adsorbent and the eluted antigens were reduced and analyzed in parallel by SDS-PAGE. The mobilities of the respective antigens are compared in Figure 1. Although peaks of
radioactivity corresponding to two major polypeptides are
observed in the CBA/N anti-CBA/J precipitate (upper panel),
when 6M urea is also present during reduction the peak with
slower mobility is diminished and the faster peak shows a
corresponding gain in radioactivity (not shown). Thus, the
two peaks appear to represent dimeric and monomeric forms
of the same molecule. The monomer peak has, in addition,
identical mobility to the alloantigenic polypeptide of H-2
(lower panel) over a wide range of acrylamide gel concentrations (7.5-12.5%, unpublished observations), indicating that
the two antigens are similar in size (mol. wt. 45,000). However, unlike H-2, a β_2 microglobulin-like component is not
observed with the antigen immunoprecipitated with CBA/N anti-
CBA/J serum. In accordance with the experimental findings
to be described below, we have defined this 45,000 dalton
antigen as Lyb-6.

Properties of the Cells Which Bear Lyb-6. In preliminary
studies the recovery of Lyb-6 by immunoprecipitation was determined after extensive absorption of the antiserum with
tissue from various organs of Lyb-6 positive mice. These
studies revealed that prior absorption with splenocytes abolished the precipitating capacity of the antiserum, whereas
absorption with brain, kidney, liver or skin tissue had no

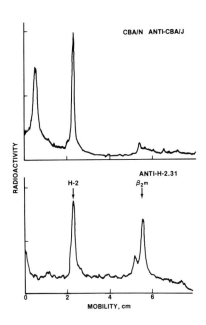

FIGURE 1.   SDS-PAGE comparing mobilities of antigens
immunoprecipitated with CBA/N anti-CBA/J serum (upper panel)
and anti-H-2.31 serum (lower panel).

effect.   In ensuing experiments, Lyb-6 was isolated quantitatively from equal numbers of cells from different lymphoid
organs. Maximum recoveries were obtained from unfractionated
(red cell-depleted) spleen and Peyer's patch cells and somewhat lower amounts from peripheral lymph nodes. Lyb-6 could
not be detected on thymocytes or cortisone-resistant thymocytes. Thus, the former studies indicated that the antiserum
reacted with a lymphoid cell-associated antigen. The latter
experiment provided evidence that the antiserum reacted selectively with an antigen on some class or subclass of lymphoid
cells, and whose recovery corresponded roughly to the proportion of B cells in the different lymphoid organs.
     A more direct analysis of the cell type bearing Lyb-6
was performed by determining its presence or absence on purified B cell and B cell-depleted populations. Spleen cells
from CBA/J mice were stained with fluorescein-conjugated goat
antibodies against mouse Ig and the cells were separated into
surface Ig$^+$ and surface Ig$^-$ fractions with the FACS. Equal
numbers of cells in the two fractions were then radioiodinated (similar specific activities were obtained) and mouse Ig

and Lyb-6 were then analyzed after sequential immunoprecipita-
tions with the respective antisera. As shown in Figure 2,
Lyb-6 was only detected in the surface Ig$^+$ fraction, indicating that the antigen is a B cell marker.

    Because Lyb-6 was defined with an antiserum made in
CBA/N mice, it was important to determine if this antigen was
further restricted to a subclass of B cells. The presence or
absence of Lyb-6 on (CBA/N x DBA/2)F_1 male mice would serve
as a crucial indicator, since these mice exhibit the same B
cell maturational arrest as CBA/N mice and the restriction of
Lyb-3 and Lyb-5 was established on this basis (3, 4). Equal
numbers of splenocytes from CBA/N, (CBA/N x DBA/2)F_1 male, F_1
female, and DBA/2 mice were radiolabeled under identical conditions, and Lyb-6 was isolated quantitatively from the respective cell lysates. The recovery of Lyb-6, expressed as
the percent of immunoprecipitable radioactivity, is shown in
Table I and clearly demonstrates the presence of Lyb-6, albeit
in substantially reduced amounts, on the F_1 male cells. Analysis of the immune precipitates by SDS-PAGE confirmed these
differences in quantitative expression (not shown). The intermediate recovery of Lyb-6 from immunologically normal F_1
female mice further suggests that Lyb-6 is present on these

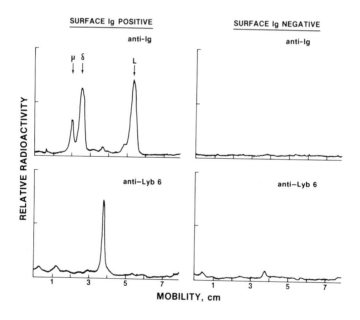

    FIGURE 2. SDS-PAGE showing amounts of both Ig and Lyb-
6 immunoprecipitated sequentially from FACS sorted surface
Ig positive and negative fractions.

TABLE I

QUANTITATION OF LYB-6 ON INBRED MICE AND F_1 HYBRIDS

Mice[a]	% Immunoprecipitable Lyb 6 Radioactivity[b] (Mean $\pm$ S.E.)
DBA/2	0.587 ± 0.047
(CBA/N x DBA/2)F_1 ♀	0.484 ± 0.016
(CBA/N x DBA/2)F_1 ♂	0.372 ± 0.015
CBA/N	0.256 ± 0.007[c]

[a]Each group contained four mice.
[b](Acid precipitable cpm in immune precipitate
÷ acid precipitable cpm in lysate) x 100.
[c]Background level.

cells as a codominant allele. Thus, production of antibodies against Lyb-6 after immunization of CBA/N mice with CBA/J splenocytes reflected primarily the recognition of genetic differences rather than maturational differences between the two strains.

Genetic Characteristics of Lyb-6. As a first approach to genetic characterization, the distribution of Lyb-6 among more than 30 inbred and congenic mouse strains was determined. A pattern of allelic polymorphism was revealed which permitted the designation of this antigen as the Lyb-6.1 allele. Strains possessing this allele included CBA/J, DBA/2, I/St, and SWR. Included among the negative strains were CBA/N, C3H/HeJ, C57BL/6, B10.D2, B10.BR, BALB/c, and SJL. This pattern ruled out any simple association with H-2 haplotype, Ig allotype, coat color, and a large number of other loci. There was, however, a remarkable similarity to the previously published distributions of both Lyb-2 (6) and Lyb-4 (7). This observation raised the possibility of linkage or identity of these antigens and made necessary a further evaluation of their genetic relationships.

The transmission of genes determining the specificities of Lyb-6, Lyb-2, and Lyb-4 was followed in (C57BL/6 x DBA/2)F_1 hybrids backcrossed with C57BL/6 mice. Lyb-2.1 and Lyb-4.1 were assayed serologically in accordance with procedures that originally defined these antigens, while Lyb-6.1 was again determined by immunoprecipitation. The results of analyses of 90 backcross mice are summarized in Table II and clearly demonstrate the linkage of these genes. The existence of recombinants among these B cell markers establishes

TABLE II

SEGREGATION OF LYB-6 WITH LYB-2 AND LYB-4 IN
(C57BL/6 x DBA/2)F₁ x C57BL/6 BACKCROSS MICE

	Lyb-2.1 (+)	Lyb-2.1 (−)	Lyb-4.1 (+)	Lyb-4.1 (−)
Lyb-6.1 (+)	42	2	43	1
Lyb-6.1 (−)	2	44	2	44

further that the genes controlling these specificities are
distinct. In most instances these recombinants have subsequently been backcrossed again with C57BL/6 mice and preser-
vation of the recombinant phenotype has been demonstrated in
their progeny. Based on the patterns of inheritance of the
three specificities, the results are consistent with the
notion that the order of linkage of the respective genes is
Lyb-2-Lyb-4-Lyb-6. A tentative recombination frequency of
3-5% has been calculated between the Lyb-2 and Lyb-6 genes,
but finalization awaits confirmation of all the recombinant
mice by progeny testing.

DISCUSSION

Although the antiserum which has been used to define
Lyb-6 was produced in immune-defective CBA/N mice, it is
clear that production of antibodies against this marker on
CBA/J B cells was due primarily to the recognition of allelic
differences between the two strains. The identification of
Lyb-6 on spleen cells of (CBA/N x DBA/2)F₁ male mice indicates that this antigen is not restricted to the population
of mature B cells which is apparently absent in these mice.
Supporting this conclusion is the finding that normal DBA/2
spleen cells which have been depleted of Lyb-5-bearing cells
by treatment with anti-Lyb-5.1 serum plus complement also
bear Lyb-6 (11). A strong histoincompatibility has been reported between various sublines of CBA mice, in particular,
the CBA/H and CBA/J sublines (21), despite the absence of
any serologically detectable differences. CBA/N mice are
derived from the former subline (22).

The linkage of genes controlling the specificities of
Lyb-2, Lyb-4, and Lyb-6 permits the tentative organization
of a small region of the chromosome on which these genes reside. Recently, the linkage of Lyb-2 on the centromeric side
of the major urinary protein (Mup-1) locus on chromosome 4

was reported and a recombination frequency of approximately 6% was calculated between the two loci (23, 24). The smaller recombination frequency observed here between the Lyb-2 and Lyb-6 loci, along with the proposed order of the Lyb-2, -4, and -6 genes, plus results of our linkage studies with Mup-1 in BxD recombinant inbred strains (11) and backcross analyses (unpublished observations), all serve to locate this gene cluster to the left of the Mup-1 locus. The significance of this genetic relationship is unclear, since correlative functional data for these antigens is not yet available. Other workers have located a gene controlling responsiveness to lipopolysaccharide (a B cell function) in C3H/HeJ mice to the right of the Mup-1 locus (25), although a structural analogue on the cell membrane has not been found. It is possible that more B cell-associated loci may exist here and that this chromosome region may play a role in B cell development or in the regulation of certain B cell functions.

A matter of equal significance concerns the possible structural homologies of the Lyb-2, -4, -6 gene products both to each other and also to H-2 antigens and a number of other 45,000 dalton polypeptides genetically linked to H-2 on chromosome 17 (13-16). The present study was restricted to an examination of these Lyb antigens using the assays with which these antigens were originally defined. A thorough analysis of the immunochemical and serological relationships of these antigens will be reported elsewhere. Insofar as structural homologies with H-2 antigens are concerned, we expect that such relationships may be revealed by comparative peptide and sequence analyses which are currently in progress.

ACKNOWLEDGMENT

We wish to thank Mrs. Janie P. Kaczmarowski for the editorial assistance.

REFERENCES

1. Melchers, F. H., Van Baehmer, H., and Phillips, R. A. (1975). Transplant. Rev. 25, 26.
2. Scher, I., Ahmed, A., and Sharrow, S. O. (1977). J. Immunol. 119, 1938.
3. Huber, B., Gershon, R. K., and Cantor, H. (1977). J. Exp. Med. 145, 10.
4. Ahmed, A., Scher, I., Sharrow, S. O., Smith, A. H., Paul, W. E., Sachs, D. H., and Sell, K. W. (1977). J. Exp. Med. 145, 101.

5. McKenzie, I. F. C., and Snell, G. D. (1975). J. Immunol. 114, 848.
6. Sato, H., and Boyse, E. A. (1976). Immunogenetics 3, 565.
7. Freund, J. G., Ahmed, A., Budd, R. E., Dorf, M. E., Sell, K. W., Vannier, W. E., and Humphreys, R. E. (1976). J. Immunol. 117, 1903.
8. Subbarao, B., Mosier, D. E., Ahmed, A., Mond, J. J., Scher, I., and Paul, W. E. (1979). J. Exp. Med. 149, 495.
9. Scher, I., Ahmed, A., Sharrow, S. O., and Paul, W. E. (1977). In "Development of Host Defenses" (M. Cooper and D. Dayton, eds.), pp. 55-74. Raven Press, New York.
10. Kessler, S. W., Ahmed, A., and Scher, I. (1978). Fed. Proc. 37, 1584.
11. Kessler, S., Ahmed, A., and Scher, I. (1979). In "B Lymphocytes in the Immune Response" (M. Cooper, D. Mosier, I. Scher and E. Vitetta, eds.), in press. Elsevier North-Holland, New York.
12. Tung, J. S., Michaelson, J., Sato, H., Vitetta, E. S., and Boyse, E. S. (1977). Immunogenetics 5, 485.
13. Nathenson, S. G., and Cullen, S. E. (1974). Biochim. Biophys. Acta 344, 1.
14. Vitetta, E. S., Artzt, K., Bennet, D., Boyse, E. A., and Jacob, F. (1975). Proc. Natl. Acad. Sci. 72, 3215.
15. Anundi, H., Rask, L., Östberg, L., and Peterson, P. A. (1975). Biochemistry 14, 5046.
16. Michaelson, J., Flaherty, L., Vitetta, E. S., and Poulik, M. D. (1977). J. Exp. Med. 145, 1066.
17. Kessler, S. W. (1975). J. Immunol. 115, 1617.
18. Kessler, S. W. (1976). J. Immunol. 117, 1482.
19. Laemmli, U. K. (1970). Nature 227, 680.
20. Laskey, R. A., and Mills, A. D. (1975). Eur. J. Biochem. 56, 335.
21. Carnaud, C., Viallat, J., and Colombani, J. (1977). Immunogenetics 5, 171.
22. Amsbaugh, D. F., Hansen, C. T., Prescott, B., Stashak, P. W., Barthold, D. R., and Baker, P. J. (1972). J. Exp. Med. 136, 931.
23. Sato, H., Itakura, K., and Boyse, E. A. (1977). Immunogenetics 4, 591.
24. Taylor, B. A., and Shen, F. W. (1977). Immunogenetics 4, 597.
25. Watson, J., Kelly, K., Largen, M., and Taylor, B. A. (1978). J. Immunol. 120, 422.

WORKSHOP SUMMARY: Markers of T- and B-Cell Differentiation. Samuel Strober, M.D., Stanford University School
of Medicine, Stanford, California 94305 and Aftab Ahmed,
Ph.D., Naval Medical Research Institute, Bethesda,
Maryland 20014

The workshop was divided into three sections: 1) Markers
of Normal T-Cell Differentiation, 2) Markers of Normal B-Cell
Differentiation, and 3) Markers of T- and B-Cell Tumor Lines.
Murphy introduced the section on normal T-cell differentiation by reviewing the markers, function, and interactions
between T-cell subsets. Recent evidence concerning the division of Ly-1$^+$ cells into Qa-1$^+$ and Qa-1$^-$ subsets was discussed. The former cells are involved in interacting with B
cells to amplify antibody responses and with Ly-1$^+$, 2$^+$, 3$^+$ to
provide feedback suppression. The latter cells interact with
B cells, but are not active in feedback suppression. The
Ly-1$^+$, 2$^+$, 3$^+$ subset involved in feedback suppression appears
to express both the Qa-1 and I-J gene products. Eardley provided evidence for the expression of I-J determinants on Ly-
1$^+$, 2$^+$, 3$^+$ cells which induce the production of Ly-2$^+$, 3$^+$
antigen-specific suppressor cells in a system designed to
assay for feedback suppression in the antibody response to
sheep red blood cells. In this system both the Ly-1$^+$, 2$^+$, 3$^+$
and the Ly-2$^+$, 3$^+$ cells in the feedback loop bear the I-J
markers.
Rothenberg summarized recent work on the biochemistry of
the thymus-leukemia (TL) antigens. A 45,000-dalton TL species was found in normal thymocytes in the cytoplasm, but not
on the surface. Pulse chase experiments suggested that the
latter molecule may be the precursor of two surface TL moieties with apparent molecular weights of 46,000 and 48,000
daltons. β_2 microglobulin was associated with all three
forms. Experiments with Endo-H digestion of the various molecules suggested that post-translational glycosylation occurs
before the TL molecules are expressed on the cell surface.
Although cortisone-sensitive thymocytes bear the usual TL
antigens, as judged by gel analysis, cortisone-resistant
thymocytes contained a different polypeptide chain which was
precipitated with anti-TL antisera. The nature of the latter
molecule is being investigated and may represent the product
of a new Qa gene locus.
Further studies on markers of different subpopulations
of thymocytes were discussed by Levy, McMichael and Pepersack.

Both Levy and McMichael developed monoclonal antisera in mice
against human thymocytes. The hybridoma reagents stained
cortical but not medullary thymocytes and did not stain human
peripheral T cells. Thus, the reagents had reactivities similar to that of murine anti-TL antisera. However, the size of
the molecules precipitated by these reagents was not identical
to those discussed by Rothenberg. Pepersack showed that cortical and medullary thymocytes differ in their expression of
terminal deoxynucleotidyl transferase (TdT) and 20α-hydrox-
ysteroid dehydrogenase (20α-SDH). The cortisone-sensitive
thymocytes express TdT but not 20α-SDH, whereas the cortisone-
resistant thymocytes show the opposite pattern. Both
Pepersack and Mathieson discussed T-cell tumor lines which
expressed one enzyme or the other as a stable marker. The
functional and lineal relationship of the two subpopulations
of thymocytes was reviewed with regard to precursory product
versus parallel, but separate differentiation schemes. No
firm evidence was forthcoming to decide between the two
alternatives.

Finally, Pichler summarized recent data to demonstrate
that the Fc receptors (FcR) for IgM or IgG on human T cells
are not stable markers of peripheral T-cell subpopulations.
In particular, he showed that after Tγ cells are identified
using the technique of rosette formation, the FcR(γ) is capped
off and the FcR(μ) appears. The latter cell can be identified
as a Tμ cell by rosetting procedures. Thus, a single T cell
may have the ability to express either the FcR(γ) or FcR(μ),
depending upon events which modulate the cell surface.

The B-cell surface markers were introduced by S. Kessler
and B. Huber. It was suggested that the Lyb alloantigens
could be used to distinguish functional subpopulations of B
cells or may inherently represent candidates of cellular interactions. It was made clear that not all of the Lyb alloantigens were detected by conventional cytotoxicity reactions.
While anti-Lyb-1, 2, 4, and 5 are defined by their cytotoxic
potential, anti-Lyb-3 was defined by a fluorescence assay,
anti-Lyb-6 by biochemical means, and anti-Lyb-7 by its ability
to block the *in vitro* response of spleen cells to dinitro-
phenyl-lysyl-Ficoll (DNP-Ficoll). Kessler described Lyb-6 in
detail and characterized it as a 45,000-dalton polypeptide,
which is distinct from H-2, and does not contain β_2 microglobulin or actin. It is predominantly expressed on B cells, and
genetic studies mapped Lyb-6 to chromosome 4 to the right of
Lyb-4 and to the left of Mup-1. Huber described Lyb-3 as a
68,000-dalton polypeptide, which is present on 50% of adult
splenic B cells, and suggested that Lyb-3 could be a receptor
for the triggering of B cells, since anti-Lyb-3 can enhance
B-cell response to suboptimal antigen doses. Anti-Lyb-3 does

not show allelic distribution, whereas Lyb-5, which is a cytotoxic antisera also present on 50% of adult splenic B cells,
does show allelic distribution. It is not known whether Lyb-3
and Lyb-5 are present on the same B cells; however, it is
postulated that Lyb-3 may represent the constant portion and
Lyb-5 the variable portion of the molecule. A new marker was
also described by Huber, which was described on the basis of
an antisera raised by immunizing (CBA/N ♀ x C57BL/6)F$_1$ ♂ mice
with C57BL/6 spleen cells, which resulted in the cytotoxicity
of 25-30% of B6 spleen cells. This marker was found to be
strain restricted and linked to the I-A subregion of the H-2
complex. Subbarao described the Lyb-7 alloantigen, which was
found to be present in Lyb-5 alloantisera. This alloantisera
is defined functionally in its ability to block the *in vitro*
response of spleen cells to DNP-Ficoll. Genetic studies showed its linkage to the immunoglobulin V$_H$ region genes.

Mond described the use of the fluorescence activated cell
sorter (FACS) as a means to study B-cell heterogeneity on the
basis of Ia density. The CBA/N mice had a large number of
cells with high Ia density, but lacked cells bearing low-to-
intermediate density of Ia.

Sitia presented data that suggested the ability of anti-δ
serum to inhibit the binding of erythrocyte-antibody complement (EAC) by 40% and anti-Ia, which inhibits the binding of
EAC by 20%. Based on these data and the assumption that every
antisera against all surface markers will interact with its
neighbor, a model was presented for the putative cell-surface
association of IgM, FcR, Ia, complement receptor (CR), and
membrane IgD.

IgM ⟵⟶ FcR ⟵⟶ Ia ⟵⟶ CR ⟵⟶ IgD

Finkelman described the occurrence of serum IgD in mice by the
ability of mouse serum to block the staining of membrane IgD
on spleen cells with FITC allospecific rabbit antimouse IgD
using the FACS. These inhibition studies showed that serum
IgD appears between 14-21 days and peaks at 6 weeks. Further,
infection with parasites, such as malaria, causes a significant increase in serum IgD. Krco reported the differential
cytotoxicity patterns seen with Ia alloantisera on cells from
mouse Peyer's patches (PP). While anti-Ia (A, B, J, E, and C)
was cytotoxic for 45% of the cells, Ia antisera against the
I-A or I-E subregions was cytotoxic for only 30% of the cells,
and I-C alloantisera was minimally cytotoxic. These studies
were performed to analyze the role of PP cells in the Ir gene
control of IgA synthesis, and in this light it was shown that
the glass-adherent cells of the PP did not present antigen.

Mathieson introduced the topic of B- and T-cell tumor
lines and suggested that these cell lines could be used to
predict differentiation stages of normal cells. Panels of

T-cell lymphomas were typed for the presence of Ly antigens, and most of them were found to be Ly-1$^+$. Thymocytes were found to be 90% Ly-1$^+$, 2$^+$, 3$^+$ and 10% Ly-2$^-$, suggesting that not all Ly cells differentiate from Ly 1$^+$, 2$^+$, 3$^+$ cells. Mathieson proposed at least two lines of T-cell differentiation from a pre-T cell:

$$\text{Pre-T cell} \left\langle \begin{array}{l} \longrightarrow \text{Ly 1}^+, \text{ cort. resist., TL}^-, \text{ Thy-1 , 20}\alpha\text{-SDH}^+ \\ \longrightarrow \text{Ly 1}^+,2^+,3^+, \text{ cort. sens., TL}^+, \text{ Thy-1 , TdT}^+ \end{array} \right.$$

Various BALB/c lymphoma lines were examined by Kim for membrane immunoglobulin. All μ^+ lymphomas also had detectable δ, as detected by immunoprecipitation with rabbit antimouse δ. These tumors were fused with IgG$_{2b}$ myeloma and the resulting hybridomas could secrete IgM, but not IgD. One-third of the B-cell lymphomas were positively stained with antipolyvalent Ig sera, but not with class-specific reagents. Kanellopoulos-Langevin examined the interaction of FcR and alloantigens on these BALB/c lymphoma lines and found: a) they had Ig FcR, but not IgM FcR; b) they were all Ig$^+$; c) they were CR$^-$; and d) the μ^+ lymphomas all had certain amounts of δ. When testing these lymphomas for inhibition of EA rosette formation with anti-H-2^d, anti-Ia, or anti-LyM-1, they found that while normal spleen cells are inhibited about 60% with all three reagents, cell line K-46 was inhibited 85%, 61% and 95% with anti-H-2^d, Ia, and LyM-1, respectively; cell line A-20 2%, 84% and 95%, respectively; and cell line M-12 3%, 0% and 91%, respectively, suggesting differential expression or distribution of these markers on these B lymphoma lines.

A variety of other data were presented from Dr. Warner's laboratory which suggested that Abelson virus-transformed murine bone marrow could be used as a tumor model of pre-B cell as they were Ig$^-$, Ia$^-$, but Lyb-2$^+$, and that plasmacytomas could be categorized to represent various stages of maturational arrests of B-cell differentiation. Further, similar evidence was presented for T-lymphoma cell lines in that they expressed less Thy-1 antigen as compared to thymomas and that the Qa antigens were identified on discrete T-cell tumor types.

BIOCHEMISTRY OF LYMPHOCYTE COMMUNICATION

James Watson, Diane Mochizuki, and Marilyn Thoman[*]

Department of Microbiology
University of California, Irvine
Irvine, California 92717

[*]Department of Immunopathology
Scripps Clinic and Research Foundation
North Torrey Pines Road
La Jolla, California 92037

ABSTRACT   Humoral factors secreted by T lymphocytes
and macrophages appear to play a role in cell communication leading to the triggering of immune responses.   A factor has been purified from the culture supernatants of Concanavalin A-activated murine
spleen cells with helper T cell-replacing (TRF)
activity in three assay systems: (i) stimulation of
antibody responses to erythrocyte antigens in T cell-
depleted cultures, (ii) amplification of production
of cytotoxic T cells in thymocyte cultures, and
(iii) stimulation of mitogenic responses to Con A in
thymocyte cultures where the cell density is too low
to support responses to Con A alone.   The biologic
activity has been purified by salt precipitation,
gel filtration, ion exchange chromatography, and isoelectric focusing (IEF).   TRF activity is found in
protein-containing molecules with a Stokes radius
corresponding to a globular protein of 30-35,000
daltons molecular weight, and a pI ranging from 4-5.
Quantitative assays reveal this material is active
at concentrations of less than 10^{-9} M in each lymphocyte response system used.   The production of TRF
requires the presence of T cells, and limiting dilution analyses reveal one in 20,000 spleen cells are
capable of producing TRF.   When produced in conditions of limiting dilution, the TRF show a segregation of biologic activities as revealed by an ability
to stimulate immune responses to one erythrocyte
but not another.   These results indicate that TRF
produced in Con A-treated spleen cultures may have
antigenic specificity.

In an attempt to develop cloned cell lines that produce TRF, antigen-specific helper T cells have been
established in continuous culture. These cells require TRF for proliferation. This finding raises the
question of whether there exists one or two factors
in the TRF preparations, a T cell growth factor (TCGF)
and a helper T cell replacing factor (TRF). The identification of the molecules required for each of these
biological assays may lead to an understanding of the
nature of specific and nonspecific helper T cell-
replacing factors.

INTRODUCTION

Antigen-sensitive cells recognize antigen in association with a cooperating cell system which has several cellular components, helper T cells, and adherent cell types
commonly referred to as macrophages. The key regulatory
element in the induction of antigen-sensitive cells is the
delivery of a signal from the cooperating cell system.
How this intercellular communication process is effected
is unknown. There are three questions to be considered.
First, what cell types comprise the cooperating system?
Second, what is the nature of the antigen-binding receptor
utilized by these cells? Third, how is information transmitted to the antigen-sensitive cell?
A number of factors have been derived that replace
the requirement for helper T cells in the induction of
antibody synthesis (1-6). Little is known concerning the
chemical structure of these factors, but the biological
activities they express suggest they are molecules involved in the communication process between B and T cells.
In order to study the mechanism of helper T cell function,
we have been purifying a class of soluble factors that stimulates immune responses to heterologous erythrocyte antigens in T cell-depleted murine spleen cultures (6). These
T cell-replacing factors (TRF) are secreted by mouse
spleen cells which have been activated in culture by the
polyclonal T cell mitogen, Concanavalin A (6-10).
In this paper we compare the molecular and biological
properties of Con A factors on (i) the induction of in
vitro antibody synthesis in nude spleen cultures, (ii)
mitogenic responses to Con A in thymocyte cultures, and

(iii) the induction of CTL responses by thymocytes. The molecules responsible for biological activity in each assay system show identical behavior upon gel filtration, ion-exchange chromatography, and isoelectric focusing. We utilize partially purified preparations of TRF to establish helper T cell lines in culture.

MATERIALS AND METHODS

Mice. BALB/c and C57BL/6 mice were obtained from the Jackson Laboratory, Bar Harbor, Maine. Nude mice partially backcrossed to BALB/c (BALB/c.nu) or C57BL/6 (C57BL/6.nu) were from our breeding colony, University of California, Irvine (6).

Purification of Biologic Activity from Culture Supernatants. Spleen cells were cultured in the presence of Con A (2 µg/ml) at a density of 5×10^6 cells/ml in a RPMI-1640 medium (Grand Island Biological Company, New York) supplemented with 1% FCS, 5×10^{-5} M 2-mercapto-ethanol, 1 mM glutamine, 50 units/ml penicillin, and 50 µg/ml streptomycin. The cultures were incubated at 37°C for 16-18 hours in a gas mixture of 7% oxygen, 10% carbon dioxide, 83% nitrogen, and then harvested (6).

Purification Procedures. Ammonium sulphate precipitation, all chromatography, and isoelectric focusing were performed at 4°C using sterile buffers as detailed elsewhere (6,7,11). Protein determinations were made as shown elsewhere (12).

Microculture Assay for T Cell-Replacing Activity. Antibody synthesis was measured in the microculture system described by Lefkovits (13,14). Spleen cells from BALB/c.nu mice were resuspended in RPMI-1640 supplemented with 20% fetal calf serum at a density of 10^7 cells/ml and then distributed into microculture trays (Falcon Plastics 3034) in 10 µl aliquots yielding cell concentrations of 1.0×10^5 cells/well. These wells also contained 0.05% SRBC or HRBC as antigen. The cultures were incubated for 5 days, and the supernatants from each microculture were assayed using a spot test, and the fraction of responding cultures determined (14). The two stage microculture used is also detailed elsewhere (15).

Induction of Mitogenic Responses to Con A in Thymocyte Cultures. Thymocytes were resuspended in the RPMI-1640 described above with 5% FCS, at a density of

10^6 cells/ml. Microcultures containing 0.1 ml (10^5 cells) were dispensed in Microtest II plates (Falcon Plastics). Factor preparations were then added in 10 μl aliquots. The cultures were incubated for 72 hours and then 0.25 μCi [^{3}H] thymidine (5 C/mmole) was added to give a final thymidine concentration of 0.5 μM for 6 hours.

Induction of CTL Responses by Thymocytes. CBA/J-thymocytes and irradiated P815 cells were cultured in 96 well microtitre trays from Linbro Scientific, Handen, Connecticut, in the presence of allogeneic cells as described elsewhere (7).

Unit of Factor Activity. When Con A supernatants are diluted into the microculture system to assay the induction of antibody synthesis, the number of positive cultures, as determined by the presence of a lytic spot, decrease. We quantitate factor activity by defining a unit of activity as the amount of factor that produces 1/3 (0.33) of the maximal response as detailed elsewhere (6). To quantitate factor in thymocyte response assays, a unit of activity is defined as the amount of factor that produces 1/3 of the maximal response. The maximum response was determined in each experiment by the use of control cultures which contained a titrated amount of factor, known to be saturating.

RESULTS

BALB/c spleens were used to prepare 200 ml of Con A supernatant, and the biologic activity was recovered in the 40-80% (NH_4)$_2SO_4$ fraction as described elsewhere (6). This fraction was applied to a Sephadex G-100 column and eluted in 0.1 M NH_4HCO_3 (Fig. 1A). Fractions were collected, lyophilized and dissolved in BSS for assay in the thymocyte and nude spleen culture systems. The active fractions in each assay system (fractions 28-34, Fig. 1A) were identical, and corresponded in size to molecules from 30,000 to 40,000 daltons.

The Sephadex G-100 fractions from the experiment of Figure 1A were then pooled, dialyzed against water, lyophilized, and then dissolved in 0.05 M ammonium acetate (pH 7.6). This material was applied to DEAE-ion exchange column, and eluted with a salt gradient from 0.05 M - 0.5 M ammonium acetate (pH 7.6). The fractions collected were lyophilized, dissolved in 0.9% NaCl and assayed for activity in the thymocyte and nude spleen culture system.

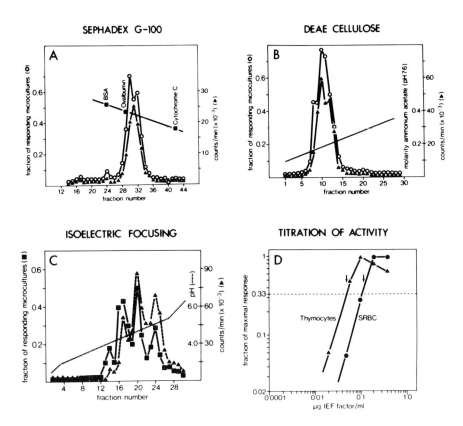

Figure 1. Purification of Con A factor. (A) Sephadex
G-100 chromatography of Con A factor. The 40-80% $(NH_4)_2SO_4$
precipitate from 200 ml Con A supernatant was dissolved
in 10 ml 0.1 M NH_4HCO_3, dialyzed twice against 100 volumes
of the same buffer before fractionation. Column fractions
were lyophilized and redissolved in 1 ml BSS for assay.
(B) DEAE ion exchange chromatography of Con A factor. The
fractions from the Sephadex G-100 column containing T cell-
replacing activity (fractions 28-34) were redissolved in
0.005 M ammonium acetate (pH 7.6), pooled and applied to a
DEAE column equilibrated in the same buffer. A gradient
from 0.005 M to 0.5 M ammonium acetate (pH 7.6) was used
for elution. (C) Isoelectric focusing of factor activity.
The activity from the DEAE column was pooled and electrophoresed in a pH gradient from 3-6. (D) The specific
activity of IEF-purified factor. The factor activity
located in the pH range of 4.0-5.0 was pooled, the protein
concentration determined, and then assayed for the stimulation of thymocyte and nude spleen culture responses.

Again, the active factors in each assay were identical
(Fig. 1B), and eluted from DEAE in these conditions in the
range from 0.15 M - 0.2 M ammonium acetate (pH 7.6). The
DEAE fractions that exhibited activity were pooled, dialyzed against water and lyophilized.
    Isoelectric focusing was used to further examine the
relationship of the biologic activities in the Con A factors. Sephadex G-100 pooled factor prepared as described
for the experiment of Figure 1A was applied to a horizontal
layer of Ultradex designed to give a pH gradient from 3.0 -
6 at equilibrium (see Methods). When biological assays
were performed after electrophoresis, most activity in
spleen and thymocyte culture assays was observed in the
pH range of 4-5 (Fig. 1C). Quantitative determinations of
activity in nude spleen and cultures were performed using
the pooled factor recovered in the pH range of 4-5 following isoelectric focusing (Fig. 1C). The protein concentration was determined (12), but it should be remembered that, even after dialysis, small amounts of ampholines
may still be present. In the thymocyte assay, 50 ng IEF-
purified factor yielded 1 unit of activity (Fig. 1D). In
nude spleen cultures, 100 ng IEF-purified factor gave
1 unit (Fig. 1D). Factor activity that stimulates the
generation of cytotoxic lymphocytes in thymocyte cultures
followed exactly the same profile (7).

    Cellular Origin of TRF. While T cells are required
for the production of TRF, it is not formally known
whether these cells synthesize and secrete TRF. One
approach to the cellular origin of TRF is to determine
the frequency of TRF-producing cells in mouse spleen,
using a two stage microculture procedure devised by
Lefkovits and Waldmann (15), which is outlined in Figure 2.
Spleen cells from normal BALB/c mice were distributed in
microculture master trays in 15 μl or 16 μl aliquots at
cell concentrations varying from 1 x 10^4 cells/well to
1 x 10^5 cells/well. Con A was present always at a concentration of 2 μg/ml. Each microculture master tray
(60 microwells) was incubated at 37°C for 24 hours. After
this time six 2 μl aliquots of culture supernatant were
sampled from every one of the master wells and transferred to fresh recipient microculture wells containing
either 1.2 x 10^5 BALB/c.nu spleen cells and 0.05% of the
test erythrocyte antigen. After incubation of the
recipient microcultures for 5 or 6 days, all cultures
were assayed for specific anti-RBC antibody by using the
spot test.

FIRST STAGE   SECOND STAGE   SPOT TEST

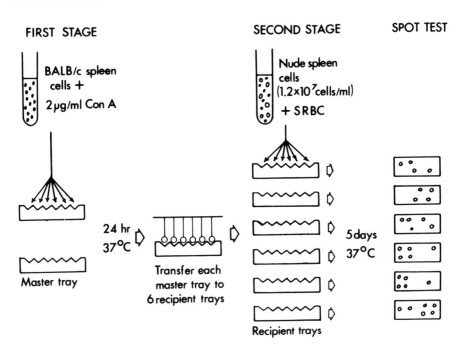

Figure 2. Concanavalin A stimulates mouse T lymphocytes to
release factors which have the biologic activity of inducing immune responses to erythrocyte antigens in spleen cultures that lack functional T cells, and the activity can be
measured in a two-stage culture assay. Spleen cells from
BALB/c mice were distributed in microculture master trays
in 16 µl aliquots of cell concentrations varying from
1×10^4 cells/well to 1×10^5 cells/well. Con A was present always at a concentration of 2 µg/ml. Each microculture master tray (60 microwells) was incubated at 37°C
for 24 h. After this time six 2 µl aliquots of culture
supernatant were sampled from every one of the master wells
and transferred to fresh recipient microculture wells containing 1.2×10^5 BALB/c.nu spleen cells and 0.05% of the
test erythrocyte antigen. After incubation of the recipient microcultures for 5 days, all cultures were assayed for
specific anti-RBC antibody by using the spot test (15).
Wherever culture supernatant from a master well induced a
response in a recipient culture, that supernatant must have
contained the Con A factor and therefore the cells of that
master culture must have contained at least one factor-
producing T cell. Thus, the number of wells in the master
tray making T cell-replacing factors must be at least
equivalent to the number obtained by integrating the
responses from all the test recipient cultures.

The experiment shown in Figure 3 summarizes the anti-SRBC responses of BALB/c.nu microcultures stimulated by supernatants transferred from <u>master</u> trays containing 1 x 10^5 cells/well, 5 x 10^4 cells/well, 2.5 x 10^4 cells/well, and 1.25 x 10^4 cells/well prepared from normal BALB/c spleen cells. Wherever culture supernatant from a <u>master</u> well induced a response in a <u>recipient</u> culture, that supernatant must have contained the Con A factor, and therefore, the cells of that <u>master</u> culture must have contained at least one factor-producing T cell. Thus, the number of wells in the <u>master</u> tray producing T cell-replacing factors must be at least equivalent to the number obtained by integrating the responses from all the test <u>recipient</u> cultures. A Poisson plot of active supernatants from the <u>master</u> wells has the features of a single hit curve (Fig. 3). The implication is that the supernatant products of only a single cell in the <u>master</u> tray are sufficient to restore immune responsiveness to SRBC in T cell-depleted cultures. The frequency of cells which, under these conditions, respond to Con A producing factors can be estimated to be one in 45,000 spleen cells (Fig. 3). This estimate is within the frequency range published elsewhere (15), and varies in the range of 1:20,000 to 1:50,000.

<u>Specificity of Monoclonal Factor</u>. Under limiting dilution conditions, it is apparent that the products of single factor producing cells are being analyzed (16). The specificity of these monoclonal factors can be considered in two ways. Firstly, the factor may have activity that could be termed <u>antigen-nonspecific</u>. The interaction of factor with cells does not involve binding to antigen. Second, the factor may have an <u>antigen-specific</u> mode of action, requiring a direct interaction with antigen to exert biologic activity. Thus, only those B cells binding antigen would be capable of responding to these factors. The Con A supernatants prepared under conditions of limiting T cells were examined for specificity by assaying for the stimulation of immune responses to two different erythrocyte antigens in BALB/c.nu spleen cultures. Because the frequency of antigen-reactive B cells for HRBC and BRBC were similar, these antigens were utilized. Master trays containing 5 x 10^4 cells/well, 2.5 x 10^4 cells/well, and 1.25 x 10^4 cells/well were incubated with 2 µg Con A for 24 hours at 37°C. Samples from each <u>master</u> well were transferred in 2 µl aliquots to six <u>recipient</u> microcultures containing 1.2 x 10^5

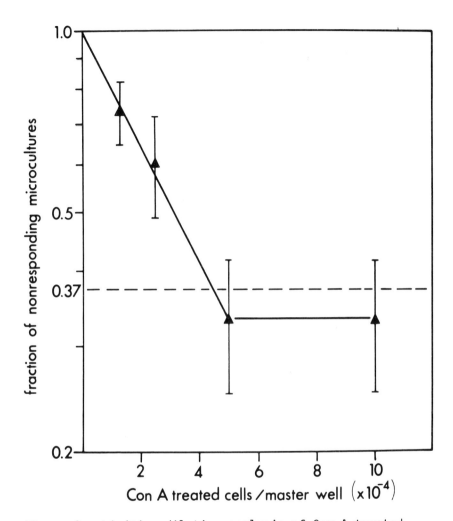

Figure 3. Limiting dilution analysis of Con A-treated
spleen cells. Master trays containing 1.25×10^{-4} to
1.0×10^{-5} cells/well were incubated for 24 h with 2 µg/ml
Con A. Each well was then transferred to six recipient
microcultures and assayed for the stimulation of immune
responses to SRBC in BALB/c.nu spleen cells. Each point
represents the fraction of master well culture supernatants that do not stimulate immune responses to SRBC.
Two master trays (120 microcultures) were assayed for
each point. The 95% confidence levels are presented.

BALB/c.nu spleen cells and a combination of 0.05% HRBC and
0.05% BRBC. The results of a typical experiment are shown
in Table 1.

TABLE 1

SPECIFICITY OF SUPERNATANT ACTIVITY PREPARED FROM

CON A-TREATED BALB/c SPLEEN CELLS

Number Master Wells Tested	Cells/ Master Well	Test Antigen		Total Positive Master Wells	Number Double Responder Wells
		HRBC	BRBC		
120	50,000	66	40	84	22
120	25,000	44	21	55	10
120	12,500	16	6	19	3

As the factor-producing cells in the master wells
decrease from 5×10^4 to 1.25×10^4, the total number of
wells in which TRF can be detected decreases from 84 to
19. However, the number of master wells that produce
TRF capable of stimulating antibody responses to both
HRBC and BRBC decreases from 22 (of 84 total) to 3 (of
19 total).

The data presented in Figure 4 summarize three similar
experiments. The fraction of the total master wells in
which TRF is detected that yield responses to both HRBC
and BRBC antigens decreases as the cell number of each
master well decreases (Fig. 4). Thus 'monclonal' factor
exhibits, under these conditions, antigen-specificity
in its mode of action (16).

Growth of Helper T Cells in Continuous Culture.
The limitation of the two stage microculture system is
that while it may be a technique for producing monoclonal
TRF, it is not feasible to purify TRF from such small
culture volumes. We therefore attempted to establish
T cell lines in continuous culture as a basis for isolating monoclonal TRF. While it is not known

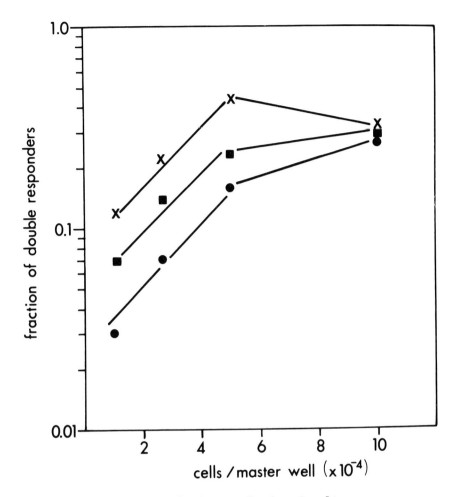

Figure 4. Limiting dilution analysis of culture supernatants prepared from Con A-treated BALB/c spleen cells.
Each master well was assayed in six microcultures containing a mixture of HRBC and BRBC antigens. Three
separate experiments are presented. In each, the number
of master wells that yielded double-responder (BRBC and
HRBC positive) supernatants was expressed as a fraction
of the total factor-producing master wells.

whether T cells synthesize and secrete TRF, if these
molecules are the products of helper T cells, an interesting paradox emerges. Are TRF molecules required for
the induction of helper T cells, and can TRF be used
to maintain the growth of helper T cells in culture?

Cell cultures exhibiting helper T cell activity
have been prepared in the following way. Mice were
irradiated (850 R) and reconstituted with 10^8 thymocytes
and heterologous red blood cells (SRBC or HRBC) as antigen.
After 7 days, mice were sacrificed and spleen cells cultured at a density of 10^6 cells/ml, 10 units/ml TRF,
antigen, and 10^5 irradiated syngeneic nude spleen cells/ml.
Each 3-4 days, this growth medium was replaced. The TRF
used was a pool of Con A-free, Sephadex G-100 purified
material (6). After 3-4 weeks in culture, growing cells
were maintained by passaging at a seeding density of 10^4
cells/ml. A number of cell lines have been established
in culture and maintained for periods of up to 40 weeks.
All cell lines exhibit a strict dependence upon the TRF
preparations for growth.

At various intervals, the cells growing in culture
have been assayed for helper T cell activity. Here, the
T cells are titrated into the microculture system of
Lefkovits (13), containing either BALB/c.nu or C57BL/6.nu
spleen cells, and either SRBC or HRBC as antigen to determine the frequency of cells that exhibit antigen-specific
helper activity.

The data summarized in Figure 5 show the results of
limiting dilution experiments to determine the frequency
of T^H_{SRBC} derived from C57BL/6J mice at various times
after culturing. At the time cell cultures were initiated
the frequency of T^H_{SRBC} in the activated spleen cell population was 1:4000. After 10 days in culture, the frequency of T^H_{SRBC} was 1:200, and after 4 weeks the frequency was 1:10 - 1:20. This probably reflects the upper
limit of sensitivity of the microculture assay, and may
be a reflection that most cells growing in culture
possess helper activity.

The antigenic and H-2 specificity of the helper
activity from these cultured cells is described in the
experiment of Figure 6. C57BL/6J T^H_{SRBC} were assayed
using either C57BL/6.nu or BALB/c.nu spleen cells, with
either SRBC or HRBC as antigen. The C57BL/6 T^H_{SRBC} show
a marked helper preference for C57BL/6.nu spleen cells
with SRBC. Little helper activity was exhibited in cultures containing C57BL/6.nu spleen cells and HRBC, or

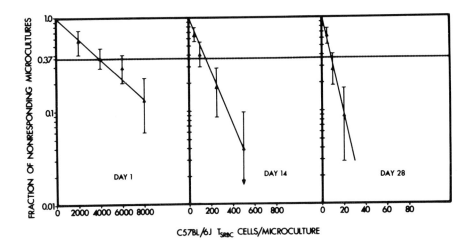

Figure 5. Frequency of SRBC-specific T helper cells at various times after transfer to cell culture. C57BL/6J T$_{SRBC}$ cells were incubated in microwell cultures containing 1 x 10^5 C57BL/6.nu spleen cells with 0.05% SRBC as antigens.

BALB/c.nu spleen cells with SRBC or HRBC. Therefore, the
cells growing in culture appear to exhibit both antigenic-
specificity and H-2 restriction in their mode of action.

A detailed analysis of these cell lines is presented
elsewhere (17). Cells have a doubling time of 20-30 hours,
and rapidly die if cultured in complete medium not supplemented with TRF. All cells growing in culture bear Thy-1
antigens, and therefore are identified as T cells (17).

DISCUSSION

T Cell-Derived Factors. The observation that supernatants from mixed lymphocyte cultures contained TRF has
resulted in the finding that, in culture, the activation
of T cells results in the production of TRF. In general,
three types of culture procedures are employed to generate
TRF. These are mixed lymphocyte cultures or allogeneic
interactions, antigen-stimulated lymphocyte cultures or
Concanavalin A-treated lymphocyte cultures. While it is
difficult to prove formally that these factors are secreted
by T cells, T cells are required for TRF production.
Further, the phenotype of the cell involved in TRF production appears to be Ly-1$^+$, which is that of the helper
class of T lymphocytes.

Are these TRF identical in structure, do they belong
to the same family of molecules, or are they different
molecular species? This issue cannot be resolved until
each TRF has been chemically purified. However, there are
several striking similarities in the mode of action of
these various factors. First, most TRF do not exhibit
antigen specificity (1-7). Secondly, the TRF have no
effect on the induction of antibody synthesis in the
absence of antigen. The TRF molecules are strictly
antigen-dependent in their mode of action. The implication of these findings to the induction is important.
The B cell requires two signals to complete the inductive
stimulus. It must first bind antigen which must result
in the initiation of a set of intracellular biochemical
events. The B cell must also receive a helper cell
signal which acts synergistically with the antigenic
signal to complete the inductive stimulus (16).

As described here, Sephadex G-100 and DEAE cellulose
ion-exchange chromatography, followed by isoelectric
focusing result in purified TRF. These purification
methods in conjunction with ^{125}I-radiolabeling, provide
a very sensitive means of detecting small quantities of
material and have allowed PAGE analysis of the molecular

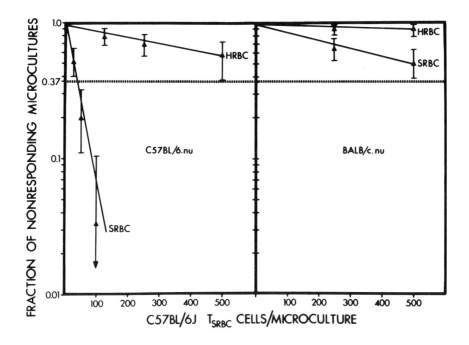

Figure 6. Antigenic and H-2 specificity of C57BL/6J helper T cells. C57BL/6J T$_{SRBC}$ cells were titrated in cultures containing: (a) C57BL/6.nu spleen cells supplemented with 0.05% SRBC and HRBC; (b) BALB/c.nu spleen cells supplemented with 0.05% SRBC and HRBC.

weight and subunit composition of TRF generated by Con A
stimulation of murine spleen cells. Preliminary experiments have shown that TRF is composed of a single polypeptide chain of approximately 70,000 daltons molecular
weight (18).

We have demonstrated that three biological activities
copurify following salt precipitation, gel filtration,
ion-exchange chromatography and isoelectric focusing (7);
these activities stimulating antibody synthesis in T cell-
depleted spleen cultures, the generation of cytotoxic
lymphocytes to allogenic tumor cells in thymocyte cultures, and the stimulation of mitogenic responses to Con
A or PHA in thymocyte cultures where the cell density is
too low to support mitogenic responses to the lectin
alone (8-10).

Origin and Specificity of TRF. The identity of TRF
has been approached by examining the specificity of their
biologic activity:

First, the factors may have activity that could be
termed hormonal. By this we mean that factors, secreted
by one cell interact directly with a receptor site on
another cell. This mode of action is antigen-nonspecific
in that the interaction of factor with cells and signal
delivery does not depend on the presence of antigen.
This cell may be a B or T lymphocyte that has bound
antigen or mitogen.

Alternatively, the factor may require a direct interaction with antigen to exert biologic activity. Thus,
only those B cells binding antigen, or T cells binding
mitogen, would be capable of responding to these factors.
This mode of action implies the factors possess antigen-
specificity.

The remarkable feature of the two-stage culture system
used in this limiting dilution analysis is that it enables
the accumulated products of single T cells to be assayed
for their B cell inducing properties (15). A previous
study that led to this work has revealed that small numbers (one out of 19,000) of spleen cells produces TRF
capable of inducing immune responses to SRBC in nude
spleen cultures (15). The basic observations reported
here are as follows:

a. If we consider the single hit curve in the
limiting dilution plots of Figure 3, we are led to conclude that one out of some 45,000 spleen cells is capable
of producing factors that restore immune responses to
SRBC. Similar numbers of spleen cells produce factors

that restore immune responses to HRBC and BRBC (data not shown).

b. When the spleen cell numbers were decreased in the master wells, there was a definite trend in the biologic activities of the Con A supernatants. In master wells containing 10^5 spleen cells, of all wells that were found to contain positive supernatants when tested with two different erythrocyte antigens (HRBC and HRBC), only some 30% stimulated immune responses to both (Fig. 4). As the number of spleen cells treated with Con A is decreased to 1.25×10^4 microwell, the number of supernatants found to be positive on two antigens also decreases. Using HRBC and BRBC as the pairs of test antigens, the number of master wells containing 1.25×10^4 cells capable of stimulating two responses is generally in the range of 3% to 13% (Fig. 4). We consider three possible explanations of these findings have different merits:

i) Subsets of Lymphocytes. In general, a supernatant from a master well was unable to activate every one of the B cell precursors in the second stage assay. There exists, therefore, heterogeneity in the B cell response. The original explanation for the heterogeneity in recipient responses was that at the level of both B and T cells there exist subsets (15). In the case of T cells these may represent cells which vary in the quantity or quality of the factors they make. In the case of B cells, activation with such factors would only occur if appropriately matching B cells interacted with the correct T cell subsets (15).

ii) Sensitivity of Lymphocytes to TRF. A direct explanation for the segregation of TRF specificities is that, under conditions of limiting dilution, the amount of TRF produced in supernatants is decreased. B cell and T cell precursors that respond to TRF, show different sensitivities with respect to the concentration of TRF required for cell activation. One obvious reason for the different sensitivities of lymphocytes to TRF lies in the synergistic mode of action with antigen or mitogen. Precursor cells will have different bind affinities for the same antigen, or mitogen, therefore the endogenous levels of cellular signals received from these interactions may vary considerably. The ability of TRF to complete an inductive signal may depend on the 'level' of the antigenic signal. When TRF concentrations are limiting, a very heterogeneous response to any antigen may be observed.

iii) <u>Antigenic Specificity of TRF.</u> Since the frequency of helper T cells specific for these erythrocyte antigens is similar to the frequency of active supernatants, the implication is that we are assaying an antigen-specific product in the culture supernatant from Con A-treated cells. The only class of molecules with this property likely to be present in these supernatants would be part of the antigen-binding receptor of T cells (19). The mitogenic activation of helper T cells may be causing the secretion of part, or all, their antigen-binding receptors. Since Con A is a polyclonal T cell mitogen, the culture supernatants will contain a polyclonal array of these receptors. The nude spleen cells used to detect TRF activity may contain an accessory cell type, perhaps a macrophage, which binds cytophilically the TRF or putative antigen-binding receptor from T cells. The interaction of antigen with the receptor bound to this accessory cell type may result in signal that is delivered to B cells. When produced in bulk cultures (i.e., high cell numbers), no antigen specificity is observed; however, when these receptors are produced in limiting dilution conditions, their specificities will emerge in the immune response assay. Thus, in Con A-treated cultures, as the cell number is decreased to less than one antigen-reactive helper T cell per culture, supernatants with activities towards one erythrocyte antigen but not another will begin to emerge.

<u>Monoclonal Sources of TRF.</u> Since the two-stage culture procedure led to experiments that imply TRF found in Con A-activated spleen cell supernatants is a mixture of factors, another approach is required to produce monoclonal TRF in quantities that can be biochemically characterized. A procedure is described here for the establishment of continuous cultures of T cells. Antigen-specific helper T cells have been maintained in culture for more than 40 weeks. Some of the characteristics of these cell lines are shown in the experiments of Figures 5 and 6, however, two issues should be emphasized:

a. All T cell lines established in culture have a strict requirement for a factor found in the Con A supernatant preparations from which TRF is purified. Selection for antigen-specificity was achieved by <u>in vivo</u> activation of thymocytes to either SRBC and HRBC. A detailed analysis of the growth and biological activity of T cells with helper functions is presented elsewhere (17).

The issue we now face concerns whether these cells contain or secrete T cell-replacing factors, either specific or nonspecific, for the induction of antibody synthesis.

   b. The limiting dilution analyses (Figs. 2,3) imply TRF has antigen-specificity. The question arises as to the relationship between TRF and the antigen-binding receptor of T cells (19). However, since TRF preparations also stimulate the growth of T cells, in the absence of antigen or any filler cell types, a property not expected for the T cell receptor, the question arises as to whether TRF preparations is composed of molecules with one or two biological activities.

   Implications of One or Two Factors.
   a. If TRF preparations contain one factor that possesses T cell-replacing activity as well as T cell growth activity, it appears likely that this factor mediates its biological effects via the direct activation of T cells or their precursors. This means that such a factor is unlikely to exhibit any antigen specificity. The limiting dilution experiments may reflect the activation and clonal expansion, by TRF, of antigen-specific precursors of T helper cells present in nude spleen cultures, rather than the interaction of TRF with antigen.
   b. If TRF preparations contain two factors, a T cell growth factor (TCGF) and a T cell-replacing factor (TRF), the biological activities we have discussed may result from different modes of action. TCGF may act directly on T cells, and may stimulate the clonal proliferation of any T cell that has been activated by antigen or mitogen. TCGF thus would stimulate growth of T cells in culture, and stimulate T cell responses to Con A or alloantigens under culture conditions limiting for mature T cells. TCGF exerts, therefore, an antigen-nonspecific or hormonal effect on T cells. On the other hand, TRF may replace T^H cells in the induction of antigen-sensitive cells. TRF may exhibit an antigen-specific activity, as revealed by the limiting dilution analysis (Table 1, Fig. 4), and may be secreted by T cells but bind cytophillically to another cell type in the cooperating system, to provide helper activity (17). This implies TRF is part, or all, the antigen-binding receptor of T cells (19).

   It is clear that only further molecular analysis of the biologically active entities will resolve these issues. Cloned T cell lines may also provide the tools for the generation of monoclonal factors which are necessary for further detailed structural and functional study

of T cell receptors, and the molecules used in the communication process between lymphocytes.

ACKNOWLEDGMENTS

The work described here has resulted from many fine
collaborative efforts. In particular, I can only express
gratitude for the interests and work of Drs. Ivan Lefkovits,
Lucien Aarden, and Vern Paetkau.

REFERENCES

1. Sjoberg, O., Andersson, J., and Moller, G. (1972)
    J. Immunol. 109, 1379.
2. Harwell, L., Kappler, J. W., and Marrack, P. (1976)
    J. Immunol. 116, 5.
3. Lefkovits, I., Quintans, J., Munro, A., and Waldmann,
    H. (1975) J. Immunol. 28, 1149.
4. Lefkovits, I., and Waldmann, H. (1977) J. Immunol.
    32, 915.
5. Hubner, L, Muller, G., Schimpl, A., and Wecker, E.
    (1978) J. Immunochem. 15, 33.
6. Watson, J. D., Aarden, L., and Lefkovits, I. (1979)
    J. Immunol. 122, 209.
7. Watson, J., Aarden, L., Shaw, J., and Paetkau, V.
    (1979) J. Immunol., in press.
8. Shaw, J., Monticone, V., Miller, G., and Paetkau, V.
    (1978) J. Immunol. 120, 1974.
9. Shaw, J., Monticone, V., and Paetkau, V. (1978)
    J. Immunol. 120, 1978.
10. Paetkau, V., Mills, G., Gerhart, S., and Monticone,
    V. (1976) J. Immunol. 117, 1320.
11. Schalch, W., and Braun, D. G. (1978) In "Research
    Methods in Immunology," (I. Lefkovits and B. Pernis,
    eds.), Academic Press, New York, in press.
12. Bradford, M. M. (1976) Analytical Biochem. 72, 248.
13. Lefkovits, I. (1972) Eur. J. Immunol. 2, 360.
14. Lefkovits, I., and Kamber, O. (1972) Eur. J. Immunol.
    2, 365.
15. Lefkovits, I., and Waldmann, H. (1977) Immunol. 32,
    915.
16. Watson, J. D. (1979) Trends in Biochem. Sci. 4, 36.
17. Watson, J. (1979) (Submitted for publication.)
18. Thoman, M., and Watson, J. (1979) (Submitted for
    publication.
19. Marchalonis, J. J. (1975) Science 190, 20.

MECHANISM OF SURFACE MEMBRANE EXPRESSION IN MURINE B-LYMPHOCYTE CELL LINES[1]

Peter Ralph, Christopher J. Paige, and Ilona Nakoinz

Sloan-Kettering Institute for Cancer Research
Rye, New York 10580

ABSTRACT Two murine B lymphomas adapted to culture do not express mature B-lymphocyte properties, but have cytoplasmic immunoglobulin (Ig) and can be induced for surface Ig by incubation with LPS and dextran sulfate (DxS). Line 70Z/3 and clone 12 are also enhanced in binding of mouse antibody-coated RBC (EA-Mo) by LPS but not DxS. Binding of rabbit antibody-coated RBC remains low under all conditions tested. Another clone, 70Z/3.1, retains sensitivity to DxS, but cannot be induced for sIg by LPS. Induction of surface μ chains by LPS is not blocked by toxic concentrations of actinomycin D, cordycepin, puromycin, or cycloheximide, indicating new RNA and protein synthesis may not be necessary for sIg expression in these cells. However, expression of κ chains is inhibited under these conditions. BUdR or actinomycin D alone induces EA-Mo binding but not sIg. These results show that two different mitogens can act on the same B cell and that mitogen receptors are present prior to surface Ig expression. These cell lines may be useful models for studying the pre-B to early B-lymphocyte transition process.

INTRODUCTION

We previously described a B-lymphoma cell line 70Z/3 staining for cytoplasmic but not surface Ig by immunofluorescence, suggesting that it was derived from a population of pre-B lymphocytes (1). However, surface Ig (sIg) could be induced in the culture line by incubation with LPS or DxS. "Induction" is used in this paper to refer to the expression of a given characteristic after exposure to a mitogen or other agent, without implying any specific mechanism. The present paper examines the mechanism of induction of surface membrane

[1]This work was supported by National Institutes of Health grant CA 24300 and AI 12741.

143

expression and places this cell line and a similar line, 70Z/2, on the threshold of maturation to immature sIg+ B lymphocytes.

METHODS AND MATERIALS

Tumor lines 70Z/2 and 70Z/3 induced by methyl nitroso-urea in thymectomized BDF_1 mice were obtained from P. Baines (2). Although the two lines are remarkably similar in many respects, 70Z/2 grows in mice s.c. as solid tumors and i.p. as ascites, whereas 70Z/3 tends to grow mainly in the spleen regardless of injection site (G. Tarnowski, personal communi-cation). The lines were adapted to growth in culture in RPMI 1640 medium plus 10% fetal calf serum with obligatory require-ment for 5×10^{-5} M 2-mercaptoethanol (1,3). Surface and cytoplasmic Ig were assayed by immunofluorescence (1). sIg was also assayed by *Staphylococcus* protein A-conjugated (4) RBC (SpA-E) binding: B cells were incubated with polyvalent rabbit anti-Ig (RaIg) serum at dilutions of 1:100 or 1:1000 for 20 minutes at room temperature, washed, and incubated with 20 times as many SpA-E five minutes 37° and centrifuged five minutes at 100 g. Cells with three or more attached RBC were scored as sIg positive. Fc receptors were assayed by binding of RBC coated with subagglutinating amounts of rabbit IgG anti-sheep RBC (Cordis Laboratories, Dade, Fla.) (EA-R) or with hyperimmune BALB/c anti-sheep RBC (EA-Mo) as for SpA-E rosetting. Control for EA-R or EA-Mo was >90% rosette forma-tion by macrophage cell line RAW264 which expresses avid Fc receptors (5). LPS (*Salmonella typhosa* WO901) was obtained from Difco, Detroit, Mich.; dextran sulfate (500,000) and other drugs from Sigma, St. Louis, Mo., except for some lectin preparations (see Results).

RESULTS

Induction of sIg in 70Z/2 and 70Z/3 Cell Lines. It was previously found by immunofluorescence techniques that $sIgM\kappa$ expression on the murine cell lines 70Z/3 (1) and 70Z/2 (3) can be induced by incubation with LPS. We now confirm and extend this observation in the parent lines and in clone 12 of 70Z/3 by means of rosetting techniques using *Staphyloccus* protein A-coupled RBC. The two cell lines normally express very little sIg (range 0-30% by immunofluorescence, 0-42% positive cells by SpA-E rosetting), but are induced by 1 or 10 µg/ml LPS and 50 µg/ml DxS concomitant with a partial in-hibition of cell growth (Table 1). In contrast to 70Z/2 and parent 70Z/3, clone 70Z/3.12 is relatively resistant to LPS toxicity and these cells can be grown continuously in 10 µg/ml LPS with constant expression of sIg. This confirms that LPS

TABLE 1

INDUCTION OF sIg IN 7OZ/2 AND IN CLONES OF 7OZ/3

| | % sIg$^+$ | | % sIg$^+$ | |
	SpA-E	IF	SpA-E	IF
	7OZ/2		7OZ/3	
Control	14	19	8	2
LPS 1 µg/ml	95	100	64	92
LPS 10 µg/ml	60	100	66	99
DxS 50 µg/ml	26	61	76	70
	7OZ/3.1		7OZ/3.12	
Control	7	2	40	31
LPS 1 µg/ml	3	0	62	91
LPS 10 µg/ml	8	0	75	99
DxS 50 µg/ml	ND	76	68	63

Cell cultures were initiated at 10^5/ml plus 0, 1 or 10 µg/ml LPS or 50 µg/ml DxS, and assayed at day 2 for sIg by SpA-E rosette formation using RaIg at 1:100 dilution or immunofluorescence (IF) using Fab$_2$ goat anti-µ (1).

toxicity is not necessary for sIg induction (1). Another clone, 7OZ/3.1, is no longer sensitive to induction of sIg by LPS but remains sensitive to DxS stimulation.

Induction of sIg by a *Lotus* Lectin Preparation is Due to an LPS-Like Contaminant. Since fucose binding proteins have been reported to be B-lymphocyte mitogens (6), we tested several commercial samples of *Lotus* and *Ulex* lectins available from Sigma, Calbiochem, and Miles/Yeda. One *Lotus* preparation consistently induced sIg in 7OZ/3. However, the sIg-inducing properties of this preparation could be dissociated from its fucose-dependent agglutination of human type O-RBC. The sIg-inducing component, like LPS, was resistant to boiling, co-incubation with L-fucose, or absorption on type O-RBC, whereas hemagglutination was abolished by these treatments (Table 2). Coincubation with polymyxin B, on the other hand, inhibited induction of sIg by both the LPS and lectin preparations with no effect on hemagglutination. Thus, the hemagglutinating

TABLE 2

sIg INDUCTION BY *LOTUS* SAMPLE DUE TO LPS-LIKE CONTAMINATION[a]

		sIg (% SpA-E rosettes)			
		100	1000	100	1000
		Untreated		10' 100o[b]	
Resistant to boiling	Control	24	21		
	LPS	77	53	78	49
	Lotus	66	29	71	29
	HA titer[e]	2		>500	
		Untreated		0.1 M fucose[c]	
Resistant to L-fucose	Control	30	12	21	6
	LPS	53	43	51	48
	Lotus	45	42	46	40
	HA titer	4		>500	
		Untreated		Absorbed[d]	
Resistant to O-RBC absorption	Control	20	8	14	10
	LPS	52	38	49	35
	Lotus	57	20	40	21
	HA titer	2		125	
		Untreated		10 µg/ml PMB[c]	
Sensitive to polymyxin B	Control	42	7	38	3
	LPS	84	52	51	12
	Lotus	76	42	36	29
	HA titer	2		2	

[a]70Z/3.12, 1 day incubation, 10 µg/ml LPS, 50 µg/ml *Lotus* (Miles/Yeda), rosetting with RaIg at 1:100 and 1:1000.

[b]LPS 1 mg/ml and *Lotus* 5 mg/ml stock solutions boiled 10 min before use.

[c]L-fucose (1/10 volume of 1 M) or polymyxin B added to cultures or hemagglutination assays.

[d]For absorption, 0.1 ml packed human type O-RBC were incubated 20'23° with 0.2 ml phosphate-buffered saline containing 0, 1 mg/ml LPS, or 5 mg/ml *Lotus* lectin.

[e]Hemagglutination titer (µg/ml) of *Lotus* sample on O-RBC.

properties are that of a fucose-binding lectin, and are completely dissociated from the sIg-inducing moiety with properties similar to LPS.

    Specific Inhibition of LPS Induction of sIg by Poly-
myxin B. DxS was shown to induce sIg in 70Z/3 independently
of LPS-like molecules by virtue of its resistance to alkali
treatment (1). Further demonstration of the distinct nature
of DxS in inducing sIg is given by its resistance to polymyxin B inhibition under conditions in which LPS is completely
inhibited (Table 3). Polymyxin B binds to the lipid A portion
of LPS and blocks its mitogenic activity for B lymphocytes
(7,8), but does not affect DxS.

TABLE 3

SPECIFIC INHIBITION OF LPS INDUCTION OF sIg BY POLYMYXIN B

Inducer μg/ml	PMB μg/ml	% sIg 100	% sIg 1000	% Rosettes EA-Mo
-	-	22	3	13
	2	29	0	10
	5	24	2	12
LPS 1	-	62	20	26
LPS 1	2	14	6	15
LPS 10	-	77	40	50
LPS 10	2	58	40	ND
LPS 10	5	30	13	ND
LPS 10	10	17	5	24
DxS 50	-	37	24	8
DxS 50	10	44	25	ND

    70Z/3.12 at 10^5/ml, assayed after 2 days incubation for
% sIg (SpA-E rosettes with RaIg at 1:100 or 1:1000) and EA-Mo
rosettes; ND = not done

LPS Enhancement of 70Z/3.12 Expression of Receptors for Mouse Ig Assayed by EA-Mo Rosettes. 70Z/3 cells express very few surface receptors for immunoglobulin Fc region or for complement, assayed by EA and EAC rosette formation, and receptor activity was not enhanced significantly by LPS incubation (1). These assays were performed with erythrocytes coated with rabbit IgG or IgM antibody, respectively. When erythrocytes were sensitized instead with mouse antibody (EA-Mo), 70Z/3 cells formed easily detectable rosettes, and the fraction of rosetting cells was enhanced by LPS incubation in parallel with induction of sIg (Tables 3 and 4). Although DxS could induce sIg expression, it did not enhance EA-Mo binding.

It has been reported that greater than 50% of splenic IgM secreting cells induced by LPS *in vivo* are producing IgM antibody to mouse IgG, measured by plaque formation on EA-Mo IgG (9). Since there is a rough correlation between the number of 70Z/3 cells positive for sIgM and EA-Mo rosette formation, we considered the possibility that the cells bound EA-Mo through an antibody function of their sIgM rather than via a classical Fc receptor. Evidence against the hypothesis of 70Z/3.12 membrane IgM with antibody activity towards mouse Ig is given by the failure of DxS to stimulate EA-Mo binding despite induction of sIg expression (Table 4), sensitivity of sIg but not EA-Mo rosette formation to trypsin, and BUdR induction of EA-Mo binding but not sIg (Table 5).

Effects of Metabolic Inhibitors on 70Z/3.12 Surface Membrane Expression. Inhibition of growth with DMSO, butyrate

TABLE 4

LPS ENHANCES 70Z/3.12 EXPRESSION OF RECEPTORS FOR MOUSE Ig

	Inducer µg/ml	sIg (% SpA$^+$) 100	1000	% Rosettes EA-Mo	EA-R	E
Exp. 1	-	4	4	30	16	2
	LPS 10	74	58	78	17	1
	DS 50	49	36	31	20	4
Exp. 2	-	22	8	37	4	ND
	LPS 10	52	38	58	6	ND
	DS 50	27	20	31	4	ND

70Z/3.12 at 10^5/ml, 2 day incubation

TABLE 5
BUdR AND ACTINOMYCIN D INDUCE 70Z/3.12 EA-Mo BINDING

Drug	Cells/ml x 10^{-5}	% sIg	% Rosettes EA-Mo	EA-R
-	5.5	10	22	2
LPS	6.1	59	62	8
LPS + BUdR	5.4	63	80	ND
LPS + AM	2.2 sick	39	86	ND
BUdR	5.4	12	82	5
AM	2.3 sick	14	59	ND
-	16.2	36		
LPS	14.6	67		
LPS + Td	6.9	64		
Td	6.7	26		

Cultures initiated at 2×10^5/ml and assayed at day 1 for sIg by SpA-E rosettes using RaIg at 1:100. LPS 10 μg/ml, BUdR 10^{-5} M, actinomycin D (AM) 0.5 ng/ml, thymidine (Td) 10^{-4} M.

or N,N-dimethylformamide (1), fucose (Table 2), thymidine or actinomycin D did not induce sIg, and the latter three agents did not interfere with LPS induction of sIg (Table 5). Unexpectedly, toxic concentrations of actinomycin D alone greatly increased EA-Mo rosetting. Binding of EA-Mo by a majority of 70Z/3.12 cells was also induced by exposure to 10^{-5} M BUdR after one day (toxic at two days) (Table 5) or to 10^{-6} M BUdR after two days.

DISCUSSION

The properties which we have described for 70Z/2 and 70Z/3 cells, both in Results and previously (1), suggest that these lines are representative of pre-B cells at the threshold of maturation to sIg + B lymphocytes. As measured by immunofluorescence, they contain cytoplasmic μ chains and can be induced to express sIg by the B-cell mitogens LPS and DxS. The small fraction of cells which already possess sIg, FcR, or CR may be indicative of a small degree of maturation ongoing in our cultures. While the majority of clones analyzed (9 for 70Z/2 and 20 for 70Z/3) are similar to the parent lines

and thus confirm that background levels of sIg expression are
not due to separate coexisting lineages, two clones are distinct. 70Z/3.1 is insensitive to LPS induction although it
remains responsive to DxS. This confirms the independence of
induction by these two mitogens as suggested by the selective
inhibition of LPS by polymyxin B (Table 3) and alkali treatment (1). Clone 70Z/3.12 is induced by LPS but is no longer
sensitive to the toxic effects which this mitogen has on the
parent line and other clones. Thus DxS-induced parent cells
and LPS and DxS-induced 70Z/3.12 cells can be maintained as
sIg$^+$ lines when continuously cultured in the presence of inducer. Surface Ig expression is reversible, however, as the
cells revert to an sIg$^-$ state upon removal of the mitogen.

In addition to an increase in sIg expression, exposure
to LPS also leads to an increase in Fc receptors as measured
by rosetting with SRBC coated with mouse anti-SRBC. Binding
of EA-Mo to 70Z/3 can be blocked by human IgG but formal proof
that this binding is via Fc receptors will require inhibition
by Fc fragments or use of Fab anti-RBC reagents. Consistent
with previous results (1), SRBC coated with rabbit antibodies,
in contrast to mouse antibodies, formed only very few rosettes
with 70Z/3 cells, either induced or uninduced. While macrophage lines form strong rosettes with either agent, these
results may indicate that pre-B cells have a very low affinity
for rabbit antibody. It will be important to determine if
this selectivity is typical of normal immature B lymphocytes.

In addition to LPS, ubiquitin, cyclic AMP and other agents
have been shown to effectively induce B-cell maturation using
selected populations of bone marrow cells (10,11). We have
been unable to induce sIg in 70Z/3 cells with ubiquitin or 8-
bromocyclic AMP ± theophylline. Similarly, DMSO, N,N-dimethyl
formamide, and butyric acid failed to induce sIg expression
even at cytostatic concentrations. On the other hand, LPS
induction of sIg is not blocked by actinomycin D (0.5 ng/ml),
cordycepin (10^{-6} M), puromycin (0.5 µg/ml) or cycloheximide
(1 µg/ml) at toxic concentrations that inhibit growth at 24
hours and kill most cells by 48 hours. This suggests that
some expression of sIg is independent of new RNA and protein
synthesis. When immunoglobulin chains were analyzed by immunofluorescence, puromycin and cycloheximide were found to
inhibit LPS-induced κ but not µ surface expression (C.J.P.
et al., manuscript in preparation). This suggests that preformed µ chains can be translocated and displayed but light
chains must be newly synthesized during LPS induction. Unfortunately, the inhibitors were not used at sufficiently
high concentrations to block macromolecular synthesis completely as such drug doses would kill the cells in the 16-24
hours required for LPS induction. Therefore, these experiments do not completely distinguish between exteriorization

TABLE 6

PROPERTIES OF MURINE B LYMPHOMA CELL LINES[a]

Name	Strain	Etiology	cIg	sIg	Fc	Ia	C'	DM	Toxicity Td	LPS
70Z/2	BDF$_1$	MNU	μ	μκ[b]	+[b]	-	-	$<10^{-7}$	$<10^{-4}$	1
70Z/3	BDF$_1$	MNU	μ	μκ[b]	+[b]	-	(-)	$<10^{-7}$	$<10^{-4}$	10
WEHI 231	CxNZB	OIL		μκδ	(+)	+		$<10^{-7}$	$<10^{-4}$	>100
WEHI 279	NZC	Spont		μκδ	+	+		$<10^{-7}$	$<10^{-4}$	>100
38C-13	C3H/eB	DMBA		μκ	+	+	-	$<10^{-7}$	$<10^{-4}$	>100
BCL[c]	BALB/c	Spont		μλδ	+	+	-	$<10^{-7}$	$<10^{-4}$	>100
Myelomas								$>10^{-5}$	10^3	>100

[a]Mouse strains: BDF$_1$ = C57BL/6xDBA/2, C = BALB/c; Fc = receptor for Ig; Ia = Ia surface antigen assayed by SpA-rosettes using ATH anti-ATL antiserum; C' = complement receptor; toxicity: molar concentration of dexamethasone (DM), thymidine (Td) or LPS (μg/ml) inhibiting growth 50% over two days.

[b]μκ and Fc receptor induced or stimulated by LPS.

[c]In culture two months.

of constitutive cytoplasmic molecules and induction requiring
new protein synthesis. Scheid *et al.* have evidence that new
protein synthesis is not required for sIg expression induced
by LPS in a minor population of bone marrow cells (12).

Stimulation of cell surface Fc receptors by the nonspecific metabolic deregulators, actinomycin D and BUdR,also
suggests that these moieties may exist preformed in 70Z/3 and
that the cells may be simply caused to exteriorize them.
Stimulation of EA-Mo rosetting in myeloma cells by colcemid
was described by Harris (13).

Other murine B-cell lines studied show more mature B-
lymphocyte properties than the 70Z lines (Table 6). In addition to μ and light chains, lines WEHI 231, WEHI 279 (13),
and BCL (14) show surface δ by SpA-E rosetting using hybridoma
antibody (15), and Ia antigen by ATH anti-ATL sera and SpA-E
rosetting. The latter result will have to be checked by absorption to rule out contaminating specificities. Line 38C-13
is reported to have surface μκ (16); it forms direct rosettes
with SpA-E so its sIg presumably belongs to that subgroup of
IgM molecules that bind SpA protein (17). None of these B-
cell lines or others recently reported (18-22) are known to
have receptors for complement, believed to be a marker for
certain mature B-lymphocyte populations (10,11).

Sensitivity to low concentrations of corticosteroids is
a property of thymocytes and related T tumors; antibody-producing cells and plasmacytomas are generally resistant (13,
23,24). Corticosteroids block induction of B lymphocytes to
antibody-producing cells, and there is evidence that accessory
cells rather than the B cells are the site of inhibition (25,
26). All of the B tumor lines tested were very sensitive to
killing by the corticosteroid dexamethasone which suggests
their relative immaturity within the B-lymphocyte lineage.
They are also killed by low concentrations of thymidine, which
among other hematopoietic tumor cell lines affects only T
lymphomas (13,23,27).

The 70Z tumor lines sensitive to induction of sIg and Fc
receptors by B-cell polyclonal activators, and cloned sublines
with altered sensitivity to LPS (Table 1), are attractive
models for studying the biochemistry and regulation of the
transition from pre-B to B lymphocyte.

REFERENCES

1. Paige, C. J., Kincade, P. W., and Ralph, P. (1978). J. Immunol. 121, 641.
2. Baines, P., Dexter, T. M., and Schofield, R. (1979). Leukemia Res. 3, 23.
3. Paige, C. J. (1979). Doctoral Thesis, Cornell University Graduate School of Medical Sciences, New York City.
4. Gronowicz, E., Coutinho, A., and Melchers, F. (1976). Eur. J. Immunol. 6, 588.
5. Raschke, W. C., Baird, S., Nakoinz, I., and Ralph, P. (1978). Cell 15, 261.
6. Schumann, G., Schnebli, H. P., and Dukor, P. (1973). Int. Arch. Allergy Appl. Immunol. 45, 331.
7. Jacobs, D. M., and Morrison, D. C. (1977). J. Immunol. 118, 21.
8. Smith, E., Hammarström, L., and Coutinho, A. (1976). J. Exp. Med. 143, 1521.
9. Dresser, D. W. (1978). Nature 274, 480.
10. Hämmerling, U., and Chin, A. F. (1977). Eur. J. Immunol. 7, 533.
11. Hämmerling, U., Chua, R., and Hoffmann, M. K. (1978). J. Immunol. 120, 750.
12. Scheid, M. P., Goldstein, G., and Boyse, E. A. (1978). J. Exp. Med. 147, 1727.
13. Harris, A. W. (1978). In "Protides of the Biological Fluids" (H. Peters, ed.), 25, 601.
14. Slavin, S., and Strober, S. (1978). Nature 272, 624.
15. Oi, V. T., Jones, P. P., Goding, J. W., and Herzenberg, L. A. (1978). In "Lymphocyte Hybridomas" (F. Melchers, N. L. Warner, and M. Potter, eds.), pp. 102-107. Springer-Verlag, Basel.
16. Bergman, Y., Haimovich, J., and Melchers, F. (1977). Eur. J. Immunol. 7, 574.
17. Howell-Saxton, E., and Wettstein, F. O. (1978). J. Immunol. 121, 1334.
18. Premkumar, E., Potter, M., Singer, P. A., and Sklar, M. D. (1975). Cell 6, 149.
19. Pratt, D. M., Strominger, J., Parkman, R., Kaplan, D., Schwaber, J., Rosenberg, N., and Scher, C. S. (1977). Cell 12, 683.
20. Lanier, L. L., Lynes, M., Haughton, G., and Wettstein, P. J. (1978). Nature 271, 554.
21. Kim, K. J., Kanellopoulos-Langevin, Merwin, R. M., Sachs, D. H., and Asofsky, R. (1979). J. Immunol. 122, 549.
22. Siden, E. J., Baltimore, D., Clark, D., and Rosenberg, N. E. (1979). Cell 16, 389.

23. Horibata, K., and Harris, A. W. (1970). Exp. Cell Res. 60, 61.
24. Ralph, P. (1973). J. Immunol. 110, 1470.
25. Lee, K.-C., Langman, R. E., Paetkau, V. H., and Diener, E. (1975). Cell. Immunol. 17, 405.
26. Mishell, R. I., Bradley, L. M., Chen, Y.-H. U., Grabstein, K. N., Mishell, B. B., Shigi, J. M., and Shigi, S. M. (1978). J. Reticuloendothel. Soc. 24, 439.
27. Ralph, P. (1976). In "Concanavalin A as a Tool" (H. Bittiger and H. P. Schnebli, eds.), pp. 613-621. John Wiley and Sons, London.

ANTIBODY AFFINITY IN CBA/N MICE

Kathryn E. Stein[1], James J. Mond, Carole Brennan
Olli Mäkelä and William E. Paul

Laboratory of Immunology
National Institute of Allergy and Infectious Diseases
National Institutes of Health, Bethesda, Maryland 20014
and
University of Helsinki, Helsink 29, Finland

ABSTRACT. The CBA/N mouse carries an X-linked trait which results in a profound inability to respond to thymus independent antigens of the TI-2 class. It has been suggested that its B cell defect might also lead to an inability to produce high affinity antibody in response to immunization with thymus-dependent antigens. We have studied the anti-hapten response to hapten-protein conjugates at various times after immunization. Defective (CBA/N x DBA/2N)F_1 male and control (DBA/2N x CBA/N)F_1 male mice were immunized with DNP_{10}-KLH and bled at 2, 4 and 6 weeks after immunization. They were boosted at 6 weeks or 6 months after primary immunization. The affinity of anti-DNP antibodies was measured in an ammonium sulfate precipitation assay using ^{3}H-DNP-lysine. We found no significant difference in the affinity of anti-DNP antibodies in defective and control mice at any of the times tested. For example, at 6 weeks following primary immunization the mean affinity of anti-DNP antibodies was 6.4×10^6 M^{-1} in defective mice and 4.6×10^6 M^{-1} in control mice while for animals boosted 6 months after priming and bled 1 week after boosting it was 59×10^6 M^{-1} in defective mice and 32×10^6 M^{-1} in control mice. Similarly, defective F_1 male and control F_1 female mice immunized with NBrP-CGG or ABA-HOP-CGG developed anti-hapten antibodies of similar relative affinity as measured by a haptenated-phage inactivation assay. We conclude that CBA/N mice are capable of producing high affinity antibodies to haptens on protein carriers and that within the period studied, the appearance of high affinity antibody occurs with the same time course in defective and control animals.

[1]Supported by USPHS National Research Service Award #7F32CA05328-03

ISBN 0-12-069850-1

INTRODUCTION

The CBA/N mouse strain carries an X-linked gene (xid)
(1) that results in a profound inability to mount an immune
response to thymus-independent antigens, such as dextran,
levan and haptenated ficoll, which have been classified as
TI-2 antigens (2). This deficiency is associated with an
absence of B lymphocytes that express the cell surface antigens Lyb5 (3) and Lyb3 (4). These lymphocytes are thought
to represent a mature or late-developing subset of B cells
which are lacking in neonatal mice (2,5). Based on the
finding that CBA/N mice lack a mature subset of B lymphocytes, investigators have been led to question whether or
not, in addition to the failure to respond to TI-2 antigens,
abnormalities of the response to thymus-dependent (TD)
antigens might also be found in CBA/N mice. Indeed, Scher
et al. (6) have recently found that the early IgG anti-
sheep erythrocyte (SRBC) response is profoundly depressed
in CBA/N mice. Furthermore, Gershon and Kondo (7) have
reported that CBA/N mice that were hyperimmunized with SRBC
failed to produce a cross-reacting antibody to horse
erythrocytes (HRBC) which was found in high titer in the
hyperimmune sera of control mice and which was of high
avidity (8). It was proposed that the absence of this
cross-reacting antibody might be due to a general inability
of CBA/N mice to produce high affinity antibodies to TD
antigens. We have studied this question by immunizing mice
with haptens coupled to protein carriers and directly
measuring the affinities of the anti-hapten antibodies
produced. Our results show that the CBA/N defect does not
result in an inability to produce high affinity antibodies
to haptens on protein carriers.

METHODS

Mice. All mice were obtained from the Small Animal
Section, National Institutes of Health, and were immunized
at 8-12 weeks of age.
Immunizations. Anti-dinitrophenyl (DNP) antibodies
were raised by immunization with 100 μg DNP_{10}-Keyhole limpet
hemocyanin (KLH) in complete Freund's adjuvant (CFA) in
the hind footpads (0.05 ml/footpad) and subcutaneously behind the neck (0.1 ml). The mice were boosted at 6 weeks
or 6 months after priming with 50 μg DNP_{10}-KLH in in-
complete Freund's adjuvant (IFA) given intraperitoneally.
Anti-(4-hydroxy-5-bromo-3-nitrophenyl) acetyl (NBrP) antibodies were raised by immunization with NBrP-chicken
gamma globulin (CGG) as previously described (9); anti-

azobenzenearsonate-5-hydroxyphenylacetyl (ABA-HOP) antibodies were produced by immunization with ABA-HOP$_8$-CGG as previously described (10). Animals received a secondary challenge eight weeks after primary immunization and were bled eight weeks later.

    Antibody Determinations. Antibody to DNP was measured by the ammonium sulfate precipitation method using ^{3}H-DNP-lysine (10^{-8}M) as the hapten, as described (11). Results are reported as ABC-33, which is 1/dilution of serum required to bind 33% of added ligand multiplied by the bound concentration of ligand (0.33 x 10^{-8}M). Equilibrium constants were also determined by an ammonium sulfate precipitation method (12). Titer and avidity of antibodies to NBrP and ABA-HOP were measured by inhibition of haptenated phage inactivation (HPI) using NBr-P-caproate and ABA-HOP as haptens, as described (9,10).

FIGURE 1

EQUILIBRIUM BINDING OF ^{3}H-DNP-LYSINE BY ANTI-DNP ANTIBODY FROM (CBA/N X DBA/2)F$_1$ MALE [♂,DEFECTIVE] AND (DBA/2 X CBA/N)F$_1$ MALE [1/♂, NORMAL] MICE

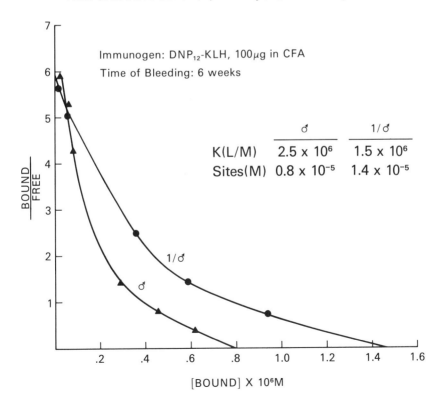

Immunogen: DNP$_{12}$-KLH, 100µg in CFA
Time of Bleeding: 6 weeks

	♂	1/♂
K(L/M)	2.5 x 10^6	1.5 x 10^6
Sites(M)	0.8 x 10^{-5}	1.4 x 10^{-5}

[BOUND] X 10^{6}M

RESULTS

Scatchard plots of the equilibrium binding of ^{3}H–DNP–lysine to anti–DNP antibodies from individual defective (CBA/N x DBA/2)F_1 and normal (DBA/2xCBA/N)F_1 male mice are illustrated in Figure 1. Association constants were calculated from the relation

$$B/F = K_o (Ab_o - B)$$

where B = bound ligand concentration; F = free ligand concentration; K_o = average intrinsic association constant; Ab_o = total concentration of antigen-binding sites. K_o is determined when half of the combining sites are occupied, i.e. when B = 1/2 Ab_o.

As is obvious, there is very little difference between the affinity of the anti–DNP antibody produced by the normal and defective individuals; however, when the number of sites is measured by extrapolation to infinite ligand concentration (as B/F approaches 0), the normal individual does have a somewhat higher serum antibody concentration.

Table 1 presents summary data from a large number of individual normal and defective mice. Over a period from two weeks to six months after primary immunization with 100 µg DNP-KLH (the latter after a secondary challenge), no substantial difference in mean K_o is noted between anti–DNP antibody from normal and defective mice. Both groups show the time-dependent increase in affinity which is characteristic of the normal "maturation" of the immune response (13). This is also illustrated by following the equilibrium constants of individual (CBA/N x DBA/2)F_1 male and (DBA/2 x CBA/N)F_1 male mice throughout primary and secondary responses to DNP-KLH (Table 2).

As noted in the Scatchard plot presented in Fig. 1, the mean serum titer of anti–DNP antibodies is somewhat lower in defective mice than in normals (Tables 1 & 2).

The relative affinity of anti–NBrP and of anti–ABA–HOP antibodies produced by immunization of (CBA/N x BALB/c)F_1 males (defective) and females (normal) with CGG conjugates of these haptens was also determined. This was done by measuring the concentration of hapten required to cause 50% inhibition of haptenated phage inactivation by antibody. In such an assay, the relative affinity is inversely related to the concentration of hapten required for 50% inhibition. No difference in the relative affinity of anti–NBrP antibody produced by the two groups was noted nor was there any significant difference in the relative amount of antibody (50% inactivation titer) (Table 3). The analysis

TABLE 1

AMOUNT AND AFFINITY OF ANTI-DNP ANTIBODY

	ABC-33 $(10^{-8}M)$		K x 10^{-6}(L/M)	
	$\male$[a]	$1/\male$[b]	$\male$	$1/\male$
1° Response				
2 weeks	2.9 ± 0.6[c]	6.1 ± 1.6	2.6 ± 0.3	3.2 ± 0.9
4 weeks	— [d]	—	3.9 ± 1.3	4.9 ± 1.0
6 weeks	23.3 ± 4.0	40.8 ± 8.5	6.4 ± 1.5	4.6 ± 2.9
2° Response (boosted at 6 weeks)				
8 days	30.8 ± 0.8	54.5 ± 13.5	11.3 ± 6.2	9.2 ± 0.7
2 weeks	41.6 ± 1.3	65.5 ± 26.5	—	—
4 weeks	—	—	25.1 ± 10.1	18.4 ± 6.4
2° Response (boosted at 6 months)				
8 days	—	—	58.5 ± 12.4[e]	32.1 ± 10.1[f]

a (CBA/N x DBA/2)F$_1$ $\male$; defective; 2 to 7 mice per time point
b (DBA/2 x CBA/N)F$_1$ $\male$; normal
c arithmetic mean $\pm$ SE
d — $\equiv$ not done
e (CBA/N x BALB/c)F$_1$ $\male$; defective
f (CBA/N x BALB/c)F$_1$ $\female$; normal

of the anti-ABA-HOP response indicated that the defective mice made antibody of a somewhat higher affinity than did the normals, although the difference did not reach statistical significance. No difference in the 50% inactivation titers were noted (Table 4).

The results presented thus far reveal no difference in affinity of antibody produced by defective and normal mice immunized with hapten conjugates of KLH and CGG. Since hapten conjugates of these proteins may be regarded as strong immunogens, we have initiated a set of experiments aimed at determining the affinity of antibody produced under more limiting conditions of immunization. In still pre-liminary experiments, (CBA/N x DBA/2)F$_1$ and (DBA/2 x CBA/N) F$_1$ males were immunized with a low dose (1 μg) of DNP-KLH or with DNP on a relatively weak carrier (bovine serum

TABLE 2

AMOUNT AND AFFINITY OF ANTI-DNP ANTIBODY PRODUCED BY INDIVIDUAL MICE

| | ABC-33 (10⁻⁸M) | | | | K x 10⁻⁶(L/M) | | | |
| | σ[a] | | $1/\sigma$[b] | | σ | | $1/\sigma$ | |
Individual Mice	#1	#2	#2	#4	#1	#2	#6	#9
1° Response								
2 weeks	3	4	3	14	3.3	2.0	2.1	2.4
4 weeks	— [c]	—	—	—	3.7	1.8	2.4	4.3
6 weeks	28	20	33	46	—	—	7.6	—
2° Response (boosted at 6 weeks)								
8 days	32	30	43	66	—	17.5	11.0	8.9
2 weeks	40	43	39	92	—	—	—	—
4 weeks	—	—	—	—	—	24.0	—	12.4

a (CBA/N x DBA/2)F$_1$ σ; defective
b (DBA/2 x CBA/N)F$_1$ σ; normal
c — ≡ not done

TABLE 3

AMOUNT AND AFFINITY OF ANTI-NBrP ANTIBODY

	σ[a]	$\female$
Antibody Concentration		
50% Inactivation Titer [(1/dilution) x 10⁻³]	532 $\overset{x}{\div}$ 1.3[b]	712 $\overset{x}{\div}$ 1.2
Antibody Affinity		
[NBrP-cap] for 50% Inhibition of haptenated phage inactivation [nmoles/ml]	6.8 $\overset{x}{\div}$ 1.1	7.7 $\overset{x}{\div}$ 1.2

a (CBA/N x BALB/c)F$_1$ σ (defective) and $\female$ (normal) mice, 5 mice per group
b geometric mean $\overset{x}{\div}$ S.E.

TABLE 4

AMOUNT AND AFFINITY OF ANTI-ABA HOP ANTIBODY

	♂[a]	♀
Antibody Concentration		
50% Inactivation Titer [(1/dilution) x 10^{-3}]	75.6 $\overset{\times}{\div}$ 1.7[b]	69.4 $\overset{\times}{\div}$ 1.3
Antibody Affinity		
[ABA-HOP] for 50% Inhibition of haptenated phage inactivation [nmoles/ml]	26.6 $\overset{\times}{\div}$ 1.3	77.5 $\overset{\times}{\div}$ 2.5

a (CBA/N x BALB/c) F, ♂ (defective) and ♀ (normal) mice,
   5 mice per group
b geometric mean $\overset{\times}{\div}$ S.E.

albumin-BSA). Our initial results do not reveal any substantial difference between normal and defective individuals
but additional results will be necessary to substantiate
these findings.

DISCUSSION

It is well known that in the course of immune responses
to a variety of antigens, the affinity of the antibody produced increases with the duration of time after immunization (13). The cellular dynamics of this process are still
poorly understood but recent work has suggested that the
memory cells which are the precursors of high affinity antibody-producing cells have a distinctive complement of immunoglobulins on their surface when compared to precursors of
low affinity antibody-secreting cells. The difference in
the two populations is that the "low affinity precursors"
possess membrane IgD while the "high affinity precursors"
appear to lack IgD (14). The possibility that high affinity
antibody production is a function of a specialized sub-

population of B lymphocytes has also been raised by the
findings of Gershon and Kondo (7) that mice with the CBA/N
defect fail to produce the high avidity anti-SRBC antibody, cross-reactive with HRBC, which is a feature of the
normal response. Because of these studies, we thought it
important to determine whether mice with the CBA/N defect
fail to produce high affinity antibody when immunized with
a series of defined antigenic determinants borne on protein
carriers. Our results indicate that mice with the CBA/N
immune defect make anti-DNP, anti-NBrP, and anti-ABA-HOP
antibodies which are indistinguishable in affinity from
those produced by appropriate normal controls at various
times in the course of primary and secondary immune responses.
Studies indicate that this is true even under limiting conditions of immunization. Our results do not rule out the
possibility that affinity maturation is a function of a
specialized B lymphocyte population; however, if this
function is uniquely expressed in a B cell subpopulation, it
must be one possessed by mice with the CBA/N defect.

REFERENCES

1.   Berning, A., Eicher, E., Paul, W.E., and Scher, I.
     (1978). Fed. Proc. 37, 699.
2.   Mosier, D.E., Zitron, I.M., Mond, J.J., Ahmed, A.,
     scher, I. and Paul, W.E. (1977). Immunol. Rev., 37,
     89.
3.   Ahmed, A., Scher, I., Sharrow, S.O., Smith, A.H.,
     Paul, W.E., Sachs, D.H., and Sell, K.W. (1977). J.
     Exp. Med. 145, 101.
4.   Huber, B., Gershon, R.K., and Cantor, H. (1977). J.
     Exp. Med., 145, 1.
5.   Paul, W.E., Subbarao, B., Mond, J.J., Sieckmann, D.G.,
     Zitron, I.M., Ahmed, A., Mosier, D.E. and Scher, I.
     In "Cells of Immunoglobulin Synthesis" (B. Pernis and
     H.J. Vogel, eds.). (In press).
6.   Scher, I., Berning, A.K. and Asofsky, R. (1979). J.
     Immunol. (In press).
7.   Gershon, R.K. and Kondo, K. (1976). J. Immunol.
     117, 701.
8.   Gershon, R.K. and Kondo, K. (1972). Immunology, 23,
     321.
9.   Imanishi, T. and Mäkelä, O. (1975). J. Exp. Med. 141,
     840.
10. Mäkelä, O., Julin, M. and Becker, M. (1976). J. Exp.
     Med. 143, 316.
11. Paul, W.E., and Elfenbein, G.J. (1975). J. Immunol.
     114, 261.

12. Stupp, Y., Yoshida, T., and Paul, W.E.   (1969).   J.
     Immunol., 103, 625.
13. Siskind, G.W. and Benacerraf, B. (1969). Adv.
     Immunol., 10, 1.
14. Black, s.J., Van Der Loo, W., Loken, M.R., and
     Herzenberg, L.A. (1978). J. Exp. Med. 147, 984.

POSSIBLE ANTIGEN SPECIFIC T CELL HELP IN POKEWEED
MITOGEN STIMULATED HUMAN PERIPHERAL BLOOD CELL CULTURES[1]

Eric M. Macy and Ronald H. Stevens

Department of Microbiology and Immunology
UCLA, Los Angeles, California 90024

ABSTRACT Limiting dilution analyses using human T and B
cells from the peripheral blood of individuals recently
(2 to 6 weeks) boosted with a combination of diptheria
and tetanus toxoids were performed in order to investigate the specificity of T cell help during in vitro pokeweed mitogen (PWM) stimulation. Limiting dilutions using
B cells were first performed in order to determine the
number of potential Ig producing B cells of a variety of
specificities activated by PWM induced T cell stimulation. The precursor frequency for total IgG production
was 1.3×10^{-3} with approximately 10% of the B cells directed against tetanus toxoid and 3% directed against diptheria toxoid two weeks after boosting. Limiting numbers
of irradiated T cells were then added to an excess of B
cells and their ability to help IgG anti-tetanus toxoid
(Tet-IgG) and IgG anti-diptheria toxoid (Dip-IgG) antibody production were compared. The helper activity for
the Tet-IgG did not dilute out in parallel with help for
Dip-IgG. Wells were observed at limiting dilutions of
added helper T cells which produced only Tet-IgG or Dip-
IgG but not both even though sufficient potential specific IgG producing B cells for each antigen were present.

INTRODUCTION

Pokeweed mitogen (PWM) has been widely used to study the
T cell dependent activation of human peripheral blood B cells
(1-2). This in vitro activation results in the differentiation of a proportion of the circulating B cells into cells
which secrete IgM, IgG or IgA (3).
     At least two general mechanisms may be postulated which
could account for the PWM induced T cell-B cell interactions
which result in immunoglobulin (Ig) production. The activa-

[1]This work was supported by National Cancer Institute
grant #CA-12800, National Foundation, March of Dimes grant
#6-147, NIH training grant #GM-7185-04 and American Cencer
Society grant #IN-131.

tion could be a non-specific interaction in which a single T
cell or several T cells in concert activate multiple B cell
clones. Alternatively T cells may be stimulated to provide
help through the recognition and interaction with antigen
specific B cell counterparts. This latter hypothesis would
predict that PWM induced generation of a specific antibody in
vitro would require the presence in the culture of antigen
specific helper T cells, as well as B cells.

Distinction between these two alternatives could provide
greater insight into the mechanism of action of PWM and would
allow a broader interpretation of the wealth of data obtained
in normal (4) and immune deficient individuals (5) whose
lymphocytes have been studied with this mitogen.

One approach to resolve these alternatives is a limiting
dilution analysis in which data pertaining to the frequency,
specificity and complexity of specific cells and interactions
in a functionally defined population can be obtained. When
the addition of a single specific cell to a culture containing
an excess of the other necessary cellular components for the
production of immunoglobulin changes a negative culture to a
positive one, then a Poisson analysis of the percent negative
cultures at each dilution of cells provides an estimate of
the relative frequency of the specific reactive cells.

If PWM stimulation of T cells leads to non-specific help
then the production of Tet-IgG or Dip-IgG should dilute out at
the same point as helper T cells are titrated when excess B
cells are present. If T cell help has specific component after
PWM stimulation then as the T cells are diluted certain cultures will produce only Tet-IgG or Dip-IgG but not both. The
latter case is observed and we propose a mechanism to account
for this possible antigen specific component of PWM induced
T cell help.

MATERIALS AND METHODS

Immunizations. Donors who had not received a tetanus or
diptheria booster immunization within the past year were sele-
ted and were booster immunized intramuscularly with alum precipitated tetanus and diptheria toxoid (DT). The prepackaged
DT used was intended for adults and contained only 1/10 the
childhood immunizing dose of diptheria toxoid.

Lymphocyte Separation and Culture. Human peripheral
blood leukocytes were prepared by Ficoll-Hypaque differential
sedimentation (6). T and B cell fractions were separated by
density sedimentation of spontaneous rosettes formed by T
lymphocytes and sheep red blood cells (SRBC) (7). T cell fractions were irradiated (3000 R) to reduce suppressive effects.

The T cell population contained 89-99% E-rosette positive
cells, less than 2% Ig positive cells and 1-2% α-naphyl esterase positive cells. The cultures were set up in a final volume of 0.20 ml of RPMI medium containing PWM and 15% FCS in
round bottom microculture plates. The cultures were incubated
in a humidified atmosphere with 5% CO_2 at 37° for 9 days.

   Radioimmunoassays. The quantitative radioimmunoassays
for Tet-IgG, Dip-IgG and total IgG, IgA, and IgM synthesized
in vitro were performed in a flexible microtitre plates (8).
Samples of 0.08 ml were used for the antigen specific antibody assays. Samples of 0.05 ml were used for the isotype
specific assays. With a specific activity of 4000 cpm/ng for
the second antibody and a background of 500 cpm/well, 0.03 ng
of Tet-IgG would be detectable. Even in the absence of cell
division the PWM stimulated plasma cells which appear 4 days
after in vitro culture and produce approximately 1 pg IgG/
cell/hr (9)   could individually produce 0.12 ng of specific
antibody.

RESULTS

   Though the primary thrust of this investigation was to
look at the specificity of the helper T cells generated in
vitro with PWM it was necessary to first quantitate the indicator cells. The basic protocol to determine the percentage
of B cells activated by PWM and T cells was to add limiting
numbers of B cells to 2-5 x 10^5 irradiated T cells in the presence of PWM. A summary of the results of such experiments is
presented in Table 1.
   A maximum of 1 of 60 B cells was activated to produce
detectable Ig in our system. This assumes that 60% of the
cells in our B cell fraction are B cells, the rest being monocytes (up to 40%), and contaminating T cells (1-2%). The
majority of the stimulated cells produced IgM (59%), with
those producing IgA or IgG being 27% and 13% respectively.
   Antigen reactive B cells producing Tet-IgG or Dip-IgG
circulated with precursor frequencies of 1.3 x 10^4 and
4.2 x 10^{-5} respectively and accounted for 10% and 3% of the
total IgG producing cells. The linearity of the dilution
curves obtained from Figure 1 and the sensitivity of the Ig
assays would argue that this is in fact a reasonable estimate
of the number of B cells stimulated by PWM and T cells.
   Since about 1 cell in 20,000 in the B cell fraction produced Tet-IgG or Dip-IgG, 10 times this number of B cells were
used as the indicator cells in the T cell titrations to ensure
an excess. Irradiated T cells were added at concentrations
ranging from 6 x 10^4 to 1 x 10^3 cells per well. As with the B
cell titrations twenty replicate wells were set up at each

TABLE 1

THE MEAN PRESURSOR FREQUENCIES OF PWM STIMULATED T CELL
DEPENDENT Ig PRODUCING PERIPHERAL BLOOD B CELLS

Donor	IgA	IgM	IgG	Tet-IgG	Dip-IgG
C.T.	1.2×10^{-3}	4.5×10^{-3}	2.8×10^{-4}	-	-
E.M.	1.5×10^{-3}	2.4×10^{-3}	6.7×10^{-4}	-	-
E.M.	5.9×10^{-3}	4.0×10^{-3}	1.6×10^{-3}	-	-
B.K.	2.4×10^{-3}	1.5×10^{-2}	3.4×10^{-3}	-	-
M.T.	9.1×10^{-4}	3.8×10^{-3}	1.4×10^{-3}	-	-
M.T.*	-	-	4.2×10^{-4}	1.1×10^{-4}	5.5×10^{-5}
D.H.*	-	-	4.8×10^{-4}	9.1×10^{-5}	4.0×10^{-5}
A.F.*	-	-	2.0×10^{-3}	3.2×10^{-4}	3.2×10^{-5}
Mean	2.7×10^{-3}	5.9×10^{-3}	1.3×10^{-3}	1.3×10^{-4}	4.2×10^{-5}
SD	2.2×10^{-3}	5.1×10^{-3}	1.1×10^{-3}	5.8×10^{-5}	1.1×10^{-5}

*Two weeks post DT boost

Table I. All titrations were set up with 2 to 5×10^5 T
cells per well. Twenty replicate cultures were set up at
each dilution.

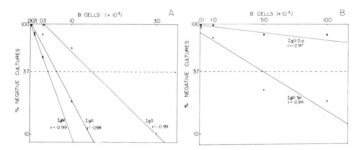

Figure 1. Limiting dilution of B cells in the presence
of 5×10^5 irradiated T cells. In experiment A, donor E.M.,
ten wells were assayed at each dilution of added B cells for
total IgM (●), IgG (0), and IgA (X). In experiment B, donor
A.F., twenty wells were assayed for total IgG, Tet-IgG (X),
and Dip-IgG (●).

dilution. Zero levels for T cell dependent Tet-IgG and Dip-
IgG production were established based on 10 to 20 replicate
wells containing 2×10^5 B cells. The mean plus two times the
standard deviation of the counts bound by these wells was
determined. This value was modified by refiguring it to ex-

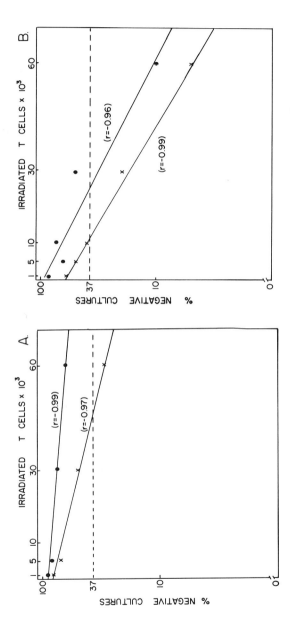

Figure 2. Limiting dilutions of irradiated T cells in the presence of 2 x 10⁵ B cells. All cultures were positive for total IgG at all dilutions of T cells. Curve A, donor D.H., is at three weeks post DT boost. Curve B, donor M.T., is at four weeks post DT boost. Twenty cultures at each dilution of added T cells were assayed for the presence of total IgG, Tet-IgG (X), and Dip-IgG (●).

clude those wells which fell outside the mean plus two standard deviations of the group. If more than 20% of the wells
containing only 2 x 10[5] B cells were outside the two standard
deviations of the mean then the experiment was discarded.

   The two dilution curves in Figure 2 are representative of
nine independent experiments. The T cells responsible for
providing Dip-IgG help consistantly diluted out more rapidly
than the help for Tet-IgG. Figure 3 shows that as increasing
numbers of T cells were added there was a 2.5 to 9 fold increase in the amount of specific IgG. The number of antigen
specific wells at each dilution of T cells is shown in Table
2. With low numbers of added T cells the majority of the positive cultures produced either Tet-IgG or Dip-IgG but not both.

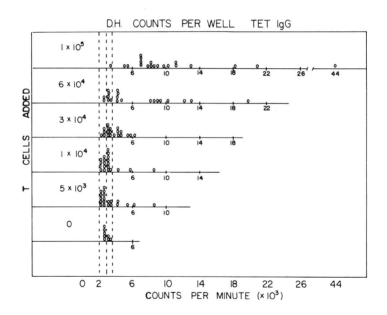

   Figure 3. Counts per well at each T cell dilution. The
center vertical line represents the mean of the counts bound
by the wells used to determine the background produced by B
cells alone in this assay. The other two lines are the range
covered by $\pm$ 2 standard deviation of the mean. All wells
at each dilution are shown as open circles. Each dilution of
T cells was added to 2 x 10[5] B cells. Counts shown are Tet-
IgG specific and indicate that increased addition of T cells
results in both more positive cultures as well as increased
antibody per culture.

antibodies. As more T cells were added the percentage of cultures producing both antibodies increased. This indicates
that at limiting numbers of T cell, the stimulation of one set
of antibody producing cells can occur while other sets of
clones remain unproductive.

TABLE 2

ANTIGEN SPECIFIC IRRADIATED HELPER T CELLS

Donor (time)	No. of wells	Added T cells	No. of positive wells		
			Tet-IgG	Dip-IgG	Both
D.H.	20	6×10^4	9	2	5
(3 weeks)	20	3×10^4	7	2	3
	20	1×10^4	3	3	0
	20	5×10^3	4	1	2
	20	1×10^3	4	2	0
	10	0	1	0	1
A.F.	20	6×10^4	5	2	2
(3 weeks)	20	3×10^4	4	1	2
	20	1×10^4	6	1	1
	20	5×10^4	5	0	0
	20	1×10^4	1	3	1
	20	0	1	3	0
M.T.	20	6×10^4	2	1	17
(4 weeks)	20	3×10^4	6	0	10
	20	1×10^4	9	2	3
	20	5×10^3	6	3	4
	20	1×10^3	4	1	2
	20	0	3	4	0
M.K.	20	6×10^4	9	0	9
(4 weeks)	20	3×10^4	4	2	11
	20	1×10^4	7	2	5
	20	5×10^3	6	3	2
	20	1×10^3	2	2	1
	10	0	2	1	0

Table 2. Antigen specific irradiated helper T cells.
Irradiated T cells (5×10^5) were added to a series of cultures containing 2×10^5 B cells. Time indicates the time
after DT boost the particular experiment was set up. After 9
days in culture each well was assayed for both Tet-IgG and
Dip-IgG and the wells were scored as Tet-IgG positive, Dip-IgG
positive, or positive for both Tet-IgG and Dip-IgG. The data
from donor D.H. at three weeks post boost and donor M.T. at
four weeks post boost are also plotted in Figure 3.

TABLE 3

THE MEAN PRECURSOR FREQUENCY OF PWM STIMULATED
IRRADIATION RESISTANT HELPER T CELLS AFTER DT BOOST

Donor	Tetanus frequency	Diptheria frequency	Ratio
M.K.*	1 in 1.9 x 10^4	1 in 8.0 x 10^4	4.21
M.T.*	1 in 1.3 x 10^4	1 in 2.8 x 10^4	2.15
D.H.[+]	1 in 4.9 x 10^4	1 in 1.7 x 10^5	3.47
A.F.[+]	1 in 1.7 x 10^5	1 in 3.9 x 10^5	2.29
Mean	1 in 6.3 x 10^4	1 in 1.7 x 10^5	2.70

*4 weeks post DT   [+]3 weeks post DT

Table 3. The mean precursor frequency of PWM stimulated
irradiation resistant helper T cells after DT boost as derived from a Poisson analysis of a limiting dilution of irradiated T cells in the presence of 2 x 10^5 B cells.

The helper T cells frequencies obtained from four donors
are given in Table 3. The ratio between the two values indicates that different numbers of helper T cells may arise in
the circulation after immunization with different antigens.

DISCUSSION

We have previously shown that the PWM stimulated in vitro
synthesis of Tet-IgG and Dip-IgG have an obligatory requirement for recent in vivo booster immunization with the corresponding antigens (2). This lead us to suggest that those B
cells which secrete measurable Ig after PWM induced T cell
stimulation represent B cells which enter the circulation
shortly after an antigenic rechallenge. The analysis of the
percentage of peripheral blood B cells devoted to the production of the three major isotypes shows that not all B cells
are activated in our system and instead, a combined maximum of
about 1 in 60 B cells in the peripheral blood of normal per-
sons appeared to be stimulated to high rate Ig production by
PWM and T cells. The limiting dilutions of B cells in Figure
1 all have correlation coefficients of less than -.93. This
linearity, the sensitivity of the Ig assays, and the quantitative increases in counts bound with increasing B cells contribute to our belief that we are detecting all of the B cells
stimulated in our system.
To determine the specificity of T cell help, two simultaneous in vivo antigenic stimuli were employed and the precursor frequencies of T cell help which stimulated Tet-IgG or

Dip-IgG production in vitro were determined. Although each culture had B cells which could synthesize Tet-IgG and Dip-IgG, T cell help for these antibodies did not dilute out at the same rate.

The correlation coefficients of the lines presented in Figure 2 are all less than -.95 and thus, according to the Poisson analysis there does not appear to be a multicomponent helper function in the T cell fraction and the activity of a single helper T cell may be expected to produce a positive well. This does not rule out the possibility that the T cells may be interacting with other intermediate cells before the B cells are stimulated, this merely shows that the T cells are limiting and all other components are at excess.

At limiting numbers of T cells, cultures could be detected which synthesized Tet-IgG or Dip-IgG, but not both. As the quantity of T cell help was increased, the percentage of cultures producing individual antibody specificities declined, with a concommitant increase in the number of cultures producing both antibodies. These results strongly suggest that PWM activation of antibody synthesis is not a random interaction between helper T cells and B cells but a certain degree of specificity exists. This specificity could be accounted for in several ways. It could result from functional subpopulations of T lymphocytes being restricted to collaboration with corresponding B cell subpopulations and be independent of an antigen specific component. Alternatively antigen or antigen fragments may be responsible for the restricted cooperation between B cells and helper T cells. This would be consistent with a number of other observations.

First, in vitro synthesis of Tet-IgG or Dip-IgG requires in vivo booster immunization. Without this immunization, there are very low numbers of active circulating B and T lymphocytes which can assist in the PWM generated production of specific antibodies. Secondly, these activities are present only transiently in the circulation, peaking around 4 weeks and being gone by 6-8 weeks.

We would view in vivo booster immunization of individuals as an event which results in antigen "armed" populations of specific T or B cells. These may be generated directly in the circulation or alternatively be released from antigen stimulated lymph nodes. These cells appear incapable of cooperating in vitro without an additional stimulus which is supplied by PWM. PWM could act in several ways to favor this cooperation. First it could directly promote release of specific helper factors from T lymphocytes which had previously been "armed" with antigen. These factors could then seek our their antigen specific B cell counterparts and initiate antibody synthesis.

Suggestions for this possible type of mechanism come from the antigen specific, and non-specific factors generated by Mudawwar, et al., following in vitro stimulation of human T cells with tetanus toxoid (10). Although tetanus toxoid antibody and non-specific helper factors are generated, the latter can be made specific for diptheria toxoid by addition of soluble diptheria toxoid. This would be one step removed from our postulated in vivo arming.

A second alternative would be that PWM stimulates an additional population of regulatory cells which would then in turn promote the collaboration of the specific helper T cells and B cells.

Finally it is unlikely that circulating monocytes carry the antigenic recognition signal. Although our B cell fractions contain 20-40% monocytes and may be in excess at all times in our cultures, these monocytes have a half-life of less than a week in circulation and it would be difficult to envisage the antigen specific activity residing in the circulation up to 6-8 weeks were these cells responsible.

REFERENCES

1. Greaves, M.F., and Roitt, I.M. (1968). Clin. Exp. Immunol. 3, 393.
2. Stevens, R.H., and Saxon, A. (1978). J. Clin. Invest. 62, 1154.
3. Keightly, R.G., Cooper, M.D., and Lawton, A. (1976). J. Immunol. 117, 1538.
4. Fauci, A.S., Pratt, K.R.K., and Whalen, G. (1976). J. Immunol. 117, 2100.
5. Wu, L.Y.F., Lawton, A.R., and Cooper, M.D. (1973). J. Clin. Invest. 52, 3180
6. Boyum, A. (1968). Scand. J. Clin. Lab. Invest. Suppl. 97, 77.
7. Saxon, A., Feldhaus, J.L., and Robbins, R.A. (1976). J. Immunol. Methods. 12, 285.
8. Zollinger, W.D., Dalrymple, J.M., and Artenstein, M.S. (1976). J. Immunol. 117, 1788.
9. Warner, N., and Potter, M. (1974). UICC Technical Report Series 13,53.
10. Mudawwar, F.B., Yunis, E.J., and Geha, R.S. (1978). J. Exp. Med. 148, 1032.

INDUCTION OF T-CELL PROLIFERATION BY ANTISERA TO THE T-CELL SURFACE[1]

Barry Jones, Hazel Dockrell,[2] and Charles A.Janeway, Jr.

Department of Pathology, Yale University School of Medicine
New Haven, CT 06510
and
Department of Immunology, Middlesex Hospital Medical School
London, England

ABSTRACT Rabbit anti-mouse brain serum was found to be
mitogenic for T-cells. The proliferative response required the presence of an ancillary cell, but there was
no necessity for identity at the H-2 locus between T-
cells and the ancillary component. The target antigen
for mitogenic antibody was shared by T-cells and brain
tissue. Antibodies against other T-cell determinants
were not active in triggering blastogenesis.

INTRODUCTION

Recent evidence suggests that T-cells are the recipients
of a number of signals transmitted by other cells in the immune system. For instance, the proliferative response of T-
cells to specific antigens or mitogens requires interaction
with macrophages (1), or in some cases, soluble factors produced by macrophages (2). Furthermore, the observation that
feedback loops exist between T-cell subsets (3) raises the possibility that multiple sites exist in the T-cell membrane for
the reception of modulating signals.
   In this paper preliminary evidence is presented which suggests that brain associated T-cell membrane determinants may
be involved in the reception of stimulatory signals, since
their perturbation with antibody results in a rapid phase of
proliferation.

[1]This work was supported by grant AI-14579 from the National Institute of Health, and a grant from the Cancer Research Campaign of Great Britain.
[2]Present address: Department of Immunology, Middlesex
Hospital Medical School, London, W1P 9PG, England.

METHODS

Antisera. Anti-mouse brain serum was prepared in rabbits as described by Golub (4). Rabbit anti-mouse thymocyte serum was obtained from Microbiological Associates (Maryland). The antisera were routinely absorbed three times with mouse liver (4). The absorbed anti-mouse brain sera will be referred to as rabbit anti-brain associated Thy 1 (anti-BaThy1) sera.

Preparation of Mouse Splenic T-Cells. Purified T-cells (<1% surface Ig positive) were prepared by passage of whole spleen cells (after lysis of contaminating erythrocytes by hypotonic shock) through Ig-anti-Ig glass bead columns (5).

Assay for Mitogenisis. $2-5 \times 10^7$ whole spleen or purified T-cells were incubated with anti-BaThy1 serum (30 min at 37° C), washed three times, and cultured in flat bottomed (5mm dia) microtitre plates. $1-10 \times 10^5$ cells have been cultured per well. After 24-29h the cutures were pulsed either for a further 16h with $1\mu Ci[^{125}I]UdR$ or $[^3H]TdR$ (60 Ci/m mole) for 3 h. The mean proliferative response induced by anti-BaThy1 in four replicate cultures (x) was compared with the background (y) in controls treated with normal rabbit serum (NRS). Results have been expressed as either the stimulation index $(SI = \frac{x}{y})$ or Δcpm (x-y). Incorporation of $[^3H]TdR$ was far greater than incorporation of $[^{125}I]UdR$.

RESULTS

BALB/c spleen cells were treated with anti-BaThy1 and after washing to remove unbound antibody were put into culture.

TABLE 1
INDUCTION OF BLASTOGENESIS BY ANTI-BaThy1

Experiment no.	Treatment	% Blast cells	SI[a]
1	Anti-BaThy1	23	2.9
	NRS	3	
2	Anti-BaThy1	18	2.9
	NRS	2	
3	Anti-BaThy1	30	4.2
	NRS	5	

[a]Stimulation index calculated from $[^{125}I]UdR$ incorporation.

TABLE 2

ROLE OF T-CELLS IN THE MITOGENIC RESPONSE TO ANTI-BaThy1

Mouse	Pretreatment[a]	Stimulating serum	$[^{125}I]$UdR incorporation (dpm $\pm$ SD)
Normal	Anti-Thy 1.2 + C'	Anti-BaThy1	2,904 $\pm$ 48
BALB/c	C'		11,500 $\pm$ 341
	None		13,444 $\pm$ 384
	None	NRS	2,745 $\pm$ 146
NU/NU[b]	None	Anti-BaThy1	1,650 $\pm$ 95
BALB/c		NRS	2,249 $\pm$ 178
Normal lit-	None	Anti-BaThy1	13,333 $\pm$ 457
ter mate		NRS	2,368 $\pm$ 227

[a]Spleen cells were depleted of T-cells with anti-Thy 1.2
+ C' prior to stimulation with anti-BaThy1.
[b]Congenitally athymic nude mice.

Incorporation of $[^{125}I]$UdR peaked between 25 and 40h, and was
accompanied by the appearance of blast cells (Table 1). Mitogenic activity has been found in all seven batches of anti-Ba-
Thy1 serum tested.

In the experiment of Table 2, anti-BaThy1 failed to stimulate spleen cells depleted of T-cells by AKR anti-Thy 1.2 and
complement (C') or cells from congenitally athymic mice.
Therefore T-cells are required for mitogenesis. However, Ig
anti-Ig column purified T-cells were incapable of responding
alone and appeared to require the presence of ancillary cells
(A-cells) present in mitomycin C treated whole spleen (Table
3). This result was analogous to the requirement for A-cells
in the proliferative response of primed T-cells to antigen (6),
but was distinguished by the absence of the requirement for
compatibility at the H-2 locus between responder T-cells and
A-cells (Table 3). It should be noted that these responses
were measured at 29h, that is, before significant allogeneic
stimulation was apparent.

The specificity of mitogenic activity was investigated by
a series of absorptions with Thy 1.2 positive or negative
cells. In Table 4 activity was specifically removed by absorption with thymocytes or the EL4 T-lymphoma, and consequently mitogenic activity was not due to contamination of the
antiserum with non-specific mitogens. The antibody responsible for mitogenesis could be directed against a unique T-cell
surface component involved in blastogenesis, or on the contrary, antibody against any T-cell antigen may be active simply

TABLE 3
RESPONSE OF PURIFIED SPLENIC T-CELLS TO ANTI-BaTh1

Responder strain[a]	Ancillary cell strain[b]	$[^3H]$ TdR incorporation Δcpm[c]
CBA	CBA	65,856
	DBA/2	71,457
	C57BL6	49,559
	None	2,037
C57BL6	CBA	60,767
	DBA/2	76,199
	C57BL6	35,514
	None	0

[a] 1.3×10^5 purified T-cells pretreated with anti-BaThy1.
[b] 5×10^5 mitomycin C treated spleen cells were added to the T-cells in micro-well cultures.
[c] Control CPM subtracted were from T-cells treated with NRS and added to the same spleen cells in each case. Thus, allogeneic stimulation is controlled for.

by providing a bridge between T-cells and A-cells via Fc receptors in the A-cell membrane. The experiment of Table 5 was designed to test this point. Rabbit anti-mouse thymocyte serum could stimulate T-cells to proliferate. However, absorption with brain tissue removed mitogenic activity. Since the brain absorbed antiserum was still capable of binding T-cells as judged by indirect immunofluorescence (Table 5), and

TABLE 4
ABSORPTION OF MITROGENIC ACTIVITY FROM ANTI-BaThy1 SERUM
BY Thy 1.2 POSITIVE CELLS

Absorption[a]	$[^{125}I]$ UdR incorporation $\overline{\Delta cpm}$
None	3,845
Thymocytes	-167
EL4 lymphoma	-240
NSI plasmacyloma	3,192
NPEC	4,495
P815 mastocyloma	3,936

[a] In addition to routine liver absorption, anti-BaThy1 serum was absorbed 3 times with packed cells (1:3), and tested at 1/20 dilution.

TABLE 5

MITOGENIC ACTIVITY OF RABBIT ANTI-MOUSE THYMOCYTE SERUM

Absorption	Serum dilution	[^{3}H] TdR incorporation Δcpm[a]	% T-cells stained[b]
Liver	1/10	25,514	100
	1/20	8,568	100
	1/40	4,699	100
Liver and brain	1/10	330	100
	1/20	192	100
	1/40	197	100

[a] 2.5×10^5 anti-thymocyte serum treated, purified T-cells were incubated with 5×10^3 mitomycin C treated whole spleen cells and pulsed at 29h.

[b] Before culture, binding of rabbit antibody to T-cells was tested using a second layer of fluorescinated sheep anti-rabbit Ig.

cytotoxicity assays (data not shown), the results suggest that antibodies to a discrete determinant shared between thymus and brain are required for mitogenic activity.

DISCUSSION

The results indicate that rabbit anti-mouse brain serum is mitogenic for T-cells. Both negative selection experiments with AKR anti-Thy 1.2 and C', and positive selection by passage through Ig anti-Ig bead columns strongly suggest that T-cells are the responsive lymphocyte class. The positive selection experiments demonstrate the requirement for an additional ancillary cell type present in whole spleen, but not in the column fractionated T-cells. The ancillary cells did not need to proliferate since they were functional after treatment of whole spleen cells with mitomycin C. At the present time it is only possible to speculate on the nature of the A-cell. By analogy to studies with antigen (6) and PHA (2) induced proliferative responses of T-cells it can be hypothesized that macrophages are required. If this is the case it is likely that they recognize the Fc portion of the antibody bound to T-cells. Such cells would presumably bind to the mouse Ig-rabbit-anti-mouse-Ig complexes on the columns.

Absorption studies suggested that the mitogenic activity of anti-brain serum was due to antibody directed against T-cell specific antigen(s). Obviously Thy 1.2 is a candidate for the relevant antigen, and the results obtained with the

anti-thymocyte serum are pertinent to this point. All the
mitogenic activity of the anti-thymocyte serum could be absorbed with brain tissue, while substantial T-cell binding activity remained and could be detected by immunofluorescent and
cytotoxicity tests. Therefore only certain T-cell antigens
are able to trigger blastogenesis after binding antibody. The
relevant determinants are shared with brain, and experiments
are in progress to determine whether they include the surface
molecule of 25,000 MW described previously (7) and shown to be
recognized by anti-brain sera, and to carry the Thy1 antigens
(8).

REFERENCES

1. Thomas, D. W., Clement, L., and Shevach, E. M. (1978). Immunol. Rev. 40, 181.
2. Rosenstreich, D. L., and Mizel, S. B. (1978). Immunol. Rev.
   40, 102
3. Eardley, D. D., Hugenberger, J., McVay-Boudreau, L., Shen,
   F. W., and Gershon, R. K. (1978). J. Exp. Med. 147, 1106.
4. Golub, E. S. (1971). Cell Immunol. 2, 253.
5. Wigzell, H. (1976). Scand. J. Immunol. 5 (Suppl 5), 23.
6. Rosenthal, A. S. (1978). Immunol. Rev. 40, 136.
7. Trowbridge, I. S., Weissman, I. L., and Bevan, M. J. (1975).
   Nature. 256, 652.
8. Morris, R. J., Letarte-Muirhead, M., and Williams, A. F.
   (1975). Eur. J. Immunol. 5, 282.

WORKSHOP REPORT: Early Events, Triggering, and Tolerance

E. Gronowicz
Immunology Division
Stanford University
School of Medicine
Stanford, California

D. Lucas
Department of Microbiology
University of Arizona
Health Sciences Center
Tucson, Arizona

F. Melchers
Institute for Immunology
Basel, Switzerland

G. Möller
Immunobiology, Karolinska Institute
Stockholm, Sweden

The session began with a statement that the activation of T and B cells have many common characteristics. Perhaps much progress could be made by investigating what might be common processes of activation. For example, is binding to surface V region products followed by mitogenic signals (polyclonal activators, factors) a common process for activating either T or B cells. The major differences between T and B cell activation might reside only in the substance delivering the signals. It was suggested that T and B cells exist in a resting state and become fully responsive only after some initial change. It might be of value to explore whether this model can be universally applied.

In respect to early events in activation, D. Lucas proposed that cAMP had to be localized to deliver an activation signal and that non-localized cAMP production was negative. Data concerning positive signalling by cGMP and a role for calcium in activation was also mentioned. No conclusions in this area were possible. The simultaneous functioning of different subpopulations in cultures, for example one activated to produce a factor and another responding to the factor, makes it difficult to define biochemical signals until experiments can be performed with pure cell populations and well-defined conditions.

Ken Smith's model for Con A activation of T cells, requiring Con A produced receptivity of cells followed by delivery of a second signal (TCGF) by a second cell, was referred to at several points in discussion of early events and consequences of Ig receptor activation. Although some urged this model as one of universal application for both B and T cell activation there was not unanimous acceptance of this model.

The question was asked whether the Ig receptor can transmit a positive signal leading to activation of B cells. The stimulation by anti-Ig reagents was discussed. It seemed evident that not all anti-Ig reagents could be stimulatory and that stimulation only led to increased DNA synthesis and not to Ig secretion. However, the data of D. Parker showed that anti-Ig in combination with a supernatant from Con A stimulated cells was capable of activation to both clonal proliferation and IgM secretion. The question was posed whether anti-Ig stimulates resting cells, and whether stimulation requires helper cells. Evidence for an independence of T cells and macrophages was mentioned, as well as that the stimulated cells are Ig positive. The inhibition of polyclonal activation of B cells by anti-Ig was discussed. The significance of these findings seem unclear. It was proposed that for future studies, purified cell populations and well characterized and purified antisera should be used. The value of affinity purified or monoclonal hybridoma antibody was stressed.

The session continued with discussions on criteria for stimulation by polyclonal B cell activators (PBA). A model was proposed by A.J. Rosenspire and D.M. Jacobs implying that PBA molecules deliver a transmembrane signal via a mitogen receptor and that this signal is sufficient for stimulation. The Ig receptor was proposed to be able to modulate the signals delivered by PBA. The question was raised whether PBA activation is ever independent of the Ig receptor. Other unclear points were brought up, such as the capacity of PBAs to activate resting cells and the possibility that PBA activation may require accessory cells. Data were referred to which suggested that, at least in certain conditions, PBAs can cause direct activation of B cells. Thus, the data of M. Wetzel and J.R. Kettman showed that single cells in culture proliferated when stimulated by LPS and DXS together. The proliferating cells were Ig positive, but did not secrete Ig. Another line of evidence was the experiments using B cell tumors. C.J. Paize and Y. Lifter used a pre B cell like tumor 702/3, which contains IgM in the cytoplasm, but lacks surface IgM. This tumor could be activated by PBAs to insert μ alone or μK in the cell membrane. E. Gronowicz used BCL_1 adapted to tissue culture. This cell line secretes IgM when stimulated by PBAs. The discussion on PBA activation was closed by the conclusion that more well-defined systems should be used for future studies. It was suggested that the use of tumor cells to study PBA activation would be useful.

A brief discussion on the evidence for clonal deletion of B cells as a mechanism of experimentally induced tolerance concluded the session. Evidence against clonal deletion was presented by D. Primi, G.K. Lewis and J.W. Goodman. They could activate B cells, tolerized with FITC-D-(G,L), with LPS, to produce anti-FITC antibodies. It was not resolved whether mostly low affinity antibodies were activated or whether a different subpopulation of B cells were activated by LPS than the one tolerized with FITC-D-(G,L).

ANTIGEN-DRIVEN ALTERATION IN SURFACE Ig ISOTYPES ON ANTIGEN BINDING CELLS[1]

Susan Kanowith-Klein, Jean E. Merrill,[2]
Ellen S. Vitetta and Robert F. Ashman

Department of Microbiology and Immunology
University of California, Los Angeles, California and
Department of Microbiology, University of Texas
Southwestern Medical School, Dallas, Texas

ABSTRACT Antigen-driven events on the cell surface of sheep erythrocyte-specific antigen binding cells (SRC-ABC) were investigated in vivo and in vitro. Spleen cells from non-immune mice cultured with SRC in vitro exhibited an antigen-specific expansion of SRC-ABC, due to cell division and maturation. Both T and B ABC were maximal on day 4 of culture. An increase in ABC on day 1 was attributable to T ABC. Surface Ig (sIg) phenotypes were revealed by inhibition of antigen binding with antisera specific for μ, δ, or γ heavy chains. SRC-ABC from non-immune animals were primarily $\mu^+\delta^+\gamma^-$ or $\mu^-\delta^-\gamma^-$, the latter group including T ABC. After immunization in vivo or in vitro, the proportion of ABC with sIgM remained constant while ABC with sIgD declined and ABC with sIgG appeared. The appearance of $\mu^+\delta^+\gamma^+$ ABC on day 3 in vitro and in vivo suggested that sIgG first appeared on cells already bearing sIgM and sIgD. After day 3, the % of $\mu^+\delta^+\gamma^+$ ABC declined. In vivo $\mu^+\delta^-\gamma^+$, $\mu^+\delta^-\gamma^-$ and $\mu^-\delta^-\gamma^+$ ABC appeared or increased by day 5, whereas in vitro most B ABC on days 4-6 were $\mu^+\delta^-\gamma^+$. Low concentrations of BUdR, effective in preventing the expression of gene products typical of differentiated cells, also prevented the increase in T and B ABC, the appearance of sIgG, and even the loss of sIgD.

[1]This work was supported by grant T32-CA-09120 (NCI,DHEW) and a fellowship in Cancer Immunology from Cancer Research Institute, New York to SK-K, by NIH training grant AI-07126-01 to JEM, grants AI-11851 and AI-12789 to ESV, NIH grants CA-12800 (NCI) and AI-14922 from NIAID to RFA, and by Center for Interdisciplinary Research in Immunological Diseases grant AI-15332 (NIAID, DHEW).
[2]Present address: Department of Virology, Karolinska Institute, Stockholm, Sweden.

INTRODUCTION

Murine lymphocytes which bind sheep erythrocytes (SRC-ABC) are a distinct antigen-specific population which increase 10-20 fold after *in vivo* immunization (1). Both T and B SRC-ABC populations (2) contain immunologically relevant cells, including precursors of specific antibody producing cells (3), helper cells (4), suppressor cells (5), and cytotoxic T cells (6).   Thus the antigen-binding property identified a cell population in which antigen-driven differentiation events should be taking place. The primary *in vitro* response to SRC provides a system in which these early events can be analyzed. We have now formally shown that most of the antigen-driven expansion of SRC-ABC *in vitro* is continuously dependent on cell division, except for the early increase in T ABC.

By adoptively transferring cells selected by their surface Ig (sIg) isotypes, it has been shown that cells bearing sIgM and sIgD are precursors of both IgM and IgG secreting cells, whereas sIgG bearing cells are precursors only of IgG secreting cells (7). This result predicts that the B cells reacting to antigen might undergo corresponding changes in their sIg isotypes. By blocking SRC binding to ABC *in vivo* and *in vitro* with μ, γ, or δ specific antisera and with combinations of these sera, we have shown that non-immune B ABC mainly bear sIgM and sIgD, and that SRC induces the appearance of sIgG on SRC-ABC and the loss of sIgD.

METHODS

Primary Responses In Vivo and In Vitro. For *in vivo* responses spleen cell suspensions were prepared as previously described (8). Briefly, cells were prepared from CBA ♀ non-immune mice, or from mice immunized with 10^8 SRC intraperitoneally 5 days previously. After 37°C incubation on cotton wool columns, these suspensions contained <5% dead cells, and <2% microphages, as judged by acridine orange fluorescence. The *in vitro* primary response to SRC was studied by the Mishell-Dutton culture technique (9), using C57Bl/6 ♀ spleen cells without macrophage removal. SRC-ABC were prepared by 50 x g centrifugation of an 8:1 mixture of SRC and lymphocytes at 4°C (8). These cells have previously been shown not to form plaques (10), but to contain the precursors of *in vitro* plaque forming cells (PFC) (11 and unpublished observations).

Enumeration of T and B ABC. T and B ABC were scored independently by indirect immunofluorescence of preformed ABC, using polyspecific rabbit anti-Ig absorbed with thymocytes and SRC, and rabbit anti-mouse thymocyte serum absorbed with liver powder, nude spleen cells, SRC and mouse IgG and IgM solid

absorbents. Fluorescein-conjugated goat anti-rabbit Ig was
the second reagent. The % Ig^+ plus the % T^+ lymphocytes
equalled the 90-95% stained with both reagents together. The
sum of Ig^+ and T^+ ABC was 100%.

Autoradiography. The percent of ABC which synthesized
DNA in vitro during daily 17 hour periods was analyzed auto-
radiographically by pulsing Mishell-Dutton cultures with 1
µCi/culture of ^{3}H-thymidine (^{3}H-TdR) and then forming SRC-ABC.
Cultured cells were smeared on subbed slides, fixed, dipped in
Ilford K2 nuclear emulsion, exposed at 4°C for 4 days, and
developed in Kodak D19 developer. The slides were stained
with Camco Quick Stain and examined at 1000 x magnification.
Cells with 20 grains/nucleus were scored as positive, as no
cells carried 5-20 grains.

Determination of Surface Isotypes on ABC by Inhibition of
Antigen Binding. Details of the preparation, absorption, and
specificity-testing of the rabbit anti-mouse isotype sera
(IgG anti-µ, (Fab)'$_2$ anti-γ, and anti-δ) have been published
(7, 12). These serum batches were identical to those used to
study the precursor functions of cells bearing different sIg
isotypes (7, 13).

Inhibition of ABC by anti-isotype sera was performed by
incubating 2.5 x 10^6/ml non-immune or immune CBA cells for 30
min. at 4°C with normal rabbit serum (NRS) or antibody to
µ,γ,δ, µ+γ, µ+δ, γ+δ, or µ+γ+δ, all at optimal inhibitory concentrations. Then the cells were washed once in cold Hanks'
medium, and ABC were prepared and counted with lymphocytes on
the same hemocytometer. The ABC count in tubes incubated with
NRS was taken as 100%. The inhibition of in vitro ABC was the
same except that the cells were incubated with antiserum at 4°
C for 10 min., then 37°C for 30 min. (capping conditions). Preliminary experiments showed no significant difference in blocking between capping and non-capping conditions.

Use of BUdR In Vitro. 5-bromo-2'-deoxyuridine (BUdR,
Sigma Chemical Co.) was added to cell cultures 24 hours prior
to harvest. Cultures were incubated in the dark.

RESULTS

In Vitro Primary SRC-ABC Response. From the total ABC/
culture and the proportion of T and B ABC determined by indirect immunofluorescence it was shown that both T and B ABC par-
ticipated in the antigen-driven expansion of the ABC population (Fig. 1). In cultures with SRC, T ABC increased significantly in the first day, whereas B ABC did not increase until
the third day. By day 4 both T and B ABC reached maximal

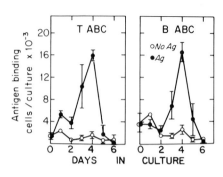

Figure 1. Absolute numbers of T and B cells in a 1° SRC response in vitro calculated from proportions of T and B ABC determined by indirect immunofluorescence and total absolute numbers of ABC/culture. Points with standard error brackets denote triple determinations.

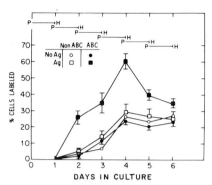

Figure 2. Autoradiography of cells pulsed 17 hr. with 1 µCi ^{3}H-TdR immediately before harvest. P=pulse, H=harvest. Percent cells labeled is number of labeled ABC/total ABC or number labeled non-ABC/total non-ABC. Standard errors shown.

numbers, representing a 4-fold increase in B ABC and a 10-fold increase in T ABC. Between days 1 and 3 about 60% of the ABC were T cells; but from day 4 on about 60% of the ABC were B cells, changes not shared by non-ABC or unstimulated ABC (not shown). This ABC response was antigen-driven; it failed to occur in cultures containing burro or ox erythrocytes. It was also antigen-specific; ABC for other erythrocytes did not increase (not shown). Only IgM anti-SRC PFC were detected.

Generation of ABC. Autoradiography experiments indicated that cell division and cell maturation contributed to the in vitro 5-fold increase of ABC. Figure 2 shows the percent of labeled ABC and non-ABC in cultures with and without SRC, pulsed each day with ^{3}H-TdR. In antigen-stimulated cultures, labeled ABC increased from 0% of the total ABC population on day 1 to 60% on day 4, the peak of the ABC response. Although the percent of cells labeled in control cultures increased somewhat, probably due to mitogenic components in the medium, antigen preferentially stimulated ABC to divide as soon as day 2. Hydroxyurea inhibition experiments (not shown) provided further evidence that continuous DNA synthesis was necessary for the generation of most new ABC.

In another set of experiments (Fig. 3), cells labeled with ^{3}H-TdR during the first 24 hours of culture were chased with cold thymidine throughout the remainder of the culture

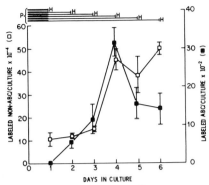

Figure 3. Autoradiography of ^{3}H-TdR pulse-chased cells.
Cells pulsed with 3 µCi ^{3}H-TdR,chased with 25 µg/ml cold TdR.
P=pulse, H=harvest. Standard deviations shown.

period. During the first 24 hours, not one labeled ABC was
observed, while at the peak of the ABC response about 3,000
ABC/culture were labeled, suggesting that cells at first not
detectable as ABC later matured into detectable ABC. Furthermore, since T ABC increased significantly during the first 24
hours of culture (Fig. 1) and since no ABC were dividing during this period (Fig. 2), it follows that some T ABC must have
arisen without cell division. Thus both cell division and
cell maturation contributed to the increase in specific ABC
observed in vitro .

ABC Isotypes: sIgM, sIgD, sIgG. Alterations in the receptor isotype of ABC were examined by exposing non-immune
cells and cells immunized both in vivo and in vitro to a range
of concentrations of anti-µ, -δ, or -γ before ABC were prepared. The proportion of ABC inhibited by anti-µ remained
50-60% throughout the early response (Table 1). Anti-δ
blocked about 50% of all ABC through day 2; then the percentage of ABC blocked by anti-δ decreased,reaching 0% for in vitro
stimulated cells (day 4-6). In contrast, ABC inhibited by
anti-γ did not appear until day 3 and then increased to
approximately 55% of the total ABC, both in vitro and in vivo.
The appearance of sIgG in vitro occurred only in SRC-contain-
ing cultures, but the FCS-containing medium sufficed to cause
sIgD loss, showing that these two cell membrane events could
be dissociated.

sIg Phenotypes. If two isotypes, A and B, each occurred
on 50% of ABC, one would expect that if A and B were on the
same cell, inhibition by anti-A and anti-B would also be 50%,
but if they never shared the same cell, it would be 100%.
Using similar logic, Dr. Edward Korn, Dept. of Biomathematics,

TABLE 1

PERCENT INHIBITION OF ABC WITH ANTI-ISOTYPE SERA
DURING PRIMARY SRC RESPONSE

	Immunized In Vivo (CBA)			Immunized In Vitro (C57B1/6)		
With:	anti-μ	anti-δ	anti-γ	anti-μ	anti-δ	anti-γ
Inhibition on day						
0	61	54	0	51	45	0
1	-	-	-	50	48	0
2	56	55	-7	51	46	0
3	52	35	32	57	27	41
4	-	-	-	58	0	55
5	65	28	45	47	0	59
6	-	-	-	45	0	55
12	43	9	55	-	-	-
36	26	12	49	-	-	-

Before binding antigen, cells were incubated with anti-μ, -δ, or -γ. Each percent represents the mean of at least 3 experiments. The standard errors ranged from 2-8% of the mean. Anti-μ and anti-γ were used at final concentrations of 5.7 and 24 μg precipitating antibody/ml, respectively. Anti-δ was used at 1:2 and 1:5 dilutions for in vivo and in vitro ABC, respectively. In control cultures without antigen, anti-μ and anti-δ continued until day 6 to block ABC to the same extent as in day 0 cultures, whereas anti-γ did not block.

UCLA School of Medicine, developed formulas for converting the percent inhibition of ABC by all the possible combinations of antibody to 1, 2, or 3 isotypes into the percent of ABC expressing various combinations of isotypes. A full explanation and justification of these formulas has been published (8).

The 2-isotype results showed that sIgD was expressed mainly on ABC bearing sIgM, and that for immune ABC the same was true for sIgG(Fig.4a). With the 3-isotype analysis (Fig. 4b), the major populations of non-immune ABC were $\mu^+\delta^+\gamma^-$ and $\mu^-\delta^-\gamma^-$ (P<.05). Five days after in vivo immunization, $\mu^+\delta^+\gamma^-$ ABC had decreased, but $\mu^+\delta^-\gamma^-$ and $\mu^-\delta^-\gamma^+$ ABC had appeared (P<.05). On day 3 of the in vitro or in vivo response there were still 33±11% $\mu^+\delta^+\gamma^+$ ABC (P<.05) and from day 4 on there were significant numbers of $\mu^+\delta^-\gamma^+$ ABC (48-64% in vitro). These 2 ABC types were also probably present at day 5 in vivo (0.05 <P<0.1)(Fig. 4b). A significant $\mu^-\delta^-\gamma^-$ ABC population was found on every day both in vivo and in vitro. By indirect immunofluorescence, most of these were shown to be T ABC.

Effect of BUdR. A selective inhibitor of the expression of genes coding for proteins characteristic of differentiated cells (14), BUdR was added to cell cultures to determine its

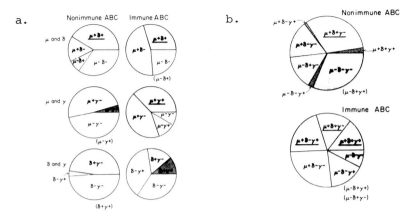

Figure 4. Estimated proportions of ABC expressing: a. pairs of isotypes, b. combinations of 3 isotypes calculated from binding inhibition data (8). Phenotypes of ABC with more than 1 isotype and P<0.1 are underlined. Phenotypes in parentheses are absent. Stippled areas are doubtful phenotypes with P>0.1.

effect on differention events in ABC, such as the generation of T and B ABC and isotype alterations on B ABC. When cells in culture were exposed to 10 μg/ml BUdR (shown not to affect cell viability or recovery and total DNA, RNA, or protein synthesis) B ABC at the peak of the response were reduced by 88%, and T ABC by 71% (Table 2a). T and B non-ABC were not affected (not shown).

Depending on the day of assay, from 20-40% of the ABC were BUdR resistant (Table 2a). These ABC were subjected to the anti-isotype inhibition (Table 2b) to determine what isotypes were present on these ABC. Although BUdR had little effect on the proportion of IgM$^+$ ABC, it prevented the appearance of IgG$^+$ ABC from day 3 on, and permitted the reappearance of IgD$^+$ ABC at a time when IgD$^+$ ABC were not normally observed (Table 2b).

DISCUSSION

We have described events occurring during the antigen-driven generation of splenic SRC-ABC, including ABC proliferation and alteration of sIg isotypes on ABC. Both cell division (Fig. 2) and BUdR-sensitive differentiation processes (Table 2a) contributed to the in vitro expansion of the T and B ABC populations, which both peaked on day 4 (Fig. 1). In the first day, an antigen driven increase in T ABC (Fig. 1) was not dependent on cell division (Fig. 2), nor was it BUdR-sensitive. Maturation without cell division also contributed

TABLE 2

BUdR EFFECTS ON ABC FROM PRIMARY SRC RESPONSE IN VITRO

a. Absolute Numbers of T and B ABC per Culture x 10^{-3}

Harvest day	T ABC		B ABC	
	Control	BUdR	Control	BUdR
2	3.5±0.9	2.0±0.5	2.0±0.6	5.0±1.0
4	15.5±0.3	4.5±0.3	16.8±1.8	2.0±0.6
6	1.0	0.5±0.3	1.0±0.4	0.5±0.3

b. Percent of ABC blocked by:

Harvest day	Anti-μ (5.7 μg/ml)		Anti-γ (24 μg/ml)		Anti-δ (1:5)	
	Control	BUdR	Control	BUdR	Control	BUdR
0	51±10	N.D.	0	N.D.	57±6	N.D.
3	30	35	49	0	8	11
4	37±5	50±13	43±5	-20±19	-11±5	45±7
5	25±10	23±5	68±10	-20±20	-10±6	50±15

T and B ABC were identified by immunofluorescence, in
cultures containing 10^7 SRC with or without 5 μg/ml BUdR added
1 day prior to harvest. Numbers with standard deviations are
the average of 3 experiments; the rest are single determinations. N.D.=not done. μg/ml=precipitating antibody.

to ABC expansion, since some ABC between days 3 and 5 derived
from dividing cells not detectable as ABC on day 1 (Fig. 3),
perhaps because they possessed too few receptors.
    Among the significant maturation events in B ABC is the
antigen-induced progression of sIg changes, observed in vivo
and in vitro. Non-immune B ABC resembled other splenic B
cells in displaying both sIgM and sIgD but not sIgG (8, 15
and Fig. 4). Such cells resemble the $\mu^+\delta^+$ precursors of primary IgM responses described by Zan-Bar, et al. (7). Five
days after in vivo immunization, $\mu^+\delta^+$ B ABC have increased
4-fold in absolute numbers, but the proportion of δ^+ ABC has
actually decreased by half. In vitro where stimulation by
mitogenic FCS was added to that of SRC, this decline in sIgD
was complete by day 3 (Table 1). A 24 hour pulse of BUdR in
vitro restored the original proportion of $sIgD^+$ ABC on day 4
and 5 (Table 2b). Two equally likely explanations may be
offered, based on the action of BUdR in other systems: 1) BUdR
may have permitted the reexpression of the δ gene previously
"turned off" during differentiation (14) or 2) BUdR may have
prevented the expression of a differentiated cell product
(16), perhaps a proteolytic enzyme that clears sIgD off the
membrane, as suggested by Bourgois, et al. (17).

sIgG appeared on ABC 3 days after antigen both in vivo and in vitro (Table 1), mainly on cells expressing sIgM. On day 3 both in vivo and in vitro, most B ABC were $\mu^+\delta^+\gamma^+$. Thereafter, in vitro, most B ABC were $\mu^+\delta^-\gamma^+$, whereas in vivo $\mu^+\delta^-\gamma^-$ and $\mu^-\delta^-\gamma^+$ ABC were also prominent (Fig. 4b). The $\mu^+\gamma^+$ ABC may include the precursors of secondary IgM responses, whereas $\mu^-\gamma^+$ ABC have been associated with secondary IgG precursor function (18). Thus our results suggest that antigen drives the maturation of the B ABC population from a predominantly IgM-precursor state through a $\mu^+\delta^+\gamma^+$ transition state to a predominantly IgG-precursor state in vivo, but to a secondary IgM-precursor state in short term culture.

sIgG failed to appear on ABC incubated with BUdR in vitro on the 3rd, 4th or 5th culture day (Table 2b) when this isotype was usually detected (Table 1), an effect analogous to the prevention of the expression of other specialized products of differentiated cells by BUdR (14).

The high proportion of ABC bearing more than one isotype suggests that blocking antigen binding with antibody to one isotype should seriously underestimate the proportion of ABC bearing that isotype. Clearly it would be advantageous to compare our results to those obtained using methods which directly detect the presence of an isotype on the ABC surface. By FACS analysis and lactoperoxidase catalyzed surface iodination of gradient-purified SRC-ABC (15), Kenny and coworkers have shown 5 days after SRC immunization in vivo that the proportion of IgM+ ABC remained constant (approximately 60-70%), that the proportion of IgG+ ABC increased from <10% to 50%, and that sIgD decreased relative to sIgM+ on ABC. This agreement between independent methods increases our confidence in the estimates produced by the binding inhibition method.

ACKNOWLEDGMENTS

We thank Thomas Fehniger for his excellent technical assistance and Emma Hollins for typing this manuscript.

REFERENCES

1. Ashman, R.F. (1975). Eur. J. Immunol. 5, 421.
2. Greaves, M.F. (1970). Transplant. Rev. 5, 45.
3. Wilson, J.D. (1971). Immunol. 21, 233.
4. Elliott, B.E., and Haskill, J.S. (1975). J. Exp. Med. 141, 600.
5. Maoz, A., Feldmann, M., and Kontiainen, S. (1976). Nature 260, 324.
6. Elliott, B.E., Haskill, J.S., and Axelrod, M.A. (1975). J. Exp. Med. 141, 584.
7. Zan-Bar, I., Strober, S., and Vitetta, E. (1977). J.

Exp.Med. 145, 1188.

8. Kanowith-Klein, S., Vitetta, E., Korn, E., and Ashman, R.F. (1979). J. Immunol., in press.

9. Mishell, R.I., and Dutton, R.W. (1967). J. Exp. Med. 126, 423.

10. Kenny, J.J., Merrill, J.E., and Ashman, R.F. (1978). J. Immunol. 120, 1233.

11. Nossal, G.J.V., and Pike, B.L. (1976). Immunol. 30, 189.

12. Vitetta, E.S., Forman, J., and Kettman, J.R. (1976). J. Exp. Med. 143, 1055.

13. Zan-Bar, I., Vitetta, E., and Strober, S. (1977). J. Exp. Med. 145, 1206.

14. Rutter, W.J., Pictet, R., and Morris, P. (1973). Ann. Rev. Biochem. 46, 601.

15. Kenny, J.J., Kessler, S.W., Ahmed, A., Ashman, R.F., and Scher, I. (1979). J. Immunol., in press.

16. Biquard, J.M., and Aupoix, M. (1978). Nature 272, 284.

17. Bourgois, A., Abney, E.R., and Parkhouse, R.M.E. (1977). Eur. J. Immunol. 7, 210.

18. Yuan, D., Vitetta, E.S., and Kettman, J. (1977). J. Exp. Med. 145, 1421.

HIGH FREQUENCY OF SPECIFIC ANTIGEN BINDING CELLS IN PROTEIN ANTIGEN STIMULATED LYMPH NODES[1]

J. A. Clarke, L. Adorini[2], J. Couderc,
A. Miller, and E. E. Sercarz

Department of Microbiology, University of California,
Los Angeles, Los Angeles, California 90024

ABSTRACT. After primary immunization with hen egg-white lysozyme (HEL) in complete Freund's adjuvant, draining lymph node cells were rosetted with HEL coupled goat red blood cells and then fixed with glutaraldehyde. Using this method to assess antigen binding, the following was determined: (1) A high frequency (5-15%) of antigen binding cells can be generated 7-10 days after antigen injection. (2) Antigen binding is antigen specific and can be inhibited with soluble antigen. (3) All antigen binding cells appear to be surface immunoglobulin positive, but a substantial (>50%) fraction also bear T cell antigens. (4) After priming with two antigens, independent antigen binding cell populations are observed. Either the cells involved in antigen binding generate their own receptors or if these cells bind via cytophilic receptors, the receptors are acquired non randomly. (5) B10 mice which do not give an antibody response or T proliferative response to HEL also do not generate large numbers of antigen binding cells (<.2%). However, B10 mice primed with the closely related ring-necked pheasant lysozyme do generate large numbers of antigen binding cells that are crossreactive with HEL.

INTRODUCTION

The interplay of many different cell types in immune responses has become increasingly apparent. With this has come the realization that any single measurement of the effect of immunogen can grossly underestimate the induced perturbation of the immune system. The shock waves follow-

[1]This work was supported by USPHS AI 11183.
[2]Recipient of a Cancer Research Institute Postdoctoral fellowship.

ing the introduction of immunogen lead to expression of antigen-specific T and B cell functions as well as expansion of such indirect elements as idiotype-bearing lymphocytes. Within this complex network, it is of importance to document those cells which are involved in the binding of native and altered antigen and to assign them a position in the hierarchy of cell types involved in the overall response.

To accomplish this end, we have employed hen egg-white lysozyme (HEL), a stable globular protein with known conformation and amino acid sequence. The Ir gene control of this antigen has been studied in extenso (1,2). Furthermore, the particular value in choosing this antigen is that we have carefully investigated the specificity of T_h, T_s, and B cells for HEL and its peptides (3,4), and therefore, just from specificity arguments alone, would be able to make an assignment to different functional subpopulations of lymphocytes.

In this initial study, we have examined the frequency of antigen-binding cells (ABC) in a lymphoid compartment (the lymph node) where there is considerable expansion of ABC following the injection of immunogen. The properties of these ABC and their possible significance are described below.

METHODOLOGY

The antigen binding assay chosen for these studies involves binding antigen primed lymph nodes cells to HEL coupled goat red blood cells in a standard rosette assay.

Draining lymph nodes from antigen primed mice were analyzed for ABC because it was predicted that in these cases, the ABC would be amplified to a detectable number. CBA or B10.A mice were immunized with 10-100 µg HEL in complete Freund's adjuvant (CFA) intraperitoneally or subcutaneously at the base of the tail. Seven to ten days later, draining parathymic lymph nodes or pariaortic and inguinal lymph nodes (LNC) were removed and cells from these lymph nodes assessed for ABC. To form rosettes, 2×10^6 primed LNC plus 15×10^6 antigen coated goat red blood cells (AgGRBC) in 0.5 ml Click medium with 10% fetal calf serum were centrifuged 10 minutes at 100 x g. The pelleted mixture was incubated one hour on ice, and then resuspended by gently shaking or by rotating with a "Lab Quake" (5).

In order to preserve possible unstable antigen binding, the rosettes were fixed with glutaraldehyde (5). After resuspending the rosette mixture, glutaraldehyde was added immediately to a final concentration of 0.8%. After 20

minutes on ice, the fixative was washed out with water and
samples stored at 4°C until counting. Counting was facilitated by adding Giemsa stain. Only unclumped blue cells
binding four or more AgGRBC were scored as positive. 100-
150 rosettes or 30,000-50,000 total cells were scanned to
determine the frequency of antigen binding cells.

RESULTS

A High Frequency of Antigen Binding Cells is Dependent
on Specific Antigen Priming. The incidence of ABC increases
dramatically after injection with antigen in CFA. From a
background of less than 0.1%, the frequency of HEL-ABC
increases 6-8% after priming with HEL CFA. Figure 1 illustrates results from 19 experiments. In these cases, draining lymph node cells from CBA mice injected subcutaneously

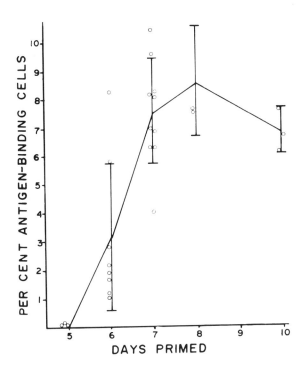

FIGURE 1. Frequency of antigen-binding cells after
antigen priming. Bars indicate mean ± standard deviation.
Circles represent individual experiments.

at the base of the tail with 10 μg HEL CFA were rosetted
with HEL coupled goat red blood cells (HEL GRBC). This
response is neither unique to HEL nor CBA mice. Priming
with other antigens (ring-necked pheasant lysozyme (REL) and
ribonuclease (RNAse)) and in other strains (A/J and B10.A)
yields comparable results.

Lymph node cells from mice primed to HEL bind only GRBC
coupled to HEL and <u>not</u> GRBC coupled to ribonuclease, another
globular protein similar in size and charge to HEL. Similarly, mice primed to ribonuclease bind only RNAse GRBC and
not HEL GRBC. This antigen binding can be inhibited specifically with soluble antigen. Inhibition was performed by
adding antigen at 500 μg/ml, 4°C, one hour before addition
of HEL GRBC (50% inhibition can be achieved with only 5 μg/
ml). Table I gives results from a representative experiment.
In this experiment, CBA mice were primed 8 days earlier with
either 10 μg HEL CFA or 100 μg RNAse CFA subcutaneously at
the base of the tail. As is shown, ABC are antigen specific
and can be only inhibited with the priming antigen.

The Majority of ABC Bear Both T and B Cell Markers.
The antigen binding cell type was evaluated by cytotoxic
treatment with antisera and complement. Table II shows a
representative experiment demonstrating that ABC include
both T and B cells. Treatment with rabbit anti-immunoglobulin and complement, but not the same serum absorbed with
normal mouse serum immobilized on affigel, removed all ABC.
Similarly, treatment with rabbit anti-mouse thymocyte serum
(absorbed with a non-secreting plasmacytoma) and both mouse
and rat anti-Thy.1 from hybridomas eliminated a substantial
proportion (from 50-90%) of ABC. ABC were resistant to the
same anti-thymocyte serum absorbed with mouse thymocytes

TABLE I
ANTIGEN BINDING CAN BE INHIBITED WITH SOLUBLE ANTIGEN

| Priming antigen | Inhibiting antigen | Per cent rosettes with | |
		HEL GRBC	RNAse GRBC
HEL	-	7.0	<0.02
	HEL	<0.01	
	RNAse	8.2	
RNAse	-	0.06	7.9
	RNAse		0.06
	HEL		10.1

TABLE II
SENSITIVITY OF REL PRIMED ANTIGEN-BINDING CELLS
TO TREATMENT WITH ANTISERA PLUS COMPLEMENT

Antisera treatment	Per cent HEL binding cells
None	9.0
Guinea pig C' alone	4.8
Rat anti-Thy.1 hybridoma	1.8
Mouse anti-Thy.1 hybridoma	1.7
Rabbit anti-mouse thymocyte	0.43
Rabbit anti-mouse Ig	0.74
Rabbit anti-mouse Ig absorbed of Ig activity	6.5

Representative experiment with B10 parathymic LNC primed 9 days i.p. with 100 μg REL CFA.

(data not shown). It appears that all ABC are surface Ig positive and a substantial fraction (>50%) bear T cell antigens.

Independent ABC Populations from Mice Primed with Two Antigens. Since all of the ABC seem to bear immunoglobulin, it was possible that the antigen binding receptors were passively acquired cytophilic immunoglobulin. If this were true it would be expected that mice primed to two antigens would have cells with two specificities of antigen-binding receptors. However, it was observed that priming with REL and RNAse, two unrelated antigens, yields largely non-overlapping populations of ABC, as is shown in Table III. Moreover, ABC of each specificity can be removed selectively on antigen coated plates. Independent antigen binding populations after priming with two antigens suggests that the cells involved had generated their own receptors or if

TABLE III
INDEPENDENT ANTIGEN BINDING POPULATIONS
FROM MICE PRIMED WITH TWO ANTIGENS

Priming antigen (B10 LNC)	Absorption with antigen coated plate	Per cent rosettes with	
		HEL GRBC	RNAse GRBC
10 μg RNAse CFA and 50 μg REL CFA	Untreated	7.2	12.9
	HEL-plate	0.34	10.1
	REL-plate	7.2	13.3
	RNAse-plate	4.8	0.02

TABLE IV
IR GENE CONTROL OF ANTIGEN-BINDING CELLS

Priming antigen	Mouse strain	Per cent HEL-binding cells ± S.D.
HEL	B10.A	6.2 ±4.4
HEL	B10	0.25±0.26
REL	B10	11.8 ±6.4

these cells bind antigen via cytophilic receptors, that the receptors had been acquired non-randomly.

The murine response to HEL is under known immune response gene (Ir) control. Unlike most other haplotypes, H-2^b (B10) mice fail to make an antibody (1) or T proliferative response to HEL under these priming conditions (6, Clarke and Maizels, in preparation) although they make a vigorous response to the closely related ring-necked pheasant lysozyme (REL). It was interesting to see whether the appearance of the characteristic large frequency of ABC was under similar Ir gene control. Antigen binding results from several experiments (Table IV) indicate that in contrast to B10.A mice, B10 mice do not generate high numbers of HEL ABC when primed with HEL. However, B10 mice make specific ABC responses to REL and RNAse (data not shown). A large proportion of rosettes in REL-primed B10 mice also bind HEL-GRBC (Table V). This is the same pattern as that seen in PFC and T proliferative responses to HEL. These features of the HEL antigen binding cell response seem to reflect immune response gene control.

TABLE V
REL PRIMED B10 LYMPH NODE CELLS CAN
FORM BOTH HEL AND REL ROSETTES

Experiment number	REL primed B10 cells rosetted with:		
	HEL GRBC	REL GRBC	RNAse GRBC
1	17.8	12.7	0.04
2	9.5	11.9	0.10
3	16.3	22.3	0.04
4	17.1	15.6	0.26

DISCUSSION

The functional cell type(s) involved in antigen binding after antigen priming is unclear but intriguing. It should be emphasized that a surprisingly large number of cells (5-15%) are involved in this antigen recognition. This incidence of ABC is considerably larger than that reported earlier by Chariere and Bach for HEL ABC (7). We believe that these authors failed to utilize optimal priming regimes. Here advantage was taken of recently primed draining lymph nodes in which the number of total lymphocytes and total ABC had been fully expanded. The extent that internal proliferation or recruitment from the circulating pool contributes to this expansion is unclear. The resulting ABC percentages are the same magnitude as those observed by Ternynck and Avrameas (8). They obtained 5% horseradish peroxidase binding cells in the popliteal lymph nodes 14 days after injection of horseradish peroxidase CFA in the hind footpads. Like HEL and RNAse ABC, peroxidase ABC are antigen specific and dependent on antigen priming. Involvement of such a large number of cells in response to antigen injection implies these ABC are immunologically relevant cells and must be considered in the context of the total immune response.

The cell surface phenotype of these ABC has been evaluated using specific antisera. These ABC are all sensitive to treatment with conventional anti-immunoglobulin serum and complement (in the presence of sodium azide). Nevertheless, a large fraction of these cells (50-90%) are also sensitive to rabbit anti-thymocyte serum or hybridoma-generated anti-Thy.1 plus complement. Thus, a large proportion of these ABC bear both Ig and T cell antigens. Since chicken anti-mouse Fab serum effectively blocks rosette formation (data not shown), it is likely that this Ig is relevant to the antigen binding. Although Ig on T cells is ordinarily not detectable with conventional anti-Ig reagents, recently, Avrameas, using an assay that carefully avoids receptor loss, has demonstrated substantial amounts of Ig on T cells with such sera (9).

It is unclear whether these ABC generate their own antigen binding receptors. The independence of the binding populations observed after priming with two antigens suggests, but does not prove, that these cells do indeed synthesize their own receptors. It is possible that receptors are obtained cytophilically, but non-randomly. For example, receptors could be acquired by direct cell-cell interaction, as might occur in a germinal center. It should be noted that stripping and resynthesis experiments have been successfully performed by others with T ABC: Owen, with idiotype binding cells (10), and Elliott, with T blasts which bind allogeneic cellular antigens (11).

There is considerable evidence that many murine T cells

prefer to respond to antigen in the context of products from
the major histocompatibility region (MHC). It is clear from
this report that T ABC are quite capable of recognition of
antigen in the absence of MHC antigens. Interaction by T
cells (12,13) with native antigen has also been reported
previously. The ABC reported here can bind antigen coupled
to goat RBC and adsorb readily to antigen coated plates.
Some suggestion of an MHC effect on idiotype binding by
idiotype-specific lymphocytes has been reported by Owen and
Nisonoff (14). Yet, with lysozyme and RNAse-coated plates
or antigen-coupled RBC, there is an absence of apparent MHC
recognition. These discrepancies may be due to the concentration or orientation of different antigens on the red cell
surface, affecting the degree of T cell binding. Therefore,
MHC antigens seem to be unnecessary for cellular recognition
of antigen but presumably are involved in cell triggering.
It is also possible that these T ABC include different T
cells that can react to native antigen, similar to B cells.
Such a cell could be important in antigen bridging between
regulatory lymphocytes.

Other investigators have observed T ABC and speculated
on their function. Elliott has shown that SRBC binding T
ABCs are not helper cells (15), but are probably cells
important in delayed type hypersensitivity (16). Eardley,
with cultured SRBC binding T cells (17), and Owen, with
idiotype-binding T ABCs (18) have evidence suggesting these
cells could be T suppressor cells. With lysozyme, B10 mice,
which are non-responders to HEL, are able to generate HEL-
specific T suppressor cells (12,13). However, large numbers
of HEL ABC were not present in HEL-primed B10 mice. After
a primary injection of antigen, T suppressor cells could be
present in small numbers, below the threshold of this ABC
assay. Preliminary results indicate that B10 mice given a
second injection of HEL do generate substantial numbers of
HEL T ABC. It could be speculated that in these boosted
mice, the incidence of T suppressor cells has been amplified
to a detectable level.

There are some preliminary specificity studies with
lysozyme which indicate that the bulk of ABC may constitute
cell types not previously described. T helper cells, T
suppressor cells, and T proliferating cells show extensive
crossreactivity for native HEL and reduced, carboxymethylated
HEL (RCM HEL) (6,19). That is, T cells from mice primed with
either HEL or RCM HEL are equally reactive with HEL. This
is despite the fact that HEL and RCM HEL show essentially no
crossreactivity at the antibody level (19). However,
priming with RCM HEL leads to generation of T cells which do
not form rosettes with HEL GRBC. On the other hand, ABC

primed with human lysozyme (HUL) show complete cross-reactivity with HEL. This is in contrast to plaque-forming cells from mice primed with HUL which are only poorly cross-reactive (<30%) with HEL. Therefore, ABC do not seem to share crossreactivity patterns with T helper, T suppressor, T proliferating, nor B cells.

The late incidence and high frequency of these ABC suggests that these cells represent an amplified end or effector stage, rather than an early regulatory event. The appearance of a large antigen-binding population to the draining lymph node would seem to answer the evolutionary need for a mechanism to react to the antigen which initiates the immune response. Such effector cells as delayed hypersensitive and cytotoxic cells have not directly been studied for their antigen-binding properties, but the rapid appearance of distinctive cellular markers may aid us in further identification of this interesting ABC population.

REFERENCES

1. Hill, S. W. and Sercarz, E. E. (1975). Eur. J. Immunol. 5, 317.
2. Sercarz, E. E., Yowell, R. L., Turkin, D., Miller, A., Araneo, B. A., and Adorini, L. (1978). Immunol. Rev. 39, 108.
3. Harvey, M. A., Adorini, L., Benjamin, C. B., Miller, A., and Sercarz, E. E. (1979). This volume.
4. Adorini, L., Miller, A., and Sercarz, E. E. (1979). J. Immunol. 122, 871.
5. Haskill, J. S., Elliott, E. B., Kerbel, R., Axelrod, M. A., and Eidinger, D. (1972). J. Exp. Med. 135, 1410.
6. Yowell, R. L., Araneo, B. A., Miller, A., and Sercarz, E. E. (1979). Nature, in press.
7. Charriere, J., Faure, A., and Bach, J-F. (1975). Immunol. 29, 423.
8. Ternynck, T., Rodrigot, M., and Avrameas, S. (1977). J. Immunol. 119, 1321.
9. Avrameas, S., Höseli, P., Stanislawski, M., Rodrigot, M., and Vogt, E. (1979). J. Immunol. 122, 648.
10. Owen, F. L., Ju, S-T., and Nisonoff, A. (1977). PNAS 74, 2084.
11. Elliott, B. E., Nagy, A., Nabholz, M., and Pernis, B. (1977). Eur. J. Immunol. 7, 287.
12. Tada, T. (1977). In "The Immune System II: Genetics and Regulation" (E. E. Sercarz, L. A. Herzenberg, and C. F. Fox, eds.), p. 345, Academic Press, New York.

13.   Krawinkel, U., Cramer, M., Imanishi-Kari, T., Jack,
      R. S., Rajewski, K., and Makela, O. (1977). Eur. J.
      Immunol. 8, 566.
14.   Owen, F. L., and Nisonoff, A. (1978). Cell Immunol.,
      37, 243.
15.   Elliott, B. E., Haskill, J. S., and Axelrod, M. A. (1973)
      J. Exp. Med. 138, 1133.
16.   Elliott, B. E., Haskill, J. S., and Axelrod, M. A. (1975)
      J. Exp. Med. 141, 584.
17.   Eardley, D. D., Shen, F. W., Cone, R. E., and Gershon,
      R. K. (1979). J. Immunol. 122, 140.
18.   Owen, F. L., Ju, S-T., and Nisonoff, A. (1977). J. Exp.
      Med. 145, 1559.
19.   Thompson, K., Harris, M., Benjamin, E., Mitchell, G., and
      Noble, M. (1972). Nature New Bio. 238, 20.

WORKSHOP SUMMARY: Role of the antigen-binding cell in immune responses. Robert F. Ashman (Dept. of Microbiology and Immunology, UCLA School of Medicine) and Alexander Miller (Dept. of Microbiology, UCLA College of Letters and Sciences) Los Angeles, California 90024.

The existence of antigen-binding cells (ABC) has tradi-tionally been considered one of the experimental pillars of the Clonal Selection Theory. Yet the early events following antigen contact with antigen reactive cells are often in-ferred indirectly from functional or mitogenic studies rather than by direct demonstration using the antigen-reactive cells themselves. One reason ABC are so seldom studied is that they cannot be equated with antigen-reactive cells without careful attention to the conditions under which ABC are assayed. It may be that under some conditions the ABC population may in-clude cells not involved in the immune response, which never-theless bind antigen via low affinity or cytophilic "recep-tors". The ABC which are antigen-reactive are a heterogeneous mixture of various T and B subpopulations. Some antigen re-active cells may have too few receptors to be scored as ABC. In view of these difficulties, the audience was urged to query speakers regarding a) the probable nature of the receptor b) specificity of ABC at the level of binding and induction c) the subpopulations included or excluded, especially T cells and non-lymphoid cells and d) the precursor functions demon-strable within the ABC, and precursor frequencies. Few if any studies have dealt with all these aspects of their ABC populations.

Four areas of active investigation were discussed at this workshop: 1) specificity restriction of receptors on ABC; 2) the heterogeneity of ABC in terms of T and B sub-populations, ontogeny, receptor density and other aspects of physiology; 3) early events of ABC responding to antigen; 4) the behavior of ABC in tolerant or congenitally unresponsive animals.

1) Specificity restriction. De Luca summarized experi-ments extending his previous work on ABC. He has shown that about ¼ of lymphoid cells from adult bone marrow or neonatal spleen bind each protein antigen tested. As much as 5% will non-competitively bind both of a given pair of antigens. Double binding ABC from marrow tend to be larger than single-binding ABC. The number of B cells binding a given antigen in adult spleen is less, as is the number of double ABC. The clonal nature of antigen binding was demonstrated by antigen binding studies of whole colonies derived from bone marrow B cells which showed clear segregation of binding capacity for different antigens. It was suggested that multiple binding ABC

are pre-B cells which give rise to clones or more restricted
binding capacity as they mature.

2) Heterogeneity of ABC. Eardley summarized her recently published work (J. Immunol. 122, 140 (1979) on generation in vitro of T cells which specifically bind sheep red
blood cells. At the peak of the ABC response, these cells are
mainly $Ly2^+$ and nylon wool adherent whereas non-immune are
are mostly by 1^+2^+, and nylon wool non adherent. Stable
hybridomas derived from these cells have been cloned by
Eardley and N. Ruddle.

Clarke summarized her work* on the formation of specific
ABC for lysozymes found at a frequency of 5-15%, 7-10 days after immunization, they are antigen-specific, show single rather
than multiple binding, and are absent when genetically nonresponding strains are immunized with the appropriate test
antigen. These ABC are all killed by anti-Ig and complement.
However, a large proportion (50-90%) are also sensitive to
rabbit anti-thymocyte sera as well as hybridoma-derived anti-
Thy 1.

Elliott described an assay for T cells activated in the
primary MLR which involved binding radiolabelled membrane
vesicles derived from the stimulator cells. He could show
that reactive cells early in the response are blasts which
later give rise to small lymphocytes and that vesicle binding
offers some promise as a method of quantifying receptor density and/or avidity.

Greenstein presented her work on FACS sorting of TNP-
binding cells through use of fluoresceinated TNP-BSA. She
reported that the parameter of cell size (measured by time of
flight) is being incorporated into their sorting procedure
and will then allow sorting of cells by density of bound
fluorochrome.

3) Early events in ABC. According to Ashman, early
events in B ABC for sheep erythrocytes (SRC) following antigen contact include capping (15 min), acceleration of phospholipid synthesis (8 hr), acceleration of receptor recovery
after pronase treatment (maximal recovery shifts from 18 hr.
to 2 hr. within a day after antigen given in vivo), proliferation, and changes in surface isotypes.

By combining hydroxyurea inhibition, autoradiography and
immunofluorescent identification of T and B ABC, Merrill has
demonstrated the continuous and major contribution of cell
division to the generation of T and B ABC in response to SRC
in vitro.* The cell division-independent rise in ABC on day
1 was attributable to T ABC. Autoradiography showed that non-
ABC dividing in the first 24 hr. after antigen gave rise to ABC
later in the response, implying maturation of denser receptor
displays.

By inhibition of antigen-binding with anti-μ, anti-γ or anti-δ, Kanowith-Klein showed that non-immune B ABC bear surface μ and δ. In contrast, day 5 ABC have lost δ and gained γ, belonging to a variety of phenotypes including $\mu^+\delta^-\gamma^-$, $\mu^+\delta^-\gamma^+$, $\mu^+\delta^+\gamma^+$ (suggested as a transition stage), $\mu^+\delta^+\gamma^-$ (reduced in proportion from before immunization), and $\mu^-\delta^-\gamma^+$. In the primary in vitro culture system, Merrill showed that the B ABC population passed through a $\mu^+\delta^+\gamma^+$ stage to become $\mu^+\delta^-\gamma^+$.

4) ABC in immunologically unresponsive animals. Desaymard reported that the induction of tolerance to thymus independent antigens in B-ABC was inhibited by a variety of agents which interfere with capping including metabolic inhibitors, cytochalasin B and colchicine, lanthanum and zinc; others remain to be tested. Capping of sIgM by anti-μ permitted lower amounts of antigen to induce unresponsiveness, but anti-δ did not show this effect. This positive relationship between capping and tolerance stands in contrast to systems such as the TNP-tolerant B cell of Ashman and Naor and the polymerized flagellin binding cell of Diener, et al. where tolerance is associated with membrane locking.

Another model of unresponsiveness is the CBA/N mouse, which is unresponsive to phosphoryl choline (PC). F_1 males share this unresponsiveness whereas females are responsive. According to Kaplan,* the males have normal numbers of PC binding cells and their T cells help PC responses normally, but PC-fowl gamma globulin fails to expand the PC-ABC population normally. The same is true for neonatal BALB/c mice, also unresponsive to PC, suggesting that an antigen-independent maturation step is lacking in CBA/N cells without which the PC-ABC cannot undergo antigen-stimulated immune induction. Scott reminded us that the fluorescein (Flu) binding cells in neonatally Flu-tolerant mice behave similarly.

Participants:

Dominic de Luca	Julia Greenstein
Jessica Clarke	Susan Kanowith-Klein
Diane Eardley	Catherine Desaymard
Ruth Kaplan	Bruce Elliott

*data presented elsewhere in this volume.

RESTRAINTS ON CURRENT CONCEPTS OF SELF-TOLERANCE

E. Diener and C.A. Waters, with the collaboration
of B. Singh

Department of Immunology and MRC Group
on Immunoregulation
University of Alberta
Edmonton, Alberta, Canada T6G 2H7

ABSTRACT We have assessed the tolerogenic potency of
human γ-globulin (HGG), bovine serum albumin (BSA) and
a synthetic peptide of defined geometry ("18") by ad-
ministering these antigens *in utero* to BALB/cCr and to
congenic C3H.A and C3H.OH mice. Maternal influences on
the outcome of these experiments were excluded. Contrary to expectation, only deaggregated HGG but not BSA
or "18", including their hapten derivatives, possessed
tolerogenicity *in utero* even though all three substances
were shown to cross the placenta and to be present in
the offspring's serum three weeks after birth at
concentrations of 10^{-6} molar. These findings put
constraints on current concepts of self-tolerance. An
alternative model based on a dual recognition system is
proposed. As for HGG, unresponsiveness in the offspring
was specific and complete for both T and B cells and
waned in parallel with loss of antigen from the circulation by 15 to 20 weeks of postnatal life. Experiments
to monitor HGG specific suppressor cells in tolerant
offspring showed that during, but not before, the postnatal period of tolerance breakdown, suppressor cells
could regularily be found.

INTRODUCTION

It appears fair to assume that the rationale behind the
work of those investigators who have contributed to the
current literature on tolerance is their desire to arrive,
by extrapolation of experimental phenomena, at a plausible
and generally applicable theory on mechanisms of self-
tolerance. However, the experimental manifestations of
tolerance to foreign antigens are so diverse that at least
three different mechanisms must be considered when
speculating about their applicability to theories on
tolerance to self.

Receptor Blockade. The term receptor blockade is best used to describe a state in B cells whereby surface receptors become immobilized by a lattice of a multivalent ligand. Ideally, such a lattice forms most readily *in vitro* at 4° incubation of immunocompetent cells with a suitable antigen so as to allow receptor ligand cross-linking without interference from capping (1). Certain antigens, however, can also bring about unresponsiveness by receptor blockade under physiological conditions *in vivo* (2-9). In some cases, where the receptors are freed from antigen by suitable manipulation of the cells concerned, responsiveness may return (3,4,6,8,9). On occasion, however, receptor blockade induced by some antigens has also been shown to be associated with irreversible tolerance (1,2). As for the receptor blockade induced by isologous IgG it has, for example, been suggested that this may be accompanied by suppressor T cell-mediated tolerance (5). Although receptor blockade in most cases concerns B cells, the same phenomenon may also apply for T cells (5).

Clonal Deletion-Abortion. Evidence for clonal deletion has first been shown in an *in vitro* tolerance induction model (10). In contrast to an unresponsive state achieved by receptor blockade, clonal deletion-abortion is, in most cases, preceded by receptor modulation (1,11). This does not exclude the possibility that for some antigens, receptor blockade may occur as an epiphenomenon besides metabolically-mediated irreversible tolerance (1). Receptor modulation involves ligand-induced pinocytosis or, depending primarily on the size of the ligand, the shedding of ligand-receptor complexes from the surface of an immunocompetent cell. In adult B cells, such immunogen-induced receptor modulation deprives the cell of its capacity to bind antigen for a period of 8 to 24 hours, after which time new receptors reappear on the surface membrane, thus restoring the cell's recognition potential. When receptor modulation is brought about by an antigen under conditions that favor tolerance induction, re-expression of antigen recognition fails to take place (1,11). This phenomenon has been demonstrated in adult B cells (clonal deletion) (1,11) and in B cells from neonatal animals (12) (clonal abortion). The discovery that most B cells in adults bear both IgM and IgD receptors, in contrast to the large numbers of solely IgM-bearing B cells in neonates, has led to speculations concerning a functional dichotomy between IgM and IgD cell surface isotypes. It was hypothesized that IgM receptors could only convey a tolerogenic signal and that therefore the exquisite sensitivity of immature B cells to tolerance induction was due to the binding of the antigen to these receptors. The additional appearance of IgD receptors

during ontogenic maturation of such cells was seen as an
important step in the development of resistance to tolerance
induction (13,14). Experimental data on this subject, however, are not all in support of this hypothesis (15).
Attempts to find a correlation between various types of receptor modulation and the tolerogenic or immunogenic potential
of an antigen have been without success. The only visually
and functionally testable feature that distinguishes immunity
from tolerance induction at the level of the immunocompetent
cell is that in the latter case, receptors are not re-
expressed (1,11). It is of particular interest in this
context that receptor re-expression after interaction of B
cells with a tolerogenic dose of POL can be brought about by
the treatment of such cells with Colchicin. In spite of
having their antigen-binding capacity restored, however, such
cells still fail to generate an immune response to an
immunogenic dose of POL (1). This suggests that tolerance
induction under these conditions is brought about by intracellular events in addition to those which result in absence
of antigen receptors.

Cell-Mediated Suppression. By now, the concept of suppressor cell-mediated (infectious) tolerance (16) has so much
become part of an immunologist's conscience that it needs no
detailed introduction in the context of this discussion.
Suffice it to say that the evidence regarding suppressor cells
as immunoregulatory elements is strong, but it is yet unclear
whether these cells play a role in the induction and maintenance of tolerance to self.

Among the three phenomena just described, reversible
receptor blockade is least likely to play an important role
in self-tolerance, with the possible exception of those self-
antigens present in very high molar concentrations. Furthermore, under those circumstances where receptor blockade simply
represents a prelude to the induction of irreversible tolerance, i.e. the functional elimination of the cells concerned,
it ceases to be conceptually meaningful. In continuing our
discussion, clonal deletion and/or active suppression will
therefore be considered as possible mechanisms of self-
tolerance.

Most models on tolerance have derived from experiments on
adult or neonatal lymphocytes *in vivo* or *in vitro* with
antigens deliberately selected for tolerogenicity. The
possibility must therefore be considered that these systems
provide us with a rather biased spectrum of interpretations
which may have little in common with self-tolerance. In view
of these considerations, we felt it appropriate to utilize a
model system for tolerance induction which permits access of

the extrinsic test antigen to the fetus well before
immunocompetent cells arise. Thus, in terms of current
thinking, the source of the antigen is the only parameter in
our experimental system that differs from the physiological
conditions of self-tolerance. The objectives of our study
were: first, to find evidence for the presence of suppressor
cells during the state of *in utero*-induced tolerance; second,
to test whether the exposure of the ontogenically immature
immune system *in vivo* to an antigen not deliberately chosen
for its tolerogenic potential is sufficient for tolerance
induction.

MATERIALS AND METHODS

Materials and methods are described elsewhere in
detail (20).

RESULTS

Tolerance Induction *In Utero* to HGG. In the following
series of experiments, deaggregated human gamma globulin
(dHGG) was used as the antigen of choice, for it had been
shown to represent one of the most potent tolerogens in
adult and neonatal animals of various species. Furthermore,
antigen specific suppressor cells have been demonstrated by
others in association with adult tolerance to this gamma
globulin (17).

Transfer of dHGG Across the Placenta, its Concentration
and Tissue Distribution Pattern in the Offspring. To derive
at a meaningful interpretation of the postnatal immune status
of an animal after treatment *in utero* with a potential
tolerogen, the kinetics of antigen distribution and concentration in the offspring throughout its fetal and early postnatal life must be known. For this purpose, BALBc/Cr female
mice at 15 days of gestation were administered 5 mg of dHGG,
1% of which had been labeled with ^{125}I, and the fetuses recovered 48 hrs. thereafter. Half of the offspring were processed for autoradiography and the other half thoroughly
homogenized in 10% Trichloroacetic acid (TCA). After washing
of this material with 10% TCA until no more than 10% of the
total radioactive count could be found in the supernatant,
^{125}I-labeled protein in the pellet was counted. It was found
that on the average, 0.3-0.5% of the total amount of labeled
HGG injected into the mother had passed transplacentally into
each fetus (based on an average litter size of 10). As evidenced by our autoradiographic studies and in support of
studies by others on antigen distribution patterns in neonatal

animals (18), ^{125}I-HGG was found distributed throughout the entire fetus at more or less uniform concentrations, including thymus, spleen and liver. Next we determined the rate of disappearance of HGG in the serum of mice treated in utero with the antigen. HGG concentrations were individually determined by radioimmunoassay. Results from these studies show that even as late as twelve weeks of age, µg/ml amounts of HGG were still present in the sera of animals that had received the antigen *in utero*. (Figure 1).

Postnatal Tolerance to HGG in Mice after Exposure to the Antigen *In Utero*. Eight-week-old offspring from BALBc/Cr mothers that had received 5 mg of dHGG on day 14-15 of pregnancy were tested for HGG specific unresponsiveness in both T and B cells. To test T cell function, the mice were challenged with TNP-HGG and their spleens individually assayed for the presence of anti-TNP specific 7S plaque-forming cells. Similarly, in studies on B cell tolerance, numbers of anti-HGG 7S plaque-forming cells were assessed in the spleens of putatively tolerant mice after they had been challenged with HGG-coated burro erythrocytes. As a specificity control, 7S plaque-forming cells reactive to burro erythrocytes were also enumerated. Similarly, mice tested for T cell responsiveness were challenged with either TNP-chicken gamma globulin (TNP-CGG) or TNP-bovine serum albumin (TNP-BSA).

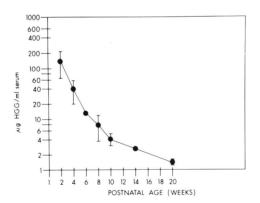

FIGURE 1. Rate of disappearance of HGG in serum of mice that had received dHGG *in utero*. Serum samples were taken from mice of various ages after tolerance induction *in utero* and HGG concentration individually determined by radioimmuno-assay. Data represent the arithmetic mean of 3 to 4 mice per group ± S.D. 6-week and 14-week ages represent data from one mouse only.

Results from these experiments show that *in utero*HGG-treated mice at eight weeks of age were specifically unresponsive to this antigen at both the level of T and B cells (Figures 2a, b; Table I). Table I also shows that during the 11-13 week period, some recovery of T and B cell responsiveness could be observed with more animals falling into response groups within 3-4 standard deviations of the control.

There have been reports indicating that under certain conditions tolerance may be induced in suckling mice by transfer of tolerogen contained in the mother's milk (19). To ascertain that in our experimental model exposure of the off-spring *in utero* was sufficient for tolerance induction, a foster nursing experiment was designed in which normal lac-tating mothers were used to foster-nurse the Caesarean-delivered babies of dHGG-treated mothers. When challenged at six weeks of age, dHGG-treated litters nursed either by their own or by foster mothers were completely unresponsive to the antigen. At 12 to 18 weeks of age, when some waning of un-responsiveness can normally be observed, both treated groups yielded a 7S plaque-forming cell response of the same magni-tude (20). Thus we may conclude that *in utero* exposure of mouse fetuses to HGG is sufficient to induce a long lasting postnatal state of tolerance. Recent observations have

TABLE I

WANING OF IN UTERO INDUCED TOLERANCE

Postnatal age (wks)	n S.D.*	% Animals responding within n S.D. of mean control PFC response	
		T cells	B cells
6-8	n = 1	–	–
	2	–	–
	3	–	–
	4	–	10
	5	9	10
11-13	n = 1	–	–
	2	–	–
	3	6	20
	4	18	30
	5	31	50
15-18	n = 1	–	–
	2	9	10
	3	25	20
	4	55	40
	5	68	40

* n = integer denoting multiple of standard deviations (S.D.) from geometric mean of normal controls.

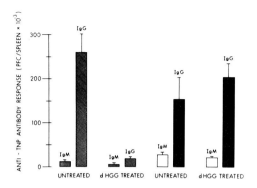

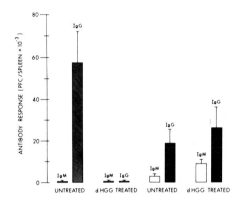

FIGURE 2a,b. T and B cell tolerance induced *in utero* to dHGG. (a) IgM and IgG PFC were enumerated in the individual spleens of 11-week-old mice treated with dHGG *in utero* and challenged with an immunogenic preparation of TNP·HGG or TNP CGG. ▨ TNP·HGG, IgG response; ▩ TNP·HGG, IgM response; ■ TNP·CGG, IgG response; ☐ TNP·CGG, IgM response.

(b) IgM and IgG PFC were enumerated in the individual spleens of 8-week-old mice treated with dHGG *in utero* and challenged with HGG coupled to BRBC. ▨ HGG, IgG response; ▦ HGG, IgM response; ■ BRBC, IgG response; ☐ BRBC, IgM response.

Data are presented as the geometric mean ± S.E. Differences between experimental and control groups p < 0.001.

established the fact that ontogenically immature immunocompetent B cells exhibit a heightened susceptibility to tolerance

induction relative to B cells from adult animals (12,21).
Based on this observation, we determined the amount of dHGG
that would minimally be required during postnatal life to
maintain this state of *in utero*-induced tolerance in the absence of mature immunocompetent cells. Mice treated *in utero*
with dHGG (5 mg administered to the mother) were given decreasing amounts (1 mg to 1 ng per animal) of dHGG beginning
at three weeks of age and continuing biweekly until immuno-
genically challenged with HGG at fifty weeks of age. A control group received no additional dHGG after birth. As
evidenced from the previous experiments, waning of HGG specific tolerance in the absence of additional dHGG progressively
increased until, by 40 weeks of age, *in utero*-tolerized
animals had recovered full responsiveness. In contrast, biweekly administration of as little as 10 µg dHGG to mice
which had received the antigen *in utero* maintained tolerance
during the 50 week postnatal period of interest (Figure 3).
It is important to note that B cells required 100fold more
dHGG (10 µg) than did T cells in order for tolerance to remain
complete (20). This agrees with observations made in experi-

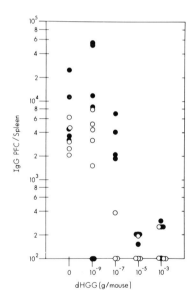

FIGURE 3. Mice treated *in utero* with dHGG were given
decreasing amounts of dHGG beginning at 3 weeks of age and
continuing biweekly until testing at 50 weeks of age. One
group was challenged with an immunogenic preparation of TNP·
HGG to assess T cell unresponsiveness (0); the other group was
immunized with HGG-coupled BRBC to assess B cell unresponsiveness (●).

ments by others on adult mice demonstrating kinetic differences in unresponsiveness between T and B cells (22).

   In Search of Suppressor Cells in Mice Rendered Tolerant
In Vivo. In the assumption that *in utero*-induced tolerance
to HGG is analogous to self-tolerance, then the presence of
HGG specific suppressor cells in such an unresponsive state
would impute active suppression as a potential element in
self-tolerance. Suppressor cells have been reported to be
associated with tolerance to HGG in adult animals (17,23,24).
The transient nature of these cells, however, has cautioned
some investigators against implicating them as the cause of
tolerance (17). For these reasons, we have examined the offspring from mothers treated with 5 mg of dHGG for the presence of suppressor cells, using admixtures of normal and
tolerant spleen cells transferred to lethally irradiated
syngeneic recipients, challenged with HGG. Significant suppression of adoptive immunity was taken to indicate the
presence of suppressor cells. Results of these experiments
appeared to reflect two distinct stages in the kinetic
pattern of the tolerant state: 1. Spleen cells from 4 to 6-
week-old mice treated *in utero* with dHGG consistently failed
to suppress normal cells even when twice as many tolerant
cells were transferred. 2. A mixture of equal numbers of
normal spleen cells and spleen cells from 14-week and older
mice treated *in utero* with dHGG resulted in a 70 per cent
reduction of the normal adoptive response (20) (Figure 4 a,b).
It is important to note that the presence in tolerant mice of
suppressor cells coincided with the period when the tolerant
state began to break down between 14 to 33 weeks of age, the
last point of testing. The suppressor population was relatively resistant to a single treatment with anti-Thy 1 antiserum and complement. It is of interest in this regard that
other investigators have described a suppressor cell expressing Ly $1^+2^+3^+$ Qal$^+$ that is also resistant to the treatment
with anti-Thy 1 and complement. Furthermore, this suppressor
cell was shown to depend on the presence of a Thy 1^+ Ly 1^+
2,3$^-$ Qal$^+$ helper cell population in order to exert a feedback
suppressor effect *in vitro*. (25,26). It appears reasonable
therefore to expect the appearance of suppressor cells in our
in vivo experiments at the time of tolerance breakdown. We
conclude from our study that the state of tolerance resulting
from *in utero* exposure of an animal to the antigen appears not
to depend on the presence of active suppression. In view of
a recent hypothesis on immune network regulation by T cell
microcircuits, an alternative explanation is possible. Thus
the regulatory circuits operating to maintain the stable phase
of tolerance would consist of cell subsets of such a limited

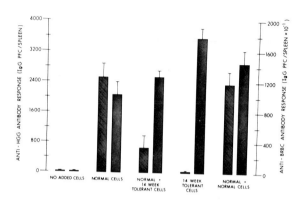

a

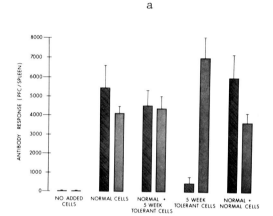

b

FIGURE 4 a,b. Active suppression is present in (a) 14-week-old, but not in (b) 5-week-old mice treated *in utero* with dHGG. Adoptive cell transfer to irradiated recipients of 7×10^7 normal or tolerant spleen cells alone or a 1:1 mixture of both populations was followed by challenge with both, heat-aggregated HGG and BRBC. After an additional challenge, mice were sacrificed and IgG PFC to HGG and to BRBC were enumerated in individual spleens. Data represent geometric means ± S.E. ▨ HGG; ▨ BRBC.
(a) 14-week-old, active suppression (p < 0.02).
(b) 5-week-old, lack of suppression.

clone size that they would escape detection. It is only
during the phase of recovery from tolerance that sufficient
help is available for induction and subsequent expansion of
the suppressor clone (27).

Do Antigens Other Than HGG Induce Tolerance *In Utero*?
None of the current models of self-tolerance in their simplest
version places any constraints upon the nature of the antigen
or its mode of presentation to the immune system. In fact,
the most popular idea at present stresses the stage in ontogenic maturation of potentially immunocompetent cells as the
decisive factor in self-tolerance induction. This implies
that any antigen, be it self or foreign, should, in appropriate concentration and overall affinity for cell surface
receptors, be equally effective in inducing unresponsiveness
provided it interacts with the immune system during the developmental phase of tolerance susceptibility. Should it
become evident that either the nature of an antigen or its
mode of presentation conditions the outcome of its encounter
with the lymphoid system, then the general applicability of
any of the current molecular models of self-tolerance would
become questionable. With these considerations in mind, we
have investigated the tolerogenic potency *in utero* of two
antigens in addition to HGG, namely bovine serum albumin
(BSA), and [GluTyrLys(GluTyrAla)$_5$]$_n$, a synthetic haptenated
peptide of defined geometry known as "18" (28). As was for
HGG in the previous experiment, the transplacental diffusion
of BSA and trinitrophenylated "18" (TNP-"18") was assessed by
both autoradiography and radioimmunoassay. BALBc/Cr females
at 14 to 15 days of gestation were injected with BSA or TNP-
"18" labeled with ^{125}I, the fetuses recovered 48 hours thereafter and their content of antigen assessed by means of TCA
precipitable material and by autoradiography. For control
reference, the same experiment was carried out but using
radio-labeled HGG. All three antigens were shown to cross the
placenta (Table II). HGG had the highest rate of transfer as
may be expected, based on our current knowledge of gamma
globulin transport. Substantial amounts of BSA and TNP-"18"
were also found in the fetuses and neonates, even though no
specific transport mechanisms for these substances are known.
TNP-"18" had a somewhat higher rate of diffusion, probably
because of its lower molecular weight (monomeric form MW
2500; polymeric form Poly-"18" MW 12,000). It is known that
the maintenance of the tolerant state depends on the presence
of the tolerogen concerned. For interpretation of our data
on tolerance induction to BSA and Poly "18" or their trinitrophenylated derivatives, it was therefore of interest to monitor the concentration of *in utero*-administered antigen in

TABLE II

TRANSPLACENTAL TRANSFER OF ^{125}I·HGG, ^{125}I·BSA
AND ^{125}I·TNP "18" AT 15 TO 17 DAYS OF GESTATION

Antigen	Specific activity TCA cpm/μg	Total protein injected	% total protein labeled	TCA cpm/ml mother serum	TCA cpm/g fetus
^{125}I·HGG	1.2×10^5	5	1.6	63.6×10^4	17.7×10^4
^{125}I·BSA	1.6×10^5	5	1.6	5.9×10^4	0.8×10^4
^{125}I·TNP· "18"	1.8×10^4	0.5	20	1.3×10^4	2.7×10^4

the serum of mice during the first few weeks of postnatal
life. As discussed earlier for HGG, monitoring of Poly–TNP–
"18" serum levels by means of radioimmunoassay has so far
been carried out. The maternally administered amount of
Poly–TNP."18" at 15 days of gestation was 1 mg. Results from
such measurements on the serum of one and three–week–old *in
utero*–treated offspring indicate the presence of the synthetic peptide in concentrations of approximately the same
molarity as that of similarly administered HGG measured in
three–week–old mice (Table III). It is of interest to note
that, for Poly "18," the serum concentrations at one and
three weeks of age did not in general significantly differ
from each other. This agrees with work by others who have
pointed out the lack of catabolic removal of antigen in the
immunologically incompetent animal (18). Autoradiographic
studies of thymus, liver and spleen of 17–day–old fetuses
and of 7–day and 35–day–old postnatal animals which had received ^{125}I.HGG, ^{125}I.BSA or ^{125}I.TNP "18" on day 15 *in utero*
indicate a similar distribution pattern in all three organs
for the three antigens. Moreover, the grain density was
comparably high in all three cases. The various antigens
tested differed drastically from HGG in their capacity to induce tolerance upon administration *in utero*. Thus, in contrast to HGG, neither "18," poly–"18," or BSA, including
their trinitrophenylated forms, were capable of inducing
tolerance (Table III, Figure 5). Although no evidence was
found for a maternal antibody response to HGG, the existence
of genetic nonresponders for "18" permitted us to more
definitively rule out maternal influences on the immune status
of *in utero* antigen–treated offspring. For "18," including
its polymeric form, genetic nonresponsiveness is recessive
and does not appear to be associated with suppressor cell
activity (28). As was the case with BALBc/Cr mice, (C3H.OH
x C3H.A)F$_1$ responder offspring from C3H.A nonresponder mated

TABLE III

"18," POLY"18" AND POLYTNP"18" FAIL TO INDUCE TOLERANCE *IN UTERO*

Mother	Father	Antigen	[Antigen] in: Mother µg/ml serum	[Antigen] in: Offspring µg/ml serum	Maternal response % antigen bound[3] IgM	IgG	Litter response % antigen bound[3] IgM	IgG
BALB/cCr	BALB/cCr	-	< 1	< 1	< 1	< 1	17.7±0.8	42.8±2.1
"	"	Poly"18" 4)	19.2 1)	1.4 1)	18.0	38.3	19.5±4.5	40.4±5.1 6)
"	"	"	19.2	4.0	22.0	38.1	17.9±0.4	40.2±5.2
BALB/cCr	BALB/cCr	-	< 1	< 1	< 1	< 1	25.3±9.8	56.6±4.3
"	"	PolyTNP"18" 4)	17.2 1)	3.8 1)	23.1	34.5	23.9±7.6	62.1±5.8 6)
"	"	"	17.2	1.8	61.6	36.0	24.3±2.5	64.9±8.3
C3H.A	C3H.OH	-	< 1	< 1	< 1	< 1	14.7±1.5	26.5±1.8
"	"	"18" 5)	15.8 1)	3.8 1)	2.4	2.3	13.4±3.9	22.1±1.2 7)
"	"	"	12.0	3.3	2.7	3.0	9.4±2.2	26.6±5.2
C3H.OH	C3H.A	-	< 1	< 1	< 1	< 1	15.0±3.6	25.1±2.3
"	"	"18" 5)	24.4 2)	4.3 2)	10.3	23.7	13.2	23.6 7)
"	"	"	25.8	2.7	7.7	20.5	9.9	22.0

1) At 1 week after birth

2) At 3 weeks after birth

3) % Antigen bound per 50 µl serum

4) 1 mg at day 15 *in utero*

5) 500 µg at day 14 *in utero*

6) Age of litter at testing, 8 weeks

7) Age of litter at testing, 6 weeks

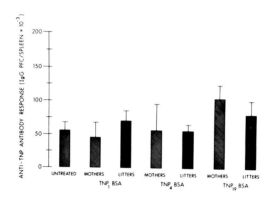

FIGURE 5. TNP-BSA fails to induce tolerance *in utero*, regardless of hapten density. IgG PFC were enumerated in the individual spleens of 8-week-old mice treated with TNP-BSA *in utero* and challenged with an immunogenic preparation of TNP-BSA. Data are presented as the geometric mean ± S.E.

with C3H.OH responder males still failed to be susceptible to tolerance induction *in utero* by "18" (Table III). These results are entirely unexpected since current thinking on tolerance induction during ontogeny of the immune system predicts no difference in the tolerogenic potential between various antigens.

DISCUSSION

Insofar as any model on self-tolerance which relies on the use of extrinsic antigens can conform to possibly peculiar structural properties or modes of presentation germane to true self-antigens, our experiments have at least ruled out interference from those regulatory effector functions which are exclusively a characteristic of immunocompetent animals. Possible maternal influences on the outcome of these experiments have also been excluded by means of foster-nursed Caesarean-delivered young, and by using genetic nonresponders as mothers of F_1 responder offspring. Two important findings have emerged from these studies, one of which we shall discuss first, since it may call into question some of the prevailing thoughts about self-tolerance; our data concerning tolerance induction via a transplacental route indicate that the tolerogenic potential of an extrinsic antigen depends on

its molecular structure rather than the developmental stage
of the immune system. When each of the three antigens, HGG,
BSA, "18", and in the latter two cases, their trinitrophenylated derivatives, were administered transplacentally to fetal
mice, only HGG but not the other antigens were capable of inducing tolerance in T and B lymphocytes of the offspring. All
three antigens did however cross the placenta and remained at
µg/ml serum concentrations in the animals for several weeks
postnatally. It is known from experiments on adult animals
that antigens differ widely in their tolerogenic potential
(29). Such differences have been attributed to the carrier
portion of an antigen rather than the nature of its epitopes
(5). Contrary to our results, at least one theory on self-
tolerance would have predicted such differences to be irrelevant within the realms of the immature system of the fetus and
the newborn (30). The clonal abortion hypothesis predicts a
phase in lymphocyte maturation when contact with antigen can
only result in immunological paralysis (31). According to the
two-signal theory on immune induction (30,32), the ability of
an antigen to convey a tolerogenic signal invariably depends
on the binding of antigen to the cell's receptors in the absence of any helper effect from T cells or macrophages. The
theory puts no constraints on the molecular nature of the
antigen other than to ask that a sufficient number of antigen-receptor complexes form on the cell surface to generate a
tolerogenic signal. Defendants of this theory may argue that,
in our experiments, the failure of BSA and "18" to induce
tolerance *in utero* could be due to the presence of sufficient
help even in the immunologically immature state of the fetus.
This argument is unlikely to be valid since we have been
equally unable to induce tolerance to these antigens even
when they were administered twice, once at a time of embryonic
development before differentiation into lymphoid tissue is
observed, and a second time four days before birth (data not
shown). From our earlier work on adult B cell tolerance *in
vitro*, we have stated that the prerequisite for an antigen to
induce tolerance resides in its multivalency, so as to effect
receptor cross-linking beyond a minimal threshold. (33). This
conclusion has been applied by others to the neonatal B cell;
multivalent dinitrophenylated derivatives of various proteins
were capable of inducing tolerance in neonatal B cells at
concentrations that were ineffective for adult B cells (21).
Contrary to our expectation, none of the multivalent forms of
"18" (TNP_2."18"; TNP_6.poly-"18") or of BSA (TNP_1BSA; TNP_4BSA;
$TNP_{19}BSA$) were capable of inducing tolerance *in utero*,
even though the binding affinities for TNP_6 poly-"18" and
for $TNP_{19}BSA$ are expected to be higher than for those
derivatives of lower substitution ratio. Our data are in

better agreement with those from another laboratory where the
tolerogenic potency of even oligovalent HGG on neonatal B
cells was demonstrated *in vitro*. The investigators pointed
out that, unlike HGG, BSA was a poor tolerogen, even for neonatal cells (12). We derive from these and our own data that
polyvalent interaction of self-antigens with surface receptors
cannot be part of the mechanism by which self-tolerance is induced. A further possible objection to our conclusions main-
tains that the absence of a tolerant state to BSA or "18" at
time of testing is due to the failure of maintaining a sufficiently high concentration of antigen in the offspring in
order to prevent spontaneous breakdown of unresponsiveness
during the period between birth and the time of immunogenic
challenge. It must be considered that all three antigens
used in our experiments, after having been administered to the
offspring *in utero*, remained in the serum in concentrations
of approximately equal molarity of between 0.3×10^6 and 1.3×10^6
during their first few weeks of postnatal life. For compari-
son, antigen dose-response studies by others for tolerance
induction in neonatal B cells to HGG *in vitro* have shown the
lowest effective concentration of the tolerogen to be between
2.5×10^{-9} and 2.5×10^{-10} M (12). It is noteworthy in this context that soluble self-antigens such as somatotropin, insulin,
ACTH, thyrotropin and others occur at serum concentrations in
the range of 2×10^{-9} to 2×10^{-10}M. Organ specific antigens are
expected to be entirely cell bound and are therefore not detected in the serum in measurable amounts. In summing up
what we have discussed so far, we feel justified in concluding
from our experiments that the ontogenic state of the lymphoid
system is not the only parameter that determines tolerance to
self. Furthermore, the encounter of an immunocompetent cell
or its precursor with antigen, in the absence of help from
either T cells or macrophages, does not appear to necessarily
lead to tolerance. It follows that the mechanism by which
tolerance to self is induced depends on either the nature of
self-antigens or their mode of presentation to the potentially
self-reactive lymphocytes. Because of the vast molecular
variety of self-antigens, the likelihood of their sharing a
common tolerogenic property is as small as for extrinsic
antigens.

As the basis of an alternative hypothesis on self-tolerance to follow, we postulate that, in analogy to our observations on extrinsic antigens, self-antigens are not *a priori*
tolerogenic to the immune system, regardless of its ontogenic
state. Most immunologists accept the fact that antigens are
converted into immunogens by macrophage-like adherent (A)
cells. This process appears to involve a series of antigen-
processing events by the A cell, resulting in the presentation

to the immunocompetent cell of antigenic determinants together with I-region products (34). Triggering of the immune
pathway is thereby facilitated by recognition of both the
antigenic determinant and the self-I-region product. Since
processing of antigens by A cells appears to be absent in
immunologically immature animals (35), conventional opinion
would predict that any extrinsic and, by analogy, any self-
antigen should induce tolerance *in utero*. Since this prediction is not verified by our data, and since we do not
assume self-antigens per se are any different in their tolerogenic properties from foreign antigens, we suggest that
in analogy with immune induction the induction of tolerance
to self also requires a dual recognition event. Consider,
for example, an organ-specific self-antigen expressed on the
cell surface. We propose that for this antigen to be tolerogenic for a self-reactive lymphocyte, it must be recognized
in association or concomitantly with another ubiquitous polymorphic self-marker designated Z. We consider it premature
in this communication to speculate about the molecular details
of such recognition. Suffice it to say, we prefer such a
self-recognition set to be seen by two separate but closely
associated receptors on the lymphocyte surface. One such
receptor is considered homologous to the V-region-determined
antigen recognition site. The other is postulated to be a
complimentary molecule to Z. It is important to note that
the association on the surface membrane of a self-antigen
with the self-marker is thought to be controlled by the cell
that synthesizes them. Therefore, any extrinsic nonself
antigen that reaches the immune system could not generally be
tolerogenic but, according to current knowledge, would be presented in an immunogenic form by specialized accessory cells
in association with I-region products. The strict exclusion
of foreign antigens from accidentally participating in
mechanisms by which self-tolerance is controlled becomes
important in the case of maternally-derived soluble antigens
of pathogenic origin, where tolerance induction to the pathogen could render the offspring unprotected from subsequent
postnatal infection. The same arguments may be extended to
the adult animal where self-tolerance is thought to be continuously acquired by newly recruited self-reactive lymphocytes. If, according to current belief, tolerance results
from an antigen recognition event involving one kind of
receptor only, lymphocytes bearing receptors specific for an
extrinsic antigen would run the risk of acquiring tolerance
should this antigen be present at that time. Aware of this
logistic problem, some immunologists have allocated the process of self-tolerance induction to the thymus where foreign
antigens are at least partially excluded from entering, due

to the blood-thymus barrier. Accordingly, an antigen administered *in utero* at the time when the blood-thymus barrier
has not yet developed should behave as a tolerogen. As indicated by our data, this is clearly not the case for BSA or
"18," in spite of these antigens having readily and uniformly
penetrated the thymic tissue. Our self-tolerance model requires self-antigens to be present as intrinsic structures
on cell surfaces, as is the case for organ-specific self-
antigens. In accordance with this and in analogy to our
results, soluble self-antigens, with the notable exception
of IgG, are not expected to be tolerogenic; for these
antigens we postulate that they are also surface associated
with the Z-bearing cells secreting them, besides being in
circulation. This, however, may not be crucial since A cells
are not expected to convert soluble unmodified self-antigens
into immunogens, due to the lack of opsonins directed against
self.

Since it appears from our work that HGG represents the
exception rather than the rule among extrinsic antigens for
induction of tolerance *in utero*, the validity of routinely
using HGG as a model for self-antigens must be questioned.
Our data on tolerance to HGG therefore do not permit us to
derive at a general conclusion pertaining to self-tolerance.
Interpreted on its own merits, our experimental system
assigns the presence of active suppression to the period when
in utero-induced tolerance breaks. This is at variance with
data by others who have implicated suppressor cells in the
induction and maintenance of tolerance in adult animals to
various antigens, including HGG (23,24). On the other hand,
there are also reports to the effect that suppressor cells
could not be found in association with tolerance even in
adult animals (36). In our view, the strongest evidence
against an obligatory role for suppressor cells in tolerance
to HGG, be it in the immunologically immature or adult
animal, derives from the demonstration that the induction of
suppressor cells, along with unresponsiveness, may be a
function of the source from which HGG is obtained (17,36).

REFERENCES

1. Diener, E., Kraft, N., Lee, K.C., and Shiozawa, C. (1976).
   J. Exp. Med. 143, 805.
2. Aldo-Benson, M., and Borel, Y. (1974). J. Immunol. 112,1793
3. Terres, G., Aldo-Benson, M. and Borel, Y. (1976) J.
   Immunol. 6, 492
4. Aldo-Benson, M. and Borel, Y. (1976). J. Immunol. 116,223.
5. Borel, Y. (1976). Transplant Rev. 31, 1.
6. Gronowicz, E. and Coutinho, A. (1975). Eur.J.Immunol. 5,413

7. Lerman, S.R., Romano, T.J., Mond, J.J., Heidelberger, M.and Thorbecke, G.J. (1975). Cell. Immunol. 15,321.
8. Romano, T.J., Lerman, S.P. and Thorbecke, G.J. (1976). Immunol. 6, 434.
9. Sjoberg, O. (1972). J. Exp. Med. 135, 850.
10. Diener, E. and Feldmann, M. (1972). Cell. Immunol. 5, 130.
11. Nossal, G.J.V., and Layton, J.E. (1976). J.Exp.Med.143,511.
12. Nossal, G.J.V. and Pike, B.L. (1975). J. Exp. Med. 141,904.
13. Cambier, J.C., Kettman, J.R.,Vitetta, E.S. and Uhr, J.W. (1976). J. Exp. Med. 144,293.
14. Vitetta, E.S., Cambier, J.C., Ligler, F.S., Kettman, J.R. and Uhr, J.W. (1977). J. Exp. Med. 146, 1804.
15. Scott, D.W., Venkataraman, M. and Jandinski, J. (1978). Immunol. Rev. 43. 241.
16. Gershon, R.K. and Kondo, K. (1971).Immunol. 21, 903.
17. Doyle, M.V., Parks, D.E. and Weigle, W.O. (1976). J. Immunol. 116, 1640.
18. Nossal, G.J.V. and Mitchell, J. (1966). In "The Thymus: Experimental and Clinical Studies" (G.E.W. Wolstenholme, and R. Porter, eds.), pp. 105-123. Churchill, London.
19. Auerbach, R. and Clark, S. (1975). Science 189,811.
20. Waters, C.A., Pilarski, L.M., Wegmann, T.G. and Diener, E. (1979). J. Exp. Med. 149, No. 5 (in press)
21. Metcalf, E.S. and Klinman, N.R. (1976), J.Exp.Med.143,1327.
22. Chiller, J.M., Habicht, G.S. and Weigle, W.O. (1971). Science, 171, 813.
23. Benjamin, D.C. (1975). J. Exp. Med. 141, 635.
24. Basten, A., Miller, J.F.A.P. and Johnson, P. (1975). Transplant. Rev. 26, 130.
25. Eardley, D.D., Hugenberger, J.,McVay-Boudreau, L., Shen, F.W., Gershon, R.K. and Cantor, H. (1978). J. Exp. Med. 147, 1106.
26. Cantor. H., Hugenberger, J., McVay-Boudreau, L., Eardley, D.D., Kemp. J., Shen, F.W. and Gershon, R.K. (1978). J. Exp. Med. 148, 871.
27. Herzenberg, L.A., Black S.J. and Herzenberg, L. A. (personal communication).
28. Singh, B., Fraga, E. and Barton, M.A. (1978).J. Immunol. 121, 784.
29. Howard, J.G. and Mitchison, N.A.(1975).Progress in Allergy, 18, 43.
30. Bretscher, P.A. and Cohn, M. (1970). Science, 169, 1042.
31. Lederberg, J. (1959). Science, 129, 1649.
32. Bretscher, P.A. (1975).Transplant, Rev. 23, 37.
33. Diener, E. and Feldmann, M.(1972).Transplant. Rev. 8,76.
34. Shevach, E.M. and Rosenthal, A.S.(1973)J.Exp.Med.138,1213.
35. Landahl, C.A. (1976).Eur. J. Immunol. 6, 130.
36. Parks,D. Doyle,M. and Weigle, W. (1978).J.Exp.Med.148,625.

EVIDENCE FOR IRREVERSIBLE INACTIVATION
OF B LYMPHOCYTES IN TOLERANCE
TO T DEPENDENT ANTIGENS[1]

D. Elliot Parks[2] and William O. Weigle

Department of Immunopathology
Scripps Clinic and Research Foundation
La Jolla, California 92037

ABSTRACT The duration of unresponsiveness to the soluble protein antigen human gamma globulin (HGG) is much
shorter in B lymphocytes than in helper T lymphocytes.
The injection of antigen along with bacterial lipopolysaccharide (LPS) stimulates responsive B cells as early
as 45 days after tolerization. However, the injection
of antigen and LPS earlier than 45 days does not elicit
plaque-forming cells (PFC) specific for HGG. LPS alone
does not stimulate significant numbers of PFC to HGG
regardless of the immune status or the time after tolerization. Removal of spleen cells from tolerant animals,
extensive washing, and transfer into lethally irradiated
recipients to circumvent any possible blockade or masking of responsive B cells by tolerogen does not alter
the kinetics of reacquisition of responsiveness in the B
cells. This is true whether reconstituted mice are
challenged with LPS alone or with LPS and antigen. The
inability to detect responsive B cells for more than 6
weeks after tolerization demonstrates that an irreversible, central unresponsiveness resulting in an intrinsic
defect in B lymphocytes can be established to this T
dependent antigen and is incompatible with antigen blockade as the mechanism of B cell tolerance to these antigens.

[1]This is publication no. 1756 from the Department of
Immunopathology, Scripps Clinic and Research Foundation, La
Jolla, California. Supported in part by United States Public
Health Service Grant AI-07007, AG-00783, and RRO-5514, and
American Cancer Society Grant IM-42I.

[2]Recipient of Junior Faculty Research Award JFRA-8 from
the American Cancer Society.

INTRODUCTION

The several theories on the mechanism of the induction and maintenance of immunologic unresponsiveness can be grouped into mechanisms by which an intrinsic defect is established in B cells either permanently inactivating or deleting responsive cells and mechanisms by which extrinsic forces temporarily inhibit the expression of responsive B cells. The theory of receptor blockade (1,2) suggests that an unresponsive state can be established by antigen which blockades the Ig receptors on responsive B cells thus preventing immunologic triggering. It has previously been demonstrated that unresponsiveness maintained by antigen blockade of cell receptors can be reversed by procedures which remove the interferring antigen (3,4) or by stimulation of inhibited cells with a polyclonal B cell activator (5,6). Subsequently, the ability to detect antibodies which bind to tolerated antigens following polyclonal B cell activation has been presented as evidence that intrinsic or central unresponsiveness has not been established to those tolerated antigens (7,8). However, the antibody response resulting from polyclonal B cell activation has been shown to differ both qualitatively and quantitatively from the antibody response elicited by the injection of specific antigen (9-11). The experiments presented here investigate both the nature of the antigen stimulated and polyclonally activated response to HGG in vivo and the ability of the polyclonal B cell activator LPS to terminate the unresponsive state to HGG, either alone or in combination with specific antigenic stimulation.

METHODS

Tolerogenic, deaggregated HGG (DHGG) and immunogenic, heat aggregated HGG (AHGG) were prepared as previously described (12,13). Primary immunization consisted of 400 µg of AHGG i.v. and a slide modification of the hemolytic plaque assay (12) was performed 6 days after immunization except in reconstituted mice that were assayed 7 days after reconstitution and challenge. Antigenic challenge was given immediately after cellular reconstitution of irradiated recipients (14). Phenol-extracted LPS from E. coli 0111:B4 obtained from Difco Laboratories (Detroit, Mich.). Polyclonal responses were elicited with 50-300 µg of LPS per mouse, whereas adjuvant responses were induced by the injection of 50 µg of LPS i.v. 3 hrs after antigenic challenge. The male A/J mice utilized in these experiments were purchased from the Jackson Laboratory (Bar Harbor, Maine).

RESULTS

Polyclonal Versus Antigen Specific Activation In Vivo.
An antibody response is stimulated to a variety of antigens
upon exposure of B cells to polyclonal activators either in
vivo or in vitro. This polyclonal B cell activation is generally most vigorous against haptenic antigens such as TNP
and least vigorous to soluble protein antigens such as HGG
(Figure 1). The hierarchy of polyclonal responsiveness paral-
lels the precursor frequencies for these antigens and may

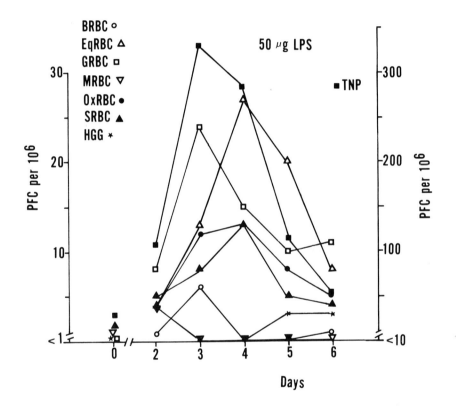

FIGURE 1. In vivo polyclonal response to LPS. Direct
plaque-forming cells to burro (BRBC), equine (EqRBC), goat
(GRBC), mouse (MRBC), ox (OxRBC), sheep (SRBC) red blood cells
and TNP heavily conjugated to indicator cells were determined
at various times after the injection of 50 μg of LPS into 8
week old mice. Both direct and indirect PFC to HGG were
determined.

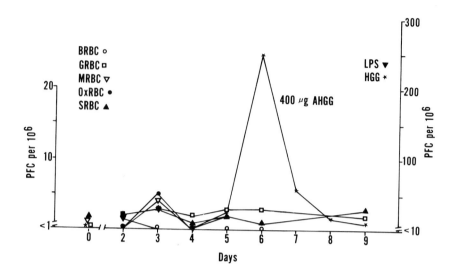

FIGURE 2.   In vivo antibody response to AHGG.   The direct
PFC responses to several red blood cells and to LPS and both
the direct and indirect PFC responses to HGG were determined
at various times after the injection of 400 µg of AHGG into
mice.

reflect precursor availability to polyclonal activation.   The
polyclonal activation of HGG reactive B cells in vivo is less
vigorous than either the polyclonal response to most erythrocyte antigens and TNP or the specific response induced by
antigen stimulation (Figure 2).   The pattern of polyclonal
responsiveness to 50 µg of LPS presented in Figure 1 remained
substantially unaltered by injecting greater quantities of
LPS up to 300 µg.

Detection of Responsive B Cells During Immunologic Unresponsiveness.   The unresponsive state induced in mice to a
single injection of deaggregated HGG has become a classic
system for the investigation of the induction and maintenance
of experimentally induced immunologic unresponsiveness to a
soluble protein antigen.   This state of complete, long-lived
and specific unresponsiveness has been extensively defined in
terms of the status and role of helper and suppressor T cells
and B cells.   Suppressor cells, although induced by tolerogenic DHGG, are not responsible for unresponsiveness in
either T or B cells (12,15,16).   Table 1 presents the tempo-
ral pattern of tolerance in these cells summarized from a

TABLE 1

TEMPORAL PATTERN OF IMMUNOLOGIC TOLERANCE TO HGG IN A/J MICE

Cells	Days of	
	Induction	Maintenance
Helper T Cells		
Thymus	< 1	120 - 135
Spleen	< 1	120 - 150
Suppressor T Cells		
Spleen	< 3	30 - 40
B Cells		
Bone Marrow	8 - 15	40 - 50
Spleen	2 - 4	40 - 50

TABLE 1. Compiled from data of A/J mice given 2.5 mg of deaggregated HGG.

number of sources including (17,18,19). Unresponsiveness is rapidly induced in the thymus and the spleen but is delayed in the bone marrow. T cells of the thymus and spleen remain completely unresponsive for at least 120 days following tolerization. In contrast to this long unresponsive state in T lymphocytes, unresponsiveness in bone marrow and splenic B cells is of relatively short duration. Therefore, approximately 7 weeks after tolerization, mice possess responsive B cells but tolerant T cells. Antigenic challenge of the intact animal during this time reveals specific unresponsiveness due to the absence of responsive helper T cells to this T dependent, protein antigen. It is at this time that termination of the unresponsive state can be accomplished by by-passing the specificity of, or the need for, T cell help as shown in Table 2. The injection of LPS and antigen into mice 80 days after tolerization leads to the production of HGG specific PFC. LPS substitutes for specific helper T cells which are unresponsive in these animals and thereby terminate the tolerant state by stimulating B cells. Although it is assumed that the effect of LPS is directly upon B cells, these experiments cannot exclude the possible role of

TABLE 2

REACQUISITION OF RESPONSIVE SPLENIC B CELLS
IN LATE TOLERANT A/J MICE

Immune Status	Antigenic Challenge	Indirect PFC/10^6
Day 36 Tolerant	AHGG	9 ± 5
Day 36 Tolerant	AHGG + LPS	2 ± 1
Normal	AHGG	132 ± 22
Normal	AHGG + LPS	746 ± 97
Day 80 Tolerant	AHGG	5 ± 4
Day 80 Tolerant	AHGG + LPS	79 ± 31
Normal	AHGG	102 ± 21
Normal	AHGG + LPS	419 ± 99

TABLE 2. Mice tolerized either 36 or 80 days previously
and age matched normal mice were challenged with 400 µg of
AHGG followed 3 hrs later by 50 µg of LPS. The mean ± standard error of the indirect PFC to HGG determined 6 days after
antigenic challenge is presented.

nonspecific T cells in this LPS response.
    A kinetic profile of the duration of and escape from
tolerance in HGG specific B cells can be obtained by chal-
lenging tolerant mice at various times after tolerization
with antigen and LPS. Responsive B cells are not detected
by this procedure until at least 45 days after tolerization
(Figure 3). Thereafter, the number of responsive B cells in
the spleen gradually increases until approximately 90 days
after tolerization, at which time the number of PFC detected
in these mice is equivalent to the number of PFC in normal
mice challenged with antigen alone. Prior to 45 days after
tolerization, HGG specific PFC cannot be detected in tolerant
animals regardless of the type of challenge. Neither antigen,
LPS, nor both antigen and LPS is capable of stimulating
splenic B cells at this time. Of special interest is the
fact that challenge with LPS alone is not able to elicit HGG
specific PFC in tolerant animals even after 45 days, when
responsive B cells are detectable by the combined challenge

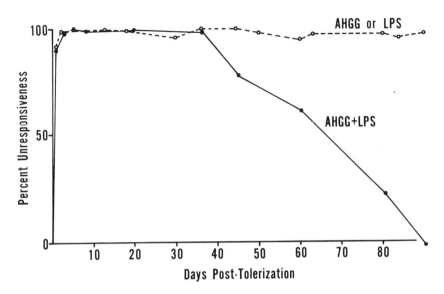

FIGURE 3. Kinetics of spontaneous reacquisition of responsive splenic B cells in tolerant mice. The indirect PFC response to HGG in tolerant mice was determined as described in Table 2. Mice received antigen and/or 50 μg of LPS. % unresponsiveness = (1-PFC/10^6 for tolerized mice ÷ PFC/10^6 for normal mice) x 100.

of antigen and LPS.

In order to exclude the possibility that tolerogen either circulating in the tolerant host or bound to B cells was blockading the antigen or polyclonal B cell activator receptors on responsive B cells in tolerant animals, the experiments reported above were repeated in mice reconstituted with tolerant cells. Spleen cells were removed from mice at various times after tolerization, washed three times in 20-100 volumes of balanced salt solution and transferred to lethally irradiated, normal recipients. This attempt to circumvent any possible blockade or masking of responsive B cells by tolerogen was unable to detect any difference in the kinetics of reacquisition of responsive B cells (Table 3). HGG specific PFC could not be demonstrated in reconstituted recipients with either antigen, LPS, or both antigen and LPS at 10 or 30 days after tolerization. Responsive B cells could be detected in the recipients of 60 day tolerant spleen cells but only when challenged with both antigen and LPS, not with either stimulus alone. These data confirm the conclusion made from the experiments reported above that the

TABLE 3

IRREVERSIBLE UNRESPONSIVENESS IN TRANSFERRED
TOLERANT SPLEEN CELLS

DONOR CELLS	CHALLENGE OF RECIPIENT	DAYS POST TOLERIZATION		
		10	30	60
TOLERANT	AHGG	2*	$<$1	5
"	AHGG + LPS	$<$1	3	43
"	LPS	$<$1	$<$1	2
NORMAL	AHGG		156	235
"	AHGG + LPS	501	303	812
"	LPS	6	$<$1	$<$1

TABLE 3. 70×10^6 spleen cells from normal mice or
mice tolerized 10, 30 or 60 days prior to sacrifice were
injected into 900 R irradiated recipients. These reconstituted mice were challenged with 400 μg of AHGG and/or 50 μg
of LPS on the day of cell transfer and indirect PFC to HGG
were determined 7 days later.

tolerant state in B cells cannot be reversed by exposure to
antigen or the polyclonal B cell activator LPS until responsive B cells have spontaneously reappeared in the bone marrow
(17) and spleen (18).

DISCUSSION

The inability to detect responsive B cells by injecting
LPS alone or along with antigen during the first 6 weeks
after tolerization strongly suggests that irreversible unresponsiveness is established in these cells following tolerization with DHGG. Challenge of tolerized mice with antigen
and LPS results in the stimulation of HGG specific PFC only
after 45 days, when responsiveness can be demonstrated in
splenic (18) and bone marrow (17) B cells by adoptive cell
transfer. In contrast, neither the injection of the antigen
(AHGG) nor the polyclonal B cell activator (LPS) alone is
capable of stimulating PFC to the tolerated antigen, even
when challenged more than 90 days after tolerization at
which time complete responsiveness has been regained in

splenic B cells (Figure 3). Furthermore, spleen cells removed
from mice at various times after tolerization, washed extensively to remove any tolerogen which may mask or blockade the
antigen receptors on the responsive B cells and transferred
into lethally irradiated recipients responded to challenge
with antigen and/or LPS in a pattern indistinguishable from
that of unmanipulated tolerant mice. Tolerant cells taken
from mice less than 6 weeks after tolerization were unresponsive to any challenge. However, cells taken from mice 60 days
after tolerization were responsive to challenge with antigen
and LPS in the reconstituted recipients. Injection of LPS
alone was incapable of stimulating responsiveness in transferred tolerant cells regardless of the time between tolerization and cell transfer indicating that polyclonal B cell
activation alone is insufficient to terminate tolerance in
unresponsive B cells.

It has been suggested that a state of reversible inhibition of B cell responsiveness can be established by blockading antigen receptors on responsive B cells with antigen (1,
2). Stimulation of blockaded responsive cells has been demonstrated in vitro with polyclonal B cell activators (5,6).
Although this theory of immunologic unresponsiveness has been
developed largely with data utilizing T independent antigens,
the implications of this theory also apply to T dependent
antigens and are contrary to irreversible mechanisms of the
induction of unresponsiveness. The tenets that all responsive B cells specific for a particular antigen are inhibited
and that this blockade can be reversed by stimulation with
polyclonal activators (5,6) were modified by Fernandez and
Moller (4,20,21) who demonstrated that certain B cells can
be irreversibly inactivated by exposure to antigen in the
presence of a polyclonal B cell activator. Cells bearing
receptors for both antigen and polyclonal B cell activator
specific for dextran were irreversibly inactivated during
exposure to that T independent antigen. These authors suggest that irreversible inactivation can be accomplished only
through interactions at both the antigen receptor and the
receptor for polyclonal B cell activation. We recently suggested that the collaboration provided B cells by helper T
cells may be analogous to the polyclonal signal provided by
T independent antigens and that exposure of T dependent B
cells possessing receptors for both antigen and T cell collaboration would be irreversibly inactivated by antigen (15).

All T dependent B cells by definition would be responsive
to the polyclonal activating signal (T cell collaboration)
and thus susceptible to irreversible inactivation by either
antigen or polyclonal activator mediated mechanisms. This
prediction was recently confirmed in mice using a polyclonal

B cell activator isolated from Con A stimulated T cells.
Primi et al. (22) suggest that their Con A induced polyclonal
B cell activator is analogous to the T cell cooperative signal
released by helper T cells. This endogenous B cell activator
stimulates polyclonal antibody to heterologous protein antigen but not to the autologous antigen murine serum albumin.
In other words, B cells responsive to self antigens are ir-
versibly inactivated by exposure to these antigens. If the
induction of unresponsiveness is accomplished in the presence
of a polyclonal B cell activating stimulus as previously suggested (23), then this stimulus must be provided by specific
T cells before they are themselves tolerized on nonspecific T
cells in the tolerant host.

The use of exogenous polyclonal B cell activators such
as LPS to probe for responsive B cells in tolerant animals
should be reassessed in view of the evidence favoring irreversible unresponsiveness. Very few PFC specific for the soluble protein antigen HGG are elicited by polyclonal B cell
activation in vivo compared to the numbers of PFC produced by
antigen specific stimulation (Figures 1 and 2). Furthermore,
the antibodies released by polyclonal activation of B cells
are of broader specificity and lower affinities than the antibodies released by antigenic stimulation (9-11). Furthermore,
polyclonal B cell activation stimulates fewer cells releasing
high affinity antibody than does activation by specific antigen (11). Therefore, the majority of the cells stimulated by
polyclonal B cell activation would appear to possess relatively low affinity Ig receptors for any particular antigen.
These Ig receptors may be below the threshold required to bind
sufficient antigen to provide either antigenic or tolerogenic
stimulation. If this postulate is correct, most of the cells
responding to polyclonal B cell activation are not inducible
to antibody production or to tolerance by antigen mediated
mechanism. For this reason, the demonstration of antigen
binding cells to self or other tolerated antigen by polyclonal
B cell activation may not represent the true level of antigen
responsiveness in the B cell population under investigation.
The bulk of antibody detected to self antigens following
stimulation by exogenous polyclonal B cell activators may be
irrelevant to the etiology of autoimmune disease and only in
rare cases in which cells and/or antibody of low affinity can
mediate autoimmune pathology would the cells detected by
polyclonal B cell activation be of danger to the host.

ACKNOWLEDGMENTS

We thank Barbara Dunbar for excellent technical assistance, Janet Kuhns for help in the preparation and composition

of this manuscript, and Karen Prescott for preparation of the
illustrations.

REFERENCES

1. Aldo-Benson, M., and Borel, Y. (1974). J. Immunol. 112, 1793.
2. Schrader, J. W., and Nossal, G. J. V. (1974). J. Exp. Med. 139, 1582.
3. Gronowicz, E., Coutinho, A., and Sjöberg, O. (1974). Eur. J. Immunol. 4, 226.
4. Fernandez, C., and Möller, G. (1978). Scand. J. Immunol. 7, 137.
5. Gronowicz, E., and Coutinho, A. (1975). Eur. J. Immunol. 5, 413.
6. Möller, G., Gronowicz, E., Persson, U., Coutinho, A., Möller, E., Hammarström, L., and Smith, E. (1976). J. Exp. Med. 143, 1429.
7. Primi, D., Smith, C. I. E., Hammarström, L., and Möller, G. (1977). Cell. Immunol. 34, 367.
8. Izui, S., McConahey, P. J., and Dixon, F. J. (1978). J. Immunol. 121, 2213.
9. Andersson, J., Sjöberg, O., and Möller, G. (1972). Transplant. Rev. 11, 131.
10. Nilsson, B. S., Sultzer, B. M., and Bullock, W. W. (1973). J. Exp. Med. 137, 127.
11. Coutinho, A., Gronowicz, E., Bullock, W. W., and Möller, G. (1974). J. Exp. Med. 139, 74.
12. Parks, D. E., Doyle, M. V., and Weigle, W. O. (1978). J. Exp. Med. 148, 625.
13. Chiller, J. M., and Weigle, W. O. (1971). J. Immunol. 106, 1647.
14. Parks, D. E., Doyle, M. V., and Weigle, W. O. (1977). J. Immunol. 119, 1923.
15. Parks, D. E., and Weigle, W. O. (1979). Immunol. Rev. 43, 217.
16. Parks, D. E., Shaller, D. A., and Weigle, W. O. (1979). J. Exp. Med. 149, in press.
17. Chiller, J. M., Habicht, G. S., and Weigle, W. O. (1971). Science 171, 813.
18. Chiller, J. M., and Weigle, W. O. (1973). J. Immunol. 110, 1051.
19. Doyle, M. V., Parks, D. E., and Weigle, W. O. (1976). J. Immunol. 116, 1640.
20. Fernandez, C., and Moller, G. (1977). J. Exp. Med. 146, 308.
21. Möller, G., and Fernandez, C. (1978). Scand. J. Immunol. 8, 29.

22. Primi, D., Hammarström, L., Smith, C. I. E., and Möller,
    G. (1978). Cell. Immunol. 41, 320.
23. Coutinho, A., and Möller, G. (1975). In "Advances in
    Immunology" (F. J. Dixon and H. G. Kunkel, eds.), pp. 113-
    236. Academic Press, New York.

SUPPRESSOR MECHANISMS IN TISSUE TRANSPLANTATION
TOLERANCE FOLLOWING TOTAL LYMPHOID IRRADIATION (TLI)[1]

Shimon Slavin

Department of Medicine A, Hadassah - Hebrew University
School of Medicine, Jerusalem, Israel

Samuel Strober

Department of Medicine and the Howard Hughes Medical
Institute Laboratory, Stanford University, Stanford
California, 94305

ABSTRACT   BALB/c mice treated with total lymphoid irradiation (TLI) consisting of 17 daily fractions of
200 rads directed to the major lymphoid organs, accepted
C57BL/Ka bone marrow without evidence of graft versus
host disease (GVHD) as well as developed permanent and
specific transplantation tolerance to C57BL/Ka skin allografts. Specific transplantation tolerance was transferred to sublethally irradiated BALB/c recipients by
intravenous injected 25×10^6 chimeric spleen cells.
Adoptive recipients were chimeric but showed no GVHD
although injection of normal C57BL/Ka spleen cells into
sublethally irradiated BALB/c mice produced lethal GVHD
in all recipients. Spleen cells from chimeric mice
obtained within one month following induction of chimerism block mixed lymphocyte reactivity (MLR) in a non
specific fashion whereas spleen cells obtained from well
established chimeras blocked specifically MLR of host
versus donor lymphocytes. The data suggest that recipients of allogeneic bone marrow cells following TLI
develop specific as well as non specific suppressor cells.

INTRODUCTION

Total lymphoid irradiation (TLI) involves exposure of the
major lymphoid organs including the thymus and the spleen to
17 daily X-ray fractions of 200 rads each, to a total of

[1]This work was supported by National Institutes of Health
grants AI 15387-01, AI-11313, the Kroc Foundation and
Israel Cancer Association grant 4/78.

3,400 rads (1-3). TLI produces a most profound and longlasting
immunosuppression of the humoral (4) as well as the cell-mediated immune responses in mice (2) as well as in man (5).
Permanent engraftment of strongly histoincompatible bone marrow (BM) allografts was accomplished following TLI in mice
(C57BL/Ka, H-2^b → BALB/c, H-2^d, 2, 3), rats (ACI, AgB^4 →
Lewis, AgB^1, 6) and dogs (Mongrel ♂ → Mongrel ♀ , 7-9). BM
recipients developed permanent and specific transplantation
tolerance to donor type organ allografts including skin (1-3,
6), perfused hearts (6), and kidney allografts as suggested
by some unpublished preliminary experiments. No graft versus
host disease (GVHD) was demonstrable in the BM recipients
despite strong histoincompatibility between the host and donor
pairs. The data obtained so far suggests that a similar approach should be furtherinvestigated for clinical BM and organ
transplantation since TLI is a potent yet safe procedure in
man as suggested by long term observations in patients with
Hodgkin's disease that underwent total nodal irradiation (10).
The mechanism by which TLI enables establishment of bidirec-
tional tolerance of host versus graft as well as graft versus
host is at present not fully understood.

Non-specific and mostly specific suppressor T cells were
already documented in BALB/c mice made tolerant to a soluble
protein antigen following TLI (11). Specific tolerance to
bovine serum albumine (BSA) was adoptively transferred by
spleen cells obtained from BSA-tolerant BALB/c mice, suggesting that specific suppressor T cells were responsible for the
tolerance to BSA following TLI (11).

In the present paper we will present data suggesting that
specific as well as non-specific suppressor cells are present
in chimeric mice following TLI. Their presence suggests that
suppressor cells may play a role in establishing or maintaining transplantation tolerance as well as the prevention of
GVHD (12).

ESTABLISHMENT OF CHIMERAS FOLLOWING TLI

Three to six months old BALB/c mice (30-35 gm) were anes-
thetized daily, five times a week, and exposed to TLI in a
lead apparatus designed to expose the major lymphoid organs
(1, 2). TLI consisted of 200 rads to a total cumulative dose
of 3400 rads. One day following termination of TLI the mice
were injected intravenously with 30x10^6 nucleated C57BL/Ka BM
cells. A full thickness C57BL/Ka skin allograft was transplanted one day following BM infusion. Chimerism was documented in 27 out of 27 mice. Permanent C57BL/Ka skin graft
survival (> 250 days) was observed in 24 out of 27 BM recipients (3). Spleen and lymph node cells obtained from these

C57BL/Ka → BALB/c chimeras were assayed for their capacity
to transfer chimerism without GVHD as well as to exert suppression of MLR.

NON SPECIFIC SUPPRESSOR CELLS

Non Specific Blocking of MLR by Suppressor Cells. Spleen
cells obtained from C57BL/Ka → BALB/c BM chimeras within one
month following induction of chimerism could efficiently block
MLR of all combinations of responding and stimulating haplotypes tested in a non specific pattern. The details of the
experiments and the assay systems are shown on table 1. The
data suggest that radioresistant non specific suppressor cells
are present immediately following TLI and therefore they may
be responsible in part for the non-specific responsiveness
following TLI.

Impairment of C57BL/Ka → BALB/c BM Chimeras to Respond in
MLR Following TLI. Lymph node and spleen lymphocytes obtained
from BALB/c mice treated with TLI alone or TLI and C57BL/Ka BM
are totally non reactive in a one way MLR within one month
following TLI (2). Chimeric lymphocytes recover their ability
to respond against unrelated lymphocutes (C_3H, $C_3H \cdot Q$), however the degree of responsiveness is somewhat impaired as compared to normal H-2 identical spleen cells (Table 2), suggesting that the non specific suppressor cells block their full
ability to respond against the allogeneic stimulating cells.

Impairment of Chimeric Spleen Cells to Stimulate in MLR.
$H-2^b$ cells obtained from the spleens of C57BL/Ka → BALB/c
BM chimeras did not stimulate responding BALB/c lymph node
lymphocytes as effectively as an equivalent number of $H-2^b$
spleen cells obtained from normal C57BL/Ka mice, suggesting
that the radioresistant non specific suppressor cells present
in the MLR system when chimeric spleen cells served as stimulators blocked the capacity of BALB/c cells as responders
(Table 2).

SPECIFIC SUPPRESSOR CELLS IN CHIMERAS

C57BL/Ka → BALB/c BM chimeras recover their ability to
respond in a one way MLR as do TLI treated BALB/c mide. The
latter recover their full capacity to respond against all allogeneic cells (i.e. against C57BL/Ka) within 70 days (2). The
former develop permanent and specific tolerance to C57BL/Ka,
i.e. they recover their ability to respond against lymphocytes
of unrelated haplotypes ($H-2^k$, $H-2^q$) and remain specifically
unresponsive to the $H-2^b$ haplotype of the BM donor. Detailed

TABLE I

SPECIFIC AND NON SPECIFIC SUPPRESSION OF ONE WAY MLR BY
SPLEEN CELLS OF YOUNG AND WELL ESTABLISHED C57BL/Ka⟶
BALB/c BM CHIMERAS[a]

Responding cells	Stimulating cells	% suppression of ^{3}H Thymidine uptake by co-cultured chimeric spleen cells	
		young chimeras $\leqslant$ 30 days	well established chimeras $>$120 days
BALB/c	C57BL/Ka	95	68
BALB/c	C$_3$H/He	95	0
BALB/c	BALB·Q	94	20
C$_3$H/H1	C57BL/Ka	97	30
BALB·Q	C57BL/Ka	90	21

[a]The degree and specificity of MLR suppression by co-cultured spleen cells obtained from chimeric spleen cells
was calculated as the mean percent of ^{3}H thymidine uptake by triplicate cultures including chimeric spleen
cells as compared to (C57BL/Ka x BALB/c)F$_1$ spleen cells
that were used as controls, since both had no ability
to respond against either parental strains (2). 1 x 10^6
cells of responding, stimulating and co-cultured cells
were plated in 0.2-ml flat bottomed microculture plates
as previously described (2, 15). Stimulating cells were
inactivated by exposure to 3000 rads. Co-cultured cells
were irradiated prior to culturing to prevent two way
MLR (young chimeras were exposed to 1500 rads, established chimeras were exposed to 3000 rads).

experiments shown on table 2 demonstrate that spleen cells
obtained from well established C57BL/Ka ⟶ BALB/c chimeras
can block the MLR of a related combination (BALB/c vs.
C57BL/Ka) in a specific way but failed to block effectively
the MLR reactivity tested in unrelated combination. It is
suggested that the specific suppressor cells constitute an
important mechanism in maintaining a state of tolerance across
major histocompatibility barriers.

TABLE II

IMPAIRED CAPACITY OF CHIMERIC SPLEEN CELLS TO RESPOND
AND STIMULATE IN MLR ASSAYS[a]

Responding cells	Stimulating cells	^{3}H thymidine uptake (C.P.M.± SD)	% reactivity
C57BL/Ka	C₃H/He	61,994 ± 3,600	100
C57BL/Ka → BALB/c (>90% C57BL/Ka cells)	C₃H/He	43,396 ± 2,188	70
BALB/c	C57BL/Ka	140,748 ± 3,308	100
BALB/c	C57BL/Ka → BALB/c (>90% C57BL/Ka cells)	67,679 ± 3,070	48

[a]10^6 Responding BALB/c lymphocytes were cultured with 10^6 irradiated (3000 rads) stimulating lymphocytes in 0.2-ml flat-bottomed microculture plates as previously described (2). Chimeric spleen cells were derived from TLI treated BALB/c mice infused with 30x10^6 C57BL/Ka BM six months prior to splenectomy. Chimeric spleen cells were typed using a microcytotoxicity assay with specific anti-H-2[b] alloantiserum and complement.

OTHER DIRECT AND INDIRECT SUPPORTIVE EVIDENCE FOR SUPPRESSOR CELLS

In Vivo Transfer of Tolerance and Chimerism into Sublethally Treated Adoptive Recipients. Indirect evidence for the presence of suppressor cells in TLI induced BM chimeras is suggested by experiments involving the adoptive transfer of the tolerance state into sublethally irradiated (550 rads WBI) syngeneic BALB/c recipients by 25x10^6 chimeric spleen cells shown to contain > 90% C57BL/Ka cells by H-2 typing. The latter developed stable chimerism but yet showed no evidence of GVHD (survival > 360 days). Similarly treated normal BALB/c mice injected with 25x10^6 normal C57BL/Ka spleen cells died uniformly from GVHD within 13 days (12, 13). Although the transfer of tolerance could be explained on the basis of passive transfer of a tolerogen by tolerant allogeneic cells, the lack of GVHD suggests the presence of an active suppressor mechanism.

GVHD Resistance by Established C57BL/Ka → BALB/c Chimeras. Although TLI protected BALB/c mice from GVHD induced by C57BL/Ka BM cells it did not provide protection against lethal GVHD evoked by 30×10^6 C57BL/Ka spleen cells (3).

Well established chimeras ($\geq$ 78 days following induction of chimerism) acquired the ability to resist six repeated injections of lethal GVHD challenges of 30×10^6 C57BL/Ka spleen cells, suggesting the development of suppressor cells in the chimeras (3).

Specific and Non Specific Suppressor Cells Following TLI in BALB/c Mice Made Tolerant to Soluble Antigens. TLI has been recently used for induction of tolerance to soluble protein antigens using a hapten carrier test system (11). The protocol used for induction of tolerance to BSA was similar to that used for tolerance induction to alloantigens except for the use of a soluble protein antigen (11). Studies on the mechanisms involved in the BSA tolerance system have clearly documented the presence of specific and non specific suppressor T cells of the host origin, (using adoptive transfer experiments), suggesting that the tolerance state following TLI involves suppressor cell mechanisms.

Inability to Generate Tolerance in NZB/NZW F_1 Female Mice. We have failed to generate tolerance to protein antigens in NZB/NZW F_1 female mice that are considered to be deficient in suppressor cell precursors (14), suggesting again that suppressor cells play an important role in the induction and maintenance of tolerance state following TLI.

CONCLUSION

Generation of antigen specific as well as antigen non specific suppressor T cells is fascilitated following TLI in mice made tolerant to protein antigens as well as alloantigens. Suppressor cells probably participate in the state of non specific unresponsiveness as well as the specific unresponsiveness in tolerant mice following TLI.

ACKNOWLEDGMENT

We are indebted to Ms. G. Garretts, C. Doss, S. Morecki & Dr. L. Mugrabi-Weiss for their valuable technical assistance.

REFERENCES

1. Slavin, S., Strober, S., Fuks, Z. and Kaplan, H.S. (1976). Science, Washington, D.C. 193, 1252.
2. Slavin, S., Strober, S., Fuks, Z. and Kaplan, H.S. (1977). J. Exp. Med. 146, 34.
3. Slavin, S., Kaplan, H.S. and Strober, S. (1978a). J. Exp. Med. 147, 963.
4. Zan-Bar, I., Slavin, S. and Strober, S. (1979). Cell. Immunol. In press.
5. Fuks, Z., Strober, S., Bobrove, A.M., Sasazuki, T., McMichael, A. and Kaplan, H.S. J. Clin. Invest. 58, 803.
6. Slavin, S., Reitz, B., Beiber, C.P., Kaplan, H.S. and Strober, S. (1978b). J. Exp. Med. 147, 700.
7. Slavin, S., Gottlieb, M., Strober, S., Hoppe, R.T., Kaplan, H.S. and Grumet, F.C. (1979c). Transplantation. In press.
8. Strober, S., Slavin, S., Fuks, Z., Kaplan, H.S., Gottlieb, M., Bieber, C., Hoppe, R.T. and Grumet, F.C. (1979). Transplant. Proc. In press.
9. Strober,S., Slavin, S., Gottlieb, M., Zan-Bar, I., King, D., Hoppe, R.T., Fuks, Z., Grumet, F.C. and Kaplan, H.S. (1979). Immunological Reviews. In press.
10. Kaplan, H.S. (1972). Harvard University Press, Cambridge. 283.
11. Zan-Bar, I., Slavin, S. and Strober, S. (1978). J. Immunol. 121, 1400.
12. Slavin, S., Zan-Bar, I. and Strober, S. (1979). Transplant. Proc. In press.
13. Slavin, S. and Strober, S. (1979a). Submitted for publication.
14. Slavin, S. and Zan-Bar. I. Manuscript in preparation.
15. Slavin, S. and Strober, S. (1979b). Submitted for publication.

GENETIC CONTROL OF EXPERIMENTAL AUTOIMMUNE MYASTHENIA GRAVIS IN MICE[1]

Premkumar Christadoss, Vanda A. Lennon, Edward H. Lambert, and Chella S. David

Departments of Immunology, Neurology and Physiology
Mayo Clinic and Medical School, Rochester, Minnesota 55901

ABSTRACT   To determine the role of major histocompatibility complex (MHC) gene products in susceptibility to experimental autoimmune myasthenia gravis (EAMG) in mice, torpedo acetylcholine receptor was injected with adjuvants into congenic mice expressing the different independent and recombinant H-2 haplotypes. The animals were screened for 1) autoantibodies to mouse muscle receptor by radioimmunoassay; 2) degree to which acetylcholine receptor in muscle was complexed with antibodies; 3) amplitude of miniature endplate potentials (a measure of postsynaptic membrane response to acetylcholine); 4) clinical signs of EAMG; and 5) T cell *in vitro* proliferative responses to torpedo acetylcholine receptor. The results suggest that H-2 linked gene(s) influence susceptibility to EAMG.

INTRODUCTION

Autoimmunity to AChR is the pathogenic cause of defective neuromuscular transmission in approximately 90% of patients with myasthenia gravis (MG) (reviewed in 1). The consistent abnormality in MG and EAMG is a low amplitude of miniature endplate potentials (mepps) due to decreased sensitivity of the postsynaptic membrane to the neurotransmitter acetylcholine. Histocompatibility studies suggest that susceptibility to MG might be genetically determined. In both sexes, onset of disease before the age of 35 is associated with an increased frequency of HLA-B8 (2). Peripheral blood lymphocytes of MG patients undergo antigen specific transformation when cultured with xenogeneic AChR (3-5). Solubilized mammalian

[1]This work was supported by grants AI-14764 (C.D.), CA-24473 (C.D.), NS-15057 (V.L.) from the National Institutes of Health; by a Research Center Grant from the Muscular Dystrophy Association (E.L. and V.L.) and by the Mayo Foundation.

muscle AChR labelled with ^{125}I α-bungarotoxin provides an antigen which detects circulating antibodies to AChR in 90% of
patients clinically diagnosed as having MG but in no subject
without MG (6).

EAMG can be induced in a variety of vertebrate species by
immunization with AChR extracted from the electric organ of
eels or torpedo rays (7) and in rats EAMG has been induced
with syngeneic muscle AChR (8). Evidence for T-cell involvement in the pathogenesis of EAMG in the rat includes the following: delayed cutaneous reactivity to AChR appears before
the onset of clinical signs of EAMG, and treatment with anti-
thymocyte serum suppresses the acute phase of EAMG (9). Experiments combining thymectomy, X-irradiation and reconstitution with selected populations of lymphocytes demonstrate that
helper T cells are required for induction of EAMG and antibody
to AChR (9,10). Immune lymph node cells can transfer EAMG to
non-immune rats (9) however no evidence has been provided that
cytotoxic T-cells play a role in the pathogenesis of EAMG.
EAMG can be passively transferred by anti-AChR antibodies of
IgG class from immunized rats to normal rats (11) and from MG
patients to mice (12). Studies in non-congenic mice by Fuchs
et al (12) indicate that strain differences exist in EAMG
susceptibility. We initiated studies using congenic inbred
strains of mice to determine whether or not MHC gene(s) control susceptibility to EAMG.

METHODS

Mice. Congenic and recombinant strains and F_1 hybrids
used in this study were produced in the mouse colony of the
Immunogenetics Laboratory at Mayo Clinic.

Antigens. Torpedo AChR protein (TAR) was isolated from
a 3% Triton X-100 extract of electric organ membranes from
torpedo californica by affinity chromatography on a conjugate
of Naja-Naja siamensis α-neurotoxin coupled to agarose (14).
For use in tissue culture, TAR was concentrated by Amicon filtration (PM30) and detergent was changed by a further step of
ultracentrifugation on a gradient of 5-20% sucrose in 0.1 M
NaCl, 0.01 M sodium phosphate, pH 7.0, 0.1% Tween-20 and
0.02% NaN$_3$ and stored at 4° until two hours before use at
which time it was dialyzed against the same buffer without
NaN$_3$. Concentration of TAR was determined by Lowry assay
using BSA as a standard and its receptor specific activity
(8.06 x 10^{-6} moles/gm) was determined by Sephadex G-100 chromatography assay of its binding capacity for ^{125}I α-bungarotoxin.

Inoculations. For EAMG challenge, mice (~8 wk old) were inoculated i.d. with TAR (20 µg) emulsified with an equal volume of complete Freund's adjuvant (CFA, composition specified in Ref. 9) and also with *B. pertussis.* Muscular weakness was scored as described elsewhere (9). Identical challenge with TAR and adjuvants was repeated 30 days after the first, and 20-40 days later, groups of mice were killed for electrophysiological studies, serum antibody assays and determination of % AChR complexed with antibody in muscle tissue. For T-cell proliferative assays, 5 male mice were injected s.c. in the base of the tail with 5 µg of TAR emulsified in CFA.

T-cell Proliferative Assays. The method of Alkans was followed (15). Seven days after inoculation, mice were killed by cervical dislocation, inguinal, lumbar and caudal lymph nodes were collected and 4×10^5 viable lymph node cells were cultured for five days in flat-bottomed microculture plates with 0.5 µg of TAR in 0.2 milliliter of culture medium. The cells were pulsed with [^{3}H]-thymidine 16 hours before harvest. Thymidine uptake is expressed as mean cpm $\pm$ S.E.M. and as stimulation indices (S.I. = $\frac{\text{cpm with TAR}}{\text{cpm with media}}$). With each strain experiments were repeated 2 to 3 times.

Assays for Antibodies and Muscle AChR-Antibody Complexes. Autoantibodies to mouse muscle AChR were measured by immunoprecipitation radioimmunoassay using solubilized AChR (from normal mice) complexed with ^{125}I α-bungarotoxin (16). AChR extracted from the carcasses of experimental mice, was labelled with ^{125}I α-bungarotoxin and % complexed *in situ* with antibody was determined by immunoprecipitation (8).

Endplate Potential Studies. The response of muscle postsynaptic membranes to acetylcholine was determined by measuring miniature endplate potentials (mepps) *in vitro.* Micro-electrode studies were done on hemi-diaphragms as described elsewhere (16). Mepp amplitudes were corrected for non-linearity of the endplate response to acetylcholine and to a membrane potential of -75 millivolts (mV).

RESULTS

Clinical and Electrophysiologic Signs of EAMG. In preliminary experiments, clinical and electrophysiological observations revealed distinct differences amongst the independent haplotypes in susceptibility to EAMG. Mice of H-2^b haplotype, whether on B10 or B6 genetic background, were highly susceptible and developed overt signs of muscle weakness and fatiga-

FIGURE 1A.   FIGURE 1B.

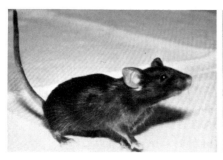 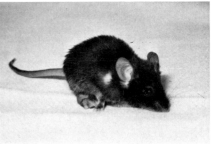

FIGURE 1A.   B10.SN ($\underline{H-2}^D$) inoculated with adjuvant alone.
FIGURE 1B.   B10.SN ($\underline{H-2}^b$) inoculated with TAR + adjuvant
with clinical sign of EAMG.

bility (Figure 1B) with mepp's of reduced amplitude.
Mice of $\underline{H-2}^k$ and $\underline{H-2}^p$ haplotypes appeared to be resistant to
EAMG induction by these criteria and mice of $\underline{H-2}^r$ and $\underline{H-2}^s$
haplotypes were of intermediate susceptibility.

Autoantibodies in Serum and Muscle and Endplate Sensitivity to ACh.   Mice of $\underline{H-2}^b$ and $\underline{H-2}^q$ haplotypes had the highest measured titers of autoantibodies (Table I).   Titers in
$\underline{H-2}^r$ and $\underline{H-2}^s$ were intermediate and $\underline{H-2}^p$ had very low antibody
titers.   AChR extracted from muscles of these mice were found
to be complexed with antibodies in direct proportion to the
amount of antibody measurable in the serum (Table I).

TABLE 1
MEASUREMENTS OF SERUM AUTOANTIBODIES, PERCENT OF MUSCLE AChR COMPLEXED WITH
ANTIBODIES AND MINIATURE ENDPLATE POTENTIAL AMPLITUDE

Strain	Haplotype	Immunogen	Serum auto-antibody+S.E.M. $(\times 10^{-10}\text{M})$	Muscle AChR complexed with antibody (%+S.E.M.)	Mepp amplitude (mV)
B6/Eg	b (n=9)[a]	TAR	112.0+38.42	51+9	n.t.[b]
B6/Eg	b (n=5)	nil	0.0+0.02	0	n.t.
B10/SN	b (n=8)	TAR	39.1+8.41	23+8	0.85+0.103
B10.S	s (n=5)	TAR	8.1+4.24	18+10	1.05+0.158
B10.S	s (n=5)	nil	0.0+0.03	0	1.47+0.060
B10.Q	q (n=10)	TAR	28.5+13.22	26+6	n.t.
B10.P	p (n=6)	TAR	1.1+0.38	3+2	1.38+0.134
B10.RIII	r (n=5)	TAR	7.2+3.76	21+8	n.t.

[a] n = Number of mice tested.
[b] n.t. = Not tested.

Mepp amplitudes of control mice of different haplotypes did not differ markedly, the mean mepp amplitudes of non-inoculated B10.S were typical of mice which were not inoculated with TAR (1.47 ± 0.060 mV, Table I). Mice of $\underline{H-2}^p$ haplotype (B10.P), inoculated twice with TAR, did not differ significantly in mepp amplitude (1.38 ± 0.134 mV) from non-inoculated controls. These findings were consistent with their very low antibody response and lack of immunoglobulin complexed with muscle AChR (Table I). B10.S ($\underline{H-2}^s$) had an intermediate reduction in mepp amplitude (1.05 ± 0.158), an intermediate titer of serum autoantibodies and approximately 18% of muscle AChR was complexed with immunoglobulin. B10/SN ($\underline{H-2}^b$), high producers of autoantibody, had the greatest reduction in mepp amplitude (0.85 ± 0.103 mV) and 23% of the muscle AChR was complexed with antibody.

TABLE 2
T-LYMPHOCYTE PROLIFERATIVE RESPONSE TO TORPEDO ACETYLCHOLINE RECEPTOR
(TAR) IN INDEPENDENT HAPLOTYPES[a]

Mouse Strain	H-2 Haplotype	Immunogen (5 µg)	Medium alone	TAR 0.5 µg	Stimulation index TAR	PPD
B6/Eg	b	nil	971±133	1110±104	1.14	38
B6/Eg	b	TAR	1069±67	38407±4305	35.9	41.1
B10/SN	b	nil	1084±52	765±34	0.70	20.2
B10/SN	b	TAR	7096±906	110284±6323	15.5	18.1
B10.RIII	r	TAR	1703±605	22808±4082	13.0	41.0
B10.WB.	j	TAR	454±22	10777±233	23.0	33.0
B10.Q	q	TAR	2762±255	25340±928	9.1	22.0
B10.M	f	TAR	3389±872	18098±707	5.34	28.6
B10.BR	k	TAR	1939±759	8569±301	4.41	43.0
B10.S	s	TAR	597±22	2947±45	4.93	25.0
B10.D2	d	TAR	570±55	1385±45	2.42	33.0
B10.P	p	TAR	2500±120	5447±188	2.17	47.0
A.BY	b	TAR	2039±142	24681±519	12.1	15.0
AKR-H-2[b]	b	TAR	772±82	34513±1937	44.0	23.8
A.SW	s	TAR	10811±935	54140±4070	5.0	19.4
Balb/C	d	TAR	462±34	802±66	1.73	21.1
B6(TL+)	b	TAR	2304±298	43772±1201	18.99	15.2
B6-H-2[bg1]	b	TAR	1860±222	33947±3190	18.25	19.5

[a] 3-5 mice of each strain were injected at the base of tail with 5 µg of TAR in CFA or with adjuvant only. Draining lymph node cells (4 x 10⁵) were cultured 7 days later with TAR (0.5 µg/0.2 ml) and with PPD (8 µg/0.2 ml). ³H-thymidine was added for the final 16 hours of culture and cells were harvested on the 5th day.

  T Lymphocyte Proliferative Response to TAR. As shown in
the Table 2 strains B10/SN ($\underline{H-2}^b$) B10.RIII ($\underline{H-2}^r$) and B10.WB
($\underline{H-2}^j$) gave S.I. between 10-25 and were classified as high
responders. B10.Q ($\underline{H-2}^q$) and B10.M ($\underline{H-2}^f$) gave S.I. between
5-10 and were classified as intermediate responders. B10.BR
($\underline{H-2}^k$), B10.S ($\underline{H-2}^s$), B10.D2 ($\underline{H-2}^d$) and B10.P ($\underline{H-2}^p$) gave S.I.
of 5 or less and were classified as low responders. To check
the background genes, several other strains were also tested.
Strains A.BY ($\underline{H-2}^b$), B6/Eg ($\underline{H-2}^b$), A.SW ($\underline{H-2}^s$), Balb/C ($\underline{H-2}^d$)
and AKR-$\underline{H-2}^b$ gave responses characteristic of their haplo-
types.
  In an attempt to map the gene(s) controlling T lymphocyte proliferative responses to TAR, several recombinant
strains were tested (Table III). B10.A(5R) having the high
responder alleles $\underline{K}^b\underline{A}^b\underline{B}^b$ and low responder alleles $\underline{J}^k\underline{E}^k\underline{C}^d\underline{S}^d\underline{G}^d$
$\underline{D}^d$ gave a high response suggesting that immune response to
TAR is controlled by gene(s) at the K end. B10.A(4R) having
low responder alleles $\underline{K}^k\underline{A}^k$ and high responder alleles $\underline{B}^b\underline{J}^b\underline{E}^b$
$\underline{C}^b\underline{S}^b\underline{G}^b\underline{D}^b$ were low responders, further narrowing the mapping
to K and A. D2.GD having low responder alleles $\underline{K}^d\underline{A}^d$ and high
responder alleles $\underline{B}^b\underline{J}^b\underline{E}^b\underline{C}^b\underline{S}^b\underline{G}^b\underline{D}^b$ were also low responders confirming the mapping. Another set of recombinants B10.F(13R)
and B10.F(14R) also confirmed the K end mapping of immune re-
sponse to TAR. Results from recombinant B10.LG ($\underline{K}^d\underline{I}^f$) suggest
that the $\underline{H-2K}$ region may not be involved, mapping the Ir gene
to the $\underline{I-A}$ subregion.

TABLE 3
GENETIC MAPPING OF Ir GENE CONTROLLING T-LYMPHOCYTE
PROLIFERATIVE RESPONSE TO TAR[ab]

Mouse strain	MHC Allele									Mean cpm ± S.D.		Stimulation index
	K	A	B	J	E	C	S	G	D	Medium	TAR 0.5 µg	
B10.F(13R)	p	p	p	p	p	p	$\underline{b}$	$\underline{b}$	$\underline{b}$	1268±137	968±40	0.76
B10.F(14R)	$\underline{b}$	$\underline{b}$	$\underline{b}$	$\underline{b}$	$\underline{b}$	$\underline{b}$	p	p	p	1117±43	22004±2024	19.7
B10.A(5R)	$\underline{b}$	$\underline{b}$	$\underline{b}$	k	k	d	d	d	d	3666±238	56690±963	15.4
B10.A(4R)	k	k	$\underline{b}$	$\underline{b}$	$\underline{b}$	$\underline{b}$	$\underline{b}$	$\underline{b}$	$\underline{b}$	1197±131	1278±218	1.06
D2.GD	d	d	$\underline{b}$	$\underline{b}$	$\underline{b}$	$\underline{b}$	$\underline{b}$	$\underline{b}$	$\underline{b}$	1524±27	3915±233	2.56
(B10/SN x B10.D2)F$_1$	b/d	b/d	b/d	b/d	b/d	b/d	b/d	b/d	b/d	2061±54	31674±1535	15.36
B10.S x B10.BR	s/k	s/k	s/k	s/k	s/k	s/k	s/k	s/k	s/k	3227±397	6196±136	1.92

[a] Methods are the same as in Table 1.
[b] High responder alleles are underlined.

An F_1 cross between a high responder and a low responder (B10 x B10.D2)F_1 gave a S.I. of 13.0, suggesting dominant control of responsiveness. A cross between two low responders (B10.S x B10.BR)F_1 gave a S.I. of 1.92 suggesting lack of complementation in this combination. Studies of backcrosses are needed to confirm the linkage study.

DISCUSSION

We are looking at several different parameters to measure susceptibility to EAMG in mice. T-cell proliferation in response to torpedo acetylcholine receptor seems to be controlled by immune response genes mapping in the K end of the major histocompatibility complex, probably in the I-A subregion. We are presently testing to see whether this response is an autoimmune response. Previous studies in other species have shown clearly that immunization with torpedo acetylcholine receptor leads to experimental autoimmune myasthenia gravis. So we would assume that at least part of this immune response at the T cell level is an autoimmune response. The mapping of gene(s) controlling this response suggests that a discrete Ir gene determines recognition of a determinant on the acetylcholine receptor.

Autoantibodies are induced in $\underline{H-2^b}$ haplotype and none in $\underline{H-2^p}$ haplotype and very low levels in other haplotypes. Since these were congenic strains the production of autoantibodies against mouse acetylcholine receptors must be controlled by MHC linked genes. It should now be possible to precisely map the genes controlling autoantibody production. There is a high correlation between the proportion of muscle AChR complexed with antibody and the titer of serum autoantibody. The reduction in mepp amplitude, which is a measure of the defect of neuromuscular transmission, was large in the $\underline{H-2^b}$ haplotype, which develops high autoantibody titers and high T-cell proliferative responses. The mepp amplitude in $\underline{H-2^p}$ haplotype, which had low levels of autoantibody as well as low T cell proliferation to AChR, was similar to that of control animals which were not inoculated with TAR.

Clinical evidence of EAMG, i.e., muscular weakness which was worsened by exercise, was pronounced in 3 out of 17 mice of the $\underline{H-2^b}$ haplotype immunized with TAR. On the other hand, none of eleven $\underline{H-2^p}$ haplotype mice developed clinical signs of EAMG. Hence, on the basis of all the different criteria tested, $\underline{H-2^b}$ haplotype seems to be most susceptible to EAMG whereas $\underline{H-2^p}$ haplotype is least susceptible. Studies of immunological and electrophysiological parameters in recombinant strains will give us a much clearer picture of how MHC genes control or regulate susceptibility to EAMG.

ACKNOWLEDGEMENTS

We are grateful to Suresh Savarirayan for maintaining
the high standard of husbandry in our mouse colony; and
Millie Thompson, Stephen Holmes, Renee McGovern and Dale
Witzel for technical assistance; and Sharon Ames for skillful
preparation of the manuscript.

REFERENCES

1. Lennon, V.A. (1978). *Human Path. 9*, 541.
2. Safwenberg, J. (1978). *Tissue Antigens 12*, 136.
3. Abramsky, O., Aharonov, A., Webb, C., and Fuchs, S. (1975).
   Clin. Exp. Immunol. 19, 11.
4. Richman, D.P., Patrick, J., and Arnason, B.G.W. (1976).
   New Eng. J. Med. 294, 694.
5. Richman, D.P. (1979). *Neurology 29*, 291.
6. Lindstrom, J.M., Seybold, M.E., Lennon, V.A., Duane, D.D.,
   and Whittingham, S. (1976). *Neurology 26*, 1054.
7. Lennon, V.A. (1976). *Immunol. Commun. 5*, 323.
8. Lindstrom, J., Einarson, B., Lennon, V.A., and Seybold, M.E.
   (1976). *J. Exp. Med. 144*, 726.
9. Lennon, V.A., Lindstrom, J.M., and Seybold, M.E. (1976).
   Ann. N.Y. Acad. Sci. 274, 283.
10. Lennon, V.A. (1978). *In* "International Symposium on Organ
    Specific Autoimmunity" (P.A. Miescher, ed.), pp. 178-198.
    Schwabe & Co. AG, Basel, Stuttgart.
11. Lindstrom, J.M., Engel, A.G., Seybold, M.E., Lennon, V.A.,
    and Lambert, E.H. (1976). *J. Exp. Med. 144*, 739.
12. Toyka, K.V. (1977). *New Engl. J. Med. 296*, 125.
13. Fuchs, S.S., Nevo, D., Tarrab-Hazdai, R., Yaar, G. (1976).
    Nature 263, 329.
14. Lindstrom, J., and Patrick, J. (1974). *In* "Synaptic Trans-
    mission and Neuronal Interactions", pp. 191-216. Raven
    Press, New York.
15. Allan, S.S. (1978). *Eur. J. Immunol. 8*, 112.
16. Lambert, E.H., Lindstrom, J.M., and Lennon, V.A. (1976).
    Ann. N.Y. Acad. Sci. 274, 300.

WORKSHOP TITLE: DISCRIMINATION BETWEEN SELF AND NON-SELF

CONVENERS: William O. Weigle, Department of Immunopathology,
Scripps Clinic and Research Foundation, 10666 North Torrey
Pines Road, La Jolla, California, U.S.A. 92037, Alastair J.
Cunningham, Ontario Cancer Institute, University of Toronto,
500 Sherbourne Street, Toronto, Ontario, Canada M4X 1K9 and
Elisabeth H. Lasarow, Department of Microbiology & Immunology,
UCLA, CHS43-239, Los Angeles, California, U.S.A. 90024

It was suggested that the points to be discussed were the
mechanisms of induction, maintenance and termination of immunological tolerance to both foreign and self antigens. The
discussions were opened by W.O. Weigle who gave a hypothetical
model for the induction and maintenance of tolerance to self
antigens and described a maneuver which could result in the
termination of self tolerance. For this model the assumption
was made that tolerance (or lack of tolerance) to self antigens was dependent solely on their concentration in the microenvironment of potential self reactive lymphocytes and not on
the nature of the antigen. The assumption was also made that
the induction and maintenance of tolerance in T cells require
considerably lower concentrations of self antigens than that
required for B cells. In fact, those B cells with low affinity receptors may escape tolerance induction with most, if not
all, self antigens. It was suggested that although polyclonal
activation of such low affinity reactive B cells does not result in autoimmune diseases, such a mechanism may be involved
in rheumatoid arthritis in which the Epstein-Barr virus has
been implicated. In vitro this virus also has been shown to
be a potent polyclonal activator of human B cells, resulting
in the production of anti (IgM) IgG. Despite the low avidity
of this antibody the complexes that it forms with IgG are
biologically active in that they readily fix complement. In
the cases where tolerance resides in only the T cells, in the
presence of competent B cells, procedures which bypass the
need for specific T cells were suggested as a mechanism of
autoimmunity. Direct activation of T cells and B cells could
occur when self-antigens are present in such low concentrations in the body fluid that tolerance is not maintained in
either T cells or B cells. In this model suppressor T cells
would play a regulatory role mainly as a "fail-safe" mechanism
and probably would not be a controlling factor with self antigens in which a solid tolerant state is present in the T cells.
    The question was raised concerning the role of suppressor
T cells in maintenance of tolerance. Elliot Parks presented
data which demonstrated the lack of requirement for suppressor
cells in tolerance induced in adult A/J mice to human gamma
globulin (HGG). Suppressor cell activity was generated with

certain preparations of deaggregated HGG, but not with others,
while tolerance was induced with all DHGG preparations. Even
when suppressor cell activity was induced, it was only transient, while the tolerant state persisted in the absence of
such suppressor activity. Furthermore, injection of colchicine with tolerogen inhibited the generation of suppressor
activity, but did not interfere with the induction of tolerance. Using adoptive transfer of suppressor cells to examine
the kinetics of the generation of suppressor activity in mice
made tolerant at the T cell level to DNP, Claman also reported
a transient appearance of specific suppressor cells. Suppressor cells peaked 7 days after tolerization with DNP and then
rapidly declined, whereas tolerance persisted. Thymectomy and
in vivo treatment with cyclophosphamide removed suppressor
cell activity, but did not interfere with induction of tolerance. These suppressor cells affected the afferent but not
the efferent levels of this response. Similarly, Dr. G.
Hashim reported that suppressor cells interfered with the
initiation of experimental allergic encephalomyelitis, but had
little effect once the disease had developed. It was pointed
out by Av Mitchison that the strongest evidence in favor of
suppression in the maintenance of self tolerance is the work
of Harvey Cantor and Dick Gershon, who showed that irradiated
mice reconstituted with lymphocytes deficient in the suppressor phenotype developed autoimmune disease. On the other
hand, Mark Greene stated that there was no evidence that in
vivo inactivation of suppressor cells with anti I-J serum
resulted in autoimmune disease. Michael Feldman suggested
that one should make a distinction among the various self
antigens and the mechanism involved in their tolerant state.
In response to a question as to the role of suppressor cells
in the autoimmune disease of New Zealand mice, Norm Talal
stated that in the last 1-2 years there has been evidence of
polyclonal B cell activation as a mechanism of these auto-
immune states, but that more than one mechanism may be involved. Dr. P. Hevele reported that the nature of tolerance
induced in chimeric chickens depended on the stage of the
development of the embryo at the time of injection of the
allogeneic cells. If chimeras were made at days 12-15 of the
embryonic development, the adult chickens failed to develop
either circulating antibody or a graft vs. host response.
These chimeras were also negative for suppressor cells to the
allogeneic cells. Al Cunningham suggested that suppressor
cells may interfere with the differentiation of precursor
cells from stem cells and that such suppressor cells may keep
background responses to self antigens from getting out of
control.
      Dr. N. Cohen described homograft studies with frogs which

are relevant to mechanisms of acquisition of self-tolerance. Intact eye primordia were removed bilaterally from tailbud embryos of <u>Xenopus</u> and "parked" in sibling embryos. At a later stage, when development of the lymphoid system of these eyeless frogs had begun, one of their eyes was returned. This was in most cases rejected. Control experiments were done as in the classical work of Triplett; if a single eye was removed and later returned, rejection usually did not occur. In a second series of experiments, it was shown that thymectomy in premetamorphis larvae prevented the establishment of tolerance to outbred parental-strain grafts in <u>Xenopus</u>.

An active role for thymocytes in the establishing of tolerance was also suggested by work presented by Dr. J. Phillips-Quagliata (New York University Medical School), who showed that neonatal thymectomy of rats prevented the subsequent development of tolerance to 20 mg BSA. Injecting thymocytes, but not T cells from other tissues, to the thymectomized animals restored their ability to develop tolerance. It was interesting to note that suppressor T cells could not be demonstrated in this tolerance system, indicating that suppression need not be overt even in a case where, by other criteria, the active participation of thymus lymphocytes is necessary to generate a tolerant state.

A brief discussion of the direct "blockade" tolerance of B cells followed, to which the main contributors were Elliot Parks and David Scott. It was decided that such central inhibition of B cells does occur in states when B cells are also susceptible to this kind of effect (Parks) which may result in lowered numbers of antigen binding cells (Scott).

Dr. Y. Kong showed that repeated injection of mouse thyroglobulin to certain strains of mice ("high responders" e.g., C3H), will result in thyroid lesions and autoantibody; Dr. G. Hashim (St. Lukes Hospital Center, New York) discussed the possibility that, in cases like this, the autoantigen may be altered (away from "self") by handling before injection.

Dr. C. Waters briefly discussed work presented earlier, in the plenary session, by her colleague Dr. E. Diener. They found that HGG, BSA, and a synthetic polymer "TNP-18", when injected into pregnant female mice, all crossed the placenta and appeared in high concentrations in the foetuses; however, only HGG induced tolerance. It was speculated that the molecular nature of the antigen might be critical in tolerance and that a "self-marker" might be important (the Fc part of HGG), a suggestion which was quashed by Dr. Av Mitchison who felt that valid comparisons between these 3 antigens were not possible without more knowledge of the amounts persisting in the young mice at different times after their initial exposure to tolerogen. A possible tolerogenic role for the Fc part of

foreign Ig was also postulated by Dr. S. Friedman who found
that either the whole rabbit Ig molecule or its Fc part alone
were tolerogenic in mice, while the Fab fragment was immunogenic. This was considered to cast some doubt on the usefulness of foreign Igs as general models for tolerance induction,
an aspersion which was vigorously refuted by W.O. Weigle on
the grounds that the important difference between the toleri-
zing properties of Fab and whole Ig lies in their very difer-
ent half lives in mice (approximately 12 hours and 7 days,
respectively).

IR GENE COMPLEMENTATION IN THE MURINE T-LYMPHOCYTE
PROLIFERATIVE RESPONSE

Ronald H. Schwartz, Alan M. Solinger, Michiel E. Ultee,
Emanuel Margoliash, Akihiko Yano, Jack H. Stimpfling,
Chuan Chen, Carmen F. Merryman, Paul H. Maurer,
and William E. Paul

Laboratory of Immunology, NIAID, NIH
Bethesda, MD. 20014
Department of Biochemistry and Molecular Biology
Northwestern University, Evanston, Il. 60201
The McLaughlin Research Institute
Great Falls, MT. 59401
Department of Biochemistry, Jefferson Medical College,
Philadelphia, PA. 19107

ABSTRACT. The immune responses to poly($\text{Glu}^{55}\text{Lys}^{36}\text{Phe}^{9}$) [GL$\phi^9$], poly($\text{Glu}^{57}\text{Lys}^{38}\text{Tyr}^{5}$) [GLT^5], and pigeon cytochrome c are controlled by two major histocompatibility (MHC)-linked immune response (Ir) genes, one mapping in the I-A subregion, the other in the I-E/C subregion. In the case of pigeon cytochrome c, the major antigenic determinant has been localized through cross-stimulation experiments involving species variants and cyanogen bromide-cleavage fragments of the molecule. The determinant was shown to be composed of at least three amino acids, Ile-3,Gln-100 and Lys-104, which lie adjacent to one another in a linear array on the back surface of the molecule. Therefore, two complementing Ir genes control the response to a single antigenic determinant. Furthermore, in one cross-reaction, that obtained with tobacco hornworm moth cytochrome c, the stimulation was greater than that achieved with the immunogen, thus demonstrating for the first time a heteroclitic T cell response.

The cellular sites of expression of these complementing Ir genes has been examined in several ways. Reconstitution of lethally irradiated high responder F_1 mice with a mixture of bone marrow cells from both low responder parental strains failed to generate chimeras which could respond to GLϕ^9. This suggested that at least one cell type involved in the immune response had to express both gene products. That the antigen-presenting cell (APC) was one such cell type was demonstrated by presenting GLϕ^9 to primed F_1 T cells on nonimmune spleen cells. Only high responder F_1 spleen cells could

261

ISBN 0-12-069850-1

present; low responder parental spleen cells, possessing
only one of the two high responder alleles, failed to
present even when both parental types were added together.

However, possession of a high responder genotype was
not always sufficient to generate a response. In the
case of GLT^5, gene dosage effects appeared to prevent the
B10 and B10.A strains from complementing to produce a
responder F_1 strain. In the case of $GL\phi^9$, histocompatibility restrictions limited antigen presentation. Genetic identity at the I-A subregion was required between
the T cells and the APCs but identity at I-E/C was not
required. B10.A(5R) responder T cells could be stimulated by $GL\phi^9$-pulsed spleen cells from F_1 progeny of B10
crossed with B10.A, B10.BR, B10.D2, B10.P, and B10.RIII
but not B10.Q, B10.M and B10.BSVS. This pattern corre-
lates with the data of others on the serological presence of Ia.7 and the biochemical presence of an I-E/C
subregion gene product in these strains. The data
suggest that the Ia.7-bearing, I-E/C gene products of
the complementing strains are all similar and that this
molecule (presumably an $Ia_9\alpha$ chain) is critically involved
in the presentation of $GL\phi^9$. Overall the experiments
support the conclusion that both complementing Ir gene
products must interact at the molecular level in the
same APC in order to generate a T-lymphocyte proliferative response.

The mechanism of action of MHC-linked Ir genes has
puzzled immunologists for many years. The recent discovery
that some immune responses are controlled by two Ir genes,
both mapping in the I region, has suggested an additional
level of complexity in the MHC regulation of lymphocyte activation (1). In this paper we will summarize our experimental approaches to the analysis of several different dual
Ir gene controlled systems in an effort to understand how the
two gene products interact with one another to produce an
immune response.

Although the original description of Ir genes demonstrated their effects on in vivo antibody formation and delayed-
type hypersensitivity (2), subsequent studies indicated that
the genetic control was also manifest in in vitro assays
(3,4). For the murine T-lymphocyte proliferative response
[PETLES assay (5)] MHC-linked, Ir gene control has been demonstrated for responses to both protein and synthetic
polypeptide antigens (4). Dual Ir gene control has also been
demonstrated in this system for the response to the synthetic
terpolymers, poly $(Glu^{55}Lys^{36}Phe^9)$ $[GL\phi^9]$ and poly

$(Glu^{57}Lys^{38}Tyr^5)$ [GLT^5] (6,7). More recently we have observed that the T-lymphocyte proliferative response to pigeon ferri-cytochrome $\underline{c}$, is also controlled by two MHC-linked Ir genes (8). Table I is a summary of the proliferative responses of several B10.$\underline{H-2}$ congenic strains immunized with 20μg of pigeon cytochrome $\underline{c}$. Only mice bearing the $\underline{H-2}^a$ or $\underline{H-2}^k$ haplotypes were high responders. All other strains were either low or non-responders to pigeon cytochrome $\underline{c}$, although PETLES from these strains responded well to PPD. Table II shows the genetic mapping of the Ir genes controlling the response to pigeon cytochrome $\underline{c}$. B10.A is a natural recombinant between the high responder, $\underline{H-2}^k$-bearing and the non-responder, $\underline{H-2}^d$-bearing strains. Its responsiveness maps the gene(s) to the left of the $\underline{I-C}$ subregion. Similiarly, because $\underline{H-2}^q$-bearing strains are non-responders, the responsiveness of the B10.AQR PETLES maps the gene(s) to the right of the $\underline{K}$ region, solely in the $\underline{I}$ region. To map the gene(s) within the $\underline{I}$ region, the B10.A(4R) and B10.A(5R) recombinants were examined Neither strain responded. (Table II). This result indicates that the response is controlled either by a single gene which maps in the $\underline{I-B}$ subregion or by two genes, one in $\underline{I-A}$ and the other in $\underline{I-J}$ or $\underline{I-E}$. To distinguish between these two possibilities, an F_1 cross was made between the B10.A(4R) and B10.A(5R) nonresponders. As shown in Table II, PETLES from this F_1 responded to pigeon cytochrome $\underline{c}$ demonstrating that two MHC-linked Ir genes control the immune response.

Similar types of complementation experiments have been used in the past to demonstrate the dual Ir gene control of the response to $GL\phi^9$ (6) and GLT^5 (7). The advantage offered

TABLE I

MHC-LINKED Ir GENES CONTROL THE T-LYMPHOCYTE PROLIFERATIVE RESPONSE TO PIGEON CYTOCHROME c

Mouse Strain	H-2 Haplotype	Thymidine Incorporation (ΔCPM) to		Cytochrome Responsiveness
		Pigeon Cytochrome	PPD	
B10.A	a	23,600	41,900	High
B10	b	800	32,300	Non
B10.D2	d	1,600	39,400	Non
B10.M	f	6,900	105,300	Low
B10.BR	k	39,200	55,800	High
B10.P	p	1,100	49,500	Non
B10.Q	q	1,600	21,800	Non
B10.RIII	r	7,900	44,200	Low
B10.S	s	5,500	23,900	Low
B10.PL	u	1,100	161,800	Non

TABLE II

GENETIC MAPPING WITHIN THE MHC OF THE Ir GENES
CONTROLLING THE PROLIFERATIVE RESPONSE TO PIGEON CYTOCHROME c

Mouse Strain	MHC Alleles K A B J E C S G D	Proliferative Response (ΔCPM) to Pigeon Cytochrome c
B10.A	k k k k k d d d d	18,500
B10.AQR	q k k k k d d d d	15,800
B10.A(4R)	k k b b b b b b b	100
B10.A(5R)	b b b k k d d d d	2,300
(4R × 5R) F$_1$	k k b b b b b b b b b b k k d d d d	18,800

Conclusion: Two complementing Ir genes control the T-lymphocyte proliferative response to pigeon cytochrome c; one in I-A, the other in I-J or I-E.

by this new protein system, however, is the ability to localize and characterize the antigenic determinants being recognized. This has been accomplished in the case of pigeon cytochrome c through the use of species variants of the molecule
to cross-stimulate in the proliferation assay (8,9). B10.A
PETLES, which are immune to pigeon cytochrome c, do not respond when challenged with mouse cytochrome c (Fig. 1). Therefore, stimulatory activity must depend on the sequence differences between pigeon and mouse cytochromes c. These differences total 7 amino-acid residues out of 104 and are shown in
Fig. 1. To assess the immunogenic importance of each of these
substitutions, cytochromes were selected for testing which
shared a common amino acid with pigeon cytochrome c at only
one of the 7 variant positions. For example, human cytochrome c possesses a serine at position 15, similar to that
of pigeon cytochrome c but different from the mouse protein's
alanine. The failure of human cytochrome c to stimulate
PETLES immune to pigeon cytochrome c suggests that residue 15
is not a principle amino acid in the antigenic determinant.
In contrast, cross-stimulation was achieved with the cytochrome c from hippopotamus (Fig 1). Of the 7 variant amino
acids, this protein shares with the pigeon protein only the
glutamine at site 100, thus implicating this residue as part
of the antigenic determinant. However, the partial nature of

the cross-reaction suggested that other residues must be involved. This was confirmed by the complete stimulation achieved with the cytochrome c from tobacco hornworm moth (Fig. 1).
This protein possesses the glutamine at site 100, but in addition contains a C-terminal lysine similar to the pigeon protein.
Thus, both the glutamine and lysine appear to be part of the
antigenic determinant. Interestingly, the response to tobacco
hornworm moth cytochrome c was actually better than that to
pigeon cytochrome c. The maximum response achieved was 30%
higher and the concentration required to stimulate one-half the
maximum response was 10-fold lower. This heteroclitic response
may be the result of a deletion of amino acid residue 103 in
the tobacco hornworm moth protein. This deletion moves the
C-terminal lysine one residue closer to the glutamine at site
100 and perhaps creates a determinant that better fits the T
cell receptor.

Source of Cytochrome c	Amino Acid Residue at Position							Proliferative Response (Δ CPM)
	3	15	44	89	100	103	104	0 10,000 20,000 30,000
Mouse	Val	Ala	Ala	Gly	Lys	Asn	Glu	▌
Pigeon	Ile	Ser	Glu	Ala	Gln	Ala	Lys	████████████████
Human	Val	Ser	Pro	Glu	Lys	Asn	Glu	▌
Neurospora crassa	Ser	Ala	Asp	Lys	Glu	Ala	–	▌
Hippopotamus	Val	Ala	Pro	Gly	Gln	Asn	Glu	██████
Tobacco Horn Worm Moth	Ala	Ala	Pro	Asn	Gln	Lys	–	█████████████████
Chicken	Ile	Ser	Glu	Ser	Asp	Ser	Lys	███
Pekin Duck	Val	Ser	Glu	Ser	Asp	Ala	Lys	███

Fig. 1. Localization of the antigenic determinant in pigeon
cytochrome c. The table lists the amino acids found at the 7
positions at which pigeon cytochrome c differs from mouse cytochrome c. Implicated residues are underlined. The graph
shows the T lymphocyte proliferative response of PETLES from
B10.A mice immunized with 20μg of pigeon cytochrome c and
challenged in vitro with the various cytochromes c listed on
the left.

Finally, cross-stimulation experiments with cyanogen bromide-cleavage fragments of cytochrome c implicated a third residue involved in the antigenic site. As shown in Table III,
of the three non-overlapping clevage fragments, only pigeon
cytochrome c fragment 81-104 stimulated as good a proliferative
response as the whole molecule. This confirmed that the major

stimulating residues were located at the C-terminal end of the molecule. However, pigeon cytochrome c fragment 1-65 also eli- cited a small but reproducible response. This stimulation was shown not to be the result of contamination of fragment 1-65 with fragment 81-104 by experiments with the cyanogen bromide- cleavage fragments of other bird cytochromes c. Chicken cyto- chrome c fragment 1-65, which has an identical sequence to pigeon fragment 1-65, stimulated as well, even though chicken fragment 81-104 gave only a weak cross-reaction (Table III). Duck fragment 1-65, on the other hand, did not stimulate, even though duck fragment 81-104 gave a cross-reaction comparable to chicken fragment 81-104 (Table III). Duck fragment 1-65 differs from pigeon and chicken fragments 1-65 at one amino acid position. Residue 3 is a valine in duck cytochrome c, similar to the mouse sequence, whereas pigeon and chicken cytochromes c possess an isoleucine at this site. Thus, the isoleucine would appear to be a third residue involved in T cell stimulation.

Although the three amino acids discussed are not next to each other in the primary structure of the protein, in its three-dimensional form these three residues do lie next to each other in a linear array on the back surface of the molecule.

TABLE III

STIMULATION OF PETLES FROM B10.A MICE IMMUNE TO PIGEON CYTOCHROME c
WITH CYANOGEN BROMIDE CLEAVAGE - FRAGMENTS OF BIRD CYTOCHROMES c

Cytochrome Source	Fragment Residue Nos.	Proliferative Response Δ CPM ± SEM
Mouse	1-104	2,400 ± 1,200
	1-65	2,100 ± 2,100
	66-80	1,200 ± 1,100
	81-104	2,300 ± 1,100
Pigeon	1-104	27,900 ± 1,200
	1-65	8,700 ± 1,100
	66-80	1,500 ± 1,100
	81-104	43,100 ± 2,900
Pekin Duck	1-104	- 100 ± 1,100
	1-65	1,300 ± 1,100
	66-80	1,800 ± 1,500
	81-104	13,700 ± 2,100
Chicken	1-104	3,400 ± 1,100
	1-65	9,400 ± 1,600
	66-80	3,600 ± 1,100
	81-104	16,400 ± 2,800

A close up view of their spatial arrangement is shown in Fig. 2. Thus, the B10.A T cells specific for pigeon cytochrome c

appear to recognize a single topographical antigenic determinant composed of at least the isoleucine at site 3, the glutamine at site 100 and the lysine at site 104. The fact that
two Ir genes control the response to this <u>single</u> determinant
suggests that complementation is not the result of synergistic
interactions between separate cells recognizing different
determinants, each of which is under the control of a single
Ir gene.

A more direct approach to the question of whether complementation involves interactions between different cell
types, each possessing one of the two responder alleles, was
carried out in the GLϕ system. In these studies radiation
chimeras of the type A + B → (AxB)F$_1$ were prepared in which
A (B10.A) and B [B10.A(18R)] were the two low responder parents and (AxB)F$_1$ the complementing high responder strain
(10). In the chimera, all the genetic material possessed by
the F$_1$ is present but segregated into the separate cells of
the two parental types. If complementation involves cell

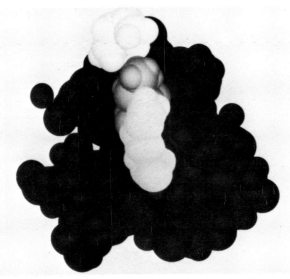

Fig. 2. The Antigenic Determinant in Pigeon Cytochrome <u>c</u>.
This is a computer simulated model of the site produced by
Richard Feldmann of the Division of Computer Research and
Technology, NIH. Using the three-dimensional structural co-
ordinates for tuna cytochrome <u>c</u>, the pigeon protein sequence
was substituted, adjusted to reduce van der Waals contacts and
modeled to maximize favorable side chain interactions. The 3
residues involved in the antigenic site are shown in lighter
tones relative to the rest of the molecule. They are from
top to bottom the Ile at position 3, the Gln at position 100
and the Lys at position 104.

interactions, then the chimeras should respond to GIɸ . However, as shown in Fig. 3, this was not the case. Although the
18R ↔ B10.A chimeras responded well to (T,G)-A--L and pigeon
cytochrome c, antigens to which only one of the two parents
was a high responder, the mice did not respond to GLɸ. Thus,
both parental cell types were functionally intact, but they
could not cooperate to generate a GL ɸ response. This failure
did not appear to result from a cryptic mixed lymphocyte reaction as 3R↔B10.A chimeras, which possess an identical I-A
region potential incompatibility, but in which one of the
parents (3R) is a responder to GLɸ, were capable of mounting
a proliferative response to GLɸ (Fig. 3). These results suggest that at least one cell type involved in the immune response to GLɸ must express both gene products.

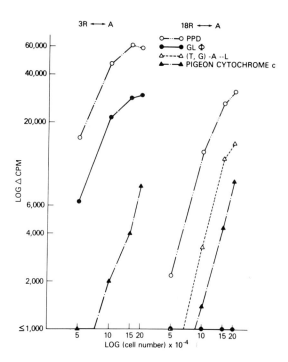

Fig. 3. The T-lymphocyte proliferative response of PETLES
from 3R↔B10.A and 18R↔B10.A chimeras. The chimeras were
immunized 6 months after irradiation and bone marrow reconstitution. Three weeks later PETLES were prepared and
cultured at various cell numbers per well of a round bottom
microtiter plate in the presence of 20μg/ml of PPD (0), 100μg/
ml of GLɸ (●), 100μg/ml of (T,G)-A--L (Δ), or 100μg /ml of
pigeon cytochrome c (▲).

The antigen-presenting cell (APC) was shown to be one such cell type. This was demonstrated by presenting GLφ to complementing (nonresponder x nonresponder)F_1 primed T lymphocytes on nonimmune spleen cells from (B10.A x B10)F_1 mice or either parental strain. As shown in Table IV neither B10 nor B10.A parental spleen cells presented GLφ, although both could present PPD. In contrast, (B10.A x B10)F_1 spleen cells could present GLφ. The failure of GLφ-presentation by either of the parental spleen cell populations could not be attributed to a general lack of presenting capacity of the parental cells, for two reasons. First, B10.A(5R) spleen cells, which possess both high responder Ir gene products, presented GLφ as well as (B10.A x B10)F_1 spleen cells, although the PPD response elicited by the B10.A(5R) cells was only equivalent to that of the parental strains. Second, mixtures of the two parental spleen cell populations did not complement to generate a GLφ response, although the response to PPD was generally enhanced. In the mixtures, as in the chimeras, there exists all the genetic material required for high responsiveness, but segregated into separate cells. These results demonstrate that both Ir gene products must be expressed in the same antigen-presenting cell. In other words, the APC must come from a high responder strain.

TABLE IV

Proliferative response of GLφ primed (B10.AxB10)F_1 PETLES to GLφ and PPD presented on parental or F_1 spleen cells

Antigen-presenting Spleen cells	Proliferative response (Δcpm±SEM)	
	GLφ-pulsed	PPD-pulsed
(B10.A x B10)F_1	16,600±2,900	27,200± 600
B10.A	1,400± 600	8,800± 900
B10	1,400± 300	12,300± 900
B10.A + B10	1,700± 900	18,400± 400
B10.A(5R)	15,600±1,100	11,800±1,000

Thus, it is essential that all the high responder genetic material be expresed in the same cell in order to obtain an immune response to antigens such as GLφ. However, there are instances in which possession of responder alleles at both controlling loci is not sufficient for a response. In some examples of two gene systems, the cross between the two types of nonresponders does not produce a complementing F_1, even though a recombinant strain, possessing both responder alleles, is a high responder (7). For example, in the proliferative response to GLT^5, PETLES from the B10.A(5R) strain show a strong response whereas PETLES from the (B10.A x B10)F$_1$ show only a weak response (Fig. 4). Both strains possess the high responder I-A^b and I-E^k alleles in the same cell; however, they differ in the number of copies they possess. The B10.A (5R) has two copies of each high responder allele whereas the (B10.A x B10)F$_1$ has only one copy of each allele. To demonstrate that this difference in gene dosage is what accounts for the difference in responsiveness to GLT^5, B10.A(5R) mice were bred to B10.A(4R) mice, a strain which does not possess any responder alleles (1). The resulting [B10.A(4R) x B10.A (5R)]F$_1$ which has only one copy of each responder allele, was a poor responder to GLT^5 (Fig. 4). The proliferative response of the (4Rx5R)F$_1$ was not significantly different from that of the (B10.A x B10)F$_1$, suggesting that the chromosomal relationship of the two responder alleles (cis vs trans) was not important, only their absolute number. Thus, gene dosage effects can mask responsiveness and in certain crosses give the impression that nonresponsiveness is dominant. These results suggest that Ir genes are co-dominantly expressed and that F$_1$ crosses, which decrease the concentration of both high responder alleles by half, can have dramatic effects in two gene systems, perhaps because the gene products must interact to generate an immune response. As a result, the concentration of the essential interaction product is decreased by 3/4, thus presumably limiting its availability.

Finally, the existence of an immune response involving genes in the I-E/C subregion has allowed us to address the question of restriction in antigen-presenting cell-T lymphocyte interaction across this subregion barrier. Although it is essential for the APC to derive from a high responder strain, not all high responder strains will suffice for presentation. As shown in Fig. 5, if GLφ-primed T lymphocytes. are obtained from B10.A(5R) mice, then spleen cells from the syngeneic B10.A(5R) high responder strain can present antigen, whereas spleen cells from the allogeneic B10.D2 high responder strain can not. The requirement for genetic identity at the I-A subregion for antigen-presentation has been demonstrated for both DNP-OVA and GAT (11,12). Thus, the failure of B10.D2 (dddddddd)* to present GLφ to B10.A(5R) (bbbkkdddd) PETLES

*Letters refer to the haplotype source of origin of the K, I-A, I-B, I-J, I-E, I-C, S, G and D regions of the MHC.

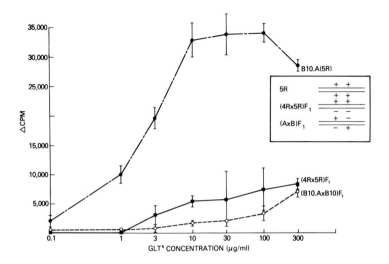

Fig. 4. Gene Dosage Effect. The three strains, B10.A(5R),
containing 2 copies of each high responder allele, (●),
(B10.A x B10)F$_1$, containing 1 copy of each high responder
allele in trans (0), and [B10.A(4R) x B10.A(5R)]F$_1$, containing 1 copy of each high responder allele in cis (■), were
immunized with 100 μg of GLT^5-PBS in CFA. Three weeks later
the PETLES were prepared from each strain and 2x10^5 cells
were cultured for 5 days in the presence of various concentrations of GLT^5-PBS. Stimulation was assessed by measuring
the incorporation of a 1μCi pulse of ^{3}H-methyl-thymidine 16
hr prior to harvesting the cultures. The responses are expressed as the difference between the antigen-stimulated
cultures and the control cultures carried out in the presence
of only medium (ΔCPM).

could result solely from the I-A subregion incompatibility.
In order to assess the contribution of the I-E/C subregion,
B10.D2 was crossed with B10 and the F$_1$ used as a source of
presenting cells. The B10 parent brings in the high respond-
er I-A^b allele, which thus makes the F$_1$ APC histocompatible
with the responding B10.A(5R) T cells at the I-A subregion.
However, the F$_1$ is still incompatible with B10.A(5R) at the
I-E subregion (I-E^k vs I-E$^{b/d}$). Despite this potential

incompatibility, the (B10 x B10.D2)F$_1$ spleen cells presented
GLφ quite well (Fig. 5).

Similar F$_1$ presentation experiments were carried out with
other GLφ-responder strains. In order to compare different
strains and to average experimental results for any given
strain, the data had to be normalized to the DNP-OVA presentation results by the formula [ΔCPM-GLφ/ΔCPM-DNP-OVA] x 100.
Because DNP-OVA presentation depends only on I-A subregion
compatibility and because presentation to B10.A(5R) T lymphocytes can only make use of the I-A^b alleleic product, all the
F$_1$s formed with B10 should theoretically be equivalent in
their DNP-OVA presentation. The data are shown in Table V.
F$_1$ crosses between B10 and B10.A, B10.BR, B10.D2, B10.P, and
B10.RIII all presented GLφ equivalently despite the fact that
the last 3 strains were histoincompatible at the I-E subregion.
In contrast, the B10 cross with B10.Q could not present GLφ
even though B10.Q is a responder to GLφ like B10.D2, B10.P
and B10.RIII. Thus, being a responder to GLφ was not sufficient for complementation. Two other strains, B10.M and

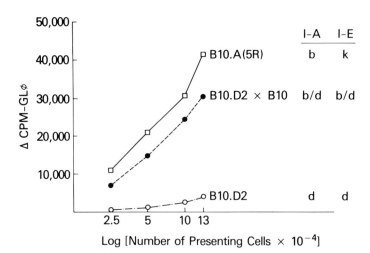

Fig. 5. The equivalence of I-E^k and I-E^d in GLφ presentation.
PETLES were prepared from GLφ-primed B10.A(5R) mice and stimu-
lated in vitro with various numbers of GLφ-pulsed B10.A(5R)
(□), B10.D2 (0) or (B10.D2 x B10)F$_1$ (●) nonimmune spleen cells.

B10.BSVS, also failed to complement, although these were both nonresponders to GLφ and might have failed to present for that reason. Analysis of the over all pattern showed one constant feature. All strains possessing a complementing form of the Ir gene at I-E, expressed Ia.7, a genetic marker of the I-E/C subregion. Furthermore, recent structural data from several laboratories (13-15) based on two dimensional gels and peptide maps of the I-E/C subregion gene products (isolated with anti Ia.7 containing sera) have indicated that the α chains from $H-2^k$, $H-2^d$, $H-2^p$, and $H-2^r$ haplotype-bearing strains are very similar (85-100%) if not in some cases identical (k vs r). In contrast, the β chains were easily distinguisable (50-60% differences in their peptide maps).

Based on these data, a simple model can be proposed which explains the failure to see genetic restriction in presentation across an I-E/C barrier. This scheme is presented in Fig. 6. If the two polypeptide chains precipitated with anti-Ia antisera are coded for by two separate genes, and if the gene products of any given pair can only associate with each other to form an active biological molecule, then complementation for presentation could be explained by

TABLE V

HISTOCOMPATIBILITY RESTRICTION AT THE I-E SUBREGION FOR GLφ PRESENTATION

Presenting Cell	MHC Alleles		B10.A(5R) Proliferation ΔCPM(GLφ/DNP-OVA) × 100	Ia.7 Bearing + α Chains Similar*
	I-A	I-E		
B10.A(5R)	b	k	33	+
B10 × B10.A	b/k	k/b	26	+
B10 × B10.BR	b/k	k/b	33	+ *
B10 × B10.D2	b/d	d/b	38	+ *
B10 × B10.P	b/p	p/b	39	+ *
B10 × B10.RIII	b/r	r/b	38	+ *
B10 × B10.Q	b/q	q/b	3	−
B10 × B10.M	b/f	f/b	3	−
B10 × B10.BSVS	b/s	?s/b	4	−

PETLES from GLφ and DNP-OVA primed B10.A(5R) mice were challenged in vitro with DNP-OVA or GLφ-pulsed nonimmune spleens from a variety of F_1 hybrids. The proliferative response to GLφ is expressed as a percentage of the response to DNP-OVA. The data represent the means for 2-5 experiments.

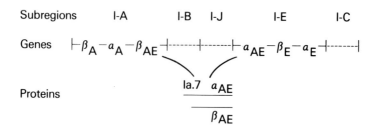

Fig. 6. A conjectural scheme for the genetic basis of Ir gene complementation. The Ia.7-bearing α_{AE} chain encoded in the I-E subregion pairs with the β_{AE} chain encoded in the I-A subregion. This pair forms the functional restriction antigen on the surface of the cell which is required for GLφ presentation.

postulating a genetic rearrangement of the murine DNA of the I region in which the genes coding for one pair of phenotypically linked α and β chains have become separated such that one lies in the I-A subregion (β) while the other lies in the I-E subregion (α). If this particular pair is required for the immune response to GLφ, then only strains carrying both genes could function. Theoretically recombination events could separate the two genes and produce only nonresponding offspring. This would seem to be a disadvantageous situation from an evolutionary point of view. However, this problem is avoided in the present situation by conserving a molecule (the Ia.7-bearing chain) which can pair with a variety of β chains to produce a functional complex. As a result many of the haplotypes which carry the gene coding for the α chain are responders ($H-2^d$, $H-2^p$, $H-2^r$ and $H-2^{i5}$). Similarly, when the T cells are primed in our experiments to recognize GLφ in association with an I region pair of gene products involving an $I-A^b$ encoded β chain, then any strain capable of donating the relatively constant α chain to a hybrid cross with B10 would be able to complement for GLφ presentation. The failure of B10.Q to complement suggests that this strain lacks the special α chain and that its response to GLφ is through a different mechanism.

    This complementation model is also consistent with all of the other experiments with GLφ as well as those with pigeon cytochrome c and GLT^5. The fact that both gene products must be expressed in the same antigen-presenting cell, requires that the complementation be intracellular and at the molecular level. The ability of two Ir genes to control the response to a single antigenic determinant is reasonable if the two gene products are required to form a unique F_1 interaction (restriction) structure which is essential for the immune response to the antigen.[5] Finally, the gene dosage effect seen in the response to GLT[5] can be explained by the concentration argument presented earlier. The mechanism by which the T lymphocyte becomes restricted to recognize such antigens in the context of F_1 interaction structures has been discussed previously (10,16). Suffice it to say that both dual receptor or single receptor models of T cell recognition could account for these observations.

REFERENCES

1. Dorf, M. E. (1978). Sem. Immunopathol. 1, 171.
2. McDevitt, H. O., and Benacerraf, B. (1969). Adv. Immunol. 11, 31.
3. Kapp, J. A., Pierce, C. W., and Benacerraf, B. (1973) J. Exp. Med. 138, 1107.
4. Schwartz, R. H., and Paul, W. E. (1976). J. Exp. Med. 143, 529.
5. Schwartz, R. H., Jackson, L., and Paul, W. E. (1975). J. Immunol. 115, 1330.
6. Schwartz, R. H., Dorf, M. E., Benacerraf, B., and Paul, W. E. (1976) J. Exp. Med. 143, 897.
7. Schwartz, R. H., Merryman, C. F., and Maurer, P. H. (1979) J. Immunol. In Press.
8. Schwartz, R. H., Solinger, A. M., Ultee, M., and Margoliash, E. (1978). In "Immunobiology of Proteins and Peptides" (M. Z. Atassi and A. B. Stavitsky, eds), Vol 1 p. 371. Plenum, New York.
9. Urbanski, G. J., and Margoliash, E. (1977). In "Immunochemistry of Enzymes and Their Antibodies" (M. R. H. Solton, ed.), p. 204. John Wiley & Sons, New York.
10. Schwartz, R. H., Yano, A., Stimpfling, J. H., and Paul, W. E. (1979). J. Exp. Med. 149, 40.
11. Yano, A., Schwartz, R. H., and Paul, W. E. (1977). J. Exp. Med. 146, 828.
12 Yano, A., Schwartz, R. H., and Paul, W. E. (1978) Eur. J. Immunol. 8, 344.
13. Jones, P. P., Murphy, D. B., and McDevitt, H. O. (1978) J. Exp. Med. 148, 925.
14. Freed, J. H. (1978). J. Immunol. 121, 1609.
15. Cook, R., Capra, J. D., Vitetta, E. S., and Uhr, J. W. (1979). Immunochemistry. In Press.
16. Schwartz, R. H., Yano, A., and Paul, W. E. (1978). Immunol. Rev. 40, 153.

MURINE MACROPHAGE-LYMPHOCYTE BINDING - SEPARATION OF
B CELL SUBSETS ON MACROPHAGE MONOLAYERS[1]

Margot O'Toole and Henry H. Wortis

Tufts University School of Medicine,
Boston, Massachusetts   02111

ABSTRACT   Spleens and lymph nodes of normal adult mice
contain cells that adhere to macrophage monolayers for
two hours or more. The majority of these binding cells
are B cells. By allowing B cells to adhere to macrophage
monolayers, and harvesting the non-adherent cells, a
population of B cells that will not subsequently bind
to macrophages can be obtained. Thus B cells can be
divided into macrophage binding and non-binding populations. The binder population is part of the previously
described Lyb3 positive B cell subpopulation. Peripheral
T cells can disrupt B cell-macrophage binding.

INTRODUCTION

The in vitro binding of lymphocytes to macrophages is a
well recognized phenomenon (1-5). Guinea pig thymocytes (3),
peripheral T and B cells (4) and murine thymocytes (6) have
been shown to bind. Several lymphocyte functions are known
to be macrophage dependent. These include helper cell and
cytotoxic T cell generation; proliferation in response to T
cell and some B cell mitogens and to antigen; and antibody
production in response to certain thymus independent antigens
(reviewed in 7). The role of macrophages in these interactions is poorly defined, although there is evidence that
they can present antigen (7), support lymphocyte viability
(8) and promote differentiation of thymocytes (9,10).
Since some lymphocyte functions are macrophage dependent,
and since lymphocytes can bind to macrophages, we wanted to
know if subpopulations of murine lymphocytes differed in their
ability to bind to macrophages.

MATERIALS AND METHODS

Mice.   CBA/Tufts and F_1 (CBA/N x CBA/Tufts) mice were

[1]This work was supported by National Cancer Institute
Grants CA 21348 and CA 16172. M. O'Toole was supported in
part by NIH Training Grant AI 00436.

bred at Tufts University School of Medicine. C57B1/6, Balb/c
and A/HeJ mice were purchased from Jackson Laboratory, Bar
Harbor, Maine.

Macrophage-Lymphocyte Binding. Macrophages were obtained
by washing the peritoneum of CBA/Tufts mice that had been
injected i.p. four days earlier with two mls of 3% thiogly-
collate. The cells were washed, suspended at 5×10^5 ml and
cultivated overnight on 5" round cover slips placed in 24 well
Falcon tissue culture plates. The medium used was RPMI 1640
(Microbiological Associates) supplemented with 0.1% bovine
serum albumin, 290 µg/ml glutamine, 100 µ/ml penicillin,
100 µg/ml streptomycin and .02M HEPES. The wells were washed.
Greater than 98% of the cells which adhered to the cover slips
took up neutral red and/or latex particles. Spleen and lymph-
node cells were suspended in medium and dead cells removed
according to the method of Von Boehmer and Shortman (11). To
test for macrophage-lymphocyte binding, 5×10^6 washed spleen
or lymph node cells suspended in 1.0 ml of medium were added
to each of three wells containing adherent cells. After
incubation, the unbound cells were removed by gentle washing
with a Pasteur pipette. It was essential that washing was
gentle and uniform. The cells were then fixed overnight at
room temperature with 0.05% glutaraldehyde in HEPES buffered
RPMI 1640 (pH 7.2). The cover slips were stained with 0.16%
crystal violet, removed from the culture wells and mounted on
glass slides. The slides were examined under a light micro-
scope using a 45x objective. The macrophages along one
diameter of each cover slip were counted with the aid of a
micrometer disc. Each macrophage was scored as having 0, 1,
2, 3 or more bound lymphocytes. Macrophages with 3 or
more   lymphocytes bound were scored as positive. Data are
expressed as percent of macrophages positive. The standard
deviation was less than 10% of the mean in 99 of a series of
100 experiments. This method of counting directly correlated
with the number of bound lymphocytes/100 macrophages, and had
the advantage of being faster.

Antisera. (N anti B6) N anti B6 serum was prepared by
B. Huber by immunizing (CBA/N x B6) F_1 male mice with B6
spleen cells according to the protocol used for preparation
of anti Lyb3 antisera. This serum identifies a new cell
surface allo-antigen that is found only on Lyb3 bearing cells
(manuscript submitted for publication). Anti-BAT (brain
associated T cell antigen) was prepared according to the
method of Golub (14). Fluorescienated rabbit anti-mouse Fab
(FlRaMFab)(a gift from B. Huber) was prepared by immunizing
with mouse Fab and affinity purifying the antisera on a mouse

Fab column.

Cell Separations. T cells were purified by the panning method of Mage (12), Wysocki and Sato (13). These cells were less than 1% surface Ig positive. Nylon wool fractionation was done using the method of Julius, et al (14) except that 1.0% bovine serum albumin was used instead of fetal calf serum. Nylon wool effluent cells were 71% Thy 1 positive, nylon wool adherent cells were 8% Thy 1 positive. B cells were obtained by treating suspensions of lymphocytes with anti-BAT serum and complement.

RESULTS AND DISCUSSION

Macrophage-Lymphocyte Binding. When suspensions of spleen or lymph node cells were overlaid on macrophage mono- layers, a large number of lymphocytes bound to the macro- phages. This was shown with syngeneic combinations of macro- phages and lymphocytes from five different strains of mice. The binding required live macrophages and was inhibited by sodium azide and EDTA. As shown in Figure 1, 86% of the spleen cells which bound to macrophages after a two hour co- incubation were surface Ig positive (B cells). When T cells were removed from the cell suspensions, (by treatment with anti-BAT and C') a large number of the BAT resistant cells were seen bound to macrophages (Figure 1, line 2). After surface Ig positive cells were removed from the cell suspen- sions, relatively few bound cells were seen (Figure 1, line 3). These findings were repeated with lymph node cells.

Purification of Non-Binding B Cells. In order to test whether (or not) all B cells can bind to macrophages, anti- BAT resistant spleen cells were incubated on macrophage mono- layers at a macrophage to lymphocyte ratio of 1:1. This was done to absorb out those cells which could bind to macro- phages. The non-bound cells are removed by gentle washing and tested for binding in a conventional assay (macrophage to lymphocyte ratio of 1:10). As controls, cells were incubated on petri dishes without macrophages. The cells harvested from macrophage monolayers did not bind to a fresh monolayer, while the cells harvested from control cultures bound as well as non-incubated control cells. It is therefore possible to purify a population of non-binding B cells by absorbing binding cells on macrophage monolayers. The non- binding cells constitute about 43% of the original anti-BAT resistant population.

Absence of Binding Cells in xid Mice. The preceding

data suggest the existence of binding and non-binding B-cell populations. The CBA/N mouse has an x-linked recessive B cell defect (x-linked immunodeficiency, xid)(16), and it has been shown by serological methods that these mice are missing a B cell subpopulation (17,18). They lack B cells bearing the surface antigens Lyb3 (17), Lyb5 (18) and the antigen defined by N anti B6 serum (B. Huber, submitted for publication). We therefore tested the macrophage binding properties of B cells from CBA/N mice and from male and female F_1 mice produced by a CBA/N x CBA/Tufts cross. (Male F_1 mice are defective, females are normal). As shown in Figure 2, the defective F_1 male mice also have a binding cell defect. Cells from the female F_1 have binding properties similar to those of the normal parent. Mice with the xid defect, therefore, lack not only the Lyb3, Lyb5 positive B cell subpopulation, but also the macrophage binding B cell population.

FIGURE 1

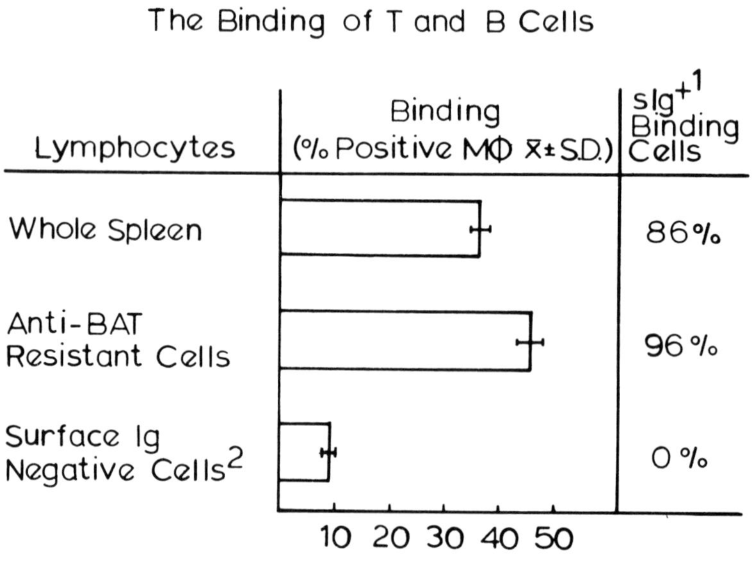

The Binding of T and B Cells

1. As judged by reaction with Fl RaMFab

2. Purified by the panning method of Wysocki and Sato (12)

FIGURE 2

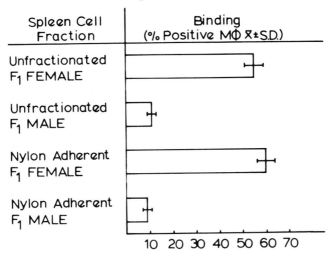

CBA/NxCBA)F₁ Males Have a Binding Cell Defect

Nylon adherent fraction refers to the B cell enriched fraction from a nylon wool column

Nylon effluent fractions from both male and female spleens were tested and had comparable (low) levels of binding

A B Cell Surface Antigen Is Restricted to Binding Cells. Since normal splenic B cells can be separated into binding and non-binding populations and CBA/N mice lack both the binding and the Lyb3 positive cells, one would predict that non-binding cells (purified from normal spleen) should be depleted of cells sensitive to treatment with the N anti B6 serum and C'. This proved to be the case. While N anti B6 antisera is cytotoxic for 55% of normal B6 spleen cells, it has no reactivity against purified non-binding cells from normal spleen B cells. Since the Lyb3 positive population appears late in ontogeny, we expected that young mice would also be deficient in binding cells. This proved to be true (data not presented).

T Cells Influence Macrophage-B Cell Binding. When suspensions of non-purified spleen or lymph node cells were incubated with macrophages, a large number of lymphocytes were
bound to macrophages after two hours (Fig. 1). If these
cultures were left for twenty four hours before termination,
very few lymphocytes remained bound (Fig. 3). (This agrees
with the findings of Lipsky and Rosenthal on antigen independent macrophage-lymphocyte binding in the guinea pig system
[19]). In contrast, when suspensions of purified B cells
(either nylon wool adherent or anti-BAT resistant cells) were
tested a large number remained bound after twenty four hours
(Figure 3, line 2). If purified T and B cells were mixed
prior to culture, the level of binding at both two and twenty
four hours resembled that of whole spleen or lymph node.
Since the initial binding does occur, and only the duration of
binding is affected by the presence of T cells, there must be
a population of T cells which causes early release of B cells
from macrophages. These we called remover T cells. Remover
cells were present in surface Ig negative spleen cell suspensions, nylon wool effluent cells and were sensitive to treatment with anti-BAT and C'. Other cells have been found to
have no influence on macrophage - B cell interactions (data
not presented).

SUMMARY

The data show clearly that mouse lymphocytes differ with
respect to their macrophage binding properties. A large proportion of B cells can bind. There are five lines of evidence
that support the conclusions that only a subpopulation of B
cells can bind to macrophages: 1)a population of non-binding
cells can be purified; 2) CBA/N mice lack a B cell subpopulation and also lack binding cells; 3) non-binding cells lack
a surface marker of a B cell subpopulation; 4) young mice have
a low frequency of binding B cells; 5) the percentage of
adult B cells that bind equals the percentage that is Lyb_3
positive and reacts with N anti-B6 serum.
As shown in Figure 1, a small number of peripheral T
cells bind to macrophages at two hours. Experiments to
further characterize this population and the remover cells
with respect to other lymphocyte markers are currently being
done. It is predicted that knowledge of the type of lymphocytes that bind will aid in the study of the functional significance of the physical interactions which occur between
macrophages and normal lymphocytes. The possible function of
remover cell activity and its mechanism of action are also
under investigation.

FIGURE 3

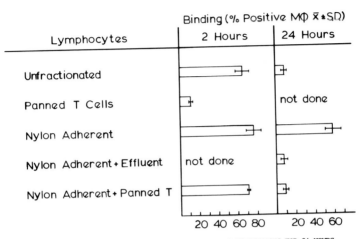

REMOVER FUNCTION IN SPLENIC T-CELLS

NYLON WOOL ADHERENT CELLS, (B CELLS), BIND TO MACROPHAGES FOR 24 HOURS. WHEN T CELLS ARE PRESENT IN CULTURES OF B CELLS AND MACROPHAGES, THE BINDING DOES NOT PERSIST. THIS IS TURE BOTH WHEN T CELLS ARE NOT REMOVED FROM SPLEEN CELL PREPARATIONS AND WHEN PURIFIED T CELLS ARE MIXED WITH B CELLS.

PANNED T CELLS = S Ig NEGATIVE SPLEEN CELLS PURIFIED BY THE PANNINING METHOD.

ACKNOWLEDGEMENTS

We thank Dr. Brigitte Huber for the generous gift of anti-sera and Peter Brodeur, Dan Gold, Kathy Hirsch, Mary Mitchell and Gerry Waneck for help in various stages of this project.

REFERENCES

1. Mosier, D.E. (1969). J. Exp. Med. 129, 351.
2. Siegal, I. (1970). J. Immunol. 105, 879.
3. Lipsky, P.E. and Rosenthal, A.S. (1973). J. Exp. Med. 138, 900.

4.   Lopez,L.R., Johansen, K.S., Radovich, J. and Talmage, D.W.
     (1974). J. Allergy and Clin. Immunol. 53, 336.
5.   Albrect,R., Hinsdill, R., Sandok, P. and Horowitz, S.
     (1978). Infect. and Immunity 21, 254.
6.   Lopez, L., Vattrer, A.E. and Talmadge, D.W. (1977). J.
     Immunol. 119, 1668.
7.   "Role of Macrophages in the Immune Response" (1978).
     Immunol. Rev. 40 (ed. Moller, G.)
8.   Nathan, C.F. and Terry, W.D. (1975). J. Exp. Med. 142,
     887.
9.   Mosier, D.E. and Pierce, C.W. (1972). J. Exp. Med. 136,
     1484.
10. Beller, D. and Unanue, E. (1977). J. Immunol. 118, 1780.
11. Von Boehmer, H. and Shortman, K. (1973). J. Immunol. Meth.
     2, 293.
12. Mage, M.G., McHugh, L. and Rothstern, T. (1977). J.
     Immunol. Meth. 15, 47.
13. Wysocki, L.J. and Sato, V. (1978). Proc. Nat. Acad. Sci.
     72, 2844.
14. Julius, M., Simpson, E. and Herzenberg, L.A. (1973).
     Eur. J. Immunol. 3, 645.
15. Golub, E. (1971). Cell. Immunol. 2, 353.
16. Amsbaugh, D.F., Hansen, C.T., Prescott, B., Stashok, P.W.,
     Barthold, D.R. and Baker, P.J. (1972). J. Exp. Med. 136,
     931.
17. Huber, B., Gershon, R.K. and Cantor, H. (1977). J. Exp.
     Med. 145, 10.
18. Ahmed, A., Sher, I., Sharrow, S., Smith, A., Paul, W.E.,
     Sacks, D. and Sell, K. (1977). J. Exp. Med. 145, 101.
19. Lipsky, P.E. and Rosenthal, A.S. (1975). J. Exp. Med.
     141, 138.

WORKSHOP SUMMARY: Role of Macrophages in the Initiation
and Regulation of the Immune Response.
Workshop Convener: P.E. Lipsky, University of Texas
Health Science Center at Dallas, Dallas, Texas 75235

The workshop explored a number of issues concerning the
role of macrophages (MØ) in the initiation of immune responses, including: 1) the uniqueness of the MØ as an antigen presenting cell; 2) the functional capabilities of various MØ
sub-populations; 3) possible mechanisms of functional interaction between MØ and lymphocytes; 4) mechanisms of "antigen
processing", and 5) genetic restrictions on MØ-lymphocyte
interaction.
    The nature of the antigen presenting cell (APC) in a num-
ber of different systems was discussed. H.B. Dickler (NCI,
NIH) characterized the murine splenic adherent cell capable of
presenting antigen for the induction of primary *in vitro* antibody responses by splenic lymphocytes and secondary proliferative responses by lymph node T lymphocytes. APC were found in
a population of glass adherent radioresistant non-T, non-B
cells that possessed Fc receptors, surface I-A and I-E/C antigens and were phagocytically active. Splenic adherent cells
were more effective APC than peritoneal adherent cells and
this appeared to correlate with the number of cells expressing
Ia antigens. Thus, 60% of splenic adherent cells expressed
I-A antigens of which about 1/3 also were positive for I-E/C,
while only 15-20% of peritoneal adherent cells were I-A or
I-E/C (+). However, this work could not rule out the possibility that more than one adherent cell was needed for effective antigen presentation since only 15-20% of the adherent
spleen cell population had all of the aforementioned criteria.
G.B. Ahmann (NCI, NIH) examined the capacity of various spleen
cell populations to present antigen or trigger the MLR. He
incubated murine spleen cells with fluoresceinated latex particles and separated them into phagocytically active and inactive populations with a fluorescence activated cell sorter.
While both populations were able to trigger the MLR, only the
phagocytic cells could function as APC. T.M. Rogoff (Southwestern Med. Sch.) studied antigen presentation by isolated
highly purified guinea pig Kupffer cells. This population
consisted of more than 95% MØ and had no identifiable dendritic cells. These cells were effective at presenting antigen
to T cells for the induction of secondary proliferative responses. They were, however, less efficient than peritoneal MØ
and this difference again correlated with the number of Ia
antigen bearing MØ present in each population.
    These data all indicated that MØ were the major APC in
the systems reported. However, it remained possible that in

other systems additional cells might function as APC or as
accessory cells necessary for the expression of immune responses. For example, J.A. Trial (Southwestern Med. Sch.) found
that mouse lymph node T cells obtained from animals sensitized by skin painting with TNCB or DNFB underwent proliferative responses *in vitro* to a variety of TNP- and DNP-antigens.
When these nylon wool-passed cells were additionally depleted
of MØ by carbonyl iron treatment, their response was not decreased. While there were no detectable esterase-staining or
latex-ingesting cells in this preparation, there was a non-
lymphoid cell with dendritic morphology. This cell comprised
10-20% of the total cell number, and was present in both
immune and control preparations. It differed from a dendritic
cell, however, in that it apparently contained Fc receptors.
The possibility that this cell was similar to the Langerhans
cell of the epidermis and might function as an APC was entertained.

Although it appeared clear that MØ could function as APC,
the possibility that different MØ populations might have differing antigen presenting capabilities was discussed. As
mentioned above, in the guinea pig, peritoneal MØ were more
effective APC than Kupffer cells, while, in the mouse, splenic
adherent cells were more efficient than peritoneal adherent
cells. K.C. Lee (U. Alberta) separated murine peritoneal MØ
by size and found that the smaller MØ were rich in Ia antigens and were effective APC, while the larger MØ consisted of
fewer Ia (+) cells and were ineffective at presenting antigen.
Splenic MØ were found to be enriched for smaller, Ia (+) APC.
Both large and small MØ secreted factors that could augment T
cell proliferation. T.B. Tomasi (Mayo Clinic) presented evidence that murine Peyer's patches contain MØ-like cells that
were unable to function as APC. Adherent Peyer's patch cells
contained about 20% B cells, 10% T cells, 15% phagocytically
active cells and 22% esterase positive cells. Although these
cells could stimulate the MLR and appeared to be Ia (+), they
were unable to function as APC.

R.I. Mishell (UCB) pointed out that responses in these
systems reflected a balance between positive and negative influences, and that peritoneal MØ from different strains may
differ in their capacity to provide positive and negative signals to T cells. He further discussed the role of non-specific MØ factors in regulating the immune system. MØ factors
could block the immunosuppressive activity of dexamethasone.
These factors were produced by peritoneal MØ including Ia (-)
MØ or MØ cell lines after stimulation by a number of agents
such as LPS. Biochemically there were two peaks of activity.

Mechanisms of functional MØ-lymphocyte interaction were
discussed. C.R. Lyons (Southwestern Med. Sch.) presented the

view that transmission of signals between antigen-bearing MØ
and T cells involved the establishment of physical contact.
In this system, antigen-primed guinea pig T cells bound to
antigen bearing syngeneic but not allogenic MØ. Antibody to
antigen did not block binding, but antibody to Ia determinants inhibited the development of this physical interaction.
 Since the primed T cells employed were Ia antigen (-), it was
concluded that the action of the alloantiserum was directed
against Ia determinants on the MØ. These data were interpreted as indicating that physical contact between MØ and T cell
is required to facilitate antigen recognition by T cells.
In addition, it appeared that native antigen was not seen by
the T cell, but rather a fragment of antigen in the context
of MØ Ia antigens was likely to be the relevant immunogenic
moiety. Finally, antigen on the surface of MØ did not appear
to be of importance in T cell antigen recognition. This
latter point was consistent with a number of previous studies
indicating that anti-antigen antibody did not inhibit the
capacity of MØ to present antigen to primed T cells. For example, S. Leskowitz (Tufts Med. Sch.) pointed out that DTH
to ABA-tyrosine was not blocked by anti-antigen antibody.
However, these conclusions appeared to conflict with the
findings of E. Shevach (NIAID, NIH), who found that antibody
to TNP blocked the capacity of TNP-modified MØ to present antigen to TNP primed T cells. He, therefore, argued that T
cells not only could see unprocessed antigen but that relevant antigen resided on the surface of the MØ. He further
suggested that the inability of previous investigators to see
this effect resulted from the low density of antigen on the
surface of MØ, and the consequent inability of antibody to
establish multivalent binding of surface antigen. The possibility that haptenation of the MØ surface allowed anti-hapten
antibody to function as an anti-MØ surface determinant antibody in this system was discussed as an alternative explanation for these findings.
     M. Feldmann (Univ. College) presented a model of helper
T cell induction in which antigen presentation is accomplished by means of a soluble factor. This factor, GRF, or genetically related factor, has a molecular weight of about
60,000 daltons and is composed of Ia antigen and a fragment
of the specific immunogen. There is no evidence that it contains heavy chain variable region determinants. The factor
binds to T cells. GRF is not generated by MØ obtained from
non-responder strains. Acid treatment can cause dissociation
of the Ia portion and the antigenic fragment of GRF. If GRFs
from two sources specific for different Ia regions and different antigens were mixed, acid treated, and then brought to
neutrality, the dissociated molecules reassociated in random

fashion yielding GRF activity specific for both Ia regions
and both antigens. It was emphasized that this particular
system had been established for the purpose of detecting
soluble factors. It should not be inferred that functional
interaction between MØ and T cells only occurs by means of
soluble factors, or that transmission of signals is not facilitated by the establishment of cell to cell contact. The production of GRF by MØ was felt, however, to be good evidence
for an antigen processing role for MØ.

The genetic restriction of functional MØ-T cell interaction was discussed by R. Hodes (NCI, NIH). Making use of
(A x B)F$_1$ → Parent A radiation bone marrow chimeras, the requirement for unprimed helper T cells to recognize MHC determinants expressed on accessory cells was examined. It was
found that helper T cells from these chimeras could cooperate
only with accessory cells expressing K or I-A region H$_2$ determinants identical to those of the host. Such restrictions
were not dependent on antigen exposure and there were no similar requirements for T-B cell interaction. These data indicated that helper T cell activation required recognition of
MHC determinants expressed on adherent cells and that T cells
were restricted to recognizing H$_2$ determinants identical to
those of the adherent cells present in the milieu in which
they developed. Feldmann reported similar findings with
F$_1$ → P chimeras but discrepancies were reported with P → F$_1$
chimeras in which genetic restriction of T cell recognition
for P MØ persisted unless F$_1$ was supplemented with the other
parent MØ. It was felt that this apparent discrepancy may relate more to the instability of the P → F$_1$ chimeras than to
genetic restrictions of MØ-T cell interaction.

In summary, MØ play a number of important roles in the
induction and regulation of immune responses. A subpopulation
of Ia antigen bearing MØ act as antigen presenting cells.
Additionally, Ia(+) and Ia(-) MØ secrete factors that augment
or in some cases suppress immune responses. Further investigation should provide additional insight into the significance of functional heterogeneity of MØ subpopulations, as
well as the role of other Ia antigen bearing non-MØ accessory
cell populations in the immune response. While it is apparent that functional interaction between MØ and T cells requires recognition of MØ Ia determinants by potentially responsive T cells, the mechanisms involved in antigen handling
by MØ and the details of signal transmission by antigen-
bearing MØ to lymphocyte populations remain to be fully defined.

WORKSHOP SUMMARY: HELPER AND SUPPRESSOR EPITOPES

N. A. Mitchison and E. E. Sercarz, University
College, Department of Tumor Biology, London WC1
6BT and the University of California at Los
Angeles, Department of Microbiology, Los Angeles,
California, 90024.

In this workshop an effort was made to understand the basis
for association of certain determinants on soluble or cellular
antigens with T cell helper effects and of others with T cell
suppression. There are at least three levels at which a
choice could be made:
1) at antigen presentation in the initial association of
    antigenic fragments with different MHC molecules;
2) at the level of the repertoire of T_H and T_S cells:
3) as a result of overriding other forces (e.g. idiotypic).

Sercarz pointed out the consequences of having a single, so-
called "suppressor determinant" on a molecule. By antigen-
bridging, T_S directed against this determinants would nullify
T_H activity against other determinants on the same molecule.
The same general process might be more effective for cell
surface antigens, where not only intramolecular, but also
intermolecular effects should occur.

In the first part of the workshop, evidence was brought forth
in a variety of systems where help vs. suppression results
from minor amino acid changes in the antigen. The second
part involved a discussion of these and other data trying
to relate these effects to cellular causes.

Adorini spoke of the control of anti-lysozyme response in
$H-2^b$ mice. These mice raise T_S against one determinant near
the N-terminal end of hen egg-white lysozyme (HEL) but T_H
against other determinants on the molecule. Whether or not
T_S are induced by a given lysozyme can be related to a single
tyr-phe switch at a known position: lysozymes like HEL with
phe, induce suppression, and are therefore non-immunogenic
for $H-2^b$ mice. The suppressor T cells affect helper or proliferative T cells. By "amputation" of the offending residues, HEL can be converted into an immunogen.

Chiller and Corradin found a similar situation with beef
cytochrome C where reactivity with one moiety of the antigen
was revealed after separation from other (putatively
suppressive) peptides of the molecule. Schwartz pointed out
that hidden proliferative T cells were not found in the pigeon
cytochrome C system; Chiller added tuna to this category. It
was agreed that it might only be possible to demonstrate this

phenomenon in special cases.

Goodman pointed out that with azobenzene arsonate, both
helpers and suppressors could be simultaneously triggered by
the same determinant. However it is possible that with
haptens, the decision may depend on the nature of neighbouring
residues.

Two instances involving myelin basic protein and the ensuing
experimental allergic encephalomyelitis (EAE) were discussed.
Swanborg described conversion of myelin basic protein from a
disease-inducing to a tolerance-inducing molecule for the rat
by change of a single crucial tryptophan on the molecule.
Hashim described a similar situation in the guinea pig, involving an amino acid sequence which, when changed, induces skin-
test reactivity rather than EAE. Chemical manipulations of
the crucial peptide can be shown radically to alter its
effect.

Dutton argued that for a single specificity (i.e. comparing
normal B6 mice with a mutant solely affecting the K cistron),
the T cell response can change markedly. Miller suggested
that such a single mutational difference may drastically
affect the cell surface.

The discussion shifted towards cell surface antigens.
Suppressor determinants on the cell surface, it was suggested,
constitute a special case. Here, separate molecules may be
linked together in a single structure, a cell membrane, and
so may remain associated together as a single antigenic
structure during processing by the immune system. In
consequence, intermolecular suppression could be detected.
Example of this type of suppression can be found in the
associations between MHC products as restriction elements and
the H-Y antigen (Simpson) or MHC products as restriction
elements and viral proteins (Zinkernagel). In both cases
there occur presentation hierarchies, in which the foreign
antigen (H-Y or viral) can associate with a given MHC product
but will abandon it in favor of another MHC product if the
second product is made available on the same cell. These
hierarchies can be explained in two ways, one of which
Simpson favors. This is that MHC products physically bind
the foreign antigens, and compete with one another for
limiting amounts of these antigens in much the same way as
antibodies might do, although with a lower degree of specificity. Swain favors an alternative view, previously formulated by Zinkernagel and Cohn. This is that both the competing associations (MHC + foreign antigen) are available

on the surface of the antigen-presenting cell, and competition occurs between lymphocyte precursors differing from one another in affinity or frequency. Mitchison argued in favor of the second alternative, at least in the context of suppression of the anti-Thy-1 response by incompatibility at H-2. The strongest evidence in favor of competition between lymphocytes here is that "deviation" of H-2 reactive lymphocytes by pretreatment with massive intraperitoneal doses of H-2 incompatible cells can abate the suppressive effect.

There was some discussion of the suppressive effects mediated by I-J which Streilein's poster had described. Mice which had been injected at birth with an appropriate number of cells foreign at I-J + D would nearly always accept skin grafts of the same foreign type late in life - an example of classical neonatal tolerance. Surprisingly, the same mouse would often reject skin grafts foreign for the same D antigen alone, and with a second set reaction. This can be explained in terms of I-J acting as a restricting element for suppressor T cells, Streilein proposes. Swain did not accept this hypothesis, having found that suppressor T cells are restricted by K and D molecules, not I-J. Simpson hesitated to accept the mouse strains used by Streilein as differing only in the way the H-2 charts indicate. In spite of these criticisms one feels that these experiments say something interesting, for only a minority of the cells in the skin grafts carry I-J molecules, and yet they seem to exert a strong local effect on neighbouring cells.

As regards the MHC restriction of suppressor T cells, some of the views expressed were strongly against restriction at the factor level and less confidently, against restriction in the cell interactions themselves.

Thus (i) Germain finds that the GAT suppressor factor is unrestricted, and that suppression works in mixtures of allogenic cells; (ii) Kontiainen finds that macrophages are not required for the production of KLH-specific or NP-specific suppressor T cells in vitro, although they are for helper T cells, and that the suppressor factors produced are not restricted; (iii) Sercarz mentioned that Araneo finds macrophage-T suppressor precursor cell interaction to be H-2 restricted.

We were then left with the following general view. A simple theory is that the decision about suppression is made at the level of the antigen-presenting cell, and depends only on whether a molecule can associate appropriately with an MHC

restriction element (I-J or K/D) or not. This would readily
explain why some determinants are suppressive and others not.
The difficulty is that there is little evidence that I-J
molecules in fact act as restriction elements in the presentation of antigen. Furthermore, as Vitetta pointed out,
there is little direct evidence for physical associations
between antigens and MHC products (except perhaps for the C-
type viruses) in spite of these associations looming so large
in immunological theories. Nevertheless even if the idea
of physical association comes to nothing, Swain emphasised
that antigen-presenting cells may still be able to make
crucial decisions. Indeed, the only coherent alternative
view was expressed by Janeway, who thinks that it is largely
a matter of regulatory circuits among T cell subsets. He
opts for a role for the existing repertoire in determining
whether suppression or help will dominate. Thus, the levels
of pre-existent idiotype-specific T cells and carrier
specific T cells collaborating for a variety of T cell
functions, would be crucial for the outcome of a particular
response.

MULTIPLE MHC LOCI CONTROLLING LYMPHOCYTE
INTERACTIONS

Tomio Tada, Masaru Taniguchi, Kyoko Hayakawa,
and Ko Okumura

Department of Immunology, Faculty of Medicine, University
of Tokyo, Tokyo, and Laboratories for Immunology, School
of Medicine, Chiba University, Chiba, Japan

ABSTRACT   Antigen-binding T cells were specifically enriched from keyhole limpet hemocyanin(KLH)-primed splenic
T cells by adsorption to and elution from KLH-coated Petri
dishes. The cells thus obtained had KLH-binding sites on
their cell surface together with I-J subregion-coded determinants. The presence of the framework structure of
immunoglobulin heavy chain V region (V_H) on antigen-binding T cells was determined by staining with anti-V_H and
fluoresceinated anti-rabbit Ig, and by the cytotoxic killing with anti-V_H and rabbit C. Anti-V_L antibody had no
cytotoxic effect on antigen-binding cells. Furthermore,
the antigen-specific suppressor T cell factor was absorbed by both anti-V_H and anti-I-J columns, and was successfully recovered in the acid eluate from them.
    The enriched population of antigen-binding T cells
was utilized to make hybridomas by fusion with a thymoma
cell line BW5147. After selection by the I-J expression
with fluorescence activated cell sorter, hybrids were
cloned to establish I-J^+ hybridoma lines. Some of these
I-J^+ hybridomas secreted the KLH-specific suppressor factor, which was also adsorbable to anti-I-J and anti-V_H.
The specific T cell factor from hybridomas having I-J-
coded determinants had a strict genetic restriction, in
that the factor could suppress the responses of only H-2
compatible strains. These results indicate that the
antigen receptor of suppressor T cells, which is released
under certain circumstances as the factor, contains two
distinct antigenic determinants, i.e., Ig V_H gene and I-J
subregion gene products, the former determining the antigen-binding specificity and the latter the genetically
determined restriction specificity.

[1] This work was supported by a grant from the Ministry of
Education, Culture and Science, Japan.

INTRODUCTION

One of the major concerns in current immunology has been centering around the structure of antigen-receptor of T cells. Whereas a number of recent reports indicate that T cell receptors for certain antigens carry idiotypic determinants shared with antibody molecules and B cells (reviewed in 1 and 2), evidence has been presented that T cells recognize not only antigenic determinants but also the products of major histocompatibility complex (3,4). At the moment, there is no clear resolution for this dichotomy.

We have sometimes been interested in this problem, since the putative antigen-receptor of suppressor T cells (Ts), namely, antigen-specific suppressor factor (TsF), possessed an antigen-binding capacity as well as an ability to distinguish the fine differences of I region gene products expressed on responding lymphocytes. In short, the factor is produced by antigen-primed Lyt-2^+,3^+ T cells and acts only on histocompatible Lyt-1^+,2^+,3^+ T cells. The critical identity of the haplotype origin of I-J subregion was found to be required in this suppressive cell interactions (5). These findings led us to postulate that the antigen-receptors of T cells are bifunctional in that they can bind antigen by one functional end, but by virtue of another functional end they would recognize the products of MHC expressed on other cell types with which they interact. The antigen-specific suppressor T cell factor would allow us to study the structures involved in above versatile nature of T cell receptors.

In this communication, we would present our view on the possible structure of the antigen-receptor of Ts, which accommodates two different specificities, i.e., antigen-specificity and genetic restriction specificity. Evidence is presented that the former is based on the structure identical or similar to V region of immunoglobulin heavy chain, and the latter is determined by I region products controlled by multiple loci closely linked to each other.

PROPERTIES OF ANTIGEN-BINDING T CELLS

We have previously reported a simple procedure to enrich antigen-binding T cells by adsorption to and elution from antigen-coated columns or Petri dishes (6,7). The method employed in the present experiment in brief is as follows: C57BL/6 or CBA mice were immunized with two injections of 100 μg each of soluble keyhole limpet hemocyanin (KLH) at a two-week interval. The spleen cells were taken two weeks after the second immunization. The cell suspension was incubated in Petri dishes coated with anti-mouse immunoglobulin to adsorb B cells. The B cell-depleted cell suspension was taken, and then the antigen-binding T cells were adsorbed onto the surface of other Petri dishes coated with KLH at 37°C. After removal of unbound cells (Fr. 1), the Petri dishes were cooled on ice, and the cells bound to the dishes (Fr. II) were removed by washing with chilled Eagle's minimal essential medium (MEM).

The properties of these two fractions of T cells are summarized in Table I. The KLH-specific suppressor activity was always enriched in Fr. II, while helper activity was detected only in Fr. I. The sonicated extract of Fr. II cells contained a very strong suppressor activity. This enrichment of Ts in Fr. II was always associated with the enrichment of $I\text{-}J^+$, Lyt-2^+,3^+ T cells (Table I).

TABLE   I

ENRICHMENT OF $I\text{-}J^+$, Lyt-2^+,3^+ SUPPRESSOR T CELLS
IN FR. II

Properties	Fr. I	Fr. II
KLH-specific suppressor T cell	−	++
KLH-specific TsF	−	++
KLH-specific helper T cell	++	−
$I\text{-}J^+$ T cell	< 5%	>30%
Lyt-1^{+*}	>45%	≃10%
Lyt-2^+,3^{+*}	≃10%	>40%

* Caliculated value.

The direct evidence that many of the Fr. II cells can bind antigen on their cell surface was obtained by observation with scanning electron microscopy (Matsuzawa et al., unpublished). Fr. II cells from C57BL/6 mice were incubated with freshly prepared KLH (M.W. approximately 8,000,000) at 37°C. After washing with MEM, the cells were rapidly fixed by freeze-drying at a critical point. KLH molecules bound on the cell surface were easily observed with scanning electron microscopy.

It was found that a number of KLH molecules were bound on the flat surface of the hemisphere of Fr. II cells (Fig. 1). The molecules were identified to be KLH by comparing with free KLH molecules fixed on a millipore membrane. Such cells were rarely found in Fr. I and unseparated splenic T cell population. If the same Fr. II cells were pretreated with anti-$I\text{-}J^b$

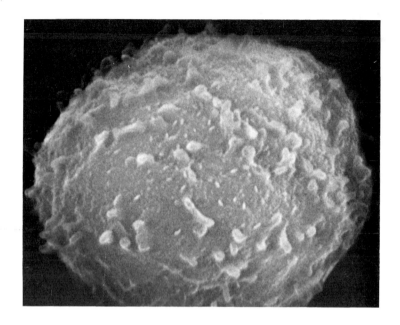

FIGURE 1.   Scanning electron microgram of antigen-
      binding T cells.   Note several KLH molecules
      bound on the flat surface of lymphocyte hemi-
      sphere.

antiserum without complement (C), very few cells bound KLH
molecules in a much smaller number.   The treatment of Fr. II
cells with normal mouse serum as well as anti-I-J^b antiserum
preabsorbed with H-2^b spleen cells did not block the antigen-
binding activity.   The results suggest that I-J determinant is
at least in close proximity to the antigen-binding site on
KLH-specific Ts, and thus the treatment of Ts with anti-I-J
antiserum can block the binding of antigen by the receptor.

PRESENCE OF IgV_H FRAMEWORK STRUCTURE ON Ts AND TsF

The second approach to the structural entity of the antigen-binding site on Ts was made possible by taking advantage
of antisera directed to the framework determinants of immunoglobulin variable regions.   The purified rabbit antibodies
against isolated variable region fragments of mouse myeloma
protein (M-315) heavy and light (λ) chains (anti-V_H and anti-
V_L) were kindly provided by Dr. David Givol of the Weizmann
Institute of Science, Rehovot, Israel.   These antibodies can

react with variable portion of a variety of heavy or light chains, and are regarded to be antibodies directed to the framework structure of V regions. The detailed description of these antibodies have been described by Ben-Neriah *et al.* (8,9).

The enriched Ts (Fr. II) from CBA mice was stained with anti-V_H and fluoresceinated anti-rabbit Ig. Even though more than 95% cells were Thy-1 antigen positive, 30 to 40% of Fr.II cells were found to be stained with anti-V_H. Only a negligible number (less than 5%) of Fr. I cells were stained with anti-V_H under the identical condition. The staining profile was sometimes 'patchy' but not 'capped' even after an incubation at 37°C for 30 min.

We then tested the cytotoxicity of fractionated T cells with anti-V_H and anti-V_L in the presence of rabbit C. The essential results are summarized in Table II. Whereas both Fr. I and Fr. II consisted of more than 95% Thy-1 antigen positive cells, about 80% of Fr. II cells were killed with anti-V_H and C. No significant killing was observed in Fr. I.

TABLE II

PRESENCE OF V_H FRAMEWORK DETERMINANTS ON ENRICHED SUPPRESSOR T CELLS

Cell fraction	Antiserum (dilution)		% killed
Fr. I	Anti-Thy-1.2	(1:30)	>95
	Anti-I-J^k	(1:20)	<15
	Anti-V_H	(1:20)	<15
	Anti-V_L	(1:20)	<15
Fr. II	Anti-Thy-1.2	(1:30)	>95
	Anti-I-J^k	(1:20)	75
	Anti-I-J^b	(1:20)	<15
	Anti-V_H	(1:20)	80
	Anti-V_L	(1:20)	<15
	Anti-mouse Igs	(1:10)	<15
	Anti-IgG$_{2a}$	(1:5)	<15
	Anti-IgM	(1:5)	<15

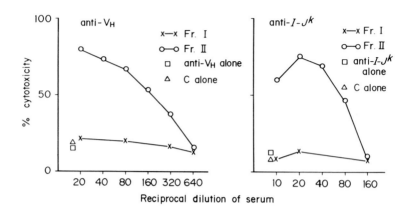

FIGURE 2.   Cytotoxicity of anti-V_H and anti-I-J
against specifically enriched suppressor T cell.

In this particular experiment, maximally 75% of Fr. II cells
were killed by an anti-I-J^k antiserum. No cytotoxicity was
observed with anti-mouse Ig isotype antisera as well as with
anti-V_L both in Fr. I and Fr. II. Fig. 2 shows the striking
parallelism between cytotoxic curves of Fr. II cells with
anti-V_H and anti-I-J. This indicates at least the majority
of Fr. II cells carry both V_H and I-J determinants. We have
recently determined that the treatment of Fr. II cells with
anti-Lyt-2 but not anti-Lyt-1 resulted in the elimination of
V_H-and I-J-bearing T cells.
     In order to learn whether or not the KLH-specific TsF
carries V_H determinants, the extract of KLH-primed splenic T
cells was absorbed with the immunoadsorbent of anti-V_H, anti-
V_L or anti-I-J^k. The results shown in Fig. 3 indicate that
the KLH-specific suppressor activity was absorbed by anti-V_H
and anti-I-J columns but not by anti-V_L. Acid eluates from
both anti-V_H and anti-I-J columns fully retained the suppressive activity, while that from anti-V_L had no activity. These
results indicate that the KLH-specific TsF carries both V_H and
I-J determinants but not V_L.

TsF PRODUCED BY I-J^+ HYBRIDOMA CELL LINES

     In order to characterize further the nature of KLH-spe-
cific TsF, we applied the cell fusion technique to obtain T
cell hybridomas which produce a larger quantity of TsF. Semipurified suppressor T cells from C57BL/6 mice, which were obtained by adsorption to and elution from the antigen-coated
Petri dishes, were fused with a thymoma cell line BW5147 of

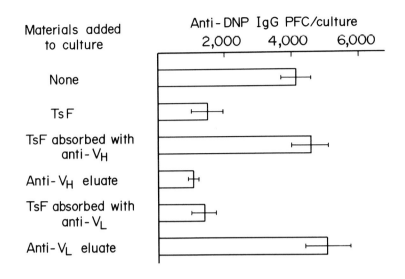

FIGURE 3.   Absorption of KLH-specific suppressor T
       cell factor with anti-V_H but not anti-V_L columns.
       Note that the acid eluate from anti-V_H but anti-
       V_L contained strong suppressor activity.

the AKR origin. After selection with HAT medium, I-J^+ hybrids
were obtained by sorting out with the fluorescence activated
cell sorter (FACS) followed by cloning with the limiting dilution. There are several I-J^+ hybridoma cell lines maintained
in our laboratory, some of which continuously display the suppressive activity in the secondary *in vitro* antibody response
either in antigen-specific or nonspecific fashion (10).
    TsF from one of the hybridoma cell lines (9F181a) has
been extensively studied (10). This cell line is transplanta-
ble to F$_1$ of H-2^b (C57BL/6) and H-2^k (AKR or C3H) mice, and
produces a large quantity of ascites which has a striking
antigen-specific suppressor activity. The extracted material
as well as ascites was characterized by the absorption with
various immunoadsorbents composed of antigens and antibodies.
Representative results of an experiment are shown in Fig. 4.
TsF in the hybridoma extract was found to be absorbed by KLH,
anti-H-2^b, anti-I-J^b and anti-V_H, but not by anti-I-J^k, anti-
Igs and anti-V_L. Similar results were obtained with the
ascites from the hybridoma-bearing F$_1$ animals. It is, therefore, obvious that some of the I-J-bearing hybridomas produce
similar molecules to those from primed suppressor T cells with
respect to the antigen-binding capacity and the I-J-coded

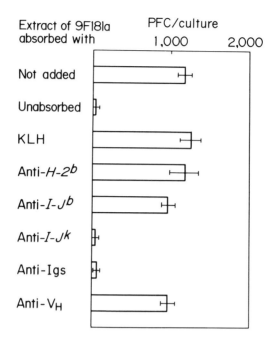

FIGURE 4.   Absorption of hybridoma-derived
        suppressor T cell factor with antigen
        and antibodies.

determinants (see Taniguchi *et al.*, in this volume).
    Another important property of TsF confirmed with the
hybridoma-derived factor is that the extracts from hybridomas
also displayed a strict genetic restriction in the suppression
of the antibody response. We have previously shown that the
suppressor factor from KLH-primed spleen cells was unable to
suppress the responses of *I-J* incompatible strains (5).   The
factor from hybridomas made between $H-2^b$ suppressor T cells
and BW5147 ($H-2^k$) could suppress the responses of C57BL/6
($H-2^b$) and (C57BL/6 x C3H)F$_1$ ($H-2^{b/k}$) mice but not that of
C3H ($H-2^k$) (10).   It is, therefore, conceivable that certain
processes of the suppressive cell interaction require the
compatibility in *I-J* subregion genes between the producer of
the suppressor factor and the target cells, supporting our
previous postulate that some of the T-T cell interactions are
mediated by *I* region gene products (5).

DISCUSSION

The results presented in this paper would allow us to consider the possible structure of antigen-receptor of T cells. It is most probable that the antigen-receptors of Ts, which are released as TsF, have both antigen-binding site and I region-coded determinants. The antigen-binding site has a structure identical or similar to V region of immunoglobulin heavy chain, while the V region of light chain has so far been undetectable. Although the antiserum used in this study is only reactive with V region of λ chains, even no minor effect was observed with this antiserum. The I region determinants, on the other hand, were clearly defined to be controlled by an I-J subregion gene, and are probably involved in the genetically restricted cell interactions.

We have shown that there is another analogous antigen-specific T cell factor determined by genes in I-A subregion, which augments the specific antibody response (11). This factor is comparable but not identical to antigen-specific cooperative or helper factors described by Taussig, Munro and Mozes, and Feldmann and Kontiainen (reviewed in 12). In our own studies, the augmenting T cell factor acts on T cells with a strict genetic restriction governed by I-A subregion genes (11).

In addition, we have demonstrated that there exist helper T cells having an I-J subregion gene product (13), which is distinguishable from the I-J product on Ts. The activity of I-J$^+$ helper T cells was found to be the direct target of TsF (described by Okumura et al., in this volume). Our more recent studies revealed that I-J determinants expressed on functionally different T cell hybridomas are antigenically different. All these results suggest that there are multiple loci in I-J and I-A subregions, which are expressed on different subsets of interacting T cells.

Our hypothetical model of antigen receptors of T cells based on the above and other findings is presented in Fig. 5. The molecule is most probably composed of two chains by a recent chemical analysis of TsF. A V$_H$ gene product is detectable by serological assays, while no known Ig constant region has been identified. It is unlikely that this V$_H$ structure has no meanings in the antigen-binding capacity of TsF. On the other hand, I region determinants encoded by genes in I-J and I-A subregions would determine the cellular consequences to lead to the suppression and enhancement. It is possible that these I region gene products by themselves have defined biologic activities as those of Fc portion of immunoglobulin molecules. Our presumption is, however, that the I region products may simply select the second cell type to be activated by virtue of their restriction specificity, and that as a

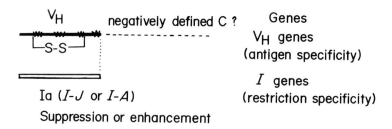

FIGURE 5.   Possible structure of T cell receptor.

consequence the whole suppressor or enhancing process is turned on by this simple selection of target cells. This is analogous to the IgE-mediated histamine release, in which IgE simply
selects the target cells with a very high affinity for the receptor, but the histamine release itself is an internal biochemical event within mast cells, which could occur even without IgE (14). The multiplicity of *I* subregion loci closely
linked to each other would be suitable devices to activate
one of the cognitive domains in the cellular network. As
these factors have both antigen-binding site and MHC-associated antigen, one can consider a sequential activation of a
series of T cells which are linked by antigen specificity
together with complementary interaction of *I* region gene products.
     The above concept of the T cell receptor can easily accom-
modate the two generally known specificities, antigen-specificity and restriction specificity. Hence, we think that *I* region products associated with the T cell antigen-binding unit
serve as self-recognizing molecules by discriminating the fine
polymorphism of other *I* region gene products so as to find out
the proper partner cells to talk with. Such a genetic restriction has been found in *I* region-controlled specific suppression and augmentation of antibody response to KLH (15) and
in MLC reaction (16). It has to be determined, however, under
what circumstances such a restriction is negated as in the
experiments reported by Kapp (17), and Kontiainen and Feldmann
(18), since we do not know whether such an ability of T cells
to discriminate self is genetically predetermined or acquired
during their ontogeny in the thymus.
     Our more recent studies indicated that not only in T-T
cell interactions but also in the T-B cell collaboration, the
I-J+ helper T cells (Th$_2$) preferentially interact with B cells
having high density of Ia antigen (see Okumura *et al.*, in this
volume). We postulate that Ia antigens on both T and B cells

are critically concerned with the accuracy of cellular interactions, which is indeed required for the stability of the
immune network system.

ACKNOWLEDGEMENTS

We wish to thank Dr. David Givol of the Weizmann Institute of Science, Israel for his generous gift of anti-V_H and
anti-V_L antibodies. We are grateful for the excellent technical assistance of Mr. H. Takahashi and Mrs. T. Fukuda, and
for the secretarial work of Ms. Y. Yamaguchi.

REFERENCES

1. Rajewsky, K., and Eichmann, K. (1977). Contemp. Topics
   Immunobiol. 7, 67.
2. Binz, H., and Wigzell, H. (1977). Contemp. Topics Immunobiol. 7, 113.
3. Zinkernagel, R.M., and Dohorty, P.C. (1977). Centemp.
   Topics Immunobiol. 7, 179.
4. Shearer, G.M., Schmitt-Uerhurst, A.M., and Rehn, T.G.
   (1977). Contemp. Topics Immunobiol. 7, 221.
5. Tada, T., Taniguchi, M., and David, C.S. (1976). J. Exp.
   Med. 144, 713.
6. Okumura, K., Takemori, T., Tokuhisa, T., and Tada, T.
   (1977). J. Exp. Med. 146, 1234.
7. Taniguchi, M., and Miller, J.F.A.P. (1977). J. Exp. Med.
   146, 1450.
8. Ben-Neriah, Y., Lonai, P., Gavish, M., and Givol, D.
   (1978). Eur. J. Immunol. 8, 792.
9. Ben-Neriah, Y., Wuilmart, C., Lonai, P., and Givol, D.
   (1978). Eur. J. Immunol. 8, 797.
10. Taniguchi, M., Saito, T., and Tada, T. (1979). Nature
    278, 555.
11. Tokuhisa, T., Taniguchi, M., Okumura, K., and Tada, T.
    (1978). J. Immunol. 120, 414.
12. Tada, T., and Okumura, K. (1979). Adv. Immunol. in press.
13. Tada, T., Takemori, T., Okumura, K., Nonaka, M., and
    Tokuhisa, T. (1978). J. Exp. Med. 147, 446.
14. Ishizaka, T., and Ishizaka, K. (1978). J. Immunol. 120,
    800.
15. Tada, T., Taniguchi, M., and David, C.S. (1976). Cold
    Spring Harbor Symp. Quant. Biol. 41, 119.
16. Rich, S.S., Orson, F.M., and Rich, R.R. (1977). J. Exp.
    Med. 146, 1221.
17. Kapp, J.A. (1978). J. Exp. Med. 147, 997.
18. Kontiainen, S., and Feldmann, M. (1978). J. Exp. Med. 147,
    110.

EFFECTIVE SUPPRESSION OF HAPTEN-SPECIFIC DELAYED-TYPE HYPERSENSITIVITY (DTH) RESPONSES IN MICE BY ANTI-IDIOTYPIC ANTIBODIES[1]

Hiroshi Yamamoto[2] and David H. Katz

Department of Cellular and Developmental Immunology,
Scripps Clinic and Research Foundation
La Jolla, California 92037

ABSTRACT   Delayed-type hypersensitivity (DTH) responses specific for the phosphoryl-choline (PC) hapten were induced in BALB/c mice by immunization with syngeneic peritoneal exudate cells (PEC) coupled with diazotized phenyl-phosphorylcholine. PC-specific DTH responses were elicited in such immunized mice following footpad challenge with PC-derivatized syngeneic spleen cells. Moreover, PEC-immune lymph node cells could passively transfer PC-specific DTH responses to naive BALB/c mice and it was possible to demonstrate that the cells responsible for such passively transferred responses were T lymphocytes. Since the T-15 idiotypic determinants displayed on the TEPC-15 PC-binding myeloma protein is known to be a dominant idiotype associated with anti-PC antibody responses in BALB/c mice, an analysis was made of the effects of anti-T-15 idiotypic antibodies on the induction and expression of murine PC-specific DTH responses. Repeated injections of anti-T-15 idiotypic antiserum, raised in A/J mice by immunization with TEPC-15 myeloma protein, into recipient BALB/c mice both immediately before and after sensitization with PC-PEC virtually abolished the development of PC-specific DTH responses. While administration of anti-T-15 antiserum effectively inhibited the *induction* phase of PC-specific DTH

[1] This is publication number 103 from the Department of Cellular and Developmental Immunology and publication number 1749 from the Immunology Departments, Scripps Clinic and Research Foundation, La Jolla, CA. This work was supported by USPHS Grant AI-13781 and Biomedical Research Support Grant RRO-5514.
[2] Supported by a Fellowship from the Cancer Research Institute, Inc.

responses, these anti-idiotypic antibodies had no suppressive activity at the *effector* phase of these responses. The inhibition observed with anti-T-15 antibodies was highly specific for the PC hapten, since the same antiserum failed to inhibit the induction of DTH responses to an unrelated hapten, trinitrophenyl (TNP) induced in BALB/c mice by immunization with TNP-PEC. Moreover, while anti-T-15 antibodies could effectively inhibit development of PC-specific DTH responses in BALB/c mice, these same antibodies had no inhibitory effects on the development of PC-specific DTH responses in A/J mice which do not express the dominant T-15 idiotype. The significance of these observations to concepts of shared idiotypic determinants on T and B lymphocytes are discussed.

INTRODUCTION

During the past few years, the biological effects of anti-idiotypic antibodies have received increasing attention due to the (i) postulated role that idiotype-anti-idiotype responses may play in both regulation and diversification of the immune system, as fostered by Jerne (1) and (ii) possible clues such anti-idiotypic reactivities might provide to the ultimate clarification and elucidation of the mystery concerning the molecular nature of T cell receptors (reviewed in 2,3). The BALB/c PC-binding TEPC-15 myeloma protein displays idiotypic determinants (T-15) which represent the dominant idiotype present on anti-PC antibodies produced by BALB/c mice. Previous investigations by others have demonstrated effective modulation of PC-specific immune responses following appropriate exposure of BALB/c mice to anti-T-15 idiotypic antibodies. These include suppression of PC-specific antibody production (4), suppression of PC-specific helper T lymphocyte activities (5) and induction of T-15 idiotype-specific suppressor T lymphocyte activities (6). We have recently established a system for the induction of PC-specific DTH responses in BALB/c mice. Studies reported here summarize the effects we have observed on such responses as a result of administration of anti-T-15 idiotypic antibodies.

BASIC EXPERIMENTAL SYSTEMS

Details of materials and methods are described elsewhere (7). Briefly, BALB/c mice were immunized subcutaneously in the hind trunk area with 20-40 x 10^6 syngeneic PEC derivatized with diazotized phenyl-phosphorylcholine, which is the active

derivative of PC. Five days after primary sensitization, animals were challenged with 20-30 x 10^6 PC-derivatized syngeneic
spleen cells (SC) into the right footpad. Footpad thicknesses
were measured at 36-48 hours after challenge. All data are
expressed as the difference in thickness of the right (experimental) and left (control) footpads.

    Anti-T-15 idiotypic serum was raised in A/J mice by the
method of Potter and Lieberman (8). Antisera were obtained
from bleedings made on days 27,35,42,49 and 56 after primary
immunization, which were pooled and adsorbed by passage
through MOPC-167 myeloma protein-conjugated Sepharose 4B to
remove anti-allotypic antibodies. The same adsorbed serum
pool was used throughout this study. In experiments involving
administration of anti-T-15, or normal A/J mouse serum (NMS)
as control, the serum was administered as follows: Recipient
BALB/c mice were injected with 50 µl of anti-Id serum or NMS
(1:20 dilution)per day for 4 consecutive days (administered
i.p. and s.c.) on days-1,0,1 and 2. All sensitizations with
PC-PEC were conducted on day 0.

RESULTS

    Induction of PC-Specific DTH Responses in BALB/c Mice
and Passive Transfer of Such Responses with PC-Immune T
Lymphocytes. Groups of BALB/c mice were sensitized on day 0
with either syngeneic PC-PEC or TNP-PEC. Five days later,
these mice and unsensitized control mice were challenged in
the right footpads with either PC-SC or TNP-SC and the development of DTH responses, as reflected by footpad thickness,
was determined on day 7. As shown in Figure 1, BALB/c mice
sensitized with PC-PEC manifested specific DTH responses upon
challenge with PC-SC (*cf*. groups II and I) but failed to respond to challenge with TNP-SC (group III). Conversely,
BALB/c mice sensitized with TNP-PEC responded to challenge
with TNP-SC (*cf*. groups V and IV) but not to PC-SC (group VI).
These data illustrate the hapten specificity of DTH responses
induced in this fashion.

    Since it has been well-established that DTH responses
are mediated by T lymphocytes, a passive transfer experiment
was conducted to confirm the requirement for T lymphocytes in
the hapten-specific DTH responses generated by immunization
with PC-PEC in BALB/c mice. Naive BALB/c recipients were
either not injected or injected intravenously with 65 x 10^6
regional lymph node cells from either normal or PC-PEC-primed
donor mice (5 days after immunization), and then challenged
shortly thereafter with PC-SC in the right footpads (day 0).
Footpad thickness was assayed on day 2. As shown in Figure 2,
uninjected control mice (group I) and recipients of normal

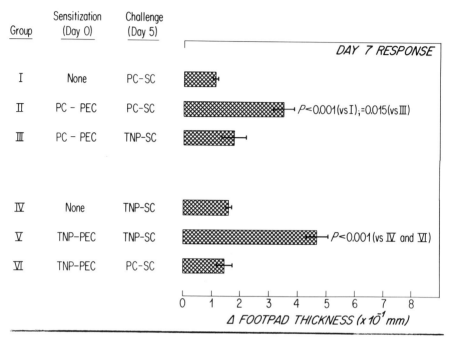

FIGURE 1

SPECIFICITY OF DELAYED-TYPE HYPERSENSITIVITY RESPONSES IN
BALB/c MICE SENSITIZED WITH HAPTEN-DERIVATIZED SYNGENEIC PEC

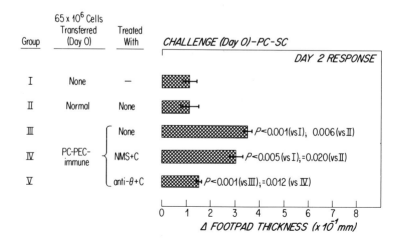

FIGURE 2

DEMONSTRATION OF REQUIREMENT OF T LYMPHOCYTES FOR SUCCESSFUL
ADOPTIVE CELL TRANSFER OF PC-SPECIFIC DTH RESPONSES IN BALB/c MICE

lymph node cells (group II) failed to develop detectable PC-
specific DTH responses. Conversely, recipients of PC-PEC-
immune lymph node cells displayed significant DTH responses
(group III). Pretreatment of PC-PEC-immune lymph node cells
in vitro with NMS + C had no appreciable effect on the ability
of such cells to positively transfer DTH reactivity (group
IV), whereas pretreatment with anti-θ + C almost completely
abolished the passive transfer of PC-specific DTH responses
(group V).

Effects of Anti-Idiotypic Antibodies on the Induction
and Effector Phases of PC-Specific DTH Responses in BALB/c
Mice. Having established that (i) PC-specific DTH responses
could be readily induced in BALB/c mice and (ii) that such
responses were, indeed, mediated by T lymphocytes, experiments
were then carried out to investigate the effects of anti-T-15
idiotypic antiserum on such responses. The experiment summarized in Figure 3 illustrates the substantial inhibitory
effects of anti-Id antibodies on the *induction* phase of PC-
specific DTH responses. Thus, BALB/c mice sensitized with PC-
PEC, and not otherwise treated, developed excellent PC-
specific DTH responses (*cf.* groups II and I), and the administration of A/J NMS immediately prior to and just after sensitization had no inhibitory effects on the development of such
responses (group III). In contrast, administration of anti-Id
significantly diminished the development of PC-specific DTH
responses (group IV).

In contrast to the ability of anti-Id administration to
diminish induction of PC-specific DTH responses (Figure 3),
anti-Id treatment just prior to and after challenge of previously sensitized mice with PC-SC was ineffective in diminish-
ing the expression of DTH reactivity. As shown in Figure 4,
this ineffectiveness of anti-Id treatment was true over 3
different doses of antiserum employed.

Specificity of Anti-Idiotypic Antiserum-Mediated Suppression of Hapten-Specific DTH Responses. Specificity of the
anti-Id-mediated suppression of murine DTH responses, as
illustrated in the preceding experiment, was analyzed both in
terms of antigen and strain specificity. The experiment summarized in Figure 5 demonstrates the specificity of anti-T-15
idiotypic antiserum treatment for DTH responses specific for
the PC hapten. This is illustrated by the fact that while
anti-Id treatment effectively inhibited induction of PC-
specific DTH responses (groups I-III), this same antiserum had
no inhibitory effects on the induction of DTH responses specific for the TNP hapten (groups IV-VI).

As mentioned above, T-15 is a dominant idiotypic marker

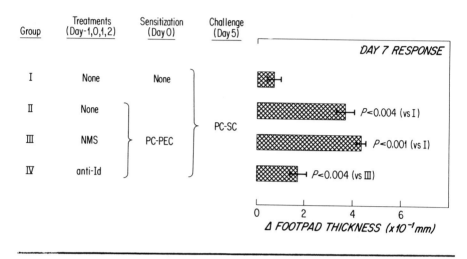

FIGURE 3

EFFECTIVE SUPPRESSION OF SENSITIZATION FOR
PC-SPECIFIC DTH RESPONSES BY ANTI-T-15 IDIOTYPIC ANTI-SERUM

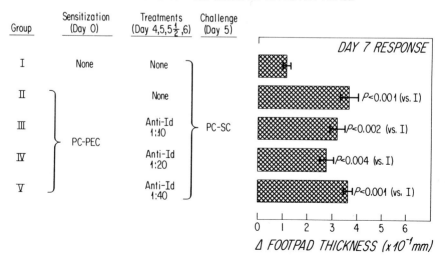

FIGURE 4

FAILURE OF ANTI-IDIOTYPIC SUPPRESSION OF
PC-SPECIFIC DTH RESPONSES AT EFFECTOR PHASE

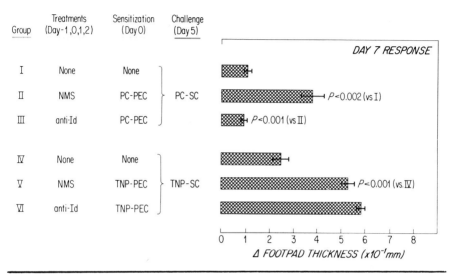

FIGURE 5

SPECIFICITY OF ANTI-T-15 IDIOTYPIC ANTISERUM-MEDIATED
SUPPRESSION OF HAPTEN-SPECIFIC DTH RESPONSES

present on anti-PC antibodies of BALB/c mice, and the expression of T-15 is closely linked to the Ig-1a allotypic marker (9). A/J mice do not display the T-15 idiotypic marker and, moreover, are capable of developing good anti-T-15 idiotypic antibodies following immunization with the BALB/c TEPC-15 myeloma protein. In order to document the anti-Id suppression observed in the preceding experiments as true idiotype-anti-idiotype interactions on the development of DTH responses, we felt it essential to ascertain the strain specificity of such suppression. In other words, a true idiotype-anti-idiotype phenomenon should be demonstrable in a mouse strain possessing T-15 as a dominant idiotype, such as BALB/c but not in a mouse strain lacking the T-15 idiotype, such as A/J. This expectation was confirmed in the experiment summarized in Figure 6. Thus, anti-Id treatment was clearly effective in inhibiting induction of PC-specific DTH responses in BALB/c mice (groups I-III), but had no inhibitory effect on the development of PC-specific DTH responses in A/J mice (groups IV-VI).

DISCUSSION

In the experiments presented above, we have illustrated

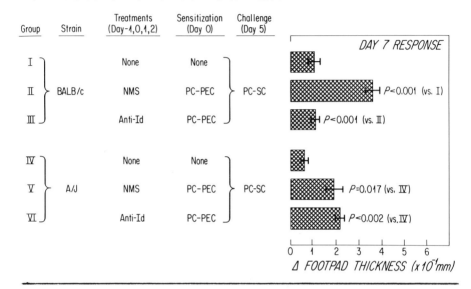

FIGURE 6

STRAIN SPECIFICITY OF ANTI-IDIOTYPIC SUPPRESSION OF PC-SPECIFIC DTH RESPONSES

the capability of inducing DTH responses specific for the PC
hapten in both BALB/c and A/J mice and to the TNP hapten in
BALB/c mice by sensitization with either PC- or TNP-derivatized syngeneic PEC. The PC-specific responses in BALB/c mice
could be passively transferred with sensitized lymph node
cells, and the capacity of such cells to passively transfer
DTH reactivity was abolished by pretreatment of such cells
with anti-Θ antibodies + C.
    The possibility of inducing DTH in mice to simple chemi-
cal haptens provides an excellent model for studies on the
specificity of T lymphocyte activities. The system we have
employed was made possible by the recent studies of Greene *et
al* (10) who were the first to demonstrate that syngeneic
macrophages coupled with TNP were highly immunogenic in terms
of inducing hapten-specific DTH responses in mice. We were
particularly interested in using the PC system in this way
for purposes of investigating idiotypic determinants on T
lymphocytes as well as obtaining insights into idiotype-anti-
idiotypic immunoregulatory mechanisms, because the T-15-PC
system has been extensively studied in terms of idiotypic determinants in BALB/c mice. As compared to certain other haptens which can easily sensitize mice by means such as skin
painting, the PC system posed considerably greater difficulties since usual derivatization with PC requires diazonium

coupling under alkaline conditions. This obstacle was overcome when, in preliminary experiments, we found that the
derivatization of spleen cells or PEC with diazonium phenyl-
phosphorylcholine could be successfully achieved at weak alkaline conditions (pH 8.2) with retention of good viability of
the derivatized lymphoid cells. This allowed us to establish
the basic experimental system described here for the induction
of PC-specific DTH, although in the course of our studies,
Bach *et al* (11) reported the induction of azobenzene arsonate-
specific DTH responses using similar procedures.

Having established the system for induction of PC-
specific DTH responses, and confirmed the hapten-specific
nature of the response, we then turned to the question concerning the effects of anti-T-15 idiotypic antibodies on such
responses. As shown herein, using an A/J anti-T-15 antiserum,
the specificity characteristics of which are described in detail elsewhere (12), we were successful in virtually abolishing the induction of PC-specific DTH responses in BALB/c mice.
Suppression of the induction phase of DTH responses by treatment with an anti-Id satisfied all criteria of antigen (Fig.5)
and strain (Fig. 6) specificity.

In terms of the mechanism(s) of successful suppression by
anti-Id antiserum in these studies, any one, or combination,
of several possible explanations could be entertained. First,
one might consider the possibility of stimulation of PC-
specific B lymphocytes following interaction with anti-Id
antibodies at the surface-bound, idiotype-containing, PC-
specific immunoglobulin receptors. This might lead to increased production of anti-PC antibodies which, in turn,
could serve as a neutralization mechanism for inhibiting development of PC-specific DTH by blocking the PC determinants
exposed on the sensitizing PC-derivatized PEC. The unlikeli-
hood of this explanation stems from the fact that BALB/c mice
normally have rather decent concentrations of PC-specific
antibodies circulating in the serum, and if such a neutralization mechanism were of any importance, one might expect to
have great difficulty in sensitizing such mice for PC-specific
DTH responses under normal circumstances. Since this is not
the case, as evidenced by the results reported here, this explanation seems unlikely. Moreover, we have demonstrated in
studies described elsewhere (12) that the anti-T-15 antibodies
employed in the present experiments *fail* to stimulate PC-
specific B lymphocytes, but rather exhibit marked suppressive
effects on such cells.

Second, it is possible that the administered anti-Id
might combine with the normally present circulating T-15-
positive anti-PC antibodies to form immune complexes. These
immune complexes, in turn, might become highly suppressive for
precursor T lymphocytes during the early phases of development

of DTH reactivity. Third, it is possible that administration
of the anti-Id generates suppressor T lymphocyte populations
which are highly specific in their reactivity with T-15 idiotypic determinant-bearing receptors on other T cells. Very
recently, Bottomly *et al* (6) reported observations that were
interpreted to illustrate the capacity of anti-idiotypic antibodies to induce suppressor T lymphocytes effective in inhibiting secondary anti-PC antibody responses in mice. We have
neither data nor logical arguments against either of these two
possibilities for explaining our present results and current
investigations should clarify the validity of this mechanism
as it pertains to the present system.

Finally, and perhaps most simply, the anti-Id antibodies
could exhibit their inhibitory effects by directly interacting
with T-15-bearing determinants present on T cell receptors for
the PC-hapten. Such reactions, in analogy to what has been
shown in other studies to be true with T-15-positive, immunoglobulin-bearing B lymphocytes, could effectively inhibit the
early differentiation stages of such cells to become mature
effector cells.

Irrespective of the primary mechanism(s) underlying the
inhibitory effects of anti-Id antibody treatment on the development of PC-specific DTH responses, it is clear from the data
presented here that the primary target of the relevant mechan-
ism(s) is the precursor of the PC-specific DTH effector T
cell. This reasoning is supported by the fact that anti-Id
was effective in inhibiting the *induction*, but not the effector, phase of the PC-specific DTH response. Indeed, this predilection of anti-Id inhibitory activity for *unprimed*, as
opposed to *primed*, T cells in the DTH system is remarkably
consistent with the known predilection of anti-Id antibody inhibitory activities for unprimed, as opposed to primed,
idiotype-bearing *B* lymphocytes as pointed out by Pierce and
Klinman (13) and Owen and Nisonoff (14). As in the case of
the B cell, this possibility as it pertains to T cells mediating DTH responses may imply that the idiotypic receptor specificities of DTH-T cells might undergo rapid selection in terms
of minor idiotypes after proper immunostimulation by the relevant haptenic determinant (15), either alone or perhaps in
conjunction with cell interaction (CI) molecules encoded by
major histocompatibility complex genes (11,16).

It should be obvious that delineation of the precise
mechanism(s) of anti-Id mediated suppression of hapten-
specific DTH responses will ultimately provide important insights on the central issue concerning the existence, or not,
of shared idiotypic determinants on antigen receptors expressed on T and B lymphocytes, respectively.

ACKNOWLEDGMENTS

We express our best appreciation to our colleagues in our laboratory who gave us continuous support and help during this work, especially to Dr. Fu-Tong Liu who kindly synthesized diazonium phenyl-phosphorylcholine and gave valuable discussions. We thank Anthea Hugus for assistance in preparation of the manuscript. Drs. Norman Klinman and Makoto Nonaka who critically commented in a most helpful way on the work and on the manuscript.

REFERENCES

1. Jerne, N.K. (1974). Ann. Immunol. (Inst. Pasteur) 125C, 375.
2. Binz, H. and Wigzell, H. (1976). Cold Spring Harbor Symp. Quant. Biol. 41, 275.
3. Krawinkel, U., Cramer, M., Berek, C., Hammerling, G., Black, S.J., Rajewsky, K. and Eichmann, K. (1976). Cold Spring Harbor Symp. Quant. Biol. 41, 285.
4. Cosenza, H. and Köhler, H. (1972). Science 176, 1027.
5. Cosenza, H., Augustin, A.A. and Julius, M.H. (1976). Cold Spring Harbor Quant. Biol. 41, 709.
6. Bottomly, K., Mathieson, B.J. and Mosier, D.E. (1978). J. Exp. Med. 148, 1216.
7. Yamamoto, H. and Katz, D.H. (1979). Submitted for publication.
8. Potter, M. and Lieberman, R. (1970). J. Exp. Med. 132, 737.
9. Lieberman, R., Potter, M., Mushinski, E.B., Humphrey, W., Jr. and Rudikoff, S. (1974). J. Exp. Med. 139, 983.
10. Greene, M.I., Sugimoto, M. and Benacerraf, B. (1978). J. Immunol. 120, 1604.
11. Bach, B.A., Sherman, L., Benacerraf, B. and Greene, M.I. (1978). J. Immunol. 121, 1460.
12. Yamamoto, H. and Katz, D.H. (1979). Submitted for publication.
13. Pierce, S.K. and Klinman, N.R. (1977). J. Exp. Med. 146, 509.
14. Owen, F.L. and Nisonoff, A. (1978). J. Exp. Med. 148, 182.
15. Mäkelä, O. and Karjalainen, K. (1977). Immunological Rev. 34, 119.
16. Miller, J.F.A.P., Vadas, M.A., Whitelaw, A. and Gamble, J. (1976). In "The Role of Products of the Histocompatibility Gene Complex in Immune Responses" (D.H. Katz and B. Benacerraf, eds.), pp. 403-415. Academic Press, New York.

ALLOHELP TO H-2K APPEARS TO DEPEND ONLY ON A MATURE LY123 T CELL[1]

Susan L. Swain, Richard W. Dutton, and Peter R. Panfili

Department of Biology, University of California, San Diego
La Jolla, California 92093

ABSTRACT The Ly phenotype of help induced by recognition of allogeneic histocompatibility antigens (allohelp) depends on the intra MHC region involved. While allohelp induced by I, *Mls*, or whole H-2 depends only on Ly1 T cells, Ly123 T cells are required for allohelp induced by H-2K alone. Studies of allohelp to an H-2K only difference between B6 and the mutant H-2^{ba} indicate that such help is due to a single limiting precursor T cell present in high frequency. It depends only on a T_2 population of T cells which are resistent to adult thymectomy and sensitive to the *in vivo* administration of ATS. This suggests that the Ly123 cell which responds to H-2K and is a mature antigen reactive cell. Ly2$^+$ T cells separated from Ly2$^-$ T cells on FACS were able to generate allohelp to H-2K. Thus there was no requirement for Ly1 cells for this help. The difference in Ly phenotype of T cells which have the same function (allohelp) but respond to different MHC antigens (K/D versus I) emphasizes the fundamental dichotomy of these two sets of MHC antigens.

INTRODUCTION

One of the more intriguing aspects of the role of the antigens of the major histocompatibility complex (MHC) in T cell response is that different T cell functions are associated with the recognition of different subregions of the MHC (1). This dichotomy is seen both in the stimulation of T cells by conventional antigen in the context of self H-2 and in their stimulation by allogeneic H-2 antigens. In the mouse, T cells which help and proliferate preferentially recognize products of the I region, while T cells which kill (and in some cases suppress (2)) recognize those of the K and D region. The reason for this association of different MHC subregions with different functions is not known.

A second dichotomy is the association of Ly phenotype with T cell function described by Cantor and Boyse (3). In general, T cells which help or proliferate express only the Ly1 antigen not Ly23, while those which suppress or develop

[1]This work was supported by USPHS AI 08795 and CA 09174 and ACS IM-1L.

into cytotoxic cells express only Ly23.

To examine the significance of this triple correlation of Ly phenotype, function, and MHC subregion in T cell responses, we have studied an exception to the association of function with MHC subregion — the case of allogeneic help induced by K only or D only differences (4). In these experiments we have measured the helper activity of T cells triggered by allogeneic B cells to sheep erythrocytes (SRBC). We have used the term allohelp to describe this activity. The first question that we asked was whether the Ly phenotype of the precursors of help would be that associated with helper function, Ly1, or that associated with K/D recognition, Ly23. We found a requirement for Ly123 cells in the response to K or D, in contrast to a requirement only for Ly1 cells in response to I, *Mls*, or whole H-2 (4,5). From our initial experiments it was not possible to determine if any cell, in addition to the Ly123 cell, was necessary for help to K/D or if both precursor and effector allohelper cells were from the Ly123 subclass. In the experiments reported here we have asked two questions: (1) Is the allohelp generated by differences at K dependent on T_1 cells, T_2 cells or both? (2) Can T cells selected to recover Ly2 positive cells generate allohelp to K or D in the absence of Ly1 cells? The results of these studies support the concept that the Ly12 cell which responds to K or D is neither an amplifier cell nor an *immature* precursor cell and that Ly1 cells are not required for allohelp to K or D. The most likely interpretation of our data is that the helper cell itself is an Ly123 cell although other interpretations are not rigorously excluded.

RESULTS

Experimental Model. T cells from mouse spleen were separated by passage through nylon wool. Suppressor T cell activity was minimized by mitomycin C treatment (2). The T cells were further fractionated and titrated into two or more populations of T cell-depleted spleen cells from normal mice which differed from the T cells at K, D, I, or at the whole haplotype. SRBC were added to all cultures and plaque forming cells determined four days later. The size of the response was taken as a measure of allohelp. The effect of various treatments of the helper population on allogeneic help to K/D versus I or whole haplotype was directly compared. For further details of the methods and reagents used see our earlier publications (4,5).

In most experiments the K difference we have used is that between B6 and the B6 mutant B6.C-H-2[ba] which differ only at H-2K.

Ly phenotype of allohelp precursors. The results of our earlier studies (4) are summarized in Table I. In these experiments T cells were pretreated with anti Lyl or anti Ly2 reagents plus complement. The depletion of allohelp to K/D with either of these reagents and the failure of the mix of the two surviving populations to reconstitute help indicated only that an Lyl2 cell was required for allohelp to K/D. We considered three possible explanations for this requirement. First, that Lyl23 cells were the precursors and effectors of allohelp to K/D. The second, that Lyl23 cells were precursors of allohelpers which differentiated into Lyl (or less likely Ly2/3) effectors. The third, that Lyl23 cells acted as amplifier cell aiding the development of mature Lyl cells. The following experiments were designed to distinguish between these possibilities.

The precursors of allohelpers to mutant K are present in high frequency and a single cell type is limiting. In general the great strength of proliferative and cytotoxic responses to allogeneic MHC has been accounted for by the large number of precursors for a given alloantigen among the T cell population. Our studies carried out in collaboration with Ivan Lefkovits[2] suggest that the frequency of precursors for allohelp is also considerably larger than that for conventional antigens. In these studies we have compared the frequency of precursors for help to SRBC, for help to a whole haplotype difference and for help to an H-2K difference. Help was determined by a limiting dilution titration of T cells into nu/nu spleen cells in the Lefkovits microculture system (6,7) and

TABLE I

LY PHENOTYPE OF HELPER CELLS REQUIRED
FOR POSITIVE ALLOGENEIC EFFECTS[a]

MHC region involved	Ly phenotype of cell required
Syngeneic (I)	1
Allogeneic: I	1
Mls	1
Whole haplotype	1
K	123
D	123

[a]Summary of conclusions on the Ly phenotype of helper cells (Swain, S. and Panfili, P. 1978, J. Immunol. 122, 383). Ly phenotype of helper precursors was determined as described in the text.

[2]Swain, S., Panfili, P., Dutton, R., and Lefkovits, I. Submitted for publication.

responses were determined by a spot test, using the replica-
tor, on day 5. A summary of the frequencies we have determined is indicated in Table II. (An example of these results
is shown in Figure 1.) Several points can be made. In all
cases the plot of the number of T cells against the logarithm
of the fraction of nonresponding cultures, gave a straight
line intercepting with the origin. Thus only one cell was
limiting for the production of help and the frequency determined from the number of T cells which gave 37% nonresponding
cultures was the frequency of that one cell. This was true
for the H-2K difference (B6.H-2^{ba} T cells titrated into B6
nu/nu cells) as well as a whole H-2 difference. The mean frequency found for this response — one in 4,800 — is high. The
frequency of allohelpers to whole H-2 differences (including
K, D, I, and sometimes *Mls*) which we know depends only on Lyl
cells, had a mean of one in 2,500, only twice as high.

Allohelp to K/D is mediated by T_2 not T_1 cells. If the
Lyl23 cells involved in allohelp to K/D are either precursor
cells (possibility two) or amplifier cells (possibility three)
it is likely that the required Lyl23 cell would be an immature
cell of the sort associated with the T_1 class of cell originally described by Raff and Cantor (8). Post thymic T cells
have been divided into T_1 and T_2 classes on the basis of several criteria. T_1 cells have been described as the short-
lived, non-recirculating T cells (8) which, because they respond more slowly to antigenic challenge (9), and do not contain memory cells (10) are thought to be "virgin." Because of
their properties they are depleted following adult thymectomy
(Tx) and are relatively insensitive to the *in vivo* effects of
anti-thymocyte sera (ATS). T_2 cells, on the other hand, are
recirculating and longer lived and thus sensitive to ATS but
not to Tx (8,11). In addition, they respond more rapidly to
antigen and thus are thought to be more mature memory population. Recently Araneo, Marrack and Kappler have demonstrated
that T_1 cells are converted T_2 cells by exposure to antigen
(11).

TABLE II
FREQUENCY OF ALLOHELP PRECURSORS

Difference	Mean frequency	
None (syngeneic, SRBC specific)	5.33×10^{-5}	1 / 18,000
Whole haplotype	4.15×10^{-4}	1 / 2,400
Mls and background	4.00×10^{-4}	1 / 2,500
H-2K (H-2^{ba} → B6)	2.08×10^{-4}	1 / 4,800

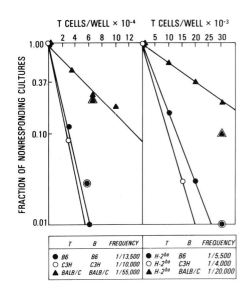

FIGURE 1. Precursor frequency for allohelp.
T cells from H-2^{ba} mice were compared with syngeneic T cells from three strains of mice: B6, C3H, and BALB. T cells were added to 7.5×10^4 B cells from nu/nu mice (regular symbols) or to 1.5×10^5 B cells (double symbols). Lines and frequencies were determined for the full titration.

In other studies which describe Ly123 cells as amplifiers (12) or as immunoregulatory cells (13) they have been shown to be T_1 cells which are depleted by adult thymectomy.

To test the contribution of T_1 and T_2 cells to allohelp, groups of B6 mice were depleted of T_1 cells by adult thymectomy or depleted of T_2 cells by treatment with anti-thymocyte sera. A summary of the ability of T cells from these mice to give allohelp to a K difference (H-2^{ba} B cells) and a whole haplotype difference (BDF$_1$ B cells) is presented in Table III. In no case did adult thymectomy result in a decrease in allogeneic help to either the K difference or to whole haplotype. Nonetheless, thymectomized mice from the same pool had many fewer Ly123 cells in the spleen on the basis of microcytotoxicity (a range of 10-50% of control). Long term thymectomized mice gave a reduced response to SRBC indicating a helper cell deficit (see legend to Table III). In contrast, mice which were treated with anti-thymocyte serum were severely depleted of allohelpers which could respond either to H-2K alone or to whole haplotype differences. The results of further experiments are shown in Figures 2 and 3. These experiments demonstrate that mixing populations of cells enriched for T_1 and T_2 (the TX-ATS mix in Figure 2, and the anti Ly2.2-ATS mix in Figure 3) does not reveal any synergy between these two populations. In Figure 3, the effect of anti Ly2.2 treatment was included to demonstrate that the cell required for allohelp to K was still Ly2 positive (presumably an Ly123 cell) even in adult thymectomized animals where the total number of Ly123 cells was small compared to normal mice. Thus the Ly123 cell

TABLE III

CONTRIBUTION OF T_1 AND T_2 CELLS TO ALLOHELP

Treatment	No. Expts.	Cells Remaining	% Control Response ± SE	
			K only	Whole Haplotype
None		T_1 and T_2	100	100
Thymectomy[a] (TX)	4	T_2	155 (37)	129 (28)
Antithymocyte[b] (ATS)	8	T_1	18 (3)	19 (5)

[a]Adult mice were thymectomized 10-30 weeks before use. Mice were examined for thymic remnants and none were seen. By 30 weeks spleen cells of mice from the same pool were able to give a primary response to SRBC that was only 10% of control age-matched mice.

[b]Mice were injected i.p. with 0.03 - 0.06 ml of ATS two days or both one and three days before sacrifice. Spleens of mice which had been thymectomized and ATS treated gave no primary response to SRBC.

involved in allohelp to a K difference (like the Lyl cell which mediates help to whole haplotype differences is a T_2 cell in the operational sense that it is insensitive to adult thymectomy and sensitive to the effects of *in vivo* administration of ATS. Our failure to detect synergy between anti Ly2.2 treated cells (enriched for Lyl cells) and cells of ATS treated animals (still containing T_1 cells) suggests that if there is an interaction between Lyl23 and Lyl cells they are both of the T_2 class.

Lyl23 cells can give help to H-2K in the absence of Lyl cells. Since our experiments showed only that T_1 amplifiers or precursors were not required for allohelp to K, a mechanism involving T_2 Lyl23 cells interacting with Lyl precursors was not ruled out. We directly tested this possibility by cell separation on the fluorescence activated cell sorter (FACS). Nylon column passed T cells of B6 mice were stained with an anti-Ly2 serum and then with fluoresceinated rabbit-anti mouse immunoglobulin. The fluorescence of these cells was analyzed on the cell sorter and fractions of bright cells (Lyl23 and Ly2/3) and dim cells (Lyl) were selected. Figure 4 indicates the fluorescence profile. Cells in fractions 250-1000 were collected as "bright" whereas those to the left of fraction 250 were collected as "dim." Under these conditions the bright fraction contained 26% of the total T cells and the

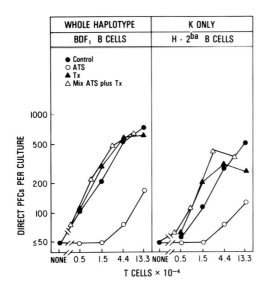

FIGURE 2. Involvement of T_1 and T_2 cells in allohelp. T_1 and T_2 cells were obtained from ATS-treated and TX mice respectively as described in Table III. T cells of control, T_1 (ATS) and T_2 (TX) mice were titrated into B cells of BDF_1 (left panel) or $H-2^{ba}$ (right panel). For the mix line, ATS and TX cells were mixed in a 1:1 ratio.

dim fraction approximately 30%. Small cells not falling within the normal distribution of cell size (approximately 15%) were discarded. This fraction presumably contains dead cells and erythrocytes. Drops with two cells (15-20%) were also discarded. After sorting, unseparated cells and the separated bright cells and the separated bright and dim cells were resuspended to 8×10^6 cells/ml and their ability to give allohelp when stimulated by a K difference and a whole haplotype difference was titrated. Results are indicated in Figure 5. When the responding B cells were from the $H-2^{ba}$ mutant the bright cells were as efficient as unseparated cells in giving allohelp. In contrast these same bright cells gave marginal, if any, help to the BDF_1 responding cells. Conversely, the dim population consisting predominantly of Lyl cells gave very little help to the responding cells differing at K. They had only 5% of the activity of either unseparated or bright cells. The same dim cell population gave help to responding B cells differing at the whole haplotype which was comparable to that of unseparated cells. Equal mixtures of bright and dim cells gave results similar to the unseparated populations. Some drop off of help activity was seen at high doses of T cells which we interpret to mean that some suppression was induced at high T cell levels. Similar results were obtained in a second experiment.

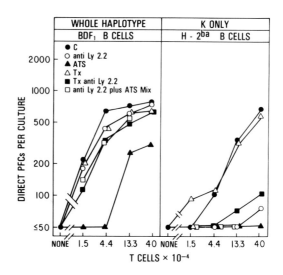

FIGURE 3.   Involvement of Ly2 positive cells of the
            T_2 class in allohelp. (See Figure 2.)

DISCUSSION

        Together these results support the hypothesis that allo-
help to K/D is mediated by a different subset of cells than
allohelp to I, *Mls*, or whole haplotype. The analysis of precursor frequencies suggests that in both cases a single cell
type is limiting. This single cell appears to be a mature
cell of the T_2 class which is sensitive to *in vivo* administration of ATS but resistant to the effects of adult thymectomy.
Separation of Ly2 positive cell from Ly2 negative cells on
FACS shows that the cell responsible for allohelp to K/D is an
Ly2 positive cell while the cell responding to a whole haplotype different (predominantly I) is an Ly1 cell. No evidence
of synergy between two populations was noted in any of the
experimental models we examined, though Ly123-Ly23 interactions are not excluded. A feedback loop of the sort described by Cantor and his colleagues in which Ly123 amplifier
cells interact with an Ly1 cells to generate Ly1 helpers (13)
does not appear to explain the Ly123 requirement in help to K
or D. Wettstein and his colleagues have shown that proliferation to a K difference depends on an Ly123 cell (14). We would
predict that it is the Ly123 cell itself that proliferates.
Bach and Alter have reported that killing to K/D depends on an
Ly123 cell (15). This might be due to the fact that the
helpers have an Ly123 phenotype or it might indicate that both
helpers and precursors of cytotoxic effectors are Ly123.

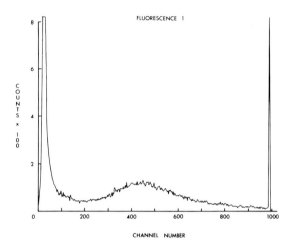

FIGURE 4.   Fluorescence profile of anti-Ly2.2 stained
            T cells.

Why then do helper precursors that respond to K/D come
from an Ly123 subclass instead of an Ly1 subclass of T cells?
Though it is not possible to answer this question at the present time several speculations might be offered.

A simple explanation might be that precursors of effectors to allogeneic K or D are still members of a less differentiated Ly123 class that differentiate prior to delivery of
their effector function as has been suggested for precursors
of TNP-killers (16) or tumor killers (17,18). Cantor,
Benecerraf and colleagues have proposed that non antigen-
stimulated killer precursors are members of the Ly123 class
(19,20). They suggest that the reason alloprecursors are
found among Ly23 cells is that they have been stimulated by
environmental antigens associated with self MHC antigens
which cross react with alloantigen. One could argue that in
the case of help or proliferation to allogeneic K or D no
stimulation has occurred because cells with these functions
are only stimulated by foreign antigens associated with I region in the autogenous situation. Although at first sight an
attractive hypothesis, this would leave several difficult
questions. Why are the non antigen-stimulated precursors not
short lived T_1 cells as would be expected? Why are there so
many precursors to some K or D antigens, such as the H-2^{ba}
mutant, if K or D antigens are never used for help in *in situ*
responses? And how can help be delivered in these *in vitro*
circumstances if help can only be stimulated by I? We are

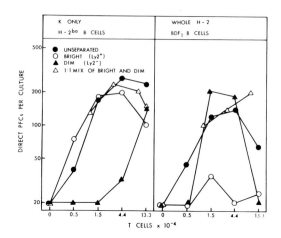

FIGURE 5. Ability of separated Ly2 positive and Ly2 negative cells to give allohelp. Unseparated, stained T, bright T (Ly23 and Ly123) and dim T (Ly1) cells described in Figure 4 were tested for ability to H-2^{ba} B cells (left panel) and DBF$_1$ B cells (right panel).

nevertheless, currently testing if memory and antigen-stimulated helpers to K or D retain the Ly123 phenotype or convert to an Ly1 phenotype.

An alternative class of explanations would involve some hypothesis in which recognition of K or D and expression of Ly2 were causally linked. One can only speculate on how this might be. One possibility is that the Ly2 gene product forms some part of the T cell receptor for the K or D molecules. A second intriguing possibility is that interaction of the T cell receptor with the K or D molecule on the target cell starts some chain reaction which eventually triggers the T cell function. It is possible that the Ly2 molecule on the T cell surface plays some essential part in this chain reaction which cannot go to completion if Ly2 is not supplied.

While none of the above speculations seems completely satisfactory, the fact that allohelp or K or D arises from a different subclass of T cells (Ly123) than help stimulated by I antigen in either syngeneic or allogeneic situations (Ly1), underlines the fundamental dichotomy between K or D and I (originally formulated by Bach and colleagues). The exception proves the rule!

REFERENCES

1. Dutton, R. W., Panfili, P. R., and Swain, S. L. (1978). Immunol. Rev. 42, 20.
2. Swain, S. L., and R. W. Dutton (1977). J. Immunol. 119, 1179.
3. Cantor, H., and Boyse, E. A. (1976). Cold Spr. Harb. Symp. Quant. Biol. 41, 23.

4. Panfili, P. R., and Dutton, R. W. (1978). J. Immunol. 120, 1897.
5. Swain, S. L., and Panfili, P. R. (1979). J. Immunol. 122, 383.
6. Lefkovits, I., and Kamber, O. (1972) Eur. J. Immunol. 2, 366.
7. Waldmann, H., Lefkovits, I., and Quintans, J. (1975). Immunol. 28, 1135.
8. Raff, M. C., and Cantor, H. (1971). In "Progress in Immunology" (B. Amos, Ed.), p. 83. Academic Press, New York.
9. Araneo, B. A., Marrack, P. C., and Kappler, J. W. (1976). J. Immunol. 117, 1233.
10. Araneo, B. A., Marrack, P. C., and Kappler, J. W. (1976). J. Immunol. 117, 2131.
11. Araneo, B. A., Marrack, P. C., and Kappler, J. W. (1977). J. Immunol. 119, 765.
12. Feldmann, M., Beverly, P. C. L., Woody, J., and McKenzie, I. F. C. (1977). J. Exp. Med. 145, 793.
13. Eardley, D. D., Hugenberger, J., Boudreau, L. M., Shen, F. W., Gershon, R. K., and Cantor, H. (1978). J. Exp. Med. 147, 1106.
14. Wettstein, P. J., Bailey, D. W., Mobraaten, L. E., Klein, J., and Frelinger, J. A. (1978). J. Exp. Med. 147, 1395.
15. Bach, F., and Alter, B. J. (1978). J. Exp. Med. 148, 829.
16. Cantor, H. and Boyse, E. A. (1977). In "T Cells, Contemporary Topics in Immunobiology" (O. Stutman, ed.), Vol. 7, pp. 47-67. Plenum, New York.
17. Shiku, H., Takahashi, T., Bean, M. A., Old, L. J., and Oettgen, H. F. (1976). J. Exp. Med. 144, 1116.
18. Stutman, O., Shen, F. W., and Boyse, E. A. (1977). Proc. Nat'l Acad. Sci. 74, 5667.
19. Finberg, R., Burakoff, S. J., Cantor, H., and Benacerraf, B. (1978). Proc. Nat'l Acad. Sci. 75, 5145.
20. Burakoff, S. J., Findberg, R., Glimcher, L., Lemmonier, F. Benacerraf, B., and Cantor, H. (1978). J. Exp. Med. 148, 1414.

T CELL RECOGNITION
OF SYNGENEIC AND ALLOGENEIC H-2 DETERMINANTS

Richard J. Hodes, Gerald B. Ahmann, Paul I. Nadler,
Karen S. Hathcock, and Alfred Singer

Immunology Branch, National Cancer Institute,
National Institutes of Health, Bethesda, Maryland 20014

ABSTRACT. The ability of T cells to recognize $\underline{H-2}$
encoded determinants expressed by subpopulations of
lymphoid cells was examined in two different
response systems. In the first of these systems,
it was demonstrated that $(AxB)F_1 \text{-->} Parent_A$ chimera
helper T cells were able to recognize the $\underline{H-2}$
determinants of $Parent_A$, but not $Parent_B$, as
measured by the ability of these T cells to
cooperate with parental (B + Accessory) cells
in primary antibody responses. It was further
demonstrated that recognition was for $\underline{K}$ or $\underline{I-A}$
encoded determinants expressed on accessory spleen
adherent cells (SAC) but not on B cells. In the
second system, it was demonstrated that T cells
responded in MLR to allogeneic $\underline{H-2}$ determinants
expressed by SAC, but did not respond to B cell
enriched or T cell enriched spleen cell populations.

INTRODUCTION

The ability of T lymphocytes to recognize major histocompatibility complex (MHC) encoded determinants has been
widely studied in a number of immune responses. T cell
recognition of MHC products was initially appreciated in
T cell mediated in vitro responses to allogeneic MHC
determinants in the mixed lymphocyte reaction (MLR), and
for the generation of cell-mediated lympholysis (CML); and
in T cell mediated in vivo graft-versus-host responses (GVH)
and allograft rejection (1). Subsequently, evidence was
accumulated suggesting that T cell recognition of MHC
determinants was also a critical feature of syngeneic cell
interactions which were required for the generation of immune
responses to a wide variety of antigens (2-6). As a result,
it has become important to determine whether T cells
differentially recognize MHC determinants expressed on
specific lymphoid subpopulations. The experiments presented
in the current report have investigated this question in
two different response systems: the T cell dependent

antibody response of murine spleen cells to soluble antigen,
in which helper T cell recognition of syngeneic H-2
determinants on cooperating B cells and accessory cells
was assessed; and the MLR response of T cells to
allogeneic H-2 antigens expressed on various lymphoid
subpopulations.

MATERIALS AND METHODS

The methods employed have been previously reported
in detail (7,8). Primary antibody responses to
trinitrophenyl (TNP) conjugated keyhole limpet hemocyanin
(KLH) were generated in microculture wells, at a total
cell density of $4-5 \times 10^5$ cells/200 uL culture (7).
Plaque-forming cell (PFC) responses were assayed on TNP-
modified sheep erythrocytes, and results presented as
the geometric mean (standard error) of triplicate
cultures (7). MLR responses were assayed in microcultures of 4×10^5 responding cells/culture and titrated
numbers of 1000R irradiated stimulating cells. Spleen
cell subpopulations employed were as follows: T cells:
nylon column nonadherent spleen cells; (B + Accessory)
cells: spleen cells treated with a T cell-specific rabbit
anti-mouse brain serum (RAMB) and complement (C);
adherent cell-depleted populations: Sephadex G-10 passed
spleen cells; B cells: Sephadex G-10 passed and RAMB+C
treated spleen cells; spleen adherent cells (SAC): glass-
adherent, RAMB+C treated, 1000R irradiated spleen cells.
Details of the preparation of these populations have been
reported elsewhere (7,8).

RESULTS

I. Analysis of Helper T Cell Recognition of Syngeneic
MHC Determinants Expressed on Accessory Cells and B Cells.

(AxB)F$_1$-->Parent Chimera Helper T Cells are Restricted in
Their Recognition of Parental H-2 Determinants. It has
previously been demonstrated that primary in vitro PFC
responses to TNP-KLH require the cooperation of three
functionally distinct cell populations: T cells, B cells,
and accessory cells (8). The ability of helper T cells to
recognize H-2 encoded determinants expressed on (B+
Accessory) cells was examined by assessing the ability
of (B10xB10.A)F$_1$ (F$_1$), (B10xB10.A)F$_1$-->B10 (F$_1$-->B10), or
(B10xB10.A)F$_1$-->(B10.A) (F$_1$-->B10.A) T cells to cooperate
with B10, B10.A, B10.A(5R), or B10.A(4R) (B+Accessory)
cells in primary antibody responses to TNP-KLH.

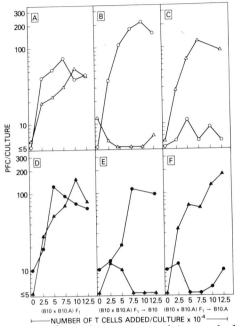

FIGURE 1. $(AxB)F_1$ --> $Parent_A$ chimera helper T cells
are restricted to recognizing K or I-A region encoded H-2
determinants of $Parent_A$. Graded numbers of either normal
or chimera T cells were added to cultures containing 10
ug/ml TNP-KLH and $4x10^5$ (B+Accessory) cells from B10
(○———○), B10.A (△———△), B10.A(5R) (●———●), or B10.A(4R)
(▲———▲). Less than 5 PFC/culture were observed either in
the absence of antigen or in cultures containing TNP-KLH
and T cells alone.

        Normal F_1 T cells cooperated equally well with B10,
B10.A, B10.A(5R), or B10.A(4R) (B+Accessory) cells
(Fig. 1 A,D). In contrast, F_1-->B10 T cells were
effective in cooperating with B10 or B10.A(5R), but not
B10.A or B10.A(4R) (B+Accessory) cells (Fig. 1 B,E); while
F_1-->B10.A T cells cooperated with B10.A or B10.A(4R),
but not B10 or B10.A(5R) (B+Accessory) cells (Fig. 1 C,F).
Thus, helper T cells of reciprocal F_1-->$Parent_A$ origin
were restricted in their abilities to recognize and
cooperate with (B+ Accessory) cells expressing K or I-A
encoded determinants of $Parent_A$ origin. Since all cell
populations employed in these experiments were derived
from unprimed animals, this restriction of helper T cell
recognition of H-2 determinants was present prior to
antigen exposure.

$(AxB)F_1$-->$Parent_A$ Chimera Helper T Cells are
Restricted in their Recognition of Parental H-2
Determinants Expressed on Accessory Cells, but Not in
their Recognition of H-2 Determinants Expressed on B Cells
Since unprimed helper T cells from F_1-->$Parent_A$ chimeras
distinguished the (B + Accessory) cells of $Parent_A$ from
those of $Parent_B$, unprimed helper T cells recognize the
H-2 encoded determinants expressed on B cells and/or
accessory cells. Further studies were conducted to
determine more precisely which of these populations was
recognized by T cells. F_1-->B10 or F_1-->B10.A T cells
were cultured with B10 or B10.A B cells and B10 or B10.A
accessory cells.

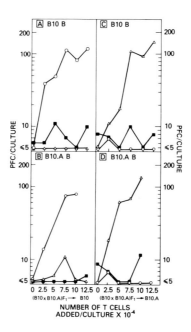

FIGURE 2. $(AxB)F_1$--> $Parent_A$ chimera T cells
cooperate with $Parent_A$ or $Parent_B$ B cells in the presence
of $Parent_A$ accessory cells. Graded numbers of chimera T
cells were added to cultures containing 10 μg/ml TNP-KLH;
$4x10^5$ B cells from either B10 or B10.A; and either no
SAC (■——■) or $4x10^4$ SAC from B10 (○——○) or B10.A
(△——△). Less than 5 PFC/culture were observed either
in the absence of antigen or in cultures devoid of B
cells.

Unprimed F_1-->Parent$_A$ T cells from either of these chimeras cooperated with Parent$_A$ but not Parent$_B$ SAC; and, in the presence of Parent$_A$ SAC, cooperated equally well with B cells of either parental origin (Fig. 2). These results suggest that unprimed helper T cells are restricted in their recognition of H-2 encoded determinants expressed by accessory cells, but are not similarly restricted in recognition of B cell H-2 determinants.

(AxB)F_1-->Parent$_A$ Chimera Helper T Cells are Only Restricted in Their Recognition of Parental H-2 Determinants on Accessory Cells in vivo. In order to determine whether these findings are unique to the in vitro system employed, or are consistent in vivo, short term adoptive transfer experiments were carried out with unprimed T cells (nylon nonadherent spleen), "B cells" (RAMB+C treated spleen), and "accessory cells" (RAMB+C treated, 1000R irradiated spleen).

Table I

(AxB)F_1-->PARENT$_A$ CHIMERA T CELLS COOPERATE WITH PARENT$_B$ B CELLS IN THE PRESENCE OF PARENT$_A$ ACCESSORY CELLS

	B10	F_1--> B10.A	Acces.	PFC/Spleen[1]	
Group	B Cells	T Cells	Cells	Expt. 1	Expt. 2
A	+	−	−	186(1.09)	159(1.09)
B	+	+	−	228(1.15)	176(1.26)
C	+	+	B10	147(1.30)	N.D.
D	+	+	B10.A	1,486(1.23)	868(1.09)
E	−	−	B10	61(1.03)	N.D.
F	−	−	B10.A	37(1.60)	78(1.22)
G	15x10^6 B10 Spleen			1,132(1.21)	937(1.42)

[1]B10 recipient mice were lethally irradiated with 850R and reconstituted with 10^7 unprimed "B" cells (RAMB+C treated spleen cells), 2x10^6 unprimed (B10xB10.A)F_1--> B10.A chimera T cells (nylon nonadherent spleen cells), and/or 10^7 B10 or B10.A "accessory" cells (RAMB+C treated and 1000R irradiated spleen cells). The irradiated mice were simultaneously reconstituted and immunized with 50 ug TNP-KLH intravenously. Six days after reconstitution, the spleens from these adoptively transferred mice were assayed for the number of anti-TNP PFC/spleen.

F_1-->B10.A T cells transferred with B10 "B cells" into lethally irradiated B10 recipients failed to provide help for the response to TNP-KLH (Table I). In this situation, chimera T cells would be expected to fail to cooperate with any accessory cells provided by either the B10 "B cell" population or the irradiated B10 recipient. Indeed, the addition of B10 "accessory cells" to F_1-->B10.A T cells and B10 "B cells" also failed to allow a response (Table I, Group C). In contrast, the addition of B10.A "accessory cells" to F_1-->B10.A T cells and B10 "B cells" (Table I, Group D) did allow a response to TNP-KLH which was equal in magnitude to that produced by unfractionated B10 spleen cells (Table I, Group G). These findings demonstrate that in vivo, as well as in vitro, F_1-->Parent$_A$ chimera helper T cells are restricted in their recognition of H-2 determinants on SAC or equivalent accessory cells, but that these same helper T cells are not similarly restricted in their recognition of B cells.

II. Analysis of T Cell Recognition of Allogeneic MHC Determinants Expressed on T Cells, B Cells, and Adherent Accessory Cells.

Responding T Cells in Mixed Lymphocyte Response (MLR) Efficiently Recognize H-2 Determinants Expressed on Allogeneic SAC, but do not Similarly Recognize B Cell or T Cell H-2 Determinants. The MLR was employed as a response system in which T cell recognition of H-2 encoded determinants expressed on allogeneic lymphoid subpopulations could be examined. B10 spleen cells were mixed with titrated numbers of irradiated H-2 congenic B10.BR cells. If the number of stimulating cells producing a given level of ^{3}H-thymidine uptake is compared, stimulating SAC were at least 50 times more efficient than unseparated spleen cells in stimulating MLR (Fig. 3). T cell-depleted (RAMB+C treated) spleen cells were comparable to unseparated spleen cells in stimulating ability. In contrast, populations depleted of adherent cells were essentially nonstimulatory, including populations enriched in B cells (Sephadex G-10 passed, RAMB+C treated) or populations enriched in T cells (nylon column nonadherent) (Fig. 3). These adherent cell-depleted populations were nonstimulatory even when SAC syngeneic to the responding population were added to cultures to avoid any deficiency in nonspecific accessory function in these cultures (data not shown). Thus, alloreactive T cells responding in MLR recognize and respond preferentially to H-2 determinants expressed on allogeneic SAC, but not to H-2 determinants on T cells or B cells.

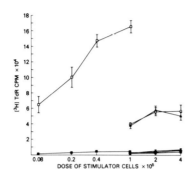

Figure 3. Responding T cells in MLR preferentially recognize H-2 encoded determinants expressed on spleen adherent cells (SAC). 4x10⁵ B10 spleen cells were mixed with titrated numbers of the following 1000R irradiated B10.BR populations: unfractionated spleen (o——o); T cells or nylon nonadherent spleen (△——▲); (B+Accessory) cells or RAMB+C treated spleen (▲——▲); adherent cell depleted or G-10 passed spleen (◇——◆); B cells or G-10 passed and RAMB+C treated spleen (○——○); spleen adherent cells (SAC) (□——□). Stimulation by syngeneic B10 control populations: unfractionated spleen (●——●); SAC (■——■).

SAC Activity in MLR Stimulation, as well as in Accessory Cell Function, is Dependent Upon an Ia+ Subpopulation of Cells. Among the H-2 encoded determinants which could serve as cell interaction structures for T cell recognition, Ia antigens have received extensive attention. In the current studies, it was therefore of interest to determine whether the SAC populations being recognized by helper T cells in antibody responses and by allogeneic T cells in MLR expressed Ia determinants. In previously reported studies it has in fact been demonstrated that the accessory function of SAC for antibody responses is dependent upon an Ia positive (Ia+) subpopulation of these cells (9). The role of Ia+ cells in the stimulation of MLR by SAC was therefore evaluated by determining the effect of treatment with anti-Ia reagent and C on MLR stimulation.

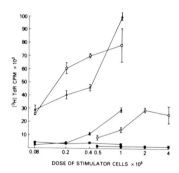

DOSE OF STIMULATOR CELLS × 10⁵

Figure 4. The MLR stimulating ability of spleen
adherent cells (SAC) is eliminated by treatment with
anti-Ia reagent and complement (C). 4×10^5 B10.D2
responding spleen cells were mixed with titrated numbers
of 1000R irradiated B10.BR stimulating cells: unfractionated spleen (○——○); medium treated SAC (□——□); normal
ascites+C treated SAC (△——△); A.TH anti-A.TL ascites+C
treated SAC (▲——▲). Stimulation by syngeneic B10.D2
control populations: unfractionated spleen (●——●); SAC
(■——■).

Untreated or control treated B10.BR SAC efficiently
stimulated responding B10.D2 cells (Fig. 4). Cells
surviving treatment of B10.BR SAC with A.TH anti A.TL
reagent and C (which lysed 60% of cells) were markedly
less efficient in stimulating MLR (Fig. 4). As was
observed for the accessory function of SAC, T cell
recognition of allogeneic H-2 in MLR is dependent upon on
Ia+ subpopulation of SAC. Additional experiments have
demonstrated that determinants encoded in the I-A
subregion as well as determinants encoded in the I-E/C
subregion are simultaneously expressed on this SAC
subpopulation (data not shown).

DISCUSSION

The present study has examined the recognition by T
cells of H-2 encoded cell-surface determinants. Such
recognition has previously been documented in a number of
immune response systems. T cell recognition of allogeneic
H-2 products has been described in MLR and cell-mediated

lympholysis in vitro, as well as in graft-versus-host
response and allograft rejection in vivo (1). More
recently, the ability of T cells to recognize both antigen
and syngeneic H-2 products has been demonstrated in T
cell-mediated cytotoxic responses (2,3). Recent
investigations have demonstrated that the ability of T
cells to cooperate with other lymphoreticular populations
in the generation of antibody or proliferative responses
depended on their ability to recognize the MHC
determinants expressed by these populations (4-6). Such
information suggests that T cell recognition of H-2
products is critical to the syngeneic cell interactions
which occur in immune responses to a wide variety of
antigens, in addition to occuring in the alloreactions
measured by parameters such as the MLR. In order to
further understand the role of H-2 recognition in immune
response, it therefore becomes important to determine
whether T cells differentially recognize H-2 encoded
determinants expressed on specific lymphoid
subpopulations. The experiments presented in the
current report have investigated this question in two
different response systems.

In studying H-2 restrictions induced in F_1-->Parent
chimeras, it was determined that for the primary PFC
response to TNP-KLH a strict requirement exists for
helper T cell recognition of syngeneic H-2 determinants
expressed on SAC accessory cells, but that no similar
requirement was observed for T cell recognition of H-2
determinants on B cells. Moreover, helper T cell
recognition of H-2 determinants on accessory cells is
required for mediation of help. It should be pointed out
that these data do not exclude the possibility that
a second helper T cell population exists which recognizes
B cell-expressed H-2 determinants, but if such a population exists it must be unrestricted by the chimera host
environment and must itself be insufficient to provide
help in the in vitro and in vivo responses studied.
Whether or not such a population exists, the present
study demonstrates that one helper T cell population
is not required to recognize the H-2 determinants
expressed on both accessory cells and B cells, if
B cell H-2 products are recognized by helper T cells
at all.

In the MLR, it was found that SAC were, on a cellular
basis, up to 50 times more stimulatory than unfractionated spleen cells. In contrast, enriched T cell or B cell
populations depleted of adherent cells had little or no
ability to stimulate MLR. The T cell, B cell, and SAC
populations employed in these experiments were identical

to those used in studies of antibody response, and the
findings in these two response systems were consistent.
T cell recognition of allogeneic H-2 determinants in MLR
was preferentially specific for H-2 determinants
expressed on SAC; the generation of antibody responses
to TNP-KLH required helper T cell recognition of syngeneic
H-2 determinants on SAC accessory cells. In neither
case was T cell recognition of either syngeneic or
allogeneic B cell H-2 determinants observed.

    The failure of helper T cells to recognize H-2
encoded determinants on B cells, and the failure of T
cells to be stimulated by B cells in MLR suggest that
either H-2 encoded determinants expressed by SAC and
B cells are intrinsically different, for which there is
no supporting evidence, or that T cells recognize H-2
determinants expressed by SAC but fail to recognize the
identical determinants as expressed by B cells. The
latter possibility cannot yet be distinguished from the
possibility that T cells can recognize H-2 determinants
expressed on both accessory cells and B cells, but are
only triggered by their interaction with accessory cells.
In either case, the findings presented in this report
suggest that T cell recognition of H-2 determinants
expressed on a spleen adherent cell population is of
unique importance to the cell interactions involved in
immune response.

REFERENCES

1. Shreffler, D.C., and David, C.S. (1975). Adv. Immunol.
   20,125.
2. Shearer, G.M., Rehn, T.H., and Schmitt-Verhulst, A.
   (1976). Transplant. Rev. 29, 222.
3. Doherty, P.C., Blanden, R.V., and Zinkernagel, R.M.
   (1976). Transplant. Rev. 29, 89.
4. Rosenthal, A.S., and Shevach, E.M. (1973). J. Exp.
   Med. 138, 1194.
5. Katz, D.H., Hamaoka, T., and Benacerraf, B. (1973).
   J. Exp. Med. 137, 1405.
6. Swierkosz, J.E., Roch, K, Marrack, P., and Kappler,
   J.W. (1978). J. Exp. Med. 147, 554.
7. Hodes, R.J., and Singer, A. (1977). Eur. J. Immunol.
   7, 892.
8. Singer, A., Hathcock, K.S., and Hodes, R.J. (1979).
   J. Exp. Med. in press.
9. Hodes, R.J., Ahmann, G.B., Hathcock, K.S., Dickler,
   H.B., and Singer, A. (1978). J. Immunol. 121, 1501.

CELL-CELL RECOGNITION AND REGULATION: C. A. Janeway, Jr. and
H. H. Wortis, Departments of Pathology, Yale University School
of Medicine, New Haven, Ct., and Tufts University School of
Medicine, Boston, Mass.

This workshop dealt with the issue of self recognition in
cellular interactions. In particular, systems were examined
that might shed light on those elements carried on self cell
surfaces that are involved in collaboration between various
sets of T cells and B cells in antibody responses. Both self
cell surface markers and their cellular localization were examined.
The first question addressed was whether helper T cells,
known to recognize antigen in association with I-A encoded
structures, required macrophages and/or B cells to carry the
appropriate I-A structure. All the participants presenting
data concurred that T cell recognition of antigen depended on
the presence of macrophages carrying the appropriate I-A encoded structures, while most of the participants found that B
cells did not need to carry the matching I-A structures. These
results were obtained primarily in in vitro systems. However,
Hodes and Singer reported that they had confirmed their results by adoptive transfer experiments in vivo. They further
reported that the irradiated recipient itself did not provide
adequate macrophage function, but that 2×10^7 irradiated spleen
cells injected in the recipient did provide adequate macrophage function. They thus questioned previous findings that T
cells and B cells needed to share I-A determinants in order to
collaborate effectively, provided the appropriate macrophage
was present in the system. No resolution of the differences
in these results was arrived at; however, it was pointed out
that other authors (Sprent; Katz; Swierkosz, Kappler and
Marrack) had used different conditions, perhaps giving different results. In particular, primed cells were used in other
experiments, while unprimed cells were tested in the experiments of Hodes and Singer. It is clear that further experimentation is required to harmonize these conflicting results.
Nonetheless, these results do illustrate the necessity of distinguishing between T-B and T-macrophage interactions in any
experimental system. The data are consistant with earlier
observations that various "thymus help replacing factors,"
whether generated by allogeneic cells or lectins, do not show
any MHC restriction. None of the experiments presented addressed the question as to whether T cells that provide Ig
(e.g. idiotype) specific help are MHC restricted. Finally,
the point was raised that none of these systems had used pure
$Lyl^+,23^-$ T helper cells, and thus suppression might account

for part or all of the restrictions seen.

A second question examined involved the ability of different subsets of T cells to interact with different subsets of B cells. Two different criteria for distinguishing subsets of B cells were presented: Okumura described B cells differing in the intensity with which they strained with anti-Ia antibodies in the FACS; this finding was confirmed by Subbarao and Mond, who find bright and dull anti-Ia staining B cells, and further, that only the brightly staining subset is present in CBA/N mice. Finally, Huber reported that she has a new antiserum, (CBA/NxC57B1/6)F1 male anti-C57B1/6, which recognizes and kills half of B cells in mice having I-A^b; this subset is missing in the CBA/N mouse and its F1 male offspring. The second criterion for distinguishing B cell sets was the type of product produced: Okumura distinguished B cells by the affinity of antibody produced, while Bottomly, Woodland, Eardley and Sercarz all used idiotype as a B cell marker. While the data presented were not conclusive, a general picture emerged that can be summarized as follows: There are specialized T helper cells performing distinct functions. In particular, there would appear to be a carrier-specific helper T cell that requires a hapten-carrier bridge, and which is required for B cell activation, at least <u>in vivo</u>. A second type of T helper cell recognizes Ig and its interactions may be restricted to particular subsets of B cells, such as those bearing particular idiotypic receptors or those of low surface I-A antigen content. A case was made by Janeway, based on his own evidence and that of Bottomly, that helper T cells recognizing Ig learn to do so from B cells or the conventional Ig pool, rather than from T cell surface idiotypes or idiotypes encountered on thymic epithelium.

Eardley presented evidence that T cell-T cell interactions can also be governed by structures encoded in or very closely linked to the VH region of the genome.

Sercarz presented evidence that different epitopes of the same antigen (hens egg white lysozyme) may preferentially trigger different subsets of T cells.

Mitchison, in summarizing the session, pointed out that T cell-macrophage interactions leading to non-MHC-restricted B cell activation can be taken as a priori evidence for the involvement of T helper factors in the interaction of T cell with B cell. Thus, he would draw the conclusion that the experiments of Hodes and Singer are most important in showing that helper factors can work in <u>in vivo</u> experiments, thus greatly reducing the problem of bringing together specific cells present at very low frequency. Secondly, he raised questions about the <u>in vivo</u> relevance of idiotype recognizing helper T cells in most antibody responses, which do not show dominance by a single idiotype.

In conclusion, it is clear that we have a great deal to learn about cellular interactions, their antigenic requirements, self restrictions and relative importance in the <u>in vivo</u> situation. Other workshops gave the hope that T cell clones of almost any specificity and function might be produced, and such clones should be the ultimate reductionist tool for resolving some of these arguments. Those pertaining to the <u>in vivo</u> situation may have to wait until such reductionist answers are available.

ON THE NATURE OF SPECIFIC FACTORS AND THE INTEGRATION OF THEIR SIGNALS BY MACROPHAGES

Marc Feldmann[1],[3], J. Michael Cecka[1], Humberto Cosenza[2],[2],
Chella S. David[3],[4], Peter Erb[4], Roger James[1], Sarah Howie[2], [8]
Sirkka Kontiainen[5], Paul Maurer[6], Ian McKenzie[7], Chris Parish[8],[9]
Anne Rees[1], Ian Todd[1], Alfredo Torano[1], Larry Winger[1], J.N. Woody[9]

1. ICRF Tumour Immunology Unit, Dept. Zoology,
University College, London WC1.
2. Basel Institute for Immunology, Switzerland.
3. Dept. Immunology, Mayo Clinic, Rochester.
4. Institute Medical Microbiology, University of Basel, Switzerland.
5. Dept. Bacteriology and Immunology, University of Helsinki, Finland.
6. Dept. Biochemistry, Jefferson Medical College, Philadelphia.
7. Dept. Medicine, Austin Hospital, Melbourne.
8. Dept. Microbiology, John Curtin School Medical Research, Canberra.
9. Immuno-Oncology Division, Lombardi Cancer Center,
Georgetown University Medical School, Washington D.C.

ABSTRACT Antigen specific helper and suppressor factors have a similar structure, which has two major sections, a 'variable region', determining antigen specificity which is probably controlled by Immunoglobulin V_H genes, with which it shares idiotype and framework determinants. Specific factors also have a 'constant region' which does not vary between strains or with the antigenic specificity of the factors, which are defined by rabbit anti- helper or anti-suppressor antisera. This region determines the biological function of the molecule. Anti-Ia antisera react with factors, but the nature and function of Ia molecules on T cell factors is unclear. The model of specific factor structure, with C and V regions resembles that of immunoglobulin, and it is thus possible that the C region of factors like the V region is Ig linked. Because there are multiple T cells, helping and suppressing antibody responses specifically, it seems improbable that all of these cells could interact directly with rare antigen-specific B cells. Thus we propose that macrophage presenting cells are the key to the integration of signals for immune induction and regulation for both T and B cells. Since Ir genes have been identified in the macrophage presenting cells interacting with both T and B cells, this suggests that macrophage Ia antigens are of importance in the integration of triggering signals for the lymphoid pool.

INTRODUCTION

Based on the profound degree of heterogeneity within the lymphoid system, the immune system is currently accepted to be composed of a network of interacting cells (1,2,3,4). There is, however no consensus about the exact composition of these networks, nor upon the mechanisms of communication or interaction of the cellular components. Certain studies have highlighted the importance of products of the major histocompatibility complex in these interactions, while others have focussed on idiotype - anti-idiotype interactions, or on allotype (5). Some experimental analyses have only investigated the lymphocyte interactions, while others have stressed the importance of the non-lymphoid accessory (macrophage-like) cells in immune homeostasis (6). Since these various concepts of the immune system are based on widely contrasting experimental systems, it is not surprising that different aspects are emphasized. But a common feature of all current analyzes of the mechanisms of immune induction and regulation is the multiplicity of interacting components.

The mechanism of interaction of the various components of the immune system is not well understood, and there are substantial conceptual differences. Some experiments suggest that cell contact is necessary for effective cell interaction (7), whereas others have indicated that cell free supernatants adequately mimick the function of the cells themselves (1,3,8,9). While it is not possible at present to interpret the experimental models unequivocably and determine the 'physiological' manner of interaction, it is evident, that as the number of interacting specific cells involved in any given reaction increases the probability of all the rare specific cells finding each other efficiently and rapidly diminishes, and so the probability that some interactions are mediated by molecules acting at a distance from the cell surface increases. Furthermore, analysis of cell free supernatants containing immunological activity derived from a certain cell population would reveal the nature of the molecules involved, regardless of whether they may function just as or more effectively while still attached to the cell membrane. Thus there appears to be substantial justification for attempts to characterize the mediators of cell interaction. This communication summarizes our attempts to analyse the nature of several antigen specific mediators of cell interaction by a variety of techniques, and discusses the relationship of such molecules to mechanisms of Ir gene action and immune regulation. Interpretations of factor structure, and of the mechanisms regulating their interactions will be suggested.

METHODS

Since all of these have been detailed elsewhere these will not be repeated here in detail (1,8,9,10).

RESULTS

Idiotype Markers on Antigen Specific Helper Factors

The several reports of shared idiotypes between B cells and T cells (11,12), have been instrumental in documenting that T cell receptors for antigen have some resemblances to immunoglobulin molecules. The extent of this resemblance is not yet clear but at least part of the variable region of T cell receptors is similar to that in B cell Ig receptors. Since there are multiple reports that antigen specific helper factors have serological cross reactivity to immunoglobulin, especially IgM, we became interested in ascertaining whether these factors shared idiotype markers with antibody molecules. For this purpose we chose the well documented Phosphorylcholine system in BALB/c mice, described by Cosenza, Kohler, Rowley and others (13,14), in which the majority of the response (approximately 95%) has an idiotype shared with a myeloma (TEPC 15). Injection of adult BALB/c mice with anti idiotype antiserum induces helper cells, suggesting that helper T cell receptors carry the TEPC 15 idiotype marker (13).

Spleen cells from mice injected with A/J anti TEPC 15 were cultured in vitro with PC-KLH for 4 days, and after washing and a further 24 hours culture with antigen the supernatants were found to have PC specific helper activity as assayed using PC-GAT as antigen. This helper factor (HF_{PC}) was analyzed on immunoadsorbents to determine its characteristics. As shown in Table 1, HF_{PC} bound to the relevant antigen, to the appropriate anti Ia antisera, and to anti-TEPC 15 columns. Thus HF_{PC} has the same basic characteristics as other helper factors analyzed in this manner, and it carried the TEPC 15 idiotype marker, suggesting that the antigen combining site region is similar to that on antibody molecules. Independent groups have recently reported analogous findings in other systems. For example Mozes has reported that a specific mouse helper factor to (T,G)-A--L shares the idiotype marker found on anti(T,G)-A--L antibodies of the same strain (15).

Determinants Controlled by the I Region on T Cell Factors

Taussig, Munro and their colleagues first demonstrated that helper factors were specifically bound by immunoadsorbent columns of the relevant anti-Ia antisera. HF_{TGAL} derived from in vivo activated T cells was mapped serologically to the I-A region (16). We have been interested in determing the nature of Ia specificities on in vitro induced HF; HF_{TGAL} mapped to I-A, confirming the results obtained with in vivo induced HF, but HF_{GAT} was mapped in I-J (17). HF_{KLH} also mapped to I-A (Kontiainen et al, In preparation) as did HF_{Strep} (Zanders et al, personnal communication). Thus as HF_{GAT} was the exception to the rule (Table 2), it was important to verify the observation, and so multiple anti I-J antisera were used, raised against both $I-J^{k}$ and $I-J^{b}$, in various strain combinations. All were reactive,

TABLE 1

PHOSPHORYL CHOLINE HELPER FACTOR

STIMULUS		Response (IgM AFC/10^6)	
Ag	Helper factor	Filtrate	Eluate
GAT	–	0	
GAT	HF$_{GAT}$	217	
PcGAT	–	0	
"	HF$_{PC}$	303	
"	" $_{PC}$ Abs CGG	213	7
"	" " PcKLH	23	167
"	" " αT15	20	227
"	" " αMOPC 167	197	33
"	" " αIa^d	27	230
"	" " DNP OA	187	42

HF$_{PC}$ generated in vitro from BALB/c mice primed with anti-Idiotype, restimulated with PcKLH. HF$_{PC}$ was used at 1% HF$_{GAT}$ at 0.1%. Absorptions and cultures performed as described (9,34). Response to GAT assayed at day 4 in Mini-Marbrook culture.

TABLE 2

GAT SPECIFIC HELPER FACTOR CONTAINS I-J

STIMULUS			Response (IgM/10^6)	
Ag	Helper factor	Absorbed with	Filtrate	Eluate
GAT	–	–	7	
"	CBA HF$_{GAT}$	–	81	
"	"	Anti-K^k	56	0
"	"	Anti-I-A^k	97	0
"	"	Anti-I-B^k	66	18
"	"	Anti-I-J^k	0	102
"	"	Anti-I-E/C^k	75	3

CBA helper cells generated by a 4 day culture with 1μg/ml of GAT. Helper factor released upon a further 24 hour culture with antigen. HF absorbed with immunoabsorbents, and eluted as described in ref. 9, 17. Responses to GAT assayed in Mini-Marbrooks.

but controls such as anti-I-J^s and various anti I-A sera were not (17). This observation indicates that the subregion assignment of helper and suppressor factors is not necessarily distinct,and that there is no rigid assignment of I subregions according to the functions of the factors (18,19).

Parish and McKenzie (eg.20) have demonstrated that rabbit antisera can be raised against mouse serum, which after absorption with dialyzed serum, were specific for Ia determinants. These were found to be inhibited by sugars and reacted with low molecular weight serum glycolipids and suggested that the I region antigens detected by this method were carbohydrate in nature, in contrast to the protein Ia antigens detected on B cells (21). It was of interest, considering that the MW of helper factors is relatively low to determine whether the Ia antigen of HF may be carbohydrate in nature. We found that HF_{TGAL} or HF_{GAT} was absorbed with rabbit anti Ia^k, and all the activity was recovered in the acid eluate. Pre-absorption of the rabbit anti Ia with whole serum, but not dialyzed serum, inhibited the binding of HF to the immunoadsorbent indicating that the relevant antibody reacted with a dialyzable product. This result suggests that the Ia product on HF may be a carbohydrate (17).

Suppressor factors have also been shown to react with anti Ia antisera, usually anti I-J (3). This is true for both suppressor factors obtained in supernatants of (22) or extracts of activated T cells (3,23). No suppressor factors have been detected which carry I-A.

Antisera to suppressor factors

Since serology is a classical method of characterizing unknown material, we have been interested in raising antisera to factors. Since different species often recognize distinct antigenic determinants, both rabbit and mouse antisera to SF_{KLH} were raised (24). Both antisera reacted with SF_{KLH} and also with other factors. Rabbit anti SF reacted with SF of all antigenic specificities and mouse strains but not helper factor, whereas syngeneic mouse anti SF only reacted with SF_{KLH} or HF_{KLH} of certain specific strains (24).

These results, illustrated in Table 3 indicated that two distinct regions of the suppressor factor molecule can be defined by serological means, a 'constant' region defined by reaction with the rabbit antiserum and a more variable region, defined by reaction with syngeneic mouse antiserum. These results have been consistently obtained with multiple batches of rabbit anti SF, and also with multiple batches of CBA anti CBA SF_{KLH} and more recently with anti SF_{GAT} using either of two experimental protocols, namely adding the antisera to cultures inhibited by SF and detecting anti SF activity by an augmentation of the response, or by coupling the antisera to beads and determining whether factor preparations were absorbed. These sera are thus valuable tools for probing the role of such factors in the immune response in vivo and in vitro, and are also helpful in our attempts to characterize these molecules.

One aspect which was investigated was the species specificity of the rabbit anti mouse SF. Certain preparations are clearly not species specific, and have absorbed out both human and monkey specific suppressor factors (unpublished data). This supports the notion that there is a portion of SF molecule which is relatively invariant, and determines its biological properties. The lack of species specificity of the antisera is compatible with, and explains the fact that both human and monkey SF suppress mouse assay systems (unpublished data).

The mouse anti SF reacts only with KLH specific factors of restricted strain distribution. The reaction with both specific HF and SF factors reactive to the same antigen suggests that both factors may employ the same combining site.

In order to determine whether the factor 'variable region' may be Ig or Ia related, a strain distribution analysis was performed to investigate allotype or MHC linkage. No associations with H-2 were noted and demonstrated that the mouse anti SF is not an anti Ia antiserum, but glimmerings of allotype association were suggested by the reaction of the CBA antiserum with BALB/c mice. However, as C3H mice did not react, allotype linkage has not been shown by strain distribution and thus back cross analysis is in progress to examine this possibility further.

Use of anti SF in vivo has begun, and the data so far is compatible with the notion that the determinants recognized by anti SF are involved in a suppressor mechanism in vivo.

The Generation of Antigen Specific Helper and Suppressor Factors from Human Peripheral Blood Lymphocytes

Significant immunological phenomena occur in analogous ways in different species. Thus it was of interest to ascertain whether specific lymphoid factors may be produced in other species and thus we have made attempts to induce human helper and suppressor cells and generate factors from them. Because methods of detecting human antibody forming cells are not yet satisfactory, we have tested the function of human factors on mouse lymphoid cells (25,26). Both specific and non-specific helper factors were detected (25,26), and more recently specific suppressor factor (27). Since the viability of the human cell suspensions which generate factors is much higher than that of the mouse cells (80% or more) the generation of human factors suggests that release of factors is a physiological process, and not merely membrane shedding from damaged or dying cells.

The nature of human specific HF has been examined using the same immunoadsorbent techniques used for characterizing mouse HF. Binding to, and elution from the appropriate antigen and anti Ia immunoadsorbents indicates that the basic structure of human factors is analogous to that of mouse factors (28).

Further development of these techniques provides an approach to the study of human Immune Response genes, and also provides tools for the study of Immune regulation in humans.

TABLE 3

EFFECTS OF ANTISERA TO SUPPRESSOR FACTOR

Stimulus HC/HF	Suppresion SF	Immunoadsorbent	Response (IgM/10^6) Filtrate	Eluate
CBA HC$_{KLH}$	-	-		309
"	CBA SF$_{KLH}$	-		100
"	"	MαSF	249	131
-	-	-		33
CBA HC$_{KLH}$	-	-		380
"	CBA SF$_{KLH}$	-		127
"	"	RαSF	240	121
-	-	-		43
CBA HF$_{KLH}$	-	-		209
"	-	MαSF	62	167
—	-	-		24

RαSF, MαSF (CBA anti CBA SF$_{KLH}$) prepared as in ref. 9,24. Absorptions as ref. 24. Data shown is 4 day response of unprimed CBA cells in Marbrook flasks to 0.1μg/ml TNP KLH (See ref. 24 for additional details).

TABLE 4

NATURE OF HUMAN HELPER FACTOR

Ag	Stimulus HF	Immunoadsorbent	Response (IgM/10^6) Filtrate	Eluate
(T,G)-A--L	-	-		0
"	HF$_{TGAL}$	-		56
"	"	(T,G)-A--L	11	45
"	"	KLH	51	9
GAT	-	-		9
"	HF$_{GAT}$	-		62
"	"	RαIa	16	62

Immunoadsorbent analysis of helper factors. Human helper cells induced by a 4 day culture with 0.1μg/ml antigen in Marbrook flasks. Human HF, a 24 hour culture supernatant was used at 1%. DNP(T,G)-A--L and DNP GAT used at 1μg/ml. (See 25, 26 for additional details). 4 day response of unprimed spleen cells.

DISCUSSION

The various approaches to the structure of antigen specific factors has led us to a synthesis which is represented in Fig. 1. Regrettably this conceptual model cannot yet be extended to encompass the biochemical features - relative proportions of protein and carbohydrate, nor the number of peptide chains etc.

The key features of the model are the existence of two major areas: the 'constant' region, defined by its reaction with rabbit antisera and its function in determining the biological properties of the molecule; and the 'variable' region, determining the binding specificity of the molecule, and its antigen specificity. The model has been drawn in monovalent form, as from analysis of the usual molecular weights of antigen specific factors (50-70,000 daltons), a divalent form is less likely but is not excluded.

Ia antigens also contribute to antigen specific factors (3,9,16,22,23) but their role is unclear. One hypothesis is that the Ia antigen contributes to, or constitutes the constant region of factors, with the I-A region involved in helper factor, and the I-J region in suppressor factor. The serological and functional invariance of the constant region could be attributed to an invariant part of the Ia molecule, which does not vary substantially between strains (or species), as some evidence exists for conservation of Ia structures between different strains and even species, as judged by serologically cross reactivity and sequence analysis (29,30). There is some evidence against this notion, based upon the finding that HF_{GAT} contains I-J determinants, which would be strengthened if it could be proven that only carbohydrate Ia structures are present on factors (17). Furthermore, if RαHF, the sera recognizing the constant region of HF were recognizing the constant, invariable part of I-A molecules, it may be predicted that they would recognize IA molecules on other cells also, such as B cells macrophages or their factors. To date that has not been found; but one could suggest that the I-A molecule is T cell specific in this case as evidence for T cell specific Ia molecules has been presented(31).

The strain specific Ia determinants do not appear to have a restricting role in the function of factors, as usually the factors do not have strain specificity although there are notable exceptions, such as suppressor cell extracts reactive to KLH (3) or helper cell extracts (32). While it is possible that there are multiple classes of antigen specific factors, differing in strain specificity the existence of non-strain specific, and non-species specific factors argues that strain specificity is not casually linked to the effector function, but must play a part, where it occurs in determining target specificity. Furthermore the Ia content of factors has no direct relationship to responder or non-responder status, has SF may be produced in both responder and non-responder strains (33). Analogous observations have

FIGURE 1.   Structure of Specific Factors
            Two basic regions, C and V with Ia determinants
            also present at a site unspecified

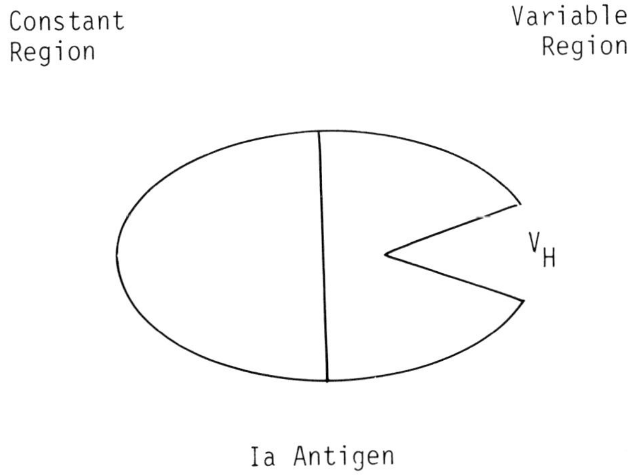

Constant   Variable
Region   Region

Ia Antigen

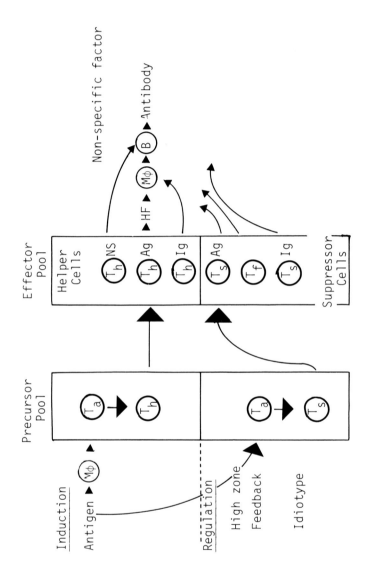

Figure 2. Complexity of Immune Networks
It is difficult to envisage that the rare specific cells could meet
with any reasonable frequency.

recently been made with helper cells. In certain chimeric mice, stem cells of a non-responder haplotype differentiate in either an irradiated (responder x non-responder)F_1 or in an allophenic mouse to yield T cells of non-responder H-2 haplotype which nevertheless are functional responders, as they respond to responder or F_1 macrophage associated antigen (34). Clearly such helper T cells of this type would generate functional HF bearing a non-responder Ia antigen. Considerations of this kind rule out T cell Ia as a contributor to the antigen specificity of factors. Thus the part of the Ia antigen which varies between strains is not of importance in the function of HF, just as noted previously for SF (33).

However, because many T cell, and also macrophage factors contain Ia determinants, some role must be envisaged, and perhaps Ia molecules are of importance in maintaining the factors in a stable, non-degraded form, or in determining the recirculation and distribution of the factors in vivo. Alternatively one could speculate a role similar to that of light chains in antibody molecules.

The two region model of factors, with constant and variable regions, is highly reminiscent of immunoglobulin (Ig) structure, and it is evident that the two classes of molecules are evolutionarily linked, just as they are functionally associated. Indeed, since antibody has a major role in regulating the magnitude and time course of antibody and cell mediated responses, one can consider a major function of antibody as a regulatory factor of B cell origin.

There is much evidence now that T cell factors are related to 'B cell factors' (Ig). The least disputed aspect is that the variable region of specific factors contains idiotypic determinants shared with Ig molecules. This has been found with HF_{TGAL} by Mozes and Haimovitch (15), with HF phosphorylcholine by Feldmann et al (35), see Table 1) with SF_{GAT} (Germain, Benacerraf, Theze, personal communication) and presumably with the syngeneic mouse anti factor sera (Table 3, ref. 24). Because T cell receptors bear idiotypic markers shared with B cells (reviewed 11,12) and the predictable, relationship (on the basis of clonal selection) of the specificity of T cell receptors and of specific T cell factors; the existence of idiotype markers on specific T cell factors had been expected. Based on the evidence discussed, it seems that the variable region of factors contains all or part of the V_H region of immunoglobulin. Does it contain anything else, such as a V_L region? Currently there is no evidence for anything else, but it will be of interest to look whether factors bearing idiotype markers which are dependent on the nature of the L chain, such as in the case of the NP idiotype marker, which is dependent on λ chains. In the same system heterocliticity of T cell receptors has been reported, and it is noteworthy that in antibody heterocliticity depends on a λ chain (36).

More controversial is the presence of other Ig determinants in factors. There are multiple reports of reaction of helper factors with anti IgM antisera, and in fact far more 'positive' than 'negative' reports. Feldmann and Basten (37), Tada and Taniguchi (38), Rieber and Riethmuller (39), used rabbit anti IgM on mouse or rat factors, while Howie and Feldmann (9) used chicken anti IgM, and there is preliminary data using rabbit anti Human IgM on monkey helper factor (Zanders et al, personal communication). Despite these reports it seems unlikely that there is a classical μ chain which would be too large since the mw of μ chain is approximately 70,000, but some cross reactive immunoglobulin domain like molecule. However all these results with anti-IgM may be misleading due to the very low molarity of factor molecules, compared to that of antibody in the assays. At present it is not possible to ascertain whether the cross reaction is in the variable or in the constant region of factors.

It is possible that some anti-immunoglobulin antisera have antibodies against the framework of the variable region, perhaps antibodies to the F_V region (40), but there may be cross reactivity to the C_{HF}, which on an 'evolutionary' basis may resemble C_μ more than any other region. Over the past few years we have used rabbit antisera against the F_V (distal end of Fab) of MOPC 315 myeloma protein prepared by Dr. D. Givol and Dr. I. McConnell. It has been found that anti-F_V inhibits the induction of helper cells, and more recently that helper factor binds to anti-F_V immunoadsorbents. It is pertinent that anti-F_{VH} is active, but not anti-F_{VL} (Feldmann et al., unpublished data). In a similar way we have used chicken anti-mouse Ig antisera, which react with HF (9). However the possibility of anti carbohydrate antibodies being responsible for the cross reaction must be considered, and the data cannot be interpreted unequivocally.

The dual regions of factors, T lymphocyte products is so reminescent of that of antibody that the possibility must be entertained that C_F regions may be associated with the immunoglobulin cluster of genes, of either the heavy or the light chain, but perhaps more logically with the former. This would suggest a V-C association mechanism for both T and B cell products, an attractive hypothesis, which could also explain the nature of T cell receptors, which are lacking in Ia antigens (11,12). Regrettably the anti factor antisera defining C_F that we have are not strain specific and thus cannot be used to map the genetic origin of C_F ie. its linkage to allotype or other markers in a back cross analysis.

It should be stressed that the specific factors discussed are not the total representation of either T cell help or suppression. Other factors eg. non-specific are implicated, but there is also the possibility that other components have not been analyzed. One dilemma concerns the difference between the common genetic restriction of T cells assayed in vivo in T-B cooperation assays and the usual lack of restriction of $\overline{HF}$ action (41,9). There are reports of strain restricted HF (32), prepared by extraction of T cells and iso electric focussing, and it is also possible that this is the more complete representation of T cell help - the non genetically restricted HF being a partly degraded form, which has lost its receptor site for

Ia. Helper factor and helper cell genetic restrictions would thus be due to the possession of both these receptors. However there are other interpretations, which are not yet possible to exclude, such that the common genetic (I) restriction of T and B cells is an experimental artefact, due to the requirement for restimulation of T cells by appropriate antigen bearing 'macrophages' and the differences of the homing patterns of injected macrophages and lymphocytes (compare 7, 42). Genetic restriction of the Mph HF-B cell interaction, not usually analyzed if anti spleen is used as the 'B cell' source may also be responsible for apparent T-B restriction.

Current models of the regulation of the antibody response envisage multiple cell interactions, with several classes of T helper cells and of T suppressor cells. For example help comprises non-specific and specific T cells, the latter contain both antigen specific and immunoglobulin specific idiotype and/or allotype specific T cells (1,3,31,43,44). Suppression involves different types of suppressor cells, specific and non-specific, those induced by high concentrations of antigen (38) and feedback suppressor cells (45) allotype suppressors and the like. The logistic problem presents itself as to how these various effects are integrated into the coherent patterns we understand as immune responses (Fig. 2).

There has been speculation over the years concerning the mechanism of the carrier effect, with its requirement for 'linked recognition' by T and B cells (46). Because determinants recognized by both cells had to be present in the same molecule major constraints were placed on mechanisms of T-B cooperation, with either direct interaction of T and B cells with an antigen bridge, or indirect interaction, via shed T cell receptor or T cell factors (37). In order to avoid the requirement of two rare antigen specific cells colliding at high frequency, the concept of helper factors, bound to common, non-antigen specific cells gained popularity (47). With the advent of additional complexity, such as the other specific helper cells recognizing idiotype rather than antigen, the problem is substantially magnified, and it is illogical to assume that 3 or more antigen specific cells have a reasonable probability of interacting. Thus an integrating cell is essential as an intermediary. In fact it is known that HF acts indirectly via macrophages (47,48), and this concept needs be only modified to incorporate the macrophage as the intermediary for other T cell signals, such as idiotype selection, and some forms of suppression. Indeed several suppressor factors have been reported to work via macrophage intermediary cells (49,50). This concept is represented schematically in Fig. 3.

The concept of the macrophage surface as the integration or signalling site for lymphocytes both T and B cells has a certain appeal, based on both numerical and experimental analysis. It could be proposed that T cells of various types shed factors which effectively increase the T cell's diameter and increase the probability of interaction with the appropriate target. However inverse square laws

FIGURE 3.   Integration of the Immune System
            Most cell interactions between rare high
            specificity cells occur via the common macrophage
            antigen presenting cell pool.

Immune Regulation Based on Macrophage-Lymphocyte Interaction

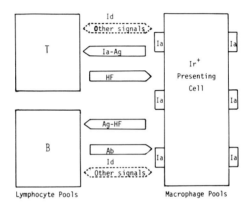

must apply at least in part and concentrations of factors would rapidly diminish as the factors migrate away from the parent cell. As Cohen and Eisen (51) have pointed out, two dimensional surfaces markedly augment effective concentration and biologically meaningful (concentration dependent) signalling would be much more efficient on cell surfaces, provided these were those not of rare antigen specific cells. Experimental analysis supports this concept based on the requirement for macrophages for both T and B cell triggering (6,10,47,52), the obvious macrophage-lymphocyte clusters which rapidly form in vitro and also, perhaps critically the dominant expression of Ir genes on the macrophage presenting cells, rather than on lymphocytes (6,48). Ir genes are significant forms of regulation and their expression on the presenting (? integrating) cell at both the T-macrophage and B-macrophage interaction (eg. 6,10,48) contributed to the development of this concept, and suggests that macrophage Ia molecules will be involved in the interactions with B cell signals. Preliminary experiments indicating that anti Ia treatment of macrophages abrogates their capacity to bind HF (Howie, Parish & Feldmann, unpublished) supports this notion.

The concept presented above leads to certain predictions, for example that interfering with macrophage surfaces would inhibit immune and induction, that multiple like signals, focussing on a single set and of receptors should 'compete' with each other. We have previously postulated that a form of 'antigenic competition' is in fact due to competition of HF of two specificities for macrophage surface receptors for HF(53). Adding fresh macrophages, or clearing cell surfaces by trypsinization abolished the inhibition, (54) supporting this concept. Another prediction is that macrophage receptors, in a form unable to induce lymphocyte activation would act as a reversible inhibitor. This experiment has been performed by Gershon, using heat killed macrophages (55). The latter experiments, together with the role of Ir genes in the integrating cells clearly imply that the integration is an active process, and that the macrophage provides more than a readily accessible membrane replete with receptors. Perhaps the crucial role of Ir genes and Ia antigens is to correlate the information content of the membrane, and to deliver the appropriate message(s) to the specific lymphocytes.

ACKNOWLEDGEMENTS

The authors thank Miss S. DeBono for typing the manuscript and Miss C. Mark for preparing the illustrations.

REFERENCES

1. Feldmann, M., Beverley, P.C.L., Erb, P., Howie, S., Kontiainen, S., Maoz, A., Mathies, M., McKenzie, I., and Woody, J. (1977). Cold Spring Harbor Symposium Quant. Biol. 41, 113.
2. Jerne, N.K. (1974). Annal. Immunol. (Inst. Pasteur) 125C, 373.
3. Tada, T., Taniguchi, M., and David, C.S. (1977). Cold Spring Harbour Symp. Quant. Biol. 41, 119.
4. Cantor, H., and Gershon, R.K. (1979). Fed. Proc. (In press).
5. Herzenberg, L.A., Okumura, K., Cantor, H., Sato, V.L., Shen, F.W., Boyse, E.A., and Herzenberg, L.A. (1976). J. Exp. Med. 144, 330.
6. Rosenthal, A.S., and Shevach, E.M. (1973). J. Exp. Med. 138, 1198.
7. Sprent, J. (1978). J. Exp. Med. 147, 1838.
8. Kontiainen, S., and Feldmann, M. (1977). Eur. J. Immunol. 7, 310.
9. Howie, S., and Feldmann, M. (1977). Eur. J. Immunol. 7, 417.
10. Erb, P., Feldmann, M., and Hogg, N. (1976). Eur. J. Immunol. 6, 365.
11. Binz, H., and Wigzell, H. (1977). Cold Spring Harbour Symp. Quant. Biol. 41, 275.
12. Eichmann, K., and Rajewsky, K. (1977). Contemp. Top. Immunobiology 7, 69.
13. Cosenza, H., Augustin, A.A., and Julius, M.H. (1977). Cold Spring Harbour Symp. Quant. Biol. 41, 709.
14. Cosenza, H., and Kohler, H. (1972). Proc. Nat. Acad. Sci. 69, 2701.
15. Mozes, E., and Haimovich, J. (1979). Nature 278, 56.
16. Taussig, M.J., Munro, A.J., Campbell, R., David, C.S., Staves, N.A. (1975). J. Exp. Med. 142, 694.
17. Howie, S., Parish, C., David, C.S., McKenzie, I.F.C., Maurer, P.H., and Feldmann, M. (1979). Eur. J. Immunol. (In press).
18. Okumura, K., Herzenberg, L.A., Murphy, O.B., McDevitt, H.O., and Herzenberg, L.A. (1976). J. Exp. Med. 144, 685.
19. Tada, T., Taniguchi, M., and David, C.S. (1976). J. Exp. Med. 144, 713.
20. Parish, C., Jackson, D.C., and McKenzie, I.F.C. (1978). In 'Ir Genes and Ia Antigens' (H.O. McDevitt, ed.) p. 243. Acad. Press.
21. Cullen, S., Freed, J.H., and Nathenson,S.G. (1976). Transplant Rev. 30, 237.
22. Feldmann, M., Howie, S., and Kontiainen, S. (1979). In 'Biology of Lymphokines' (S. Cohen, J.J. Oppenheim and E. Pick eds). p.391

Acad. Press. New York.

23. Theze, J., Waltenbough, C., Dorf, M.E., and Benacerraf, B. (1977). J. Exp. Med. 146, 287.

24. Kontiainen, S., and Feldmann, M. (1979). Thymus (In press).

25. Kantor, F. and Feldmann, M. (1979). Clin. Exp. Immunol. 36, 71.

26. Zvaifler, N., Feldmann, M., Howie, S., Woody, J., Ahmed, A. and Hartzmann, R. (1979). Clin. Exp. Immunol. (In press).

27. Feldmann, M., Woody, J., Rees, A., and Kontiainen, S., Manuscript in preparation.

28. Woody, J.N., Rees, A., Nathan, J., Zvaifler, J., Howie, S., Ahmed, A., Strong, M., Hartzman, R.J., Kantor, F., and Feldmann, M. (1979). In 'In vitro induction and measurement of antibody synthesis in man' (A.S.Fauci and R.E.Ballieux. eds). Acad. Press.

29. Blankenhorn, E., Cecka, M., Goetze, D., and Hood, L. (1979). Immunogenetics (Submitted).

30. Cecka, M., McMillan, M., Murphy, D., McDevitt, H., and Hood, L. (1978). In 'Ir genes and Ia antigens' (H.O. McDevitt ed.) p.275. Acad. Press, New York.

31. Tada, T., Takemori, T., Okumura, K., Nonuka, M., and Tokuhisa, T. (1978). J. Exp. Med. 147, 446.

32. Shiozawa, C., Singh, B., Rubenstein, S., and Diener, E. (1977). J. Immunol. 118, 2199.

33. Kontiainen, S., Howie, S., Maurer, P.H., and Feldmann, M. (1979). J. Immunol. 122, 233.

34. Erb, P., Vogt, P., Matsunaga, T., Rosenthal, A.S., Rees, A., and Feldmann, M. (1979). In 'Regulatory role of macrohages in Immunity' (A.S. Rosenthal and E.R. Unanue eds.) Acad. Press.

35. Feldmann, M., Cosenza, H., and Kontiainen, S. In preparation.

36. Makela, O., and Karjalainen, K. (1977). Immunol. Reviews 34, 119.

37. Feldmann, M. (1972). J. Exp. Med. 136, 737.

38. Okumura, K., and Tada, T. (1974). J. Immunol. 112, 783.

39. Rieber, E.P., and Riethmuller, G. (1974). Z. Immunitatsforsch. 147, 262.

40. Webb, J.V., Fudenberg, H.H. and Givol, D. (1973). Proc. Nat. Acad. Sci. 70, 1985.

41. Munro, A.J., and Taussig, M. (1975). Nature 256, 103.

42. Singer, A., Hathcock, K., and Hodes, R.J. (1979). J. Exp. Med. 149, 1208.

43. Woodland, R.T., and Cantor, H. (1978). Eur. J. Immunol. 8, 600.

44. Eichmann, K., Falk, I., and Rajewsky, K. (1978). Eur. J. Immunol. 8, 853.

45. Eardley, D., Hugenberger, J., McVay-Boudreau, L., Shen, F.W., Gershon, R.K., and Cantor, H. (1978). J. Exp. Med. 147, 1106.

46. Mitchison, N.A., Rajewsky, K., and Taylor, R.B. (1970). In 'Developmental Aspects of Antibody Formation and Structure' (J. Sterzl, ed.) p.547 Czech. Acad. Sci.

47. Feldmann, M., and Basten, A. (1972). J. Exp. Med. 136, 49.

48. Howie, S., and Feldmann, M. (1978). Nature 273, 664.

49. Zembala, M., Asherson, G.L., Munro, A.J., and Tagart, V.B. (1977). Int. Arch. Allergy Appl. Immunol. 54, 183.

50. Tadakuma, T., and Pierce, C.W. (1976). J. Immunol. 117, 967.

51. Cohen, R.J.,and Eisen, H.N. (1977). Cell Immunol. 32, 1.

52. Feldmann, M. (1972). J. Exp. Med. 135, 1049.

53. Feldmann, M., and Nossal, G.J.V. (1972). Transplant. Rev. 13, 3.

54. Schrader, J.W., and Feldmann, M. (1973). Eur. J. Immunol. 3, 711.

55. Ptak, W., Naidorf, K.F., and Gershon, R.K. (1977). J. Immunol. 119, 444.

ANTIGEN AND RECEPTOR STIMULATED REGULATION.
THE RELATIONSHIP OF IDIOTYPE AND MHC PRODUCTS
TO REGULATORY NETWORKS[1]

Mark Irwin Greene, Bruce Allen Bach, Man-Sun Sy,
Alan R. Brown,[¶] Alfred Nisonoff,[¶] and Baruj Benacerraf

Department of Pathology, Harvard Medical School, Boston, MA
and the Department of Biology, Rosenstiel Research Center,
[¶]Brandeis University, Waltham, MA

ABSTRACT Antigen-specific suppressor thymus-derived
(T) cells (T_s) are generated in A/J mice by the intravenous administration of azobenzenearsonate modified
A/J spleen cells (ABA-spl). Discrete subcellular
proteins have been obtained from ABA-specific suppressor
T cells which can limit the *in vivo* development of ABA-
specific DTH in A/J. Immunochemical analysis of such
molecules has established that T_s suppressor factor
(T_sF) bear H-2 encoded structures and determinants
recognized by anti-idiotypic antibody. Furthermore all
strains of mice tested produce ABA-specific T_s after
i.v. immunization with syngeneic ABA-spl. However, only
the A strain or the allotype congenic C.AL-20 produces
antibody with the cross-reactive idiotype (CRI) and the
idiotype bearing T_sF. B10.A ($H-2^a$) which can make T_sF
active in B10.A, produces T_sF which do not bear crossreactive idiotypic determinants. ABA T_sF, derived from
T_s, when administered to naive mice stimulates the
development of T_{s_2} capable of inhibiting ABA DTH.
Furthermore, antibodies with CRI, when coupled to
lymphocytes and administered intravenously, stimulate
the development of specific T_s. Anti CRI passively
administered also was found to elicit T_s capable of
inhibiting the DTH reaction to ABA in A/J mice.

INTRODUCTION

Several lines of evidence indicate that immunoglobulin
variable region (V) gene products are structural components

[1]This work was supported by grants CA-14723 from the
Department of Health, Education and Welfare and Grants
AI-12907, AI-12895.

of the T cell receptor for antigen. Most of the evidence to
date supporting this notion has been obtained using anti-
idiotypic antisera as probes to analyze the biological and
biochemical properties of such receptors. The evidence using
anti-idiotypic antisera has been of three sorts. First,
passively administered anti-idiotype antiserum can stimulate
functional T helper (T_H) or T suppressor (T_S) cells responsive
to the antigen to which the initial idiotype bearing antibody
was raised (1,2). Secondly, in mice and in rats, studies
employing anti-idiotype antisera indicated that the expression
of anti-major histocompatibility complex (MHC) T cell receptors on mixed lymphocyte culture (MLC) blasts is associated
with the Ig-heavy chain allotype locus (3,4) and with the MHC
locus (5). It has also been reported that T cell-derived
antigen binding material can be bound to nylon mesh, and
analysis of the fine antigen binding specificity of this T-
cell material has been correlated genetically to the appropriate Ig-1 allotype (6,7). Therefore, three separate lines
of study have suggested that T cell antigen binding products
are associated with V_H gene products. Finally, recent
studies of resistance of graft versus host (GVH) induction in
rats has suggested that idiotypes on anti-MHC receptors of a
particular MHC specificity, as detected by host T cells,
appear to be similar in several unrelated strains of rats.
This observation might indicate that the polymorphism of
these anti-MHC receptors is very limited: it has been suggested that these receptors are encoded by genes of highly
conserved loci, possibly germ line genes (8).
     The implications of all of these findings relate to the
presence of idiotypic determinants on T cell receptor(s) for
antigens, including alloantigens. The genetic origin of such
determinants in the mouse, and in some cases in the rat,
appears to be in loci closely associated with the heavy chain
allotype linkage group of genes. The presence of idiotypic
structures on functional T_S cell products has not been
studied extensively (9,10) but is an important issue since
such regulatory molecules have been found to bear MHC-encoded
determinants in many cases.

     Suppressor T Cells. The work of Eichmann and coworkers
(1,2) and Owen and Nisonoff (9) suggested that passively
administered anti-idiotypic antisera could stimulate the
development of T_S. The studies of Eichmann *et al.* indicated
that different isotypes of anti-idiotypes could sensitize
either suppressor or helper cells (2). The observation in
the ABA system that anti-idiotype administration followed by
immunization stimulated T_S which could bind to idiotype
coupled cells suggested that T_S generated by this regimen
were idiotype specific. Hence, such T_S were considered to

have anti-idiotypic receptor structures and were thought to act on idiotype[+] B or T cells (9). Recent studies using passively administered anti-idiotype in the phosphorylcholine (PCl) system have also suggested that it is possible to selectively stimulate T_S which can dampen antigen-specific responsiveness. Thus anti-idiotypic antisera can be used to probe the immunological receptor network (10) to stimulate or inhibit reactivity.

A parallel network of immune regulation has been deduced from the observations that certain I-J[+] suppressor molecules associated with antigenic fragments obtained from T_S appeared to induce second order T_{S_2} when administered to naive mice. This was the case for I-J[+] $T_S F$ operative in the response to 1) synthetic copolymers (11) *in vivo* and 2) *in vitro* (12) to 3) trinitrochlorobenzene (13) 4) to tumor antigen (14) and to other antigens (15). Second order T_{S_2} were endowed with the same operationally defined specificity as the T_S from which $T_S F$ were derived.

These sets of data could be organized according to a modified network concept. We will provide evidence that antigen-induced ABA specific T_S bear antigen-specific recognition units, which can be shown to possess definable idiotypic determinants. Suppressor molecules elaborated from such T_S are composed of polypeptides bearing idiotypic determinants mediating antigen binding and a polypeptide encoded by genes in the K + I regions of the H-2 MHC, possibly mediating cellular interactions. Such $T_S F$ can mediate inhibition of T cell-dependent immune responses, probably by limiting the generation of T_H or T-effector function (afferent inhibition). However, by virtue of the idiotypic determinant and/or bound antigen fragment which most $T_S F$ bear, these $T_S F$ are also capable of acting as immunogens to possibly stimulate 1) anti-idiotypic T_{S_2} (idiotype binding) or 2) alternatively, by virtue of the antigenic fragment, act to induce idiotype bearing T_{S_2}. We would predict that second order T_{S_2} act at a different point in the network to mediate suppression (efferent suppression), *i.e.*, at the expression of the effector T cell in T cell responses and B cells in antibody responses. We will show that anti-idiotype is capable of inducing suppressor cells endowed with the capacity to inhibit ABA specific T cell dependent responses. Furthermore, we will also demonstrate that idiotype coupled to cells covalently can be used as a probe of idiotype initiated regulatory events prior to or concomitant with antigen perturbation of the immune system.

Materials and Methods. Mice: A/J (H-2[a], Ig-1[e]), BALB/c (H-2[d], Ig-1[a]), B10.A (H-2[a], Ig-1[b]) were obtained from

The Jackson Laboratory. C.AL-20 (H-2^d, Ig-1^d) were obtained from M. Potter and maintained at Brandeis University.

Antigen: Azobenzenearsonate (ABA) coupled to syngeneic cells were prepared as described (16). ABA-specific STC were generated by the i.v. administration of 5 x 10^7 ABA-coupled syngeneic spleen leukocytes. ABA-specific DTH responses were induced by the s.c. immunization of mice with 3 x 10 syngeneic ABA-coupled cells. Challenge was done with either 25 μl of 10 mM diazonium of p-arsanilic acid or 10^7 ABA coupled spleno-cytes in the footpad 5-6 days post-immunization. The DTH response has been shown to be T cell dependent elsewhere (16). All DTH responses were measured blind by two individuals. The means and standard errors are presented with the relevant p value. ABA idiotype and anti-crossreactive idiotype (CRI) antibodies were prepared according to methods published elsewhere (17).

ABA Specific T$_s$F Bear Idiotypic and MHC Determinants.

ABA specific T$_s$ are generated in the thymuses and spleens of A/J mice given 5 x 10^7 ABA conjugated A/J cells i.v. 7 days previously. Sonicates, extracts or antigen boosted super-natants from such T$_s$ are suppressive when administered in doses of 10^7 cell equivalents/day/mouse to A/J mice primed with 3 x 10^7 ABA cells s.c. and challenged 5 days later with ABA (16). Such T$_s$F are specific inasmuch as 1) they are bound to and recoverable from ABA FGG immunoadsorbents, but are not retained by FGG immunoadsorbents, and 2) they inhibit DTH reactivity to ABA but not to TNP (18). The MW of ABA T$_s$F was also determined to be in the order of 3.3 - 6.8 x 10^4 daltons (19) by gel filtration. To analyze the antigen bind-ing structures on ABA T$_s$F, they were passed on immunoadsor-bents composed of 1) anti-CRI, 2) the prebleed normal rabbit serum (NRS) control, or 3) B10.D2 anti-B10.A anti-H-2^a (anti-K^k I-A^k I-B^k I-J^k I-E^k). The filtrates and eluates were collected, dialyzed and readjusted to original volumes and tested in A/J mice. As is shown in Table 1, T$_s$F from T$_s$ induced by ABA-cells were found to bear idiotypic determi-nants and H-2^a K-end determinants. That such structures were present in the same complex was deduced by sequential passage of T$_s$F first on anti-idiotypic columns and the acid-eluate from the first column passed on a second anti-H-2^a column and eluted (17,18). Such T$_s$F were still found to be significantly suppressive for ABA specific T cell dependent DTH responses.

Genetic Linkage Analysis of Idiotype$^+$ T$_s$F.

To ascertain the genetic relationships of ABA specific idiotype$^+$ suppressor molecules to the allotype linkage group of genes, T$_s$F were generated in BALB/c (H-2^d, Ig-1^a), C.AL-20 (H-2^d, Ig-1^d), A/J

TABLE 1

ABA SPECIFIC SUPPRESSOR MOLECULES BEAR
IDIOTYPIC AND H-2 ENCODED DETERMINANTS

Group	ABA T_sF treatment[a]	Immunization[b]	Mean footpad[c] response 10^{-3} in ± SEM	p [d]
I	T_sF untreated	ABA-A/J	3.5 ± 1.0	<.001
II	T_sF filtrate from (anti-CRI-Seph)*	ABA-A/J	8.0 ± 1.0	n.s.
III	T_sF eluate from (anti-CRI-Seph)	ABA-A/J	2.0 ± 0.7	<.001
IV	T_sF filtrate from (B10.D2 anti-B10.A Seph)	ABA-A/J	9.5 ± 1.0	n.s.
V	T_sF eluate from (B10.D2 anti-B10.A Seph)	ABA-A/J	4.6 ± 1.0	<.005
VI	T_sF filtrate from (prebleed rabbit serum-Seph)	ABA-A/J	4.0 ± 0.5	<.005
VII	T_sF filtrate from (normal mouse globulin-Seph)	ABA-A/J	4.0 ± 0.9	<.005
VIII	————	ABA-A/J	11.0 ± 0.7	————
IX	————		2.5 ± 1.0	<.001

[a] 10^7 cell equivalents/day/mouse for 5 days.
[b] 3×10^7 ABA-A/J cells subcutaneously into A/J mice.
[c] 25 μl 10 mM ABA diazonium in the footpad.
[d] Compared to positive control—after Bach et al. (18) and Greene et al. (19).
*(immunosorbent column).

($H-2^a$, $Ig-1^e$) and B10.A ($H-2^a$, $Ig-1^b$). C.AL-20 has the same
H-2 region as BALB/c but the heavy chain allotype linkage
group of genes is similar to A/J; whereas A/J has the same
H-2 haplotype as B10.A but a different allotype region. All
T_sF produced in the strains by the i.v. administration of ABA-
coupled syngeneic cells were passed on anti-CRI immunoadsorbents, the filtrates and eluates collected and evaluated
in vivo. As shown in Table 2, only C.AL-20 and A/J produced
idiotype positive T_sF, thus indicating that genes linked to
the allotype heavy chain linkage group control the expression
of idiotypic structures on these suppressor molecules.

   Idiotype$^+$ T_sF Stimulate Second Order T_{s2}. To determine
whether T_sF in this system operate in a circuit, 10^7 C.E. of
A/J T_sF were administered to naive mice/day/5 days and spleen
cells removed 7 days later. The spleen cells were adoptively
transferred to naive recipients which were immunized and
challenged with ABA. As can be seen in Table 3, ABA T_sF
stimulate the development of suppressor cells in such mice.
Thus T_{s1} derived T_sF appear capable of inducing second order
T_{s2}. It is not at present known whether such T_{s2} bear idiotypic or anti-idiotypic receptors.

   The Effect of Anti-CRI and CRI-Coupled Cells Administered
to A/J Mice. To further investigate the notion of idiotype
initiated regulation, two approaches were used. In the first
anti-CRI or NRS was administered daily to A/J mice primed
with ABA A/J cells in an attempt to stimulate T_s which on
adoptive transfer could inhibit ABA specific DTH. In a
second approach, idiotype was covalently coupled to A/J
lymphocytes as described elsewhere (20). These cells were
administered to A/J mice (i.v.). Their spleen cells were
taken 6 days later and transferred to naive A/J recipients
which were then immunized with ABA cells. As is shown in
Table 4 idiotype coupled cells when administered to naive
mice caused the emergence of transferrable T_s which suppressed
ABA DTH. Anti-idiotype antiserum, but not NRS or the $F(ab')_2$
anti-CRI, also induced a population of suppressor cells which
similarly inhibited this response.

                            DISCUSSION

   The results of these studies show that both idiotypic
determinants and MHC structures are present on ABA specific
T_s derived suppressor molecules. It is relevant that CRI
determinant expression on the T cell derived T_sF is determined by genes linked to the allotype linkage group of genes

TABLE 2

GENETIC ANALYSIS OF ORIGIN OF T_SF IDIOTYPIC STRUCTURES

Group immunized[a]	H-2	Source and treatment of ABA T_sF	Recipient immunization[b]	Footpad response[c]	p[d]
1. A/J	a	A/J T_sF	ABA-A/J	3.0 ± 1.00	<.001
2. A/J	a	A/J T_sF filtrate from (anti-CRI-Seph)*	ABA-A/J	9.0 ± 1.00	n.s.
3. A/J	a	A/J T_sF eluate from (anti-CRI-Seph)	ABA-A/J	3.8 ± .90	<.001
4. A/J	a	No factor used	ABA-A/J	11.0 ± 1.00	—
5. B10.A	a	B10.A T_sF	ABA-B10.A	2.0 ± 1.00	<.001
6. B10.A	a	B10.A T_sF filt.(anti-CRI-Seph)	ABA-B10.A	3.5 ± .70	<.001
7. B10.A	a	B10.A T_sF el.(anti-CRI-Seph)	ABA-B10.A	7.8 ± .50	n.s.
8. B10.A	a	No factor used	ABA-B10.A	9.0 ± .75	—
9. C.AL-20	d	C.AL-20 T_sF	ABA-C.AL-20	4.0 ± 1.00	<.001
10. C.AL-20	d	C.AL-20 T_sF filt.(anti-CRI-Seph)	ABA-C.AL-20	9.0 ± .75	<.05
11. C.AL-20	d	C.AL-20 T_sF el.(anti-CRI-Seph)	ABA-C.AL-20	4.2 ± .70	<.001
12. C.AL-20	d	No factor used	ABA-C.AL-20	12.0 ± .50	—
13. BALB/c	d	BALB/c T_sF	ABA-BALB/c	3.0 ± .50	<.001
14. BALB/c	d	BALB/c T_sF filt.(anti-CRI-Seph)	ABA-BALB/c	4.0 ± .70	<.001
15. BALB/c	d	BALB/c T_sF el.(anti-CRI-Seph)	ABA-BALB/c	11.0 ± .60	n.s.
16. BALB/c	d	No factor used	ABA-BALB/c	11.0 ± .50	—

[a]Mice were given syngeneic T_sF 10^7C.E. day/mouse for 5 days beginning at the time of immunization with 3×10^7 syngeneic ABA-coupled splenic lymphocytes.

[b,c,d], as in Table 1.

*(immunosorbent column).

TABLE 3

T_SF DERIVED FROM A/J T_S INDUCE T_{S2} IN NAIVE A/J MICE

Group	Treatment of Group 1	Cells transferred[b] from T_SF-treated mice Group 1 to Group 2	Immunization of Group 2	Mean footpad[c] response 10^{-3} in ± SEM	p
I	—	—	3×10^7 ABA-A/J	10.80 ± .30	—
II	10^7 C.E. T_SF/day mouse for 5 days	5×10^7 splenocytes or	3×10^7 ABA-A/J	4.60 ± .40	<.001
III	10^7 C.E. T_SF/day mouse to normal A/J	5×10^7 thymocytes from T_SF-treated mice	3×10^7 ABA-A/J	5.25 ± .75	<.01
IV	—	5×10^7 normal spleen cells	3×10^7 ABA-A/J	9.75 ± .50	n.s.
V	—	—	—	1.00 ± .50[d]	<.001

[a] 10^7 C.E. of ABA STC derived T_SF/day/mouse.
[b] 5×10^7 spleen cells or 5×10^7 thymocytes obtained from T_SF treated mice 5 days after treatment. Alternatively, normal spleen cells were transferred.
[c] Challenge with 25 μl 10 mM ABA diazonium in the footpad.
[d] Challenge only.

in correspondence with the expression of CRI[+] antibody (17). These T_S and T_SF arise as a consequence of antigen stimulated regulation. Furthermore, it is possible to initiate second order regulatory events by T_SF, an example of antigen and/or receptor initiated regulation. B cell idiotypic products coupled to lymphocytes similarly appear to induce T_S capable of inhibiting ABA specific DTH reactions and are an example of B cell receptor initiated regulation (Table 4) of T cell reactivity. Thus it is likely that T cell responses as shown herein and B cell reactivities as described elsewhere (1,2) are to some extent coordinated and regulated by receptor anti-receptor interactions initiated by the perturbation of the immune system by antigen.

Immunochemical analysis of ABA T_SF presented in depth elsewhere (18-19) has revealed that such molecules bind specifically to ABA FGG immunoadsorbents but not to FGG control columns. Furthermore, the molecular weight of this factor was determined by column chromatography to be $33 - 68 \times 10^3$ daltons. Suppressor molecules could be obtained from STC by extraction, sonication or from supernatants after antigen boosting. Since the T_S cell derived T_SF is intimately associated with MHC determinants it is not surprising that allo-antisera (anti-I-J or anti-Ia) can be shown to modulate T_S or effector cell immune reactivity (21,22).

It is clear that such suppressor molecules can themselves stimulate second order T_{S2} in naive recipients. Although T_{S2} emerges as a consequence of this stimulation it is not yet apparent whether the idiotypic determinant on the T_SF, or the antigen fragment contained within the complex (12, 13) is responsible for this action. Preliminary studies suggest A/J T_SF can suppress C57BL/6 (H-2[b], Ig-1[b]) ABA DTH, and this might suggest that the idiotypic determinant is not responsible for the induction of T_{S2}. However, idiotypic structures have been shown in other studies to initiate anti-idiotype regulation (23), and further experiments to resolve this issue as it relates to T_SF are in progress.

In this regard we have undertaken studies to use B cell idiotype coupled covalently to lymphocyte surfaces as a probe of the receptor initiated regulatory effects on immune reactivity. Such idiotype[+] lymphocytes when administered to A/J mice (i.v.) stimulated the development of suppressor cells in these animals capable of specifically suppressing ABA DTH. This is an example therefore of "receptor driven regulation" since T_S arise before the perturbation of the immune system by antigen. Similar results with respect to B cell reactivities have been obtained by Y. Dohi and A. Nisonoff (in preparation), who pretreated A/J mice with CRI coupled to thymocytes, and inhibited CRI production.

TABLE 4
THE INFLUENCE OF IDIOTYPE AND ANTI-IDIOTYPE ON THE DTH RESPONSE TO ABA

Group[a]	Pretreatment[b]	Cell transfer[c] to second recipient	Immunization[d]	% control response[e] (DTH)	p
I			3×10^7 ABA-A/J	100%	—
II	5×10^7 normal Ig coupled cells		3×10^7 ABA-A/J	85%	n.s.
III	5×10^7 CRI coupled cells		3×10^7 ABA-A/J	35%	<.001
IV	5×10^7 CRI coupled cells to naive mice	5×10^7 spleen cells from CRI cell treated mice	3×10^7 ABA-A/J	40%	<.01
V	NRS		3×10^7 ABA-A/J	90%	n.s.
VI	Anti-CRI 2 μg/IBC/day/mouse[f]		3×10^7 ABA-A/J	0%	<.001
VII	Anti-CRI 2 μg/IBC/day mouse to naive mice + 3×10^7 ABA-A/J s.c.	5×10^7 spleen cells from anti-CRI treated mice	3×10^7 ABA-A/J	30%	<.001
VIII				0%	<.001

[a] 10 A/J mice per group/pooled data of 2 experiments.
[b] Cells were coupled with protein by the carbodiimide technique (19). 1 mg protein/10^7 cells.
[c] Spleen cells obtained from first recipient and transferred to second recipients which were immunized with ABA-A/J cells.
[d] As described (18).

[e] % response = $\dfrac{x - \text{negative control}}{\text{positive control} - \text{negative control}}$ Positive control $10\text{-}12 \times 10^3$ in.
   Negative control $1\text{-}2 \times 10^{-3}$ in.

[f] IBC = Idiotype Binding Capacity as defined in (9,17).

To further complement these studies anti-idiotype (anti-receptor) was passively administered to A/J mice immunized with ABA A/J. It was found that such treatment similarly inhibited ABA specific DTH by the generation of T_S. The specificity and binding structures of these cells remains to be defined, but may be idiotypic (18) or anti-idiotypic (9).

The data suggest that antigen initiated or receptor (idiotype) stimulated regulation are components of a large regulatory circuit capable of dampening reactivity at many points in the immune response. It might be envisioned that antigenic stimulation leads to idiotypic responses, which in turn initiate anti-idiotypic reactions to limit the reactions (9). The latter notion appears to be substantiated by the observation that antigen, idiotype and anti-idiotype can all be used to initiate regulation of T cell dependent immune responses.

REFERENCES

1. Eichmann, K. (1974). Eur. J. Immunol. 4, 296.
2. Eichmann, K. (1975). Eur. J. Immunol. 5, 511.
3. Binz, H., and Wigzell, H. (1977). Contemp. Top. Immuno-biol. 7, 113.
4. Binz, H., and Wigzell, H. (1975). J. Exp. Med. 142, 1218.
5. Krammer, P.H., and Eichmann, K. (1977). Nature 270, 733.
6. Krawinkel, U., Cramer, M., Imanishi-Kari, T., Jack, R.S., Rajewsky, K., and Mäkelä, O. (1977). Eur. J. Immunol. 7, 566.
7. Reth, M., Imanishi-Kari, T., Jack, R.S., Cramer, M., Krawinkel, U., Hämmerling, G.J., and Rajewsky, K. (1977). In "Immune System: Genetics and Regulation" (E.E. Sercarz, L.A. Herzenberg and C. Fred Fox, eds.), p. 39. Academic Press, New York.
8. Bellgrau, D., and Wilson, D.B. (1978). J. Exp. Med. 234, 149.
9. Owen, F.L., and Nisonoff, A. (1978). J. Exp. Med. 148, 182.
10. Jerne, N.K. (1976). Harvey Lect. 70, 93.
11. Waltenbaugh, C., Theze, J., Kapp, J.A., and Benacerraf, B. (1977). J. Exp. Med. 146, 970.
12. Germain, R.N., Theze, J., Kapp, J.A., and Benacerraf, B. (1978). J. Exp. Med. 147, 123.
13. Greene, M.I., Pierres, A., and Benacerraf, B. (1977). J. Supramol. Struct. Suppl. 1, 204.
14. Perry, L.L., Benacerraf, B., and Greene, M.I. (1978). J. Immunol. 121, 2144.

15. Tada, T. (1977). In "ICN/UCLA Symposia on Molecular and Cellular Biology" (C.F. Fox, ed.), Academic Press, New York.
16. Bach, B.A., Sherman, L., Benacerraf, B., and Greene, M.I. (1978). J. Immunol. 121, 1460.
17. Ju, S-T., Owen, F.L., and Nisonoff, A. (1977). Cold Spring Harbor Symp. Quant. Biol. 41, 699.
18. Greene, M.I., Bach, B.A., and Benacerraf, B. (1979). J. Exp. Med. 149, No. 5.
19. Bach, B.A., Greene, M.I., Benacerraf, B., and Nisonoff, A. (1979). J. Exp. Med. 149, No. 5.
20. Miller, S.D., Wetzig, R.P., and Claman, H.N. (1979). J. Exp. Med. 148, 758.
21. Greene, M.I., Pierres, M., Dorf, M.E., and Benacerraf, B. (1977). Proc. Natl. Acad. Sci. USA 74, 5118.
22. Greene, M.I., Perry, L.L., Dorf, M.E., and Benacerraf, B. (1978). J. Immunol. 121, 1616.
23. Cazenave, P.-A. (1977). Proc. Natl. Acad. Sci. USA 74, 5122.

TWO T CELL SIGNALS ARE REQUIRED FOR
THE B CELL RESPONSE TO PROTEIN-BOUND ANTIGENS[1]

Daniel M. Keller,[2] James E. Swierkosz,
Philippa Marrack,[3] and John W. Kappler

Division of Immunology, University of Rochester
Cancer Center and Department of Microbiology,
University of Rochester,
Rochester, New York 14642

ABSTRACT We have studied the requirements for T cell
help for B cell responses to protein-bound and red blood
cell-bound antigens. Anti-protein responses need two
types of helper T cells. One, apparently Ia$^-$, is needed
early and delivers an antigen specific signal, and
another, I-A$^+$, is needed later and delivers a
nonspecific signal.

INTRODUCTION

For some years our laboratory has been studying the
ways in which helper T cells stimulate B cell responses to
antigen. Originally we made the observation that at least
two different types of helper T cells exist (1). One we
called antigen specific, because it would apparently only
help B cells respond to determinants coupled to the same
antigen as it was recognizing, and another type which we
called nonspecific, as it responded to antigen by helping B
cell responses to unrelated structures, apparently by secreting a nonspecific mediator (2). We found that this cell
type was particularly active in stimulating anti-red blood
cell (RBC) responses and had little activity in stimulating
B cell responses to determinants on unrelated proteins.

[1]This work was supported by USPHS research grants AI-
11558 and CA-11198 and American Cancer Society research grant
IM-49.
[2]Supported by USPHS Graduate Fellowship 5-T01-00592 GM.
[3]Recipient of an Established Investigator Award from
the American Heart Association.

Other investigators have supported the idea that two different types of helper T cells exist. The extensive literature on antigen specific and non-specific T cell-derived helper factors lend credence to this hypothesis. In some cases requirements for two types of helper T cells in anti-trinitrophenylated (TNP) protein responses have been demonstrated (3-5). In one series of these experiments it was shown that one of the helper T cells was $\underline{I-J}^+$ and acted by secreting a nonspecific factor(s) (5).

The results described in this paper support the hypothesis that two types of helper T cells exist and are needed for anti-TNP-protein responses. One of the helpers is $\underline{I-A}^+$ and acts relatively late in the B cell response by secreting a nonspecific factor(s).

MATERIALS AND METHODS

Mice. B10.A ($\underline{H-2}^a$), C57BL/10.Sn (B10, $\underline{H-2}^b$) and BDF_1 mice were obtained from Jackson Laboratories. B10.S, A.TH, and A.TL mice were raised in our facilities from breeding pairs kindly supplied by Dr. Chella David.

Antigens and Immunizations. Antigens were prepared and used in their unsubstituted and TNP conjugated forms as previously described (6). T cells were primed for helper activity, and B cells were primed for anti-TNP responses as we have already reported (6). A.TH anti-A.TL T cell blast serum was prepared and used as described by Hayes and Bach (8).

Preparation and Culture of Cells. B cells, MØ, and T cells were obtained from spleen cell suspensions (6). Rich populations of MØ were obtained from the peritoneal washings of normal mice. These washings were usually incubated overnight in culture medium, in the wells in which they were to be used, at $2 \times 10^5/0.5$ ml. Nonadherent cells were then removed by pipetting off the supernatant fluid and washing with gentle swirling, to leave behind a population of adherent MØ. In some cases antigen-pulsed MØ were added to cultures. These were prepared as reported before (9). Assays of T cell-B cell cooperation were done either in microculture wells (0.1 ml/well) (1) or in Linbro 76-033-05 wells holding about 0.5 ml/well (6). Helper T cell activity was titrated as previously described (6). Activities are expressed as plaque forming cells (PFC)/culture/10^6 T cells $\pm$ the standard error (SE).

Assay of PFC.   PFC were assayed directly in the microculture wells (1) or on slides (6).

Preparation of Concanavalin A Supernatant.   Supernatants
of concanavalin A activated spleen cells (Con A SN) were
prepared and absorbed as previously described (2).

RESULTS

Anti-RBC and Anti-TNP-Protein Responses Do Not Have the
Same Requirements for T Cell Help.   For some years it
has been known that a T cell-derived, apparently nonspecific
factor, found in the supernatants of activated T cells, would
stimulate responses of B cells to RBC-bound antigens (2).
There are, however, conflicting reports over the activity of
this factor in stimulating responses to protein-bound antigens.   In our own laboratory we have been unable to show
that this factor is sufficient for such responses, even when
the factor is obtained from its richest source, Con A SN
(2).   Since other experiments suggested that the factor
might only stimulate responses to membrane-bound antigen, we
therefore tested the activity of Con A SN in stimulating
responses to SRBC, TNP-KLH, and TNP-KLH bound to MØ membranes
by preincubation (9).

As shown in Table I anti-TNP-KLH responses were stimulated by KLH-primed T cells whether the antigen was added to
cultures in soluble form, or on MØ.   By contrast, Con A SN
addition had no stimulatory effect on these responses, irrespective of the mode of addition of TNP-KLH to cultures.
In control experiments Con A SN was very active in stimulating anti-SRBC responses.   Thus the defect in Con A SN
stimulation of anti-protein-bound antigen responses does not
seem to be corrected by presenting the antigen on a cell
membrane, supporting the idea that requirements for T cell
help for anti-RBC responses are different from those for
anti-protein responses.

We were curious to investigate further the differences
in B cell responses to these two types of antigen.   It has
been reported (10) that B cells go through at least the
first round of division in response to RBC antigens in the
absence of T cell help.   T cell help must be added after 24
or 48 hours of such a response to stimulate further division
and differentiation.   We investigated whether this was also
true for responses to TNP-KLH.   TNP-primed splenic B cells
and MØ were cultured with antigen, and T cells, or T cell
help in the form of Con A SN was added at various times

TABLE I
Con A SN IS NOT SUFFICIENT FOR ANTI-TNP-KLH RESPONSES

| Additions to Cultures[a] | | PFC/microculture[b] | |
Antigen	Source of T cell help	Anti-TNP	Anti-SRBC
0.1 μg/ml TNP-KLH	-	0.9±0.5	nd
0.1 μg/ml TNP-KLH	10^5 KLH-primed T cells	15.2±8.7	nd
0.1 μg/ml TNP-KLH	25% Con A SN[c]	2.5±0.8	nd
TNP-KLH-MØ[d]	-	4.4±2.3	nd
TNP-KLH-MØ	10^5 KLH-primed T cells	26.5±6.1	nd
TNP-KLH-MØ	25% Con A SN	5.0±2.8	nd
SRBC	-	nd	0.8±0.8
SRBC	25% Con A SN	nd	97.3±37.2
None	25% Con A SN	3.8±3.6	nd

[a] All cultures contained 2 x10^5 splenic, TNP-primed B cells and MØ.
[b] Average of 3 experiments ± SE.
[c] Added at 0 time.
[d] 2 x 10^4 TNP-KLH-pulsed MØ added to microcultures at 0 hr.

after the start of cultures. As shown in Figure 1, the response to BRBC on different days was the same whether T cell help in the form of Con A SN was added at time 0 or 24 hours. In contrast the response to TNP-KLH was significantly delayed by delayed addition of helper T cells. For both responses, delays occurred if antigen was added late. This experiment suggests that RBC-bound antigens can initiate B cell responses without T cell help, but protein bound antigens cannot, suggesting, again, a qualitative difference in the T cell help which the two responses need.

Anti-TNP-Protein Responses Require Two Types of Helper T Cells. Various experiments led us to hypothesize that anti-TNP-protein responses require two different helper T cells (1-5, 7), one of which delivers a signal(s) present in Con A SN to B cells. We have sought ways of proving this hypothesis. Three different methods which we have used are described here.

In the first method KLH-primed T cells were incubated on MØ monolayers with KLH for 3 days to yield preactivated T

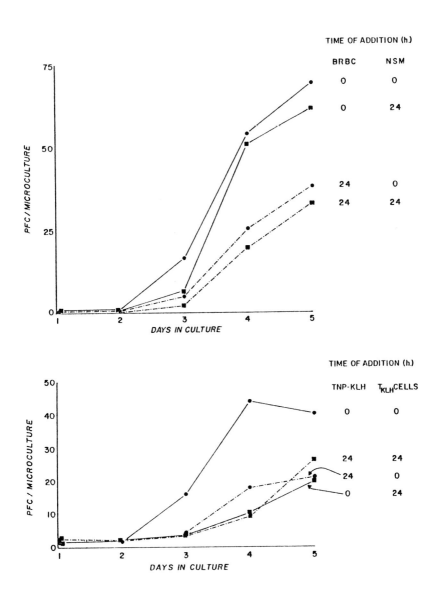

Figure 1. Kinetics of response to BRBC and TNP-KLH. 2 x 10⁵ TNP-primed splenic B cells and MØ were incubated in microcultures with BRBC or TNP-KLH as antigens, added at time 0 or at 24 hours. T cell help, in the form of 25% Con A SN or 1 x 10⁵ KLH-primed T cells, was added at time 0 or at 24 hours. Twelve identical microcultures were assayed daily for anti-TNP PFC on 5 successive days.

cells which were very much more active than before preincubation. These T cells were then titrated into microcultures
containing TNP-primed B cells and MØ, and TNP-KLH in the
presence or absence of Con A SN. Preincubated T cells had
little activity when used as the only source of T help, and
addition of Con A SN very much increased the response (Table
II). This experiment suggests that preincubated T cells
might be selectively deficient in a necessary but not totally
sufficient helper cell, and that the activity of this cell
can be supplied by Con A SN addition.

In a second type of experiment KLH-primed or GZ-primed
T cells (T_{KLH},T_{GZ}) were incubated with TNP-primed splenic B
cells and MØ and KLH or GZ (1 µg/ml) for 48 hours. Nonadherent cells were then removed by moderate washing. TNP-
primed splenic B cells and MØ were then added to these
cultures with various antigens in the presence or absence of
Con A SN. As shown in Table III no response was observed in
the absence of Con A SN. In the presence of Con A SN,
however, an anti-TNP response occurred, but only if the T
cells were responding to TNP-KLH. Bystander GZ-primed cells
failed to stimulate a response. These results suggested
that two helper signals were needed for B cell responses to
TNP-KLH. One, antigen specific, was provided by the MØ monolayer, after incubation with KLH-primed T cells and KLH. The
other, presumably nonspecific, was provided by Con A SN.

TABLE II

TWO T CELL SIGNALS IN TNP-KLH RESPONSES: ONE NONSPECIFIC

Additions to Cultures[a]		
Preactivated T cells	Con A SN	Anti-TNP PFC/ microculture
0	0	1.3
0	25% at 24 hrs	1.9
2×10^3	0	1.3
2×10^3	25% at 24 hrs	8.2
6×10^3	0	6.9
6×10^3	25% at 24 hrs	18.2

[a]All cultures contained 2×10^5 splenic, TNP-primed
B cells and MØ and 0.1 µg/ml TNP-KLH.

TABLE III
TWO T CELL SIGNALS IN TNP-KLH RESPONSES:
ONE SPECIFIC, ONE NONSPECIFIC

| Additions to Cultures[a] | | Anti TNP PFC/ |
First Culture	Second Culture[b]	Culture
None	TNP-KLH + Con A SN	3
$2x10^6$ T_{KLH} + TNP-KLH	TNP-KLH	85
$2x10^6$ T_{KLH} + TNP-KLH	TNP-KLH + Con A SN	673
$2x10^6$ T_{GZ} + GZ+TNP-KLH	TNP-KLH + Con A SN	5

[a]All cultures contained $3x10^6$ TNP-primed splenic
B cells and MØ. Antigens were added throughout at
1 μg/ml.
[b]30% Con A SN was added 24 hours after the second
cultures were set up.

In a final series of experiments the specificity of
A.TH anti-A.TL T cell blast serum was examined. KLH-primed
B10.A or B10.S T cells were incubated with this antiserum
and complement and then titrated with syngeneic B cells and
MØ in anti-TNP-KLH responses in the presence or absence of
Con A SN (Table IV). The helper activity of B10.A T cells
was eliminated by treatment with the antiserum and complement. B10.S T cells were unaffected. Addition of Con A SN
to cultures restored the activity of the defective B10.A
cells. These results prove that two types of helper T cells
are needed for anti-TNP-KLH responses, and that one of these
is replaceable by Con A SN and is Ia$^+$. In mapping experiments not shown here this T cell was shown to bear at least
I-A-encoded determinants.

TABLE IV
ConA SN REPLACES AN I-A$^+$ HELPER T CELL

Strain	Treatment of T Cells	Addition of Con A SN	Helper Activity (PFC/culture/10^6 T Cells ± SE)
B10.A	C	-	643±49
B10.A	C	30% at 24 hrs	1522±88
B10.A	αIa^k + C	-	8±49
B10.A	αIa^k + C	30% at 24 hrs	494±88
B10.S	C	-	618±61
B10.S	αIa^k + C	30% at 24 hrs	554±61

DISCUSSION

The experiments in this paper clearly define several differences in requirement for help between B cell responses to RBC-bound and protein-bound antigens. A helper factor in Con A SN was sufficient for anti-RBC responses but not for anti-TNP-KLH responses, a finding which agrees with some (2) but not all (11) literature on this subject. B cell responses to RBC antigens initiated in the absence of T cell help, as shown before (7, 10, 12), but B cell responses to TNP-KLH did not. In addition previous experiments suggested that two types of helper T cells were needed for anti-TNP-KLH responses (35, 7). Of these, one type, active in anti-RBC responses, seemed also to be necessary but not sufficient for anti-TNP-protein responses (5,7).

Since anti-RBC responses can be driven by a Con A SN nonspecific factor (2) it was not unreasonable to suppose that this might be the product of the helper cell needed for both kinds of responses. We therefore sought to show that two kinds of helper T cells were needed for anti-TNP-protein responses, using Con A SN to replace one of them. As the experiments in this paper illustrate, our hypothesis was confirmed. In three different ways, we were able to deplete KLH-primed T cells of the Con A SN-replaceable helper T

cells and still leave another type, which acted in an antigen specific fashion and which was not replaceable by Con A
SN.

We would like to suggest mechanisms for the way in
which these helper T cells cooperate and stimulate B cell
responses. To deal with the Ia$^+$, Con A SN-replaceable T
cell first, other experiments (not shown here) have suggested to us that this cell acts most efficiently by
recognizing antigen on B cell surfaces (7). This finding is
understandable if the nonspecific signal is to be delivered
at highest concentrations to the appropriate B cell. This T
cell also appears to act late in the B cell response, as
exemplified by the experiment shown in Figure 1, to stimulate differentiation and terminal division of B cells (10,
12).

The mode of action of the other, apparently Ia$^-$, type
of T cell is less easy to dissect, as we have been unable to
isolate a soluble product from this cell. If T cells were
incubated with antigen and MØ and then removed, the MØ could
subsequently communicate a T cell-derived, antigen specific
signal to B cells (Table III). This signal may therefore be
analogous to the antigen specific factors described by
Feldman and others (13), which are suggested to act by
displaying antigen on MØ surfaces to B cells. Since the Ia$^-$
T cell is apparently required early in the response and
interacts with MØ, but not with B cells (Figure 1, Table II,
and 7), it is tempting to suggest that it is involved in
initiating B cell responses by arranging antigen suitably on
MØ surfaces.

ACKNOWLEDGEMENTS

We thank Lee Harwell and Jan Moynihan for their excellent technical assistance. We thank the Animal Tumor
Research Facility and the Biostatistics Facility of the
University of Rochester Cancer Center for their help in
supplying tumor cells for anti-T cell serum absorption, and
in developing computer programs for statistical handling of
our data, respectively.

REFERENCES

1. Marrack (Hunter), P. and Kappler, J. W. (1975). J.
    Immunol. 114, 1116.
2. Harwell, L., Kappler, J. W., and Marrack, P. (1976). J.
    Immunol. 116, 1379.

3. Janeway, C. A., Jr. (1975). J. Immunol. 114, 1394.
4. Woodland, R. and Cantor, H. (1978). Eur. J. Immunol. 8, 600.
5. Tada, T., Takemori, T., Okumura, K., Nonaka, M., and Takuhisa, T. (1978). J. Exp. Med. 147, 446.
6. Kappler, J. W. and Marrack, P. (1977). J. Exp. Med. 146, 1748.
7. Marrack, P., Harwell, L., Kappler, J. W., Kawahara, D., Keller, D., and Swierkosz, J. (1979). In "Recent Developments in Immunological Tolerance and Macrophage Function" (P. Baram, C. W. Pierce and J. R. Battisto, eds.). Elsevier North-Holland, in press.
8. Hayes, C. E. and Bach, F. H. (1978). J. Exp. Med. 148, 692.
9. Marrack, P. and Kappler, J. W. (1978). J. Exp. Med. 147, 1596.
10. Hunig, T., Schimpl, A., and Wecker, E. (1974). J. Exp. Med. 139, 754.
11. Hunig, T., Schimpl, A., and Wecker, E. (1977). J. Exp. Med. 145, 1228.
12. Waldmann, H., Poulton, P., and Desaymard, C. (1976). Immunology 30, 723.
13. Feldmann, M. and Basten, A. (1972). J. Exp. Med. 136, 49.

HELPER T CELLS EXPRESSING AN *I-J* SUBREGION GENE PRODUCT

Ko Okumura, Makoto Nonaka, Kyoko Hayakawa, and Tomio Tada

Department of Immunology, Faculty of Medicine, University of Tokyo, Tokyo, Japan

ABSTRACT   The locus in the *I-J* subregion coding for a serological marker on nylon wool-adherent helper T cells (Th$_2$) was shown to be distinct from the locus which controls Ia determinants selectively expressed on Lyt-2$^+$, 3$^+$ suppressor T cells. The Ia$^+$ helper T cell (Th$_2$) showed a number of characteristics that distinguish it from the conventional Ia$^-$ helper T cell (Th$_1$). Th$_2$ was extremely sensitive to the ionizing radiation or the treatment with mitomycin C in contrast to the relative resistance of Th$_1$ against these treatment. Th$_2$ did not cooperate efficiently with B cells having low Ia antigen, while Th$_1$ stimulated B cells that were resistant to anti-Ia treatment. The effect of Th$_2$ was directly suppressible by carrier-specific suppressive T cell factor, whereas effect of Th$_1$ was not. These results indicate that the mode of help given by Ia$^+$ and Ia$^-$ helper T cells is different.

INTRODUCTION

Biologic roles and serological specificities of Ia antigens on B cells and macrophages have been widely investigated, while much less is known about T cell Ia antigens. This is largely due to the difficulty to detect T cell Ia antigens by conventional serological assays. It is, however, becomming clear that some functional subsets of T cells express Ia antigens on their cell surface, and that these molecules are playing substantial role in a variety of regulatory cell interactions.

We have recently reported that there are two types of carrier-specific Lyt-1$^+$ helper T cells which are separable by a passage through a nylon wool column (1). One type of helper T cell, which we designate Th$_1$, is not adherent to the nylon wool, possesses no Ia antigens, and can help the response of hapten-primed B cells only if the haptenic and carrier determinants are presented on a single molecule. The second type of helper T cells, Th$_2$, tend to adhere to the nylon wool, express Ia$^+$ antigen which is coded for by a gene mapped in *I-J* subregion, and can help the B cell response to a hapten coupled to a heterologous carrier upon stimulation with unconjugated relevant carrier. This communication describes some other characteristics of Th$_2$ which distinguishes it from conventional Th$_1$.

A SEPARATE LOCUS IN *I-J* SUBREGION CONTROLLING Ia ANTIGEN ON TH2

It has been established in a previous experiment that the Ia locus controlling determinants on Th$_2$ maps in *I-J* subregion (1). A question was asked as to whether or not the locus for Th$_2$ is identical to the previously described locus controlling determinants selectively expressed on suppressor T cells. To answer this, an anti-*I-J*^{k} antiserum (B10.A(3R) anti-B10.A(5R)), which had an activity to eliminate both KLH (keyhole limpet hemocyanin)-specific helper (Th$_2$) and suppressor T cells (Ts), was absorbed with Lyt-2$^+$,3$^+$ cells that had been obtained by treating the semipurified suppressor T cells with anti-Lyt-1$^+$ and C. The absorbed antiserum was tested for their residual activity to kill nylon wool adherent Th$_2$ cells. On the other hand, an aliquot of the same antiserum was preabsorbed with Lyt-1$^+$ cells, and was assayed for its ability to kill Ts and Th$_2$. Essential results are summarized in Table I. It was shown that after absorption with Lyt-2$^+$,3$^+$ cells, the antiserum was still capable of eliminating Th$_2$ activity from nylon wool adherent T cell population, while the ability to kill Ts was completely removed. After absorption with Lyt-1$^+$ cells,

TABLE   I

HETEROGENEITY OF *I-J* SUBREGION PRODUCTS EXPRESSED ON FUNCTIONALLY DIFFERENT SUBSETS OF T CELLS

Functional subsets tested	Anti-*I-J* used for treatment		
	Unabsorbed	absorbed with	
		Lyt-1$^+$ cell	Lyt-2$^+$,3$^+$ cell
Ts (Lyt-2$^+$,3$^+$)	Lost	Remained	Lost
Th$_2$ (Lyt-1$^+$)	Lost	Lost	Remained

the antiserum as unable to eliminate Th_2 but effectively killed Ts. These results indicate that the determinants expressed
on suppressor and helper T cells are different, and thereby
suggest that *I-J* subregion contains two distinct loci controlling cell surface molecules on functionally different subsets
of T cells.

DIFFERENCES BETWEEN Ia^+ TH (TH_2) AND Ia^- TH (TH_2)

It has already been reported that both Th_1 and Th_2 can
cooperate with B cell independent, while the addition of a
small number of Th_2 to the mixture of Th_1 and B cells significantly augmented the net response to the hapten carrier conjugate (DNP-KLH) (1). In this study, some cellular as well as
immunological characterization of Th_2 and Th_1 was performed
utilizing a coculture system of carrier primed Th_1 or Th_2 and
hapten (2,4-dinitrophenyl, DNP)-primed B cells in the Marbrook
culture system. KLH-primed Th_2 and Th_1 cells were obtained by
fractionation on a nylon wool column. To examine their radiation sensitivity, both Th_1 and Th_2 were exposed to different
doses of ionizing X-irradiation *in vitro*. After washing,
their helper activity was tested by coculturing with DNP-
primed B cells. As shown in Table II, helper activity of Th_2,
was eliminated by 200R of X-irradiation at a condition with
saturating dose of T cells (5×10^6). A slight enhancing

TABLE II

EFFECT OF X-IRRADIATION ON THE ACTIVITY OF TH_1 AND TH_2

Cells ($\times 10^6$)	Dose of radiation (R)	Anti-DNP IgG PFC/culture
B + Th_1	0	$1{,}430 \pm 145$
(5) (3)	400	$1{,}640 \pm 241$
	600	$1{,}456 \pm 314$
	800	$1{,}230 \pm 131$
B + Th_2	0	$1{,}786 \pm 245$
(5) (5)	100	$2{,}745 \pm 346$
	200	478 ± 78
	400	216 ± 110
B only		<50

effect was usually observed when Th2 received low dose (100R) of X-irradiation suggesting that the suppressor T cell in the nylon wool adherent population was eliminated at this dose. In contrast, even 800R of X-irradiation did not affect the helper activity of Th1.

To determine whether or not the proliferation of Th1 and Th2 is required in the help of B cell differentiation, both types of T cells were treated with 10 μg/ml of mitomycin C (MMC) in *in vitro*. After exhaustive washing, they were tested for the activity to cooperate with B cells. As shown in Table III, helper activity of Th2 was completely abrogated by the treatment with a low concentration of MMC whereas that of Th1 was unaffected. Since the major parts of helper activity in Th2 population was eliminated by anti-*I-J* and C, it is concluded that *I-J*+ helper T cell is MMC-sensitive. The results strongly suggest that cell proliferation was required for the helper activity of Th2 but not Th1.

These results collectively indicate that some of the helper T cells are radiation and MMC-sensitive, and that previously known radiation resistant helper effect (2) only represents the activity of Th1 but not Th2. This also warns us that a major conflict concerning the genetic restrictions between helper T and B cells should carefully be revisited by using two distinct helper T cells.

TABLE   III

EFFECT OF MITOMYCIN C OR ANTI-*I-J* TREATMENT ON
THE ACTIVITY OF TH1 AND TH2 CELLS

	Treatment	Anti-DNP IgG PFC/culture
B + Th1	——	1,716 ± 114
	MMC	1,279 ± 156
	C only	1,662 ± 343
	Anti-*I-J* + C	1,662 ± 254
B + Th2	——	1,725 ± 263
	MMC	85 ± 71
	C only	1,321 ± 251
	Anti-*I-J* + C	384 ± 126

In order to learn which type of helper activity is suppressed by the antigen-specific suppressor T cell factor (TsF), various doses of TsF were added in the reaction mixture of B cells and Th_1 or Th_2. As already reported, in order for the effective function of TsF, the presence of nylon wool adherent T cells (Lyt-1^+,2^+,3^+) is definitely required (3). Thus, small number (2 x 10^6) of nylon wool adherent spleen cells were added to the mixture of Th_1 and B cells. No such addition was required for testing the Th_2 activity. Results shown in Table IV indicate that a low concentration of TsF, i.e., the dose obtained from 2 x 10^6 of Ts cells, could effectively suppress the Th_2 help, while more than two fold of TsF were needed to suppress the response mounted by Th_1 and B cells even in the presence of an optimal number of nylon wool adherent T cells. We have recently shown that TsF directly suppress Th_2 in the absence of Lyt-1^+,2^+,3^+ T cells (data not shown). Thus, it is conceivable that there are two different pathways of TsF mediated suppression; a direct suppression of Th_2, and indirect (long term) suppression utilizing the intermediary of Lyt-1^+,2^+,3^+ cells to suppress Th_1 help.

TABLE IV

EFFECT OF TsF (SUPPRESSOR T CELL FACTOR) ON THE TH_1 AND TH_2 HELPER ACTIVITY

Corresponding cell number (x10^6) TsF obtained	Cells	Anti-DNP IgG PFC/culture
0	Th_1 + B	2,240 ± 238
10	Th_1 + B	2,141 ± 345
10	Th_1 + B + Ad*	762 ± 342
5	Th_1 + B + Ad*	1,634 ± 435
0	Th_2 + B	2,473 ± 86
10	Th_2 + B	141 ± 89
5	Th_2 + B	680 ± 114

* 2 x 10^6 of nylon wool adherent cells (intermediary cells) were added.

TH$_1$ BUT NOT TH$_2$ CAN HELP B CELLS WITH LOW
Ia ANTIGEN

It has been known that the density of Ia antigens on
antibody-forming cell precursors (B cells) is different among
B cell subpopulations destined to make different classes of
antibodies (4). Thus, we examined the effect of negative
selection with anti-Ia serum and C on the subsequent cooperative response with Th$_1$ and Th$_2$ cells.

T cell depleted DNP-primed B cells were treated at two
different dilutions of anti-Ia and C. They were then cocul-
tured with appropriate number of Th$_1$ and Th$_2$, respectively.
Total cell number in the culture, which affect the net response of primed B cells, was adjusted by the addition of T
cell depleted B cells from unprimed mouse. When B cells from
C3H ($H-2^k$) were treated with 1:10 dilution of A.TH anti-A.TL
(anti-Ia^k) and C, about 85% of B cells were eliminated. The
residual B cells could not mount antibody response in the
presence of either Th$_1$ or Th$_2$ to antigen (DNP-KLH). However,
when B cells were treated with 1:50 dilution of anti-Ia^k
which eliminated about 50% of B cells, remaining B cells were
able to mount substantial antibody response in cooperation
with Th$_1$ but not with Th$_2$. It was confirmed by the FACS
(fluorescence activated cell sorter) analysis that residiual
B cells after this partial killing were only dully stained by
anti-Ia antiserum. These results indicate that there are
different subpopulations of antibody forming precursor cells
whose requirement of helper T cells is different.

TABLE   V

TH$_1$ BUT NOT TH$_2$ CAN HELP B CELLS WITH LOW
Ia ANTIGEN DENSITY

DNP-primed B cells	% B cells killed	Helper T cell	Anti-DNP IgG PFC/culture
None	0	Th$_1$	1,635 ± 355
		Th$_2$	1,047 ± 119
Anti-Ia(1:50)	50	Th$_1$	1,184 ± 236
		Th$_2$	52 ± 21
Anti-Ia(1:10)	85	Th$_1$	58 ± 21
		Th$_2$	29 ± 0

ACKNOWLEDGEMENT

We wish to thank Ms. Yoko Yamaguchi for her excellent secretarial help.

REFERENCES

1. Tada, T., Takemori, T., Okumura, K., Nonaka, M., and Tokuhisa, T. (1978). J. Exp. Med. 147, 446.
2. Katz, D.H., and Benacerraf, B. (1976). In " The Role of Products of the Histocompatibility Gene Complex in Immune Response" (D.H. Katz and B. Benacerraf, eds.), p. 355. Adacemic Press, New York.
3. Tada, T. (1977). In "Immume System: Genetics and Regulation: (E. Sercarz, L.A. Herzenberg and C.F. Fox, eds.), p. 345. Academic Press, New York.
4. McDevitt, H.O., Delovitch, T.L., Press, J.L., and Murphy, D.B. (1976). Transplant. Rev. 30, 197.

PURIFICATION AND B-CELL TRIGGERING PROPERTIES OF ANTIGEN SPECIFIC T-CELL DERIVED HELPER FACTORS

C. Shiozawa, S. Sonik, B. Singh and E. Diener

Department of Immunology and MRC Group on Immunoregulation, University of Alberta, Edmonton, Alberta, Canada.

ABSTRACT In previous work soluble carrier specific helper factor (Hf) extracted from carrier primed thymus derived (T) cells has been shown to specifically trigger unprimed B cells to produce anti-hapten antibodies *in vitro* in the presence of haptenated carrier. Such factor-B cell interaction was shown to be allogeneically restricted. In this communication we show that Hf to rabbit gamma globulin (RGG) contains IA determinants. Furthermore, Hf activity has been shown not only for monomeric serum protein carriers but also for histocompatibility antigens of the chicken. Purification of Hf on Sephadex G-100 revealed three fractions, each containing carrier specific as well as nonspecific activity to various degrees and having different isoelectric points. Most of the specific Hf activity was contained in two of these three fractions. DEAE-cellulose ion exchange chromatography in a phosphate buffer gradient resolved 5 fractions, two of which contained specific activity. Stability of Hf was shown to depend on the presence of Ca^{++}.

INTRODUCTION

Cell interaction mechanisms have long been accepted as the fundamental basis of immune function; the discovery of various cell classes and their subpopulations has given impetus to the conceptualization of regulatory networks. In spite of the considerable knowledge on interaction kinetics within a network of helper, suppressor and effector cell precursors, the mechanisms of such interaction at the subcellular level are largely unknown. Theories on mechanisms of T-B cell cooperation have evolved from early views on interaction by means of antigen bridges (1) to a more recent concept where soluble T cell-derived helper factor is focused onto the antigen-binding B cell by virtue of its specificity for carrier antigenic determinants (2). On the assumption that a T cell-derived secretory product represents the physiologically legitimate mediator of

specific T cell help, we have developed an experimental model
that allows the *in vitro* assessment of carrier-specific
helper factor extracted from carrier-primed T cells for the
triggering of unprimed B cells. In an earlier report on the
subject we demonstrated that this factor interacts with
immunocompetent B cells, provided both cooperating elements
are syngeneic (3). In this communication, we shall discuss
parameters bearing on the biochemical and serological
properties of a carrier-specific T cell-derived helper
factor.

MATERIALS AND METHODS

Animals. CBA/J (H-2^k), CBA/CaJ (H-2^k) and C3H/HeJ (H-2^k)
male mice bred and maintained at Ellerslie Animal Farm,
University of Alberta, were used.

Antigens. Rabbit gamma globulin (RGG) and chicken red
blood cells (CRBC) were used for the induction of helper
factor. Antigens tested *in vitro* consisted of trinitrophenylated RGG (TNP-RGG) or CRBC. Procedures of
haptenation are described elsewhere (3).

Preparation of Crude T-Cell Derived Factor. T cell-
derived helper factor was obtained as previously described
(3), with the modification that carrier-primed T cells were
suspended in Ca^{++} and Mg^{++}-free phosphate buffered saline
supplemented with 10^{-4}M EDTA. Cells were homogenized in ice-
cold, 0.05M phosphate buffer (P.B.) at pH 7.4 at a
concentration of 0.5 to 1 x 10^8 cells per ml. Homogenization
was with a glass Teflon homogenizer for 20 min. at a speed
of 80 RPM. Thereafter, the homogenate was spun at 35,000
x g for 30 min. and the supernatant used for further
purification.

Purification of T Cell-Derived Factor. The crude
extract was purified by Sephadex G-100 (1.5 x 85 cm column)
chromatography in saline or by DEAE-cellulose in 0.05 M P.B.
Elution from DEAE-cellulose was by a linear gradient of P.B.
at a concentration range of 0.05 to 0.5 M (pH 7.4). Another
means of purification was antigen affinity chromatography
using RGG coupled to Sepharose 4B beeds. Pooled fractions
were concentrated by ultrafiltration, dialyzed against saline
and passed through Millipore filter (0.45µ Millex, Millipore
Co., Bedford, Mass.). The filtrate was diluted with sterile
saline to the specified concentration. Factor concentration
was expressed in cell equivalents/culture i.e. number of
cells from which factor was extracted.

Tissue Culture. Normal or anti-Thy-1 and C' treated spleen cells were cultured at a concentration of 10^6 cells/ 0.2 ml of Click's medium in Linbro Micro Culture plates. Mercaptoethanol at a final concentration of $5 \times 10^{-5}M$ was added to all cultures (4). For some experiments, calcium-free medium supplemented with $10^{-6}M$ D-Ca-pantothenate was used. Immune responses were expressed as antibody forming cells (AFC) per culture.

Isoelectric Focusing. After separation on Sephadex G-100, helper factor was further fractionated by isoelectric focusing (column model LKB 8100, Ampholine, Type 110 ml) according to the method of Haglund (5). The pH range was set between 2 and 8.

Antisera. Hybridoma anti-IA^k antiserum was a gift from Dr. G.J. Hämmerling (Institut Für Genetik Univ. Köln). DEAE purified rabbit anti mouse IgG was purchased from Cappel Lab. Inc. Cochranville, Pa. Anti H-2^d antiserum was a gift from Dr. T. Wegmann in our department.

RESULTS

1. The Triggering of B Cells In Vitro Against Histocompatibility Antigens of Chicken Erythrocytes by Antigen-Specific T Cell-Derived Helper Factor.

It has recently been found by colleagues in this department that mouse spleen cells are capable of generating specific humoral antibodies against allelically determined antigens of the major histocompatibility locus of the chicken (6). We have exploited this finding to initiate helper factor-dependent triggering of unprimed B cells (anti-Thy-1 and C' treated spleen cells) in vitro to the products of either the B2 or the B13 allele present on chicken red blood cells (CRBC). It was found that helper factor induced by B2/B2 CRBCs is effective in helping an immune response in the presence of B2/B2 but not B13/B13 CRBCs in culture. The degree of specificity of these responses compared favorably with that of in vitro responses to CRBCs by normal spleen cells (Table I).

Helper factor induced by B2/B2 CRBCs was successfully absorbed by B2/B2 but not by B13/B13 CRBCs. Experiments were also designed to test for the presence of mouse histo-compatibility antigens on helper factor. It was found that the biological activity of helper factor derived from CBA/J (H-2^k) T cells could effectively be removed by anti-IA^k but not by anti-H-2^d antibodies. No Ig determinants on helper factor could be recognized by means of anti-IgG antibodies (Table I).

TABLE I

Hf MEDIATED RESPONSE TO B^2/B^2 AND B^{13}/B^{13} CHICKEN ERYTHROCYTES (CRBC)

Antigen Specific Hf Replaces Specific T Cells

CRBC in Culture	CRBC in Assay	AFC/Culture (± SEM)				
		Hf to B^2/B^2 ($x10^{-6}$ cell eq/culture)				
		0	0.1	0.2	1	2
B^2/B^2	B^2/B^2	8 ± 6	268 ± 30	476 ± 11	469 ± 39	400 ± 53
B^{13}/B^{13}	B^{13}/B^{13}	8 ± 11	32 ± 23	8 ± 20	32 ± 18	48 ± 2

Control Immune Response of Normal Spleen Cells to CRBC

Antigen in Culture	AFC/Culture (± SEM)	
	Assayed on B^2/B^2	Assayed on B^{13}/B^{13}
not added	44 ± 4	48 ± 6
B^2/B^2	360 ± 23	88 ± 27
B^{13}/B^{13}	48 ± 4	168 ± 46

Hf is Absorbed by B^2/B^2 CRBC and Anti-IA^k but not by Anti-H-2^d or Anti-IgG Antiserum

Hf Absorbed by	AFC/Culture (± SEM)
Sepharose 4B	248 ± 20
CRBC B^2/B^2	60 ± 23
CRBC B^{13}/B^{13}	244 ± 30
Anti-IA^k-Sepharose 4B	12 ± 18
Anti-H-2^d-Sepharose 4B	156 ± 32
Anti-IgG-Sepharose 4B	260 ± 25

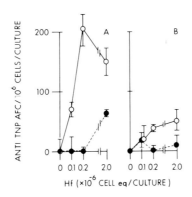

FIGURE 1. Effect of preincubating spleen cells with antigen on a Hf-mediated immune response *in vitro*. (A), CBA/CaJ spleen cells were preincubated with (0) or without (●) TNP-RGG for 30 min. at 37°, washed and cultured in the presence of Hf. In another group (B), CBA/CaJ spleen cells were cultured with (0) or without (●) TNP-RGG and Hf. Hf to RGG was prepared in CBA/CaJ mice.

2. Experimental Conditions for Helper Factor B Cell Interaction with a Soluble Antigen *In Vitro*.
    Some time ago we showed that helper factor isolated from RGG, HGG or BSA primed T cells can effectively and specifically induce unprimed B cells to generate a hapten-specific response *in vitro* in the presence of TNP-RGG, TNP-HGG, or TNP-BSA respectively (3). A systematic analysis of helper factor-B cell interaction would be greatly facilitated if it were possible to have the recognition step of antigen by the B cell separated from the events of factor-mediated help. This indeed proved feasible in experiments where spleen cells were first preincubated with TNP-RGG for 30 minutes at 37°, washed free of antigen and cultured for three days in the presence of RGG specific helper factor from RGG-primed T cells (Figure 1). Preliminary experiments suggest that the factor-B cell interaction also occurs in the absence of adherent cells. When dealing with soluble antigen as in the case of the experiments described below, the preincubation of spleen cells with antigen prior to the addition of helper factor has routinely been the practise.

3. Physicochemical Characterization of Helper Factor.
    Purification of crude helper factor from RGG-primed T cells on a Sephadex G-100 column revealed three peaks designated A, B, C which contained biological activity(Fig.2a).

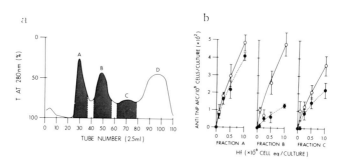

FIGURE 2 a)   Fractionation of Hf induced with RGG in CBA/CaJ mice by Sephadex G-100 chromatography. Factor activity was Found in A, B and C.   b)   Helper activity of fractions A, B and C in cultures of TNP-RGG preincubated (O) and normal spleen cells (●).

However, carrier-specific helper factor was restricted to fractions B and C while the stimulatory activity of fraction A was mainly nonspecific (Figure 2b). As determined by isoelectric focusing, the specific component in fraction A

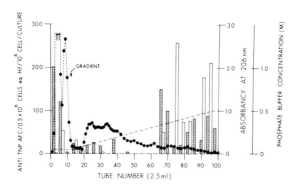

FIGURE 3. Fractionation of Hf induced with RGG by DEAE-cellulose chromatography. Elution by phosphate buffer gradient (0.05 M to 0.5 M) (−·−•−). Absorbance at 206 nm (●). Eluates were concentrated and tested for helper activity *in vitro.* ☐ Hf + TNP-RGG. ■ Hf without antigen.

had an isoelectric point (Ip) of 4.0 while the Ip of the specifically active component in fractions B and C were 4.6 and 2.5 respectively. All nonspecific components in fractions A, B and C were focused within a pH range of 5.5 to 7. Purification of helper factor by DEAE-cellulose chromatography with a phosphate buffer gradient also yielded separate antigen-specific and nonspecific factor activities. Most of the nonspecific factor passed through the column while the specific factor eluted in 0.3 to 0.4 M P.B. (Figure 3).

4. Purification of Helper Factor by Affinity Chromatography.

We have shown earlier that helper factor would only cooperate with B cells *in vitro* in the presence of the carrier to which it was induced (3). Carrier specificity of helper factor activity was reconfirmed by antigen affinity chromatography. Crude factor in saline was applied at room temperature to a saline equilibrated column containing RGG coupled to Sepharose and run at a flow rate of 10 ml per hour. After extensive washing with saline, bound helper factor eluted with 2 M NaCl at pH 6.5 or with 0.15 M Soerensen buffer at pH 2.5 was specifically active *in vitro* (Figure 4a, 4b). Unbound material contained nonspecific helper activity. It must be pointed out that, in contrast to elution by NaCl, acid elution of bound material was less complete and led to some loss of specific factor activity.

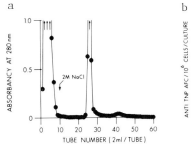 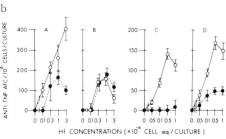

FIGURE 4 a) Purification of Hf to RGG by antigen affinity chromatography. Bound factor was eluted by 2M NaCl. b) Hf activity after purification by antigen affinity chromatography. Cultures of TNP–RGG preincubated (0) or normal spleen cells (●) in presence of (A) bound factor eluted with 2M NaCl (pH 6.5), or (B) unbound factor or (C) bound factor eluted with 0.15M Sorensen buffer (pH 2.4) or (D) bound factor eluted with 0.15M Sorensen buffer containing 0.1% BSA.

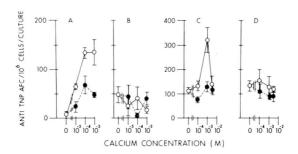

FIGURE 5. Effect of Ca^{++} on activity of helper factor.
RGG Affinity column purified Hf prepared in CBA/CaJ or C3H/
HeJ mice was pretreated with different concentrations of CaCl$_2$
and added syngeneically to cultures of TNP-RGG treated C3H/HeJ
(A) or CBA/CaJ (C) spleen cells (O). In the control group,
Hf that had not been pretreated with Ca^{++} was added to TNP-RGG
treated C3H/HeJ (A) or CBA/CaJ (C) spleen cells (●). Preincubation of Hf was with CaCl$_2$ concentrations that were 20x
the concentrations of the culture medium. Final concentration
of CaCl$_2$ present in all cultures are indicated on abscissa.
Results in Figure B and D derived from experiments identical
to those above except that an unrelated antigen TNP-OA was
used, indicating specificity of Hf for RGG.

5. Stability of Helper Factor Depends on the Presence
of Ca^{++}.

Ca^{++} is known to represent an important element in the
regulation of various cell activities and is often associated
with structural proteins of excitable membranes. We have
been able to demonstrate a dependency on Ca^{++} of helper factor
with respect to its stability and possibly its interaction
with the B cell surface membrane (Figure 5). Antigen affinity
column purified helper factor specific for RGG was reacted
for thirty minutes with various concentrations of CaCl$_2$ in
saline at room temperature before it was added to spleen cells
that had previously been incubated with TNP-RGG in Ca-free
medium for thirty minutes at 37°C and washed free of antigen.
Control cultures contained CaCl$_2$ at concentrations equivalent
to those of the experimental groups. Helper factor added to
these cultures however, had not previously been exposed to
Ca^{++}. Optimal numbers of hapten specific AFCs were generated
by those cultures that contained helper factor pre-exposed to
Ca^{++}. This effect was shown to depend on the concentration
of CaCl$_2$ used for factor pretreatment (Figure 5).

DISCUSSION

This report represents a significant improvement of a previously published experimental model for T cell-derived helper factor-B cell interaction. In the past it was necessary to utilize multi-determinant serum protein carriers conjugated to a carbohydrate backbone to achieve optimal helper factor mediated immune induction *in vitro* (3). Under the experimental conditions reported here, it has been possible instead to generate such factor-dependent responses by unprimed B cells when using the carrier protein in monomeric form. Furthermore, we have extended our antigen repertoire from soluble antigens to cell bound antigens such as histocompatibility antigens on chicken erythrocytes. As was the case for soluble antigens, *in vitro* responses to CRBC are also triggered by an antigen-specific helper factor as shown by factor absorption studies. We have also reported earlier that helper factor-B cell interaction in the presence of a multivalent carrier is allogeneically restricted (3). This finding has been extended to the use of monomeric carriers (data not shown). The demonstration of factor-associated Ia antigens is compatible with the speculation that the presence of MHC products on our helper factor may be related to its allogeneically restricted function. It must be pointed out in this context that others have described an antigen-specific helper factor that is not allogeneically restricted but also bears Ia antigenic determinants (7). In view of the increasing evidence for the existence of T-helper cell sub-populations, it is conceivable that such functional differences may reflect different T cell subclasses from which helper factor is derived. Purification of crude extracts from carrier-primed T cells by antigen affinity chromatography and column chromatography on Sephadex or DEAE-cellulose has shown the presence in such an extract of both antigen-specific as well as nonspecific helper factors. Our failure to find evidence for the presence of Ig determinants on a specific helper factor when using rabbit anti-mouse IgG is in agreement with similar experiences by other investigators (8). To clarify this point, experiments using anti-idiotype antibodies against constant region determinants in the combining site are in progress. In the past, the functional instability of T helper cell-derived products may have been the reason for the poor reproducibility of experimental data often obtained by various laboratories. The dependency of factor activity in our experiments on the presence of Ca^{++} may in part offer a solution to this problem. It is conceivable that helper

factor requires bound Ca^{++} to maintain conformational
stability. Whether it actually transports Ca^{++} to the B cell
as part of its triggering function is currently under
investigation.

REFERENCES

1. Mitchison, M.A., Rajewsky, K., and Taylor, R.B. (1970).
   In "Developmental Aspects of Antibody Formation and
   Structure". (J. Sterzl ed.), pp. 547-564. Publishing House
   of the Czechoslovakian Academy of Sciences, Prague.
2. Bretscher, P. (1972). Transplant. Rev. 11, 217.
3. Shiozawa, C., Singh, B., Rubinstein, S., and Diener, E.
   (1977). J. Immunol. *118*, 2199.
4. Click, R.E., Benck, L., and Alter, B.J. (1972).
   Cellular Immunology *3*, 264.
5. Haglund, H. (1971). *In* "Methods of Biochem. Analysis"
   (D. Glick ed.), pp. 1-104. Interscience Publishers,
   New York.
6. Longenecker, M.M., Mosmann, R.R., and Shiozawa, C.
   (1979). Immuno genetics. (manuscript submitted).
7. Taussig, M.J., Munro, A.J., Campbell, R., David, C. S.,
   and Staines, N.A. (1975). J. Exp. Med. *142*, 694.
8. Taussig, M.J. and Munro. A.J. (1978). Federation
   Proceedings *35*, 2061.

WORKSHOP SUMMARY: Mediators of Cell-Cell Interactions.

Hermann Wagner, Institute of Medical Microbiology, D-65 Mainz, Hochhaus am Augustusplatz, W.-Germany.

One of the advantages of this workshop session was the small number of attendants which in turn allowed a vivid discussion to take place. The central theme of the discussion related to soluble mediators which helped to trigger effector lymphocyte functions of either the B or T cell type. Attention was drawn on the mechanism of induction of the soluble mediator in question, as well as on its specific or non specific effects. If possible aspects of its biochemical nature were discussed.

When Dr. Kilburn (Vancouver, Canada) reported on a specific helper factor that enhances cytotoxic T cell responses to syngeneic P815 tumor cells, the target of its function became questioned. While Dr. Kilburn discussed the possibility that the factor (a complex of Ia-alloantigen and the putative T cell receptor) binds to the Ia-negative stimulator cell thereby enhancing its immunogenicity for antigen reactive prekiller T cells, others drew attention to the Munro-Taussig factor, the target cell of which appears to be the effector-lymphocyte to be triggered. It was also noted that the biological effect of the helper factor was inferior to that of the Concanavallin A (Con A) induced non specific T helper cell factor. In the latter case no antigen specificity nor H-2 restriction was observed.

Dr. Watson (Irvine, Calif.) discussed the possibility that the biological active moiety of T helper cell replacing factor (TRF) active in B cell responses, the Con A induced factor enhancing the mitogen responsiveness of thymocytes, and the T cell growth factor described by Smith and associates, and Wagner and Röllinghoff, might in fact

be identical. According to his experience all three biological
functions could not be separated by various purification schemes
applied. If so that active moiety would be composed of a single polypeptide chain of approximately 68-70 000 dalton.

Dr. Röllinghoff (Mainz, W.-Germany) alluded to the functional activity of a non specific T helper factor influencing both primary and
secondary T cell mediated cytotoxic allograft responses. Accordingly,
upon antigen specific (MLC) and non specific (Con A) activation of
Ly 1$^+$ T cells, a factor (50 000 - 60 000 dalton) is released in the
culture supernatant which triggers antigen primed Ly 23$^+$ T cells into
exponential growth. Surprisingly the proliferating cells exhibit cytolytic activity with specificity to alloantigens used for primary sensi-
tisation. When asked for the role of macrophages, it became clear
that both macrophages and Ly 1$^+$ T cells were required for the production of the T helper cell factor in question. However all available
evidence suggested that the factor is Ly 1$^+$ T cell derived. Both the
groups of Smith, Wagner and v. Boehmer have successfully used this
factor to clone cytotoxic T cell (CTL) in vitro. The lytic activity of
such in vitro propagated monoclonal CTL was found in some instances
to be extremely high (50% lysis at a ratio CTL to target of 0.02 to one).
Another point of interest was the antigen specificity pattern noted.
While most of the CTL clones exhibited a clear antigen specificity,
the lytic activity of some clones was unexpected. For example, Dr.
Wagner reported on one clone derived from a H-2^k anti H-2^d MLC.
This CTL clone lysed K^d targets, but also syngeneic cells. Third party
cells were not lysed. The question therefore was discussed whether
the lytic activity of this particular alloreactive clone towards syngeneic targets may represent H-2 restricted cytolysis specific for a yet

undefined "foreign antigen". If so H-2 restricted cytolysis versus alloreactive cytolysis would not be a function of different T cell subsets,
but rather a function of the target antigen recognised by a given CTL.

Several groups commented on the functional activity of the T helper
cell factor in primary CTL responses. The amplifying effect of the
factor in weakly antigenic system was agreed upon. The clearest data
were obtained using thymocytes as responder cells. Accordingly
peanut-agglutinin positive cortical thymocytes so far believed to be
immuno incompetent are able to mount strong CTL responses, provided
the T cell derived helper factor is added in vitro. The same finding
was reported in regard to H-2 restricted CTL responses to TNP and
sendai virus. Consequently it was argued that cortical thymocytes
contain sufficient numbers of CTL precursors, but lack T helper cells.
Moreover T helper cells were thought to act via secretion of T helper
factor, which in turn acted as second signal for CTL precursor cell
triggering. Dr. Wu (Toronto, Canada) reported on the human equivalent to the murine T helper cell factor. Basically his results were
compatible with those obtained in the murine system, except that of
the human glycoprotein appears to have 13 000 dalton, while the
murine equivalent appears to have 25 000 dalton.

Dr. Shiozawa (Edmonton, Canada) discussed his data on the biological
activity and purification characteristics of specific and non specific
T cell derived helper factors triggering B cell responses to monomeric
and polymeric antigens. Because in his system specific and non specific effects could be titrated influencing B cell responses to the same
antigens, this system was agreed upon to represent a very useful experimental model. In concluding, most of the attendants felt a need
of biochemical characterization of the various factors alluded to in
order to learn their shared biochemical and functional characteristics.

WHAT IS THE NATURE OF THE ANTIGENIC COMPLEX RECOGNIZED
BY T LYMPHOCYTES?

Ethan M. Shevach, Christina Chan, David W. Thomas[1] and
Loran Clement

Laboratory of Immunology, National Institute of Allergy
and Infectious Diseases, National Institutes of Health,
Bethesda, Maryland 20014

ABSTRACT: Macrophages modified by the trinitrophenyl
(TNP) hapten have been used to clarify the nature of
the antigenic determinant recognized by the antigen
specific guinea pig T lymphocyte. We have previously
demonstrated that the genetic restriction on the
interaction of the TNP-modified macrophage and primed
T lymphocyte was regulated by the Ia antigens of the
macrophage used for initial sensitization and that
following removal of alloreactive cells, T cells
could be sensitized to TNP-modified allogeneic
macrophages. In the present report, we will review
our recent studies which have been directed to a
further dissection of the immunogenic complex
recognized by the antigen-specific T cell. It was
relatively easy to define the role of macrophage Ia
antigens in the complex as the antigen specific
response to TNP-modified allogeneic macrophages was
eliminated by anti-Ia sera directed against the allogeneic stimulator macrophage, while anti-Ia sera
directed solely against the responder T cell produced
no inhibition of the proliferative response. Treatment of TNP-modified macrophages with anti-Ia serum
either immediately after or 24 hours after TNP modification resulted in a markedly deficient antigen-
presenting cell. As brief treatment of the TNP-
modified macrophage with anti-Ia serum did not inhibit
Ia antigen synthesis, it is possible that treatment
with anti-Ia serum resulted in removal of TNP determinants which had become associated with Ia antigens
on the macrophage surface. It has been somewhat more
difficult to clarify the contribution of antigenic
determinants to the immunogenic complex recognized by

[1]Present address: Department of Pathology, The Jewish
Hospital of St. Louis, St. Louis, Missouri, 63110

ISBN 0-12-069850-1

the T cell. A marked reduction in the stimulatory
capacity of freshly modified cells could be achieved
by brief treatment with anti-TNP serum, but the
stimulatory capacity of macrophages which had been TNP-
modified and then "aged" for 24 hours prior to addition
to primed T cells was unaffected by similar treatment.
This result initially suggested that macrophage
presentation of the TNP determinant is not simply a
surface display phenomenon and that the macrophage
must process membrane conjugated TNP in a manner so
that it is inaccessible to anti-TNP antibody to create
the relevant immunogen recognized by T cells. Recently,
we have been able to demonstrate that anti-TNP antibody
can inhibit the proliferative response induced by
aged TNP-modified macrophages provided that they have
been freshly modified with the non-cross reactive
dinitrophenyl (DNP) hapten. Under these conditions
sufficient antigen is available to allow binding of
anti-TNP antibody and a highly specific inhibition of
the proliferative response is observed. This experiment suggests that antigenic determinants are displayed
on the macrophage surface, but under normal conditions
at too low a density to allow efficient binding of
anti-antigen antibody. In order to directly investigate
the relationship between the TNP moiety and macrophage
Ia antigens, macrophages were TNP-modified, radioiodinated, and lysed in detergent. When TNP-derivatized
proteins were isolated using an anti-TNP immunoabsorbent
and the presence of TNP-derivatized antigens in the
eluted proteins determined by immunoprecipitation
techniques, no hapten modified Ia antigens were detected.
Furthermore, when Ia antigens from TNP-modified cells
were eluted from an anti-Ia immunoabsorbent, no
protein other than Ia antigens was detectable. Thus,
although the functional studies with anti-Ia serum are
strongly in favor of the model that TNP-conjugated
membrane proteins are complexed with Ia antigens on the
surface of the macrophage, we have not been able to
prove the existence of this complex by the biochemical
techniques employed. Nevertheless, a complex maintained by the integrity of an intact cell membrane
might very well exist.

INTRODUCTION

Over the past six years several different models have
been proposed to explain the role of the major histocompatibility complex (MHC) in the genetic control of immunocompetent
cell interactions. Initially, we favored a "cellular
interaction structure" model (figure 1) which proposed that I-
region genes code for specific cellular interaction structures
and homology between these structures was necessary for
effective cellular interactions (1,2). A second model was
based on the observation that mouse T cells sensitized to
hapten or virus modified cells were primarily cytotoxic for
similarly modified target cells which were H-2D or H-2K
compatible (3,4). This model was termed the "complex antigenic
determinant" model and implied that T cells do not recognize
antigens per se, but can only be sensitized to antigen modified membrane components or to complexes of antigen combined
with certain membrane molecules. The failure of allogeneic
macrophage-associated antigen to activate immune T cells in
vitro was then secondary to the fact that the T cells had
been primed in vivo only to antigen associated with syngeneic
macrophages.

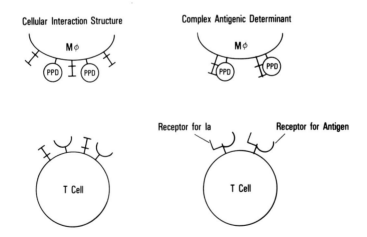

FIGURE 1. Models for Macrophage-T Cell Interaction.

The development of an assay in which guinea pig T lymphocytes could be readily primed in vitro to macrophages which
had been modified with the simple trinitrophenyl (TNP) hapten

allowed us to directly test the "complex antigenic determinant"
model. A large body of data in favor of the model was obtained from studies which demonstrated that the genetic restriction on the antigen specific T cell proliferative response
appeared to be regulated entirely by the histocompatibility
type of the macrophage used for initial sensitization (5).
Ia homology was not required for efficient T cell macrophage
interaction and T cells could be sensitized to antigen
associated with allogeneic macrophages (6). We therefore
suggested that the T cell recognizes a complex of nominal
antigen and Ia antigen which are expressed on the macrophage
surface by means of either a single receptor, specific for
determinants derived from both the nominal antigen and Ia
antigens, or two receptors, one directed against antigen and
another directed against Ia antigens. In order to apply this
model to our earlier experiments on the role of specific
immune response (Ir) genes in macrophage T cell interaction,
we proposed that the Ir gene product and the Ia antigen are
identical and that macrophages from a non-responder animal
would lack the Ia antigen which is capable of interacting
with the nominal antigen the response to which is controlled
by a specific Ir gene (8).

Although a large body of experimental evidence has been
presented which is in favor of a complex of nominal antigen
and Ia antigen on the surface of the antigen presenting cell,
little biochemical data is available to validate the existence
of such a complex. This report will review our recent
studies which have been directed at a further dissection of
the immunogenic complex recognized by the antigen-specific T
cell.

THE ROLE OF MACROPHAGE Ia ANTIGENS

Our early studies on the role of the MHC in T lymphocyte
activation demonstrated that anti-Ia sera were capable of
specifically inhibiting the in vitro proliferative response
of $(2x13)F_1$ T lymphocytes in a haplotype specific manner (9).
Although these studies were initially interpreted as demonstrating that the sera exerted their inhibitory effects by
interacting with determinants on the antigen responsive T
cell, it was impossible to precisely define the cellular
site of action of anti-Ia sera by using combinations of allogeneic macrophages and immune T cells because efficient interaction of antigen pulsed macrophages and immune T cells was
observed only when both types were syngeneic (1). Furthermore our initial attempts to demonstrate T cell sensitization

to antigen associated with allogeneic macrophages were unsuccessful because antigen-specific responses could not be detected in the presence of a mixed leukocyte reaction (MLR) (5). The development of a technique in which the MLR could be eliminated by bromodeoxyuridine (BUdR) and light treatment before priming the T cells with antigen associated with allogeneic macrophages allowed us to use anti-Ia sera directed against either the stimulator macrophage or responder T cell in order to determine against which cell type anti-Ia sera would exert their inhibitory effects (10). These studies clearly demonstrated that the antigen specific response to TNP-modified allogeneic macrophages was totally eliminated by anti-Ia sera directed against the stimulator macrophage, while anti-Ia sera directed solely against responder T cells had no effect on the proliferative response.

Although the results of these studies are strongly in favor of the concept that T cells recognize TNP determinants in association with macrophage Ia antigens, they offer no insight into the nature of this association. For example, it is possible that the TNP determinant is directly conjugated to Ia antigens to form the relevant immunogen recognized by T cells. Alternatively, the TNP may be conjugated to non-MHC membrane proteins with the simultaneous recognition by the T cell of both the TNP and Ia antigens by a dual mechanism. A third possibility is that the TNP is initially conjugated to any membrane protein with subsequent covalent or non-covalent association with Ia antigens to create the relevant antigen-MHC product complex recognized by the T cell.

If anti-Ia sera interact with non-haptenated Ia molecules and block macrophage-T cell interaction in a manner unrelated to antigen recognition, it might be expected that culturing TNP-modified macrophages with anti-Ia and removing the antiserum before adding the macrophages to the primed T cells would not result in any inhibition of the response (11). Surprisingly, TNP-modified macrophages cultured for 24 hours in the presence of anti-Ia serum (Table I) and washed before addition to TNP primed T cells were less efficient than cells cultured in normal guinea pig serum (NGPS) in stimulating a proliferative response. Furthermore, TNP-modified macrophages were sensitive to the effects of treatment with anti-Ia serum at all times following TNP-modification, as macrophages which were initially cultured for 24 hours in the presence of NGPS and then cultured for an additional 24 hours in anti-Ia serum prior to addition to primed T cells also were markedly inefficient in the induction of a TNP-specific response.

TABLE I

EFFECT OF CULTURING TNP-MODIFIED MACROPHAGES IN ANTI-Ia SERA
PRIOR TO ADDITION TO PRIMED T LYMPHOCYTES

	Time of Preculture		^{3}H-TdR ΔCPM
Exp. I	0-24 hr		
	NGPS		49,380
	Anti-Ia		13,090
Exp. II	0-24 hr	24-48 hr	
	NGPS	NGPS	33,550
	NGPS	Anti-Ia	12,190

It should be noted that this result differs from our
previous studies with macrophages that have been pulsed with
soluble protein antigens (1). Brief treatment of macrophages
after a pulse exposure to soluble protein antigens failed to
produce inhibition of T cell proliferation when the treated
macrophages were then washed and added to primed T cells in
the presence of NGPS. One explanation for the differences between the two experimental systems is that soluble protein
antigens are rapidly taken up by macrophages by a number of
pathways. Antigen that has been internalized may then be
available for processing to an immunologically relevant form
over a prolonged period of time. In contrast, when TNP is
covalently coupled to the cell surface, our studies have shown
that the majority of the TNP-conjugated proteins are probably
rapidly shed into the media and are not available for macrophage processing (12).

The results we have obtained on the effects of brief
treatment of TNP-modified macrophages with anti-Ia serum are
consistent with the model that the immunologically relevant
TNP determinants are exclusively coupled to macrophage Ia
antigens. Brief treatment with anti-Ia might lead to capping
and shedding of the TNP conjugated Ia antigens. However,
the results are also consistent with the model in which a
complex is formed between TNP-conjugated membrane antigens and
unmodified Ia antigens. Treatment with anti-Ia sera might
then lead to capping and shedding of the complex of TNP-modified membrane protein and Ia antigen. The selection of the
appropriate model for TNP-modified membrane antigens requires

a detailed biochemical analysis of the TNP-modified cell surface (see below).

THE ROLE OF ANTIGENIC DETERMINANTS

At first glance it might seem to be a somewhat rhetorical
question to ask what role antigenic determinants play in T cell
activation. The T cell must see either the entire antigen or
an immunogenic fragment in order to generate a specific immune
response. It is therefore paradoxical that while it has been
relatively easy to inhibit T cell activation with anti-Ia sera
and define the role of Ia antigens in T cell activation it has
been exceedingly difficult to inhibit T cell activation induced
by antigen pulsed macrophages with high titer antibody to
antigen. For example, Ellner et al. attempted to block primed
T lymphocyte DNA synthesis with high titer guinea pig antibody
to the 2,4-dinitrophenyl derivative of guinea pig albumin
(DNP-GPA). However, anti-DNP-GPA present continuously in the
culture did not affect the degree of proliferation induced by
DNP-GPA bearing macrophages (13). Similarly, Ben-Sasson et al.
demonstrated that antibodies to soluble protein antigens did
not inhibit the specific binding of immune lymphocytes to
antigen-pulsed macrophages even when the concentration of antibody in the incubation medium was high enough to precipitate
greater than 100 times the amount of antigen that remained
associated with the macrophage after washing (14).

TABLE II

WHY DOES ANTI-ANTIGEN ANTIBODY FAIL TO INHIBIT T CELL PROLIFERATION?

---

1. The immunologically relevant antigen is in a site inaccessible
   to antibody. (Intracellular?, Buried in the membrane?)

2. The T cell receptor recognizes an antigen-induced alteration
   of macrophage Ia and not native antigen.

3. The T cell receptor recognizes antigen fragments in
   association with macrophage Ia. The antigen fragments
   that stimulate T cells do not elicit antibody production.

A number of different explanations have been put forth in the literature to explain the failure of anti-antigen antibody to inhibit T cell activation and we have summarized them in Table II. Although each of these hypotheses could account for the observed experimental results, little solid experimental data is available to support any of them. The activation of T cell proliferation by macrophages modified by the TNP hapten seemed to us to be an ideal experimental system to re-evaluate the role of antigenic determinants in T cell activation. We assumed that the TNP determinant must be an integral part of the antigenic complex recognized by the T cell following sensitization to TNP-modified macrophages, hence the failure of anti-TNP antibody to block T cell activation could not be secondary to the fact that antibody to antigen and the T cell receptor for antigen recognize different portions of a complex antigen (Table II, point 3).

When high titer guinea pig anti-TNP sera were added to either priming cultures or secondary cultures we found substantial inhibition of the TNP-specific response (15). The inhibition was specific for the TNP determinant and not secondary to a non-specific interference with macrophage function by binding of antibody to the large number of TNP-conjugated membrane proteins, as macrophages which were simultaneously TNP-modified and pulsed with soluble protein antigens were still able to efficiently activate T cells primed to the soluble protein antigens in the present of anti-TNP serum.

Although these initial experiments suggested that anti-antigen antibody was capable of inhibiting antigen recognition by hapten primed T cells, further studies suggested more complex explanations. Ellner and Rosenthal had originally demonstrated that macrophages pulsed with soluble protein antigens retained their stimulatory capacity through several days óf in vitro culture (16). It was therefore of interest to determine if TNP-modified macrophages retained their ability to stimulate or if they rapidly lose immunogenicity as their conjugated membrane proteins are turned over. The stimulation produced by TNP-modified macrophages cultured for 24 hours prior to addition to primed T cells was 50-70% of that produced by aged unmodified macrophages that were TNP-treated immediately before addition to responder T cells. Surprisingly, anti-TNP antibody had no effect on the T cell proliferative response induced by overnight cultured TNP-modified macrophages. It thus appeared unlikely that the inhibition of the response to freshly modified cells is mediated by blocking T cell recognition of the relevant antigenic determinants. Further confirmation of this data was obtained in experiments where TNP modified macrophages were pretreated with anti-TNP

antibody prior to addition to primed T cells (Table III).
After a 24 hour preculture in anti-TNP serum, TNP-modified
macrophages were unable to stimulate an efficient T cell response. However, TNP-modified macrophages that had been cultured in NGPS for the first 24 hours and then cultured for a
second 24 hour period in anti-TNP serum were as efficient in
the activation of primed T cells as TNP-modified macrophages
that had been precultured for 48 hours in NGPS. The failure
of anti-TNP antibody to diminish the stimulatory capacity of
aged macrophages suggests that the TNP determinants are
accessible to anti-TNP antibody for a limited period of time
and do not spontaneously reappear on the macrophage surface in
a form accessible to antibody during a prolonged culture.
This result should be compared with the data shown in Table I
which demonstrated that treatment with anti-Ia sera at any
time following TNP-modification reduced the capacity of TNP-
modified macrophages to stimulate a TNP-specific response.

TABLE III

EFFECT OF PRETREATMENT OF TNP-MODIFIED MACROPHAGES
WITH ANTI-TNP SERUM

Time of Preculture		^{3}H-TdR ΔCPM
0-24 hr	24-48 hr	
NGPS		49,380
Anti-TNP		16,170
NGPS	NGPS	33,550
NGPS	Anti-TNP	37,440

We concluded from these experiments that macrophage
presentation of TNP is not simply a surface display phenomenon
and that macrophages must process membrane conjugated TNP in
a manner so that it is inaccessible to antibody to create the
relevant immunogen recognized by T cells. If the antigen
specific T cell sees a complex of TNP-modified membrane protein
and Ia antigen on the cell surface, one must postulate that the
TNP determinant must be in a covert location within this complex, hence the failure of anti-TNP antibody to block T cell
activation.

IMMUNOLOGICALLY RELEVANT ANTIGEN IS PRESENT ON THE
MACROPHAGE SURFACE

Although the studies described above favor the view that
the failure of anti-TNP antibody to block the proliferative
response induced by aged-TNP modified macrophages results from
sequestration of the relevant TNP determinants into an intra-
membranous or intracellular location, it should be pointed out
that we do not as yet fully understand the mechanism whereby
the stimulatory capacity of the freshly TNP-modified macrophage is reduced by culture in anti-TNP serum. One possibility is that anti-TNP leads to capping of TNP-conjugated membrane antigens with subsequent shedding into the media or internalization into an immunologically irrelevant intracellular
pool of antigen. Accordingly, less antigen would then be
available for macrophage processing and subsequent presentation to the T cell. If the process of inhibition of freshly
TNP-modified macrophages requires a sufficient concentration
of antibody bound to the cell surface to result in capping,
then perhaps the failure to block the aged TNP-modified macrophage is not secondary to the fact that the TNP is buried in
the membrane, but merely reflects too low a concentration of
cell surface TNP to allow binding of sufficient anti-TNP to
lead to capping and shedding of TNP-conjugated membrane proteins.

In order to evaluate this alternative explanation for our
results, we have compared the ability of macrophages modified
with different concentrations of trinitrobenzenesulfonic acid
(TNBS) to stimulate a TNP specific response and the susceptibility of that response to inhibition by anti-TNP antibody
(figure 2). Macrophages modified with 10mM TNBS, the concentration used in our earlier studies, stimulated the maximum
response which was denoted as 100% in figure 2. The response
to freshly modified 10mM TNBS treated macrophages was inhibited by about 70% when the cultures were performed in the presence of anti-TNP serum. Macrophages treated with 1.0mM TNBS
were slightly less effective as stimulators, but the resultant
proliferative response was as readily inhibited by anti-TNP
serum as that induced by 10mM TNBS modified macrophages.
Curiously, the response induced by macrophages which had been
freshly modified with 0.1mM TNBS modified cells was only 40-
50% of that induced by 10mM TNBS modified cells and was only
minimally inhibited by anti-TNP serum. Of great interest was
the observation that the percent maximal stimulation and percent inhibition of the response produced by 0.1mM TNBS modified
stimulators closely resembled the percent maximal stimulation
and percent inhibition produced when 10mM TNBS modified-aged
stimulator cells were used. This result is consistent with

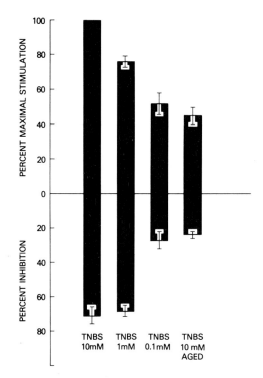

FIGURE 2. A comparison of the ability of macrophages modified with different concentrations of TNBS to induce a TNP specific response and the susceptibility of that response to inhibition by anti-TNP antibody.

the view that the failure to block the response of aged-TNP-modified stimulator cells is not the result of sequestration of the relevant TNP determinants, but merely reflects loss of TNP from the cell surface and a concomitant decrease in the amount of anti-TNP bound to the cell surface.

In order to test this hypothesis, we have developed an experimental model where a large concentration of anti-antigen antibody can be localized to the macrophage cell surface, but where only a limited number of antigenic determinants are presented to the hapten specific T cell. We have succeeded in priming T cells to macrophages modified by treatment with dinitrobenzenesulfonic acid under slightly alkaline conditions (pH 8.5) to generate DNP specific T cells and have also succeeded in priming T cells to macrophages which have been modified with the azobenzenearsonate hapten (ABA) using the methods described by Bach et al. (17). As can be seen in figure 3, the secondary T cell proliferative responses to these

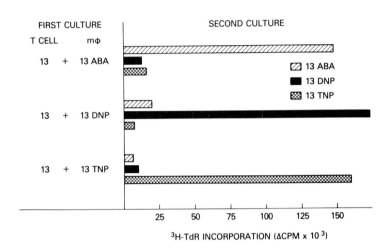

FIGURE 3. Hapten specific proliferation of guinea pig T
lymphocytes. Strain 13 T lymphocytes were primed with either
ABA, DNP, or TNP modified macrophages and then challenged in
the second culture with similarly modified cells. The resultant response is specific for the hapten used in the priming
culture.

three haptens coupled to macrophages were highly specific and
very little cross-reaction was seen. A similar situation has
been reported by Forman for the cytotoxic T cell which can
readily distinguish between DNP and TNP modified targets (18).
However, as antisera to the DNP and TNP haptens are highly
cross reactive, we now had the opportunity to study the effects
of anti-hapten antibody on macrophages which simultaneously
bore low concentrations of one hapten (aged) but high concentrations of the other (freshly modified).

The results of a typical experiment are shown in Table IV.
T cells from a non-immune guinea pig were primed by culture
in vitro for seven days with syngeneic macrophages which had
been freshly modified with 10mM TNBS. After the priming culture, the recovered cells were washed and restimulated with
different populations of macrophages as listed on the left
hand side of Table IV and then cultured for 3 days in the
presence of 5% NGPS or 5% anti-TNP serum. ^{3}H-TdR uptake was
determined during the last 18 hours of the culture. As previously noted, the response to freshly modified (10mM TNBS)
macrophages was markedly reduced by culture in anti-TNP serum,

while only minimal inhibition of the response to macrophages
which had been TNP-modified, but aged for 24 hours, was observed.   No response was seen to freshly DNP-modified macrophages.   Of great importance was the finding that the response
of TNP-modified-aged macrophages which were freshly modified
with DNP was markedly inhibited.   The same macrophage must
simultaneously bear both DNP and TNP determinants as no inhibition of the response to a mixture of TNP-Aged and DNP-Fresh
macrophages was seen.   It should also be noted that the response to macrophages which had been TNP-modified, aged, and then

TABLE IV

**INHIBITION OF TNP-SPECIFIC T CELL PROLIFERATION BY
ANTI-TNP ANTIBODY**

Macrophage Treatment	Serum	
	NGPS	Anti-TNP
0	1,125 ± 133	2,763 ± 124
TNP-Fresh	197,022 ± 11,013	74,660 ± 3,420
DNP-Fresh	1,629 ± 212	1,912 ± 565
TNP-Aged	75,266 ± 3,367	65,776 ± 5,179
TNP-Aged/DNP-Fresh	66,273 ± 1,515	16,607 ± 569
TNP-Aged/TNP-Fresh	215,645 ± 10,522	26,746 ± 1,646
TNP-Aged + DNP-Fresh	111,164 ± 5,637	99,576 ± 926

retreated with TNBS prior to addition to culture was also
markedly inhibited.   This result is again consistent with our
hypothesis that under the conditions where sufficient antibody
can bind to antigen on the macrophage surface, anti-antigen
will inhibit the T cell proliferative response.   In a large
series of experiments of similar design, the response to TNP-
modified-aged macrophages was inhibited by 22 ± 5%, while the
response to TNP-Aged/DNP-Fresh macrophages was inhibited by
78 ± 5%.   Similar results were seen when DNP primed T cells
were restimulated by DNP-modified macrophages.   Thus, the
response to DNP-modified aged macrophages was inhibited by
culture in anti-TNP sera only by 5 ± 3%, while the response
to DNP-Aged/TNP-Fresh stimulator cells was inhibited by
87 ± 7%.

Although these results are strongly suggestive that the binding of sufficient anti-antigen antibody to the cell surface leads to inhibition of the T cell proliferative response by blockade of the relevant antigenic determinants, it is critical to establish the specificity of this inhibition. For example, one might argue that TNP-modification of the aged-DNP-modified macrophage leads to derivatization of Ia antigens and the resultant inhibition of the response is secondary to blockade of TNP-modified Ia antigens by anti-TNP antibody rather than blockade of the few remaining DNP determinants present on the cell surface. The availability of a proliferative response to a third hapten on macrophage surfaces, ABA, to which neither anti-TNP antibody nor TNP-specific T cells react allowed us to perform the critical control studies (Table V). The proliferative response of T cells primed either in vivo to L-tyrosine-azobenzene-arsonate (ABA-T) or in vitro to ABA-modified macrophages was not inhibited by anti-TNP antibody when the stimulator macrophages were doubly modified with ABA and TNP. Thus, the inhibition of the DNP and TNP proliferative responses shown above is highly specific and reflects binding of antibody to antigenic determinants on the macrophage surface.

TABLE V

ANTI-TNP DOES NOT INHIBIT THE RESPONSE OF ABA-PRIMED
CELLS TO ABA/TNP MODIFIED MACROPHAGES

Exp.	Serum	Macrophage Treatment		
		0	ABA	ABA/TNP
I*	NGPS	966 ± 170	12,450 ± 394	20,833 ± 415
	Anti-TNP	1,650 ± 487	11,733 ± 451	18,944 ± 184
II*	NGPS	757 ± 141	9,127 ± 482	12,044 ± 589
	Anti-TNP	2,170 ± 478	12,973 ± 212	14,454 ± 1,589
III†	NGPS	5,588 ± 836	48,874 ± 5,923	23,014 ± 1,193
	Anti-TNP	6,734 ± 376	39,881 ± 754	18,424 ± 268

* T Cells primed to ABA-T *in vivo.*
† T Cells primed to ABA-mφ *in vitro.*

At the present time we have no further insights into the mechanism of and requirements for anti-antigen induced inhibition of T cell proliferation. Is bivalent binding of antibody required or are removal of antigenic determinants by capping and shedding necessary? It is likely that more than

mere binding of antibody is required because in the earlier
studies of Ben-Sasson et al. (14) high affinity antibodies
and heavily haptenated antigens were used in order to optimize
the conditions for binding of antibody to antigen, yet no
inhibition of the response was seen. Although all the experiments reported here have been performed with hapten modified
macrophages as the stimulator cells, similar results have
already been obtained by us in studies of the response of T
cells to macrophages pulsed with soluble protein antigens.

DOES A COMPLEX OF NOMINAL ANTIGEN AND Ia ANTIGEN EXIST ON THE MACROPHAGE SURFACE?

The studies presented thus far have demonstrated a clear
role for both macrophage Ia antigens and antigenic determinants as components of the immunogenic complex on the macrophage surface which is recognized by the antigen specific T
cell. We next attempted to demonstrate the existence of a
complex between macrophage Ia antigen and nominal antigen.
The use of TNP modified cells offers both advantages and dis-
advantages in studies designed to chemically characterize the
relationship of antigen with MHC products as the TNP determinant is covalently coupled to cell membrane components. Indeed,
one must carefully consider the possibility that the relevant
immunogen in these systems is the TNP determinant directly
coupled to an MHC gene product.
    To accomplish an analysis of MHC antigens on TNP-modified
cells, TNP-derivatized cell membrane proteins from TNBS treated, radioiodinated cells were purified and tested in immunoprecipitation experiments and by sodium dodecyl sulfate-polyacrylamide gel electrophoresis (SDS-PAGE) to determine the
extent to which membrane histocompatibility antigens were
derivatized (19,20). On cells treated with 10mM TNBS, approximately 25-30% of the radio-iodinated membrane proteins were
found to be derivatized. Analysis of specific histocompatibility antigens revealed that 15-20% of the guinea pig B.1
antigens (the guinea homologue of the mouse H-2K/D antigens)
from either strain 2 or strain 13 cells were TNP-modified.
Thus, derivatization of the guinea pig B.1 antigen was
roughly proportional to the degree to which radio-iodinated
membrane proteins as a whole were TNP-derivatized. However,
analysis of Ia antigens revealed that only 5% of strain 2 Ia
antigens were TNP-derivatized, while no TNP-derivatized
strain 13 Ia antigens were detectable. It is unlikely that
TNP derivatized Ia antigens are somehow chemically altered by
TNP conjugation such that they are no longer precipitable by
anti-Ia sera and hence escape chemical detection, as 100% of

detergent solubilized strain 13 Ia antigens treated with 10mM TNBS could be shown to be TNP derivatized yet retain Ia antigenicity.

The demonstration that strain 13 Ia antigens are not derivatized on TNP-modified cells strongly suggests that the antigenic determinant recognized by guinea pig T cells does not consist of covalently trinitrophenylated Ia antigens. Furthermore, we have recently shown that guinea pig T cells can be primed and restimulated by subcellular fractions from TNP-modified Ia-negative cells in the presence of syngeneic macrophages (21). Although it is conceivable that the murine cytotoxic T cells preferentially recognize hapten-modified H-2K or D antigens, the recent studies of Schmitt-Verhulst et al. (22) and Ozato and Henney (23) that H-2 restricted hapten specific murine cytotoxic T cells can be generated by exposure to syngeneic spleen cells which have been briefly pulse exposed to soluble hapten conjugated proteins are consistent with the view that the antigens recognized by the cytotoxic T cell may include chemically unmodified H-2 antigens.

In order to directly demonstrate a complex between TNP-modified membrane antigens and unmodified Ia, radiolabeled Ia antigens were isolated from TNP-modified cells by lentil lectin chromatography followed by anti-Ia immunoabsorbent chromatography and acid elution; substantial amounts of Ia antigens were demonstrable, but no detectable antigen was precipitable using anti-TNP serum. When the immunoabsorbent eluate was electrophoresed without specific immunoprecipitation, no protein other than Ia antigens was detectable. It is thus highly unlikely that Ia antigens are strongly bound to a TNP-modified protein in a complex which withstands solubilization of the membrane. However, a complex maintained by the integrity of the intact cell membrane might very well exist.

The only evidence we have at present for the existence of a complex are the functional studies presented in Table I. If the relevant antigen recognized by the hapten specific T cell is not hapten-modified Ia, why does treatment of TNP-modified macrophages with anti-Ia serum inhibit their ability to function as stimulator cells? One possibility is that treatment with anti-Ia leads to capping and shedding of the complex of TNP-modified membrane protein and Ia antigens. Direct proof of the existence of such a complex must await a more sophisticated biochemical approach.

REFERENCES

1. Rosenthal, A.S., and Shevach, E.M. (1973). J. Exp. Med. 138, 1194.

2. Katz, D.H., Hamaoka, T., Dorf, M.E., Maurer, P.H., and Benacerraf, B. (1973). J. Exp. Med. 138, 734.

3. Shearer, G.M., Rehn, T.G., and Garbarino, C.A. (1975). J. Exp. Med. 141, 1427.

4. Zinkernagel, R.M., and Doherty, P.C. (1975). J. Exp. Med. 141, 1427.

5. Thomas, D.W., and Shevach, E.M. (1976). J. Exp. Med. 136, 1207.

6. Thomas, D.W., and Shevach, E.M. (1977). Proc. Nat. Acad. Sci. USA 74, 2104.

7. Thomas, D.W., Yamashita, U., and Shevach, E.M. (1977). Immunological Rev. 35, 97.

8. Shevach, E.M., and Rosenthal, A.S. (1973). J. Exp. Med. 138, 1213.

9. Shevach, E.M., Green, I., and Paul, W.E. (1972). J. Exp. Med. 139, 679.

10. Thomas, D.W., Yamashita, U., and Shevach, E.M. (1977). J. Immunol. 119, 223.

11. Thomas, D.W., and Shevach, E.M. (1978). J. Immunol. 121, 1152.

12. Thomas, D.W., Forni, G., Shevach, E.M., and Green, I. (1977). J. Immunol. 118, 1677.

13. Ellner, J.J., Lipsky, P.E., and Rosenthal, A.S. (1977). J. Immunol. 118, 2053.

14. Ben-Sasson, S.Z., Lipscomb, M.F., Tucker, T.F., and Uhr, J.W. (1977). J. Immunol. 119, 1493.

15. Thomas, D.W., and Shevach, E.M. (1978). J. Immunol. 121, 1145.

16. Ellner, J.J., and Rosenthal, A.S. (1975). J. Immunol. 114, 1563.

17. Bach, B.A., Sherman, L., Benacerraf, B., and Greene, M.I. (1978). J. Immunol. 121, 1460.

18. Forman, J. (1977). J. Exp. Med. 146, 600.

19. Clement, L.T., Thomas, D.W., Kask, A.M., and Shevach, E.M. (1978). Nature. 274, 592.

20. Clement, L.T., and Shevach, E.M. (1979). Molecular Immunology. 16, 67.

21. Heber-Katz, E., and Shevach, E.M. Manuscript in preparation.

22. Schmitt-Verhulst, A.-M., Pettinelli, C.B., Henkart, P.A., Lunney, J.K., and Shearer, G.M. (1978). J. Exp. Med. 147, 352.

23. Ozato, K., and Henney, C.S. (1978). J. Immunol. 121, 2405.

IDIOTYPY AND ANTIGENIC SPECIFICITY OF T_h, T_s, AND B CELLS INDUCED BY HEN EGG-WHITE LYSOZYME[1]

M. A. Harvey[2], L. Adorini[3], Christopher D. Benjamin,
Alexander Miller, and E. E. Sercarz

Department of Microbiology, University of California,
Los Angeles, Los Angeles, California   90024

ABSTRACT   The specificity of lymphocytes induced by a
small protein antigen, hen egg-white lysozyme, has been
investigated. At the B cell level most responding mice
make antibody specific for only one region of the
molecule (N-C peptide, residues 1-17,cys6-cys127,120-
129) and these antibodies share common idiotypic
determinants. This same portion of the molecule induces
T suppressor cells in nonresponder mice (B10), and this
suppressive activity can be eliminated by treatment
with anti-idiotype and complement. In contrast,
immunization of B10 mice with a different portion of
the molecule (L_{II} peptide, residues 13-105) leads to
the induction of helper cells which are insensitive to
treatment with anti-idiotype. Immunization of responder
mice (B10.A) with the intact lysozyme molecule induces
two helper cell activities. One of these is specific
for the L_{II} peptide and the second recognizes idiotypic
determinants. These two helper activities appear to
act cooperatively in the production of an antibody
response.

INTRODUCTION

One approach to understanding the collaboration between
T and B lymphocytes has been the delineation of the specificities of these cell types. Numerous experiments exist which
indicate that in the response to a multideterminant antigen,
T cells primed to one specificity can effectively help B
cells of a different specificity (1-4). Recently, evidence
has been gathered in at least two systems that T and B
collaboration may also involve idiotypic interaction (5,6).

[1]This work was supported by USPHS AI 11183 and USPHS
CA-24442
[2]Recipient of an American Cancer Society Postdoctoral
fellowship
[3]Recipient of a Cancer Research Institute Postdoctoral
fellowship.

The nature of the interplay between idiotype and epitope recognition is still obscure as are the selection rules which lead to dominance of particular idiotypes and restricted epitope recognition on a putatively multideterminant antigen such as a protein.

In an attempt to clarify such issues, this laboratory has been investigating the murine immune response to a small protein antigen, hen egg-white lysozyme (HEL). The investigation of this response offers several advantages. Lysozyme is a small protein whose primary amino acid sequence and three dimensional structure are known. Many biological variants of lysozyme from several species of birds and mammals are available to help dissect the cellular interactions in the anti-lysozyme response. The amino acid sequences of these other lysozymes differ from that of HEL over a wide range; human lysozyme (HUL) represents the most distant relative, exhibiting 52 amino acid differences. These differences in amino acid sequence are reflected in the amount of crossreaction detected at the antibody level. For instance, ring-necked pheasant lysozyme differs from HEL at only 10 amino acids and is approximately 85% crossreactive at the antibody level, while crossreaction of anti-HEL antibody with human lysozyme is rarely detected (7). These crossreactive lysozymes and several immunologically active peptides of HEL have proven useful in determining the cellular specificities in this system.

We have demonstrated that the response to HEL is under H-2 linked Ir gene control (8). Mice of the H-2^b and H-2^s haplotypes are nonresponders, while mice bearing other haplotypes are responders. Here, we review recent studies in which we have used two peptides of HEL and anti-idiotypic antibody to delineate the specificites of various lymphoid populations induced by immunization with the intact molecule in responder and nonresponder mice.

RESULTS AND DISCUSSION

Specificity of Anti-HEL Antibodies. The antibody response to HEL in responder animals, as to most protein antigens, is heterogeneous as measured by isoelectric focusing (IEF). Initially, we attempted to restrict this heterogeneity by isolating antibody reactive with various portions of HEL to use in the generation of anti-idiotypic antibody. Figure 1 shows the primary structure of HEL and the location within the molecule of the two peptides we have used throughout this study.

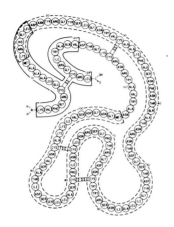

FIGURE 1. The amino acid sequence of HEL. The N-C peptide (1-17,cys6-cys127,120-129), encompassed by the solid line, is generated by mild acid cleavage. The L_{II} peptide (13-105), within the dotted line, is the mixed disulfide form of the major CNBr fragment.

Experiments using radiolabeled N-C or L_{II} peptide to stain IEF gels provided some rather surprising results. Isoelectric focusing patterns of anti-HEL antibody stained with the N-C peptide were nearly identical to the patterns obtained with HEL. In contrast, only rarely could we detect antibody reactive with the L_{II} peptide. This kind of result has been corroborated by absorption experiments which show that an N-C absorbent is capable of removing nearly all mouse anti-HEL antibodies (9). Thus, most murine anti-HEL that we have examined reacts with a determinant or determinants on the N-C peptide. This is also true of the antibody obtained from nonresponder animals, 10% of which make a restricted antibody response following immunization with HEL (8).

Production and Specificity of Anti-Idiotypic Antisera. Since most murine anti-HEL was of restricted specificity but still represented a heterogeneous array of molecules, we decided to use another method to obtain restricted antibody populations for the generation of anti-idiotypic antisera. As mentioned earlier, antibody crossreactivity between HEL and HUL is limited. Figure 2 shows the heterogeneous IEF patterns of antibody in the ascitic fluid of several Balb/c mice immunized with HUL. If these same fluids are focused in a duplicate gel and stained with ^{125}I-HEL, only a very small proportion of the antibody is observed to be HEL crossreactive.

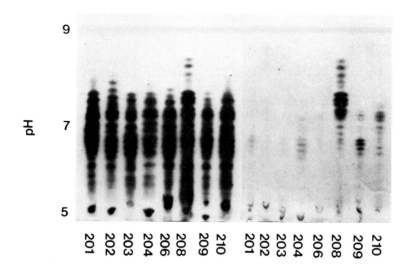

FIGURE 2.   HEL crossreactive antibody in HUL immune
ascitic fluid.   The left panel represents the autoradiograph
obtained from IEF gels in which 2 μl of Balb/c HUL immune
ascites has been focused and stained with ^{125}I-HUL.   The
right panel represents a duplicate gel which has been stained
with ^{125}I-HEL.

This HEL crossreactive antibody does not appear in every
mouse, but when it does occur, it is always more restricted
than the HUL reactive antibody. We have isolated such HEL
crossreactive antibody populations from individual HUL
immunized Balb/c mouse ascitic fluids and used these populations to generate anti-idiotypic antisera in guinea pigs
and rabbits. In addition, we have used isolated anti-HEL
responses from HEL immunized B10.A mice, which often produce
antibody which shows restricted IEF patterns. Serum from
anti-HEL immunized guinea pigs and rabbits was passed over
normal Balb/c or B10.A Ig absorbents to render them specific
for idiotypic determinants. This anti-idiotype will not
react with normal mouse Ig, mouse anti-DNP, or mouse anti-HUL
which contains no HEL reactive antibody. In contrast, these
sera will react with nearly all anti-HEL produced by mice in
response to HEL immunization. An example of a typical
result is shown in Figure 3.

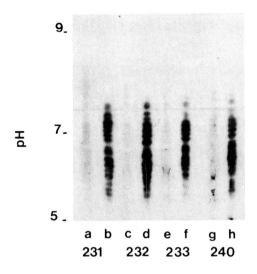

FIGURE 3. Ability of anti-idiotype to absorb Balb/c
anti-HEL antibodies. Autoradiographs of IEF gels stained
with ^{125}I-HEL. 231, 232, 233, 240 represent the ascitic
fluid from different HEL immunized Balb/C mice. a, c, e, g
are patterns obtained from 2 µl of ascitic fluid preincubated
with 10 µl of rabbit anti-idiotype. b, d, f, h are control
patterns from the same fluids preincubated with 10 µl of
saline.

We have performed most of the idiotypic analyses by
using an absorptive procedure. Anti-HEL sera to be tested
for idiotype are incubated with varying amounts of anti-
idiotypic antiserum prior to loading on IEF gels. The
formation of idiotype anti-idiotype complexes during this
incubation results in the elimination of antibody bands from
the IEF pattern relative to control samples which have been
incubated with normal serum or saline. Removal of bands can
be attributed to anti-idiotype blocking of anti-HEL antibody,
thus preventing HEL binding, or the immune complexes formed
are too large to enter the gel. This absorption procedure
offers two advantages. It allows idiotypic analysis of very
small amounts of antisera (1-2 µl are sufficient in most
cases), and it permits us to detect which portions of an
antibody response share idiotypic determinants. It is easy
with this technique to detect very minor idiotype negative
populations. As can be seen in Figure 3, nearly all of the
anti-HEL antibody from these Balb/c mice is removed by
preincubation with the anti-idiotype (at least 95% as

measured by densitometry scans of the autoradiograph). This kind of result has been found with nearly all anti-HEL antibody we have examined, regardless of the strain of mouse in which the antibody was produced (mice bearing seven different Ig allotypes have been tested).

In addition to this absorptive procedure, we have been able to demonstrate that the anti-idiotype inhibits the binding of anti-HEL to ^{125}I-HEL but has no effect on the binding of anti-HUL to ^{125}I-HUL. These data suggest that the anti-idiotype recognizes, at least in part, site associated idiotypic determinants.

Though the majority of anti-HEL antibodies we have examined react with the anti-idiotype, occasionally we have observed idiotype negative antibody. In particular, when L_{II} reactive antibody can be detected, it does not react with the anti-idiotype. Thus, it appears that in the mouse, most anti-HEL reacts with the N-C region of the molecule and this antibody shares some crossreactive idiotypic structures. More extensive data on the idiotype system will be published elsewhere (9).

<u>Specificity of HEL Induced Suppressor T Cells in Nonresponder Mice</u>. Though B10 mice are nonresponders to HEL, normal B10 spleen cells can produce a primary anti-HEL plaque-forming cell (PFC) response <u>in vitro</u> if HEL-coupled red blood cells are used as antigen in culture. Previously, we have demonstrated that preimmunization of B10 mice intraperitoneally with HEL emulsified in complete Freund's adjuvant (CFA) induces HEL specific T suppressor cells capable of eliminating this primary response (10). Comparison of the amino acid sequences from several different lysozymes has implicated the amino acid at position 3 as being instrumental in determining whether or not the molecule is immunogenic for H-2^b mice. Consistent with this view is the demonstration that the N-C peptide (which contains residue 3) is capable of inducing a population of suppressor cells in B10 mice indistinguishable from those induced by intact HEL (11). An example of this result is shown in Table I. In contrast, the L_{II} peptide (13-105), representing 70% of the molecule, induces helper cells in these "nonresponder" animals (Table II). Thus, HEL-induced suppressor cells appear to be specific for the same portion of the molecule reactive with anti-HEL. Considering the similarity in specificity between the suppressor cell population and antibody, we next attempted to eliminate HEL-induced suppressor cells by pretreatment with anti-idiotype and complement. The results in Table II show that pretreatment of HEL primed spleen cells eliminates the suppressive

TABLE I

HEL OR N-C INDUCES SUPPRESSOR CELLS IN B10 MICE

Spleen cells ($\times 10^6$) per culture from B10 mice primed with:			Anti-HEL direct PFC/culture $\pm$ S.E.
CFA	HEL-CFA	N-C-CFA	
2	-	-	158±24
-	2	-	0
-	-	2	20±5
1.9	0.1	-	16±6
1.9	-	0.1	21±10

For culture conditions, see reference 10.

activity of these populations but has no effect on the helper activity of L_{II} primed spleen cells.

TABLE II

ANTI-IDIOTYPE PLUS COMPLEMENT TREATMENT ELIMINATES
HEL-INDUCED SUPPRESSOR CELLS BUT NOT L_{II}-INDUCED
HELPER CELLS FROM B10 MICE

Spleen cells ($\times 10^6$) from B10 mice primed with:			Pretreatment of HEL* or L_{II} primed cells	Anti-HEL direct PFC/culture $\pm$ S.E.
CFA	HEL-CFA	L_{II}-CFA		
2	-	-	-	311±13
-	2	-	-	51±14
-	-	2	-	518±44
1.8	0.2	-	NGPS + C'	88±26
1.8	0.2	-	αid + C'	355±30
1.8	-	0.2	NGPS + C'	583±181
1.8	-	0.2	αid + C'	633±67

*Pretreatment of HEL or L_{II} primed spleen cells was 1/2 hour on ice with a 1:5 dilution of either normal guinea pig serum (NGPS) or guinea pig anti-idiotype (αid) followed by a 1/2 hour incubation with rabbit complement (C') at 37°C.

Similar results are found when N-C induced suppressor cells are treated with the anti-idiotype (data not shown). We conclude that HEL induces suppressor cells in nonresponding

TABLE III

SPECIFICITY OF HELPER T CELLS FROM
HEL PRIMED B10.A MICE

Cells in culture (x10⁶)		T cells from B10.A mice primed with:	T-cell absorption on plates coated with:	Anti-HEL PFC/culture
B	T			
$\frac{B}{2}$	-	-	-	1±1
-	2	HEL-CFA	-	10±7
1.8	0.2	HEL-CFA	Ribonuclease	195±38
1.8	0.2	HEL-CFA	HEL	94±31
1.8	0.2	HEL-CFA	αHEL≡Id	62±26
1.8	0.2	HEL-CFA	NMS	202±48
1.8	0.2*	HEL-CFA	*	204±51

*The T cells are a 1:1 mixture of the non-absorbed
cells from the Id and HEL plates. Culture conditions are
the same as in previous tables.

animals which display on their surface some idiotypic structures that are present on antibody from responding animals.

Specificities of Helper Cells in HEL Immunized
Responder Mice. In order to delineate the specificities of
helper cells in responding animals we have performed a
series of preliminary experiments designed to fractionate
spleen cells from HEL primed B10.A mice on antigen, peptide,
or antibody coated tissue culture plates. In the experiment
shown in Table III, the methodology for the plate absorptions was adapted from Woodland and Cantor (12). Clearly,
helper cell activity was removed on either the HEL or the
idiotype-coated plates. The reconstitution experiment shown
in the last line indicates that two different T-cell helper
populations are synergistically involved, one antigen-
specific and one idiotype-specific. Subsequent experiments
have shown that L_{II}-coated plates are just as effective at
removing the helper cell activity as the HEL-coated plates,
while N-C-coated plates are without effect. This evidence
was in accord with many experiments showing that the large
peptide fragment, L_{II}, could induce proliferation in both
responder and non-responder mice. Yet, it was noteworthy
that the predominant helper activity was directed against
part of the HEL molecule, antibodies to which seem to be
idiotypically distinct from the system we have described
here (Metzger, D. and Harvey, M., unpublished).

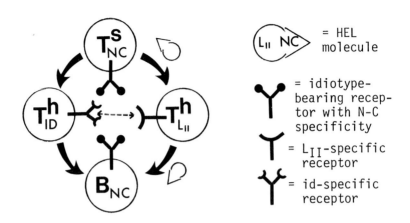

FIGURE 4. Cellular specificities and a possible network of interactions in the response to HEL. Subscripts
indicate specificity; superscripts indicate functional subset of cells. Antigen-bridging interactions occur among
the cells on the right side of the figure; idiotypic cellular
interactions occur among the cells on the left side of the
figure. An interaction between the two helper cells is
suggested by the dashed arrow.

These studies have minimally implicated four different
lymphocytes bearing complementary receptors, which could be
linked in a matrix as shown in Figure 4. HEL immunization
of B10 mice induces T-suppressor cells specific for the N-C
region. These suppressor cells potentially could interact
through idiotypic complementarity with an idiotype-specific
helper cell, or via antigen-bridging with the L_{II}-specific
T_h. The latter mechanism has been demonstrated in our
earlier work (13) but the former requires direct proof.
Finally, we have demonstrated the occurrence of N-C specific
antibody (B cells) bearing a common idiotype as the sole or
predominant specificity in secondary anti-HEL mouse responses. Anti-N-C B-cells could result from the utilization
of the two helper cells independently or in concert. With
regard to the shared idiotypy of T_s and B cells, it presumably arises from a common idiotypic stimulus at one stage,
or even from a common antigen-bridge mechanism.

Our results point to an important role for idiotypic
motifs in choosing and/or maintaining those B cells engaged
in the immune response. Furthermore, they show that antigen-
bridging mechanisms and complementary anti-idiotypic
reactions each play a vital part in B cell stimulation.

The mode of interaction of the idiotype-specific and antigen-specific helper cells is undergoing scrutiny at present.

REFERENCES

1. Mitchison, N. A. (1971). Eur. J. Immunol. 1, 18.
2. Mitchison, N. A., Rajewsky, K., and Taylor, R. B. (1970). In "Developmental Aspects of Antibody Formation and Structure" (J. Šterzl and I. Říha, eds.), Vol. II, p. 547. Publishing House of the Czechoslovak Academy of Sciences, Prague.
3. Raff, M. C. (1970). Nature 226, 1257.
4. Goodman, J. W., Fong, S., Lewis, G. K., Kamin, R., Nitecki, D. E., and Der Balian, G. (1978). Immunol. Rev. 39, 36.
5. Hetzelberger, D., and Eichmann, K. (1978). Eur. J. Immunol. 8, 846.
6. Ward, K., Cantor, H., and Boyse, E. A. (1977). In "The Immune System: Genetics and Regulation" (E. E. Sercarz, L. A. Herzenberg, and C. F. Fox, eds.), p. 397, Academic Press, New York.
7. Miller, A., Bonavida, B., Stratton, J., and Sercarz, E. (1971). Biochim. Biophys. Acta 243, 520.
8. Hill, S. W., and Sercarz, E. (1975). Eur. J. Immunol. 5, 317.
9. Harvey, M. A., Adorini, L., Miller, A., and Sercarz, E. Submitted for publication.
10. Adorini, L., Miller, A., and Sercarz, E. (1979). J. Immunol. 122, 871.
11. Adorini, L., Harvey, M. A., Miller, A., and Sercarz, E. E. Submitted for publication.
12. Woodland, R. and Cantor, H. (1978). Eur. J. Immunol. 8, 600.
13. Yowell, R., Araneo, B., Miller, A., and Sercarz, E. (1979). Nature, in press.

CELLULAR BASIS OF THE REGULATION OF PRODUCTION OF ANTI-TNP ANTIBODIES CARRYING MOPC460 IDIOTYPE

C. Bona and W.E. Paul

Laboratory of Immunology
National Institute of Allergy and Infectious Diseases
National Institutes of Health
Bethesda, Maryland 20014

ABSTRACT. An idiotype of the DNP- and TNP-binding myeloma protein MOPC460 is expressed on a small but significant proportion of anti-TNP antibodies after in vivo immunization of BALB/c mice with three T-independent TNP-antigens. In vitro experiments show that the fraction of anti-TNP-antibody secreting cells expressed the idiotype of MOPC460 (460 Id) is regulated by 460 Id suppressor T cells. These suppressor T cells are removed by dishes coated with MOPC460 myeloma protein. The suppressor activity was ablated by treatment of T cells with anti Lyt 2.2 and anti Qal sera and C. Finally, the 460 Id specific T cells were detected only in IgC_H^a mice, independently of their genetic background suggesting that the development of these suppressors may be indirectly controlled by Ig genes.

Recent studies have shown that a small fraction of anti-TNP antibodies induced by TNP-T dependent (TD) or T-independent (TI) antigens share idiotypic determinants with the DNP and TNP binding myeloma proteins MOPC460 and MPC315 [1,2].

We showed that 10-30% of the anti-TNP PFC of BALB/c mice immunized with TNP-dextran, TNP-levan (TNP-BL) or TNP-Nocardia water soluble mitogen (TNP-NWSM) secreted antibodies bearing the MOPC460 idiotype (460 Id) [3]. In further studies, reviewed here, we investigated the mechanisms which regulate the expression of clones secreting anti-TNP antibodies carrying 460 Id. These studies were focused on three major issues:
1) Specificity of the regulatory cell.
2) The phenotype of regulating cells
3) The effect of antiidiotypic antibodies on this response.

ISBN 0-12-069850-1

   1.   Expression of 460 Id on Anti-TNP Antibodies after In
Vitro Stimulation of BALB/c Spleen Cells with TNP-NWSM.   We
have previously shown that TNP-NWSM is a TI-type 1 (TI-1)
antigen which causes a primary in vitro anti-TNP response.
This response is largely independent of T lymphocyte help,
since no significant difference was noted in the number of
PFC developed in cultures of unseparated spleen cells and of
B cells purified by a two step process involving adherence
to and elution from a dish coated with purified rabbit anti-
mouse immunoglobulin followed by treatment of the eluted cells
with anti-Thy 1.2 and C (3).   The fraction of anti-TNP PFC
secreting antibody bearing 460 Id was studied by inhibition
of anti-TNP PFC by BALB/c anti-460 Id antibodies added to the
agarose in which the plaques were developed.   We found that
10-20% of the anti-TNP-PFCs produced by unseparated spleen
cells were inhibitable by anti-460 Id antibodies.   A
similar proportion of 460 Id$^+$ anti-TNP PFC was found in BALB/c
mice after in vivo immunization with TNP-NWSM.

   2.   Increase of the 460 Id$^+$ Component of the Anti-TNP
PFC Response to TNP-NWSM by Removal of T Lymphocytes.   A
comparison of the 460 Id$^+$ component of the anti-TNP response
to TNP-NWSM of unseparated and anti-Thy 1.2 and C treated
spleen lymphocytes showed that the proportion of 460 Id$^+$
PFC was substantially higher in the anti-Thy 1.2 treated
population.   This observation suggested that the population
sensitive to anti-Thy 1.2 + C treatment contained cells which
exhibited an inhibitory activity on the B cells capable of
expression 460 Id.
   This hypothesis was tested by the addition of nylon wool
purified T-cells to B-cells, obtained by anti-Thy 1.2 and
C treatment.   In such experiments, as clear inhibition of the
460 Id$^+$ component of the anti-TNP response was observed
(Table 1).   Furthermore, this inhibitory effect of nylon wool
purified T lymphocytes was ablated by pretreatment of these
cells with anti Thy 1.2 and C indicating that as suppressor
T cells could regulate the experiment of cells secreting
460 Id$^+$ anti-TNP antibodies.

   3.   Phenotype of T Cells Which Regulate the Expression
of Cells Secreting 460 Id$^+$ Anti-TNP Antibodies.   Lyt and Qal
antigens represent useful markers since they are expressed
on increasingly well-defined functional subsets of T lymphocytes.   In experiments conducted with the collaboration of
F.W. Shen and E.A. Boyse, we found that anti-Ly 2.2 and C
pretreatment ablated inhibitory activity of T cells on the
expression of 460-Id.   In some, but not all, experiments, the
suppressor activity was partially diminished by anti Lyt 1.2
and C treatment.   We have studied the Qal phenotype T

TABLE I

INHIBITORY EFFECT OF T CELLS ON THE 460 ID$^+$

ANTI-TNP PFC RESPONSE

No. of Experiment	5x10^5 B Cells Incubated With	Total Anti-TNP PFC/Culture	% of 460-Id$^+$ Anti-TNP PFC
1	$\bar{\bar{}}-$	92 ± 13	41
	5x10^5 T cells	110 ± 6	- 10
2	$\bar{\bar{}}-$	290 ± 15	58
	5x10^5 T Cells	199 ± 11	3
3	$\bar{\bar{}}-$	215 ± 48	53
	5x10^5 T Cells	223 ± 29	3
4	$\bar{\bar{}}-$	140 ± 15	38
	5x10^5 T Cells	85 ± 14	12
5	$\bar{\bar{}}-$	112 ± 10	40
	5x10^5 T Cells	146 ± 14	10
6	$\bar{\bar{}}-$	86 ± 3	69
	5x10^5 T Cells	171 ± 55	15
7	$\bar{\bar{}}-$	226 ± 29	50
	5x10^5 T Cells	295 ± 14	4
8	$\bar{\bar{}}-$	277 ± 5	50
	5x10^5 T Cells	80 ± 18	- 3

Anti Thy 1.2 and C treated BALB/c spleen cells (5x10^5/well) were cultured with nothing or with 5x10^5 nylon wool column spleen cells (T cells). Total number of anti-TNP PFC and of PFC secreting 460 Id bearing molecules were measured 4 days after stimulation with TNP-NWSM (3 μg/ml).

suppressor cells, using F_1 hybrids of BALB/c x C58/J. C58/J mice have H_2^k genetic background , IgC_H genes and at least some IgV_H genes of BALB/c mice and an allelic form of Qal which is recognized by anti-Qa sera A-T1a^b anti-ASL1. After stimulation with TNP-TD antgens C58/J mice develop 460 Id$^+$ anti-TNP antibodies (1). Treatment with antisera containing anti-Qal activity and C of T cells of (C58/JxBALB/c)F_1 mice ablated the inhibitory activity of these cells on 460 Id$^+$ component of anti-TNP response (TABLE II).

TABLE II
PHENOTYPE OF SUPPRESSOR T CELLS

	Pretreatment of T Cells	Anti-TNP PFC/Culture	
		Total	% 460 Id^{+}
A. 5×10^{5} BALB/c B Cells Incubated with:			
nil	--	226 ± 29	69
5×10^{5} T cells	--	295 ± 14	4
5×10^{5} T cells	anti-Ly 1.2+C	156 ± 28	11
5×10^{5} T cells	anti-Ly 2.2+C	240 ± 44	54
B. 5×10^{5} (C58/Jx BALB/c)F$_{1}$ B cells incubated with:			
nil	--	123 ± 18	55
5×10^{5} T cells	--	91 ± 7	15
5×10^{5} T cells	anti-Ly 1.2+C	99 ± 7	0
5×10^{5} T cells	anti-Qa1+C	105 ± 10	38

Anti-Thy 1.2 and C treated spleen cells (B cells)
(5×10^{5}/well) were cultured with nothing or with 5×10^{5} nylon
wool column passed spleen cells (T cells). The T cells were
treated with nothing or with: 1° C$_3$H/AN anti-CE/J thymocytes
(anti-Lyt 1.2) serum adsorbed on B6 Lyt 1.1 cells. 2° (C$_3$H/AN
xB6-Ly 2.1)F$_1$ anti-B6 leukemia ERLD (anti-Lyt 2.2) adsorbed
on B.6 Ly 1.2 mice cells 3° A/TL-A anti ASL.1 serum. Total
number of anti-TNP-PFC and of PFC secreting 460 Id bearing
molecules were measured 4 days after stimulation with TNP-NWSM
(3 μg/ml).

The results suggest that majority of T cells inhibit the
460 Id^{+} component of anti-TNP antibodies are Lyt 2.3^{+} and
Qa1^{+}. However, our results indicate that some of these cells
could be Ly 1.2.3^{+}, since pretreatment with anti Ly 1.2 serum
and complement slightly altered the activity of suppressor T
cells. Finally, we cannot exclude the possibility that
suppression requires the interaction of Qa1^{+} cells with
Ly 2^{+} cells.

3. Specificity of Suppressor T Cells. The results presented above indicate that 460 Id$^+$ component of anti-TNP response is regulated by suppressor T cells. The specificity of these cells was studied in plate binding experiments using dishes coated with MOPC460 and EPC109. EPC109 is an IgA$_k$ $\beta 2 \rightarrow 1$ and $\beta 2 \rightarrow 6$ fructosan binding protein which does not carry the 460 Id. In a typical experiment reported in Table III, addition of 5 x 10^5 nylon wool purified T cells to 5 x 10^5 B cells significantly decreased the expression of 460 Id. Adsorbtion of the T lymphocyte population on 460-coated dishes removed their inhibitory activity. By contrast, T cells adsorbed on E109-coated dishes retained suppressive activity. T lymphocytes which were recovered from MOPC460-coated dishes were strongly inhibitory whereas those recovered from E109-coated dishes lack inhibitory activity. These findings indicate that the suppressor T lymphocytes are specific for 460 Id and suggest that they excert their

TABLE III

SUPPRESSION OF 460 Id$^+$ ANTI-TNP RESPONSE BY T-LYMPHOCYTES
RECOVERED FROM MOPC460-COATED DISHES

B Cells (5x10^5) Incubated with T cells		Anti-TNP PFC/Culture	
T Cells	Number	Total	% 460 Id$^+$
–	0	289 ± 15	58
untreated	5 x 10^5	199 ± 11	3
ads. on E109	5 x 10^5	181 ± 2	5
rec. from E109	5 x 10^5	207 ± 16	39
ads on M460	5 x 10^5	283 ± 4	53
rec. from M460	5 x 10^5	171 ± 14	– 3
	10^5	252 ± 10	8
	10^4	250 ± 33	30

B lymphocytes (5 x 10^5) from normal BALB/c mice were cultured alone or in the presence of BALB/c T lymphocytes. The latter were either untreated or separated by incuation on plastic dishes coated with E109 or MOPC 460 (M460). Cells which fail to adhere to E109 dishes (Ads on E109) or to M460 dishes (Ads on M460) and cells which were recovered from E109 dishes (Rec. from E109) or from M460 dishes (Rec. from M460) were used. The cell mixtures were cultured in sextuplicate with TNP-NWSM (3 µg/ml) for 3 days and the number of PFC on TNP-SRBC measured in the absence of or presence of anti-460 Id.

suppressive function directly on B cells which bear 460 id
on their receptors. This direct effect of 460 Id suppressor
T cells on precursors of 460 Id anti-TNP antibody forming
cells is supported by recent experiments in which we found
that addition of Lyt 1^+ T cells did not alter significantly
the suppressor activity developed by T cells recovered
from MOPC460-coated dishes.

     5. Relationship between Occurrence of 460 Id specific
Suppressor T Cells and BALB/c IgC_H Genes. Rosenstein et al.
(1) found 460 Id^+ anti-TNP antibodies subsequent to immunization with TNP-TD antigens only in the strains having IgV_H and
IgC_H genes of the BALB/c type $(Ig1^a)$ such as B.C8 and C58/J
mice. Thus, we conducted experiments in various strains of
mice in order to establish the distribution of normally
occurring 460 Id^+ suppressor T cells. We studied the presence
of such cells in the following strains of mice: C.B20, a
BALB/c congenic strain which has IgC_H and IgV_H genes of
C_{57} Black/Ka mice $(Ig1^b)$, CAL.20, a BALB/c congenic strain
which has IgC_H and IgV_H of A.L/J mice $(Ig1^d)$, C58/J, a strain
of the H_2K type which has IgC_H and at least some IgV_H genes
of BALB/c, and BAB14 a BALB/c congenic strain which has IgC_H^b
and some IgV_H genes of BALB/c.
     The results presented in Table IV show that 460 Id
specific T cells were detected only in IgC_H^a mice independently of their genetic background. These results strongly
suggest that the occurrence of 460 Id specific suppressor T
cells is linked to IgC_H^a genes. These data are in agreement
with other findings which suggest that the expression of V_H
genes on T cells is linked to allotype (5,6), but it should
be noted that the development of these suppressors may be
indirectly controlled by Ig genes in that they may expand in
response to exposure to B cells expressing 460 Id determinants.

                      DISCUSSION AND CONCLUSIONS

     It has been proposed that idiotypic determinants express-
ed by precursors of antibody forming cells as well as by T
cells represent sites of regulation by anti-Id antibodies. In
various experimental systems used as phosphocholine, inulin,
streptococcal carbohydrate, and arsonate it has been shown
that anti-Id antibodies can modulate the functions of various
subpopulations of lymphocytes. Anti-Id antibodies exert
their suppressor effect after direct interaction with idiotype
determinants of the receptors of precursors of antibody
forming cells (7,8,9), T cells which carry idiotypic deter-

minants (10,11) or are specific for idiotypes (12).

TABLE IV

RELATIONSHIP BETWEEN NATURALLY OCCURRENCE OF 460 Id
SPECIFIC T-SUPPRESSOR CELLS AND IgC_H^a GENES

Donor Strain of 5×10^5 B Cells	Donor of T Cells			Anti TNP-PFC/Culture	
	Strain	IgC_H	IgV_H	Total	% 460 Id[+]
BALB/c	--			212 ± 4	46
	BALB/c	a	a	291 ± 11	14
	C.B20	d	d	304 ± 32	52
BALB/c	--			146 ± 14	70
	BALB/c	a	a	229 ± 15	16
	C.B20	b	b	278 ± 20	44
	CAL.20	d	d	324 ± 34	65
BALB/c	--			149 ± 8	33
	BALB/c	a	a	119 ± 13	4
	BAB14	b	a*	125 ± 18	24
C58/J	--		a**	66 ± 9	44
	C58/J	a		57 ± 4	11

5×10^5 B cells were incubated with nothing or 5×10^5 T cells.
Total number of anti-TNP PFC or PFC secreting 460 Id bearing
molecules were scored 4 days after stimulation with TNP-NWSM
(3 μg/ml).

*The BAB14 mouse is a recombinant which has IgV_H genes which
are principally of the a type but of which some are of b type.

**IgV_H region genes of C58 mice express idiotypes similar to
those of BALB/c.

Perhaps more important than the effect of intentionally
administered anti-Id antibody on the regulation of B cell
responses are recent findings that T lymphocytes can regulate
the expression of idiotypes in a given immune response.
Until now, such regulatory cells have been observed in animals
which have been immunized with antigens, antibodies or treated
with anti-idiotype antibodies. The T cells found in such

situations appear either to be specific for idiotype or to express idiotype on their receptors (13,14,15).

The general validity of the concept that lymphocyte function may be regulated through immunoglobulin determinants would be considerably strengthened by the discovery of natur- ally occuring idiotype-specific suppressor cells. We have found in BALB/c mice that the expression of cells secreting anti-TNP antibodies bearing 460 Id in response to TNP-TI$_1$ and TI$_2$ antigens is regulated by naturally occuring suppressor T cells. These suppressor T cells express the Lyt2 and Qal antigens; our present experiments cannot exclude the existence of Lyt 1^+2^+ suppressor T cells. Such regulatory T cells be- longing to the Lyt 2^- class have previously been described in mice which were intentionally pretreated with anti-idiotype (16) or anti-allotype (17) antibodies. For example, the bulk of Id specific suppressor T cells induced by treatment of A/J mice with rabbit antibody to the cross reactive idiotype of anti-arsonate are Lyt 2.3^+. However Lyt 1^+2^- cells also induce suppression in this system although whether their effects are direct or indirect has not been established (16).

Plate binding experiments described here indicate that the 460-Id specific suppressive action of T lymphocytes de- pends on a cell which binds to MOPC460 myeloma protein. Therefore, this naturally occurring suppressor T cell is specific for the 460-Id itself. BALB/c mice immunized with syngeneic anti-460 Id antibodies, and which produce in con- sequence anti [anti-460 Id] antibodies, lack 460 Id specific suppressor T cells. In addition, such mice exhibit a signi- ficant increase in 460 Id bearing anti-TNP antibodies in re- sponse to TNP-BL or TNP-NWSM immunization (18). This increase of 460 Id$^+$ molecules is very likely due to the elimination of 460 Id specific suppressor T cells by anti [anti-460 Id] anti- bodies. These results suggest that 460 Id specific suppressor T cells share Id determinants with anti-460 Id antibodies (18).

Finally, the results presented here show that the appear- ance of these naturally occurring 460 Id-specific suppressor T cells is linked to the Igl^a [BALB/c] gene complex. Such cells were not found in C.B20 or CAL20 mice which are congenic to BALB/c mice but which have an unrelated allotype.

In conclusion the data reported here demonstrated that the 460 Id$^+$ component of the anti-TNP antibody response is regulated by naturally occurring 460 Id specific suppressor T cells which can be eliminated by anti [anti-460 Id] antibodies.

REFERENCES

1. Rosenstein, R.W., Zeldis, J.B., and Richards, F.I. Immunochemistry: in press.

2. Granato, D., Braun, D.G., and Vassalli, J. (1974). J. Immunol. 113, 417.
3. Bona, C. and Paul, W.E. (1973). J. Exp. Med. 149, 592.
4. Stanton, T.H., Boyse, E.A. (1976). 3, 525.
5. Hammerling, G.J., Black, S.J., Berek, C., Eichman, K., and Rajewsky, K. (1976). J. Exp. Med. 143, 861.
6. Krammer, D. (1978). J. Exp. Med. 147, 25.
7. Kluskens, L., and Köhler, H. (1974). Proc. Natl. Acad. Sci (USA), 71, 5083.
8. Julius, M.H., Cosenza, H., and Augustin, A.A. (1978). Eur. J. Immunol. 8, 484.
9. Bona, C., Lieberman, R., House, S., Green, I., and Paul, W.E. (1979). J. Immunol. In press.
10. Eichmann, K. (1975). 5, 511.
11. Black, S.J., Hämmerling, G.J., Berek, C., Rajewsky, K., and Eichmann, K. (1976). J. Exp. Med. 143, 846.
12. Owen, F.L., Ju, S.T., and Nisonoff, A. (1977). Proc. Natl. Acad. Sci. 74, 2084.
13. Levis, G., and Goodman, J.W. (1978). J. Exp. Med. 148, 315.
14. Germain, R.N., Ju, S.T., Kipps, T.J., Beneracerraf, B. and Dorf, M.D. (1979). J. Exp. Med. 149, 613.
15. Nisonoff, A., Ju, S.T., and Owen, F. (1977). Immunol. Rev. 34, 89.
16. Ward, K., Cantor, J., and Nisonoff, A. (1977). Proc. Natl. Acad. Sci. 74, 2084.
17. Herzenberg, L.A., Okumura, K., Cantor, H., Sato, V.L., Shen, F.W., Boyse, E.A., and Herzenberg, L.A. (1976). J. Exp. Med. 149,330.
18. Bona, C., Hooghe, R., Cazenave, P.A., Leguiru, Chr., and Paul, W.E. (1979). J. Exp. Med. In press.

WORKSHOP SUMMARY: Network of Regulation. Conveners, Constantin Bona, Pasteur Institute, Paris, France and Alfred Nisonoff, Rosenstiel Research Center, Brandeis University, Waltham, MA   02154.

The focus of the workshop was on regulation of the immune response by T cells and antibodies with anti-idiotypic or anti-allotypic specificity.

Dr. C. Bona discussed evidence, obtained at the NIH, for a regulatory network involving those anti-TNP antibodies in BALB/c mice which share idiotype with the DNP- or TNP-binding myeloma protein, MOPC-460. His experiments identified a naturally occurring set of suppressor cells which regulate the expression of the idiotype. The suppressor cells have receptors with anti-id specificity and are of the Lyt-2.2 phenotype. When anti-anti-id was prepared against anti-MOPC-460 and injected into BALB/c mice it increased the fraction of anti-TNP antibodies that carries the idiotype of MOPC-460. This experiment and others in which anti-460 antibodies were injected directly into BALB/c mice indicated that anti-anti-460 antibodies inactivate suppressor cells specific for the MOPC-460 idiotype.

Dr. E. Enghofer, Institute for Cancer Research, Philadelphia, reported on studies of a mouse idiotype, U10-173, found on IgG, IgA and IgM and comprising about 1% of the normal Ig in strains expressing the idiotype. Its presence in different H chain classes and its linkage to allotype suggest that it is present in the V_H region. The idiotype has been found in all but 5 strains investigated. Strain AKR does not express the idiotype, but it can be induced in nude AKR mice by immunization with levan. Another negative strain, CWA, produces the idiotype on challenge with levan after irradiation. It was concluded that some negative strains have the potential for expressing this idiotype but are prevented from doing so by the presence of suppressor T cells.

H. M. Gebel, Washington University, St. Louis, described a system for observing the effects of various treatments on the differentiation of cell line MOPC-315. Differentiation is observed in Millipore diffusion chambers implanted into the peritoneal cavities of syngeneic BALB/c mice. The cells, which initially resemble lymphocytes, take on the appearance of plasmacytes over a period of a few days. When the mice acting as hosts had previously been primed to induce T helper activity against the MOPC-315 idiotype, the priming promoted differentiation; conversely, priming of mice so as to induce suppression of the idiotype inhibited differentiation. The system provides a unique model for studying B cell differentiation under controlled conditions. Cells enclosed in diffusion chambers could be specifically inhibited from

443

ISBN 0-12-069850-1

secreting protein 315 by the presence of idiotype-specific
suppressor T cells, whereas the presence of antiidiotypic
antibodies suppressed the appearance of protein 315 on cell
surface membranes.

G. Kelsoe, Harvard Medical School, has studied the
appearance of cells producing the T15 idiotype and anti-
idiotype (anti-T15) at various times after challenge of BALB/c
mice with the phosphorylcholine (PC) hapten. This was done
by measuring the number of plaque-forming cells specific
for PC and the amount of radioactive PC or T15 protein bound
by a fixed number of cells. It was found that there is a
biphasic curve for the number of anti-PC cells, with peaks
on days 5 and 12 after priming. Binding of labeled protein
T15, which should reflect the number of cells with anti-
idiotypic receptors, also showed a cyclic pattern, but it was
out of phase with the curve for anti-PC specific cells. The
cyclic patterns are believed to reflect suppression of idiotype-bearing cells by the products of cells which carry anti-
idiotypic receptors.

G. G. B. Klaus, National Institute for Medical Research,
London, discussed investigations of methods for enhancing
the immunogenicity of idiotypic determinants of BALB/c myeloma
proteins in BALB/c mice. The initial investigation was
carried out with protein 315, which binds the dinitrophenyl
hapten group. It was later extended to other myeloma proteins
with known antigen-binding specificity. Antigen-antibody
complexes were very effective in inducing auto-antiidiotypic
antibodies, and cooperation of idiotype-specific helper T
cells was unnecessary when complexes were used. The apparent
reason is that helper T cells against the antigen present in
complexes can substitute for antiidiotypic helper T cells.

Two reports described evidence for a role of anti-id
antibody in regulation. These are among the most direct
demonstrations of this phenomenon. E. A. Goidl, Cornell
Medical College, found that there is a 90% decrease in the
number of anti-TNP plaque-forming cells between days 4 and 7
after challenge of AKR mice with TNP-Ficoll. This was accompanied by a decrease in affinity and heterogeneity of the
antibodies released by the cells. Cells taken from mice on
day 7 could adoptively transfer a state of partial suppression
to TNP-Ficoll. An unusual effect was observed in that the
addition of hapten to the agar increased the number of plaque-
forming cells in recipients to the level in controls. It was
suggested that antiidiotype, present in day 7 serum, inhibited
plaque formation and that the addition of hapten caused the
release of the anti-id antibody from cells. When day 7
immune serum was passed over various adsorbents, the results
indicated that the inhibitory factor in serum has the

properties of anti-id antibody. Production of the inhibitory factor was not observed in nude mice, suggesting that the regulation by auto-antiidiotype is T cell dependent.

Another demonstration of a soluble inhibitory factor with the properties of antiidiotype was described by M-S. Sy, from the University of Colorado Medical Center. The system investigated involves sensitization to delayed-type hypersensitivity (DTH) as measured by ear swelling, after challenge of mice with 2,4-dinitrofluorobenzene (DNFB). It was noted that the state of DTH rapidly declines between days 5 and 9 after sensitization. Serum taken from animals on day 9 blocks the adoptive transfer of immunity by lymph node cells from mice that had been challenged with DNFB. The serum factor is an immunoglobulin which lacks anti-DNP activity although it is antigen-specific. The evidence presented suggests that the activity is antiidiotypic. However, the active serum factor lacks strain specificity. It was proposed that these antibodies are responsible for the rapid decline in delayed hypersensitivity after day 5.

Data presented by Dr. S.S. Miller, also from the University of Colorado, indicated that in the above system T suppressor cells are generated which can interfere with passive transfer of sensitivity by lymph node cells from mice which were immunized with DNFB. Two types of suppressor cells were demonstrated, 7 days and 21 days after immunization. The suppressor cells present at the earlier time were able to block DTH when co-transferred with lymph node cells from mice immunized with DNFB. Suppressor cells present at a later period did not block in a co-transfer experiment but did prevent sensitization to the DNFB hapten in recipient mice (afferent limb). The suppressor cells present at the earlier and later time periods were genetically nonrestricted and restricted, respectively, in their capacity to act on other mice.

M. Zauderer presented data supporting the concept that there are helper T cells with specificity for Ig determinants, which can act on B cells in conjunction with carrier-specific helper T cells. In vitro cultures were set up containing an excess of B cells primed to two unrelated haptens, PC and DNP, using the same carrier for each hapten. In a series of cultures the number of carrier-primed T cells was reduced until they became limiting for response. At this point each culture showed responsiveness to one or the other hapten but not to both. The implication is that there are helper T cells in addition to those specific for the carrier, and that each of these additional helper cells has specificity for one B cell type or the other but not for both. The results would be consistent with the presence of a helper cell with idiotypic specificity.

M.A. Harvey, UCLA, has observed the presence of common idiotypic determinants on antibodies and suppressor T cells. The suppressor cells were obtained by immunization of C57BL/10 mice with hen egg lysozyme (HEL) or certain normally antigenic fragments of the enzyme. C57BL/10 mice are unresponsive to HEL but produce T suppressor cells upon challenge with HEL or its active fragments. Anti-id antibodies prepared against anti-HEL from B10.A mice (a responder strain) were able to kill the suppressor cells in the presence of complement. The results are consistent with the presence of a network involving antibodies and suppressor cells with idiotypic determinants.

L.S. Rodkey, Kansas State University, has demonstrated the presence of auto-antiidiotypic antibodies in a conventionally immunized rabbit. The antigen was M. lysodeikticus and the antibodies studied were specific for carbohydrate. After an initial challenge rabbits were allowed to rest for about three months, then were challenged again. Isoelectric focusing indicated that a different group of clones had been stimulated by the secondary challenge. A radioimmunoassay using ^{125}I-labeled Fab fragments of antibodies obtained after primary immunization detected the presence of antiidiotypic antibodies in the sera of the same rabbit after the secondary challenge.

H.R. Snodgrass, University of Pennsylvania, described experiments showing the presence of cytotoxic T cells specific for allotypic determinants, which can lyse target cells with receptors having the allotype. The T cells were generated by immunizing BALB/c mice with Ig from the C57BL strain. T cells from immunized mice, when transferred to the allotype-congenic C.B-17 strain inhibited the production of the IgG_{2a} class of antibodies. Cytotoxicity in vitro against IgG_{2a}-bearing cells was demonstrated by a chromium release assay.

SPECIFIC AUTO-IMMUNITY DURING THE IMMUNE RESPONSE:
IDIOTYPES AND ANTIGEN-BINDING SPECIFICITY OF ANTI-
BODIES AND T CELL RECEPTORS

R.Andersson, H.Binz,[2] H.Frischknecht,[2] B.Jonsson,
F.W.Shen,[3] and H.Wigzell

Department of Immunology, Uppsala University Biomedical
Center, Box 582, S-751 23 Uppsala, Sweden

ABSTRACT Auto-immunity at the level of anti-idiotypes is
able at both the humoral and cellular level to enhance
or inhibit specific immune responses. The very same agent
may depending upon external conditions cause a positive
or negative impact on a particular immune reaction. Subgroups of T lymphocytes specific for allo-MHC antigens can
be shown to display distinctly different idiotypes. This
may allow interactions between T cell subsets for reasons
of anti-idiotypic reactions rather than via collaboration
through reactions against antigenic determinants present
on the same molecule or particle. Earlier work showing
enhancing ability of IgM antibodies for sheep erythrocytes
when passively administered to recipients receiving sub-
optimal doses of immunogen may also in part function via
auto-immune , idiotypic interactions. In the system of allo-
MHC reactions auto-anti-idiotypic immunity can provide a
tool for induction of specific unresponsiveness in an adult,
immunocompetent individual. Problems still to be resolved
before this approach can be used in the clinic are discussed. Finally, purified internally labelled single chains
of rat MHC type (heavy chain Ag-B and heavy and light chain
"Ia" molecules) were tested for binding abilities to immunosorbants made up of IgG allo-antibody molecules or T
cell derived molecules selected for idiotypic markers signi-
fying reactivity against a particular allo-MHC haplotype.
In the combination analyzed (Lewis-anti-DA) the allo-antibody immunosorbant columns could be shown to retain all
three DA chains (= each chain must display alloantigenic
variability) whilst failing to show binding to syngeneic
Lewis or third party BN MHC molecules. On the other hand,
the idiotypic "Lewis-anti-DA" immunosorbant constructed
from normal T cell derived molecules displayed binding for
three chains: Ag-B and Ia heavy chains of DA origin
(= strongly bound) and syngeneic Lewis heavy Ia chain
(= weakly bound). The fact that BN chains failed to express
any detectable binding proved that normal, unimmunized T
cells are indeed selected for specific binding ability for

[2]Inst.Med.Mikrobiol. der Univ. Zürich, Zürich, Switzerland
[3]Mem.Sloan-Kettering Cancer Ctr., New York,N.Y. 10021, USA

self-MHC determinants. Furthermore, as the idiotypic T
cell molecules all display strong binding ability for DA
spleen cells whilst at the same time expressing measurable anti-self-MHC reactivity one would have to conclude
that allo-reactive T cells can also react towards self-
MHC determinants using the very same receptor molecules.

INTRODUCTION

Auto-immune reactions were previously considered to be dam-
aging or at best neutral to the individual. It has lately,
however, become apparent that reactions against self-components
may be of potential benefit for the individual and that anti-
self reactions do also seem to play a significant role in the
regulation of the normal immune response. The present talk will
largely deal with highly specific anti-self reactions occurring
at different levels of the normal immune response, how such
anti-self reactions may be directly determined at the level of
the antigen-specific T cell receptor molecules and how auto-
anti-idiotypic reactions may be used in the analysis and induction of specific unresponsiveness in adult immunocompetent individuals. The reader interested in other possible uses of
controlled auto-immune reactions such as fertility vaccines
and immune reactions against normally non-immunogenic, tumor-
associated antigens is recommended to read another article
(1).

AUTO-ANTI-IDIOTYPIC IMMUNITY

General Concept of Auto-Anti-Idiotypic Regulation. It has
been convincingly shown that auto-anti-idiotypic immune reactions occur with high frequencies under normal immunization
procedures (2). Likewise, evidence from several sets of data
suggest that such auto-immune reactions may function as positive or negative interacting units in the immune machinery in
a biologically significant manner (3,4,5). Thus, it would seem
clear that there indeed exist a functional interacting network
system (6) within the idiotypic-anti-idiotypic recognitive
system. Although several pieces of evidence exist proving the
above points much is unknown of the relative importance of such
interactions at the various levels of the immune system and how
these reactions may lead to stimulation or inhibition of the
various pathways involved.

Stimulation of antigen-specific immune reactions substituting antigen with presumed anti-idiotypic antibody molecules or receptors. Several groups have reported on such findings
using various anti-idiotypic systems (3,5) but we will here
for reasons of space restrict ourselves to our own results
within this area.

a. Induction of allo-antigen specific proliferating
or killer T cells using auto-anti-idiotypic antibodies. It is
possible to induce auto-anti-idiotypic antibodies specific for
allo-MHC reactive T cells by immunization with allo-antibody
molecules or purified T receptors (7), with selected heavy
chains from such specific IgG molecules (8) or using alloreactive T blasts generated in in vitro MLC cultures and subsequently injected back with adjuvant into syngeneic recipients (9). Useful titers of anti-idiotypic antibodies will
then be produced in a minority of the animals (10). Sera from
such animals can be used for further analysis of T cell receptors and cellular functions. If such antisera are used in the
presence of complement it is possible to selectively wipe out
the immune capacity of syngeneic T cells with regard to ability
to react against the relevant allo-MHC structures (11). Using
an antiserum produced in C57BL/6 mice against C57BL/6-anti-CBA
T MLC blasts it was thus possible via absorptions on Ly-1 or
Ly-2 positive anti-CBA T blasts to selectively remove the cytolytic reactivity against either Lyt-1 positive, proliferating
anti-CBA T cells or Lyt-2 positive, anti-CBA killer T cells
(see table 1). The data presented demonstrated quite clearly
that Lyt-1 and Lyt-2 C57BL/6 T cells with specificity for CBA
MHC allo-antigens not only express the expected selective
immune capacity as to function (12) but do also express what
seems to be largely distinct, non-overlapping idiotypes (13).
Likewise, immunization with Lyt-1 and 2 positive anti-CBA T
blasts yielded similar selective reductions in immune reactivity in C57BL/6 mice against the CBA MHC antigens.
However, when such auto-anti-idiotypic sera are used in
vitro in the absence of extraneous complement we have fre-
quently instead of inhibition observed opposite effects, namely
proliferation and induction of specific functions (8). It is
thus possible to induce a second set of proliferation of T cells
in already primed MLC T blasts when adding the relevant auto-
anti-idiotypic serum. Likewise, successful induction of specific allo-reactive killer T cells were noted using as responder
cells T cells from the spleens of unimmunized mice of relevant strains (8,13). In the latter case it was in fact possible
to show that auto-anti-idiotypic antisera were superior "immunogens" than the corresponding allogeneic spleen cells allowing
purified Lyt-2 T cells to be initiated into efficient CTL:s in

the absence of helper Lyt-1 T lymphocytes (see table 2) (for details see 13). The ability of the anti-idiotypic serum to induce killer T cells under these conditions is thought provoking but should still be regarded at the level of phenomenology. It is thus possible that a few Lyt-1 T cells were still around in the supposed Lyt-2 pure population functioning as helper T cells after induction by anti-idiotypic molecules. One way to analyze this would be to absorb such antisera with the corresponding Lyt-1 anti-CBA MLC blasts and then study whether the ability to induce CTL:s was left unperturbed. Alternatively, the ability of the anti-idiotypic serum to substitute for helper T cells in the generation of CTL:s could be taken as an argument that these T cells may in fact elaborate help via anti-idiotypic specificities after having been induced by i.e. Ia alloantigens. This is at present sheer speculation but the hypothesis is easily testable using MLC supernatants under limiting conditions and proper idiotypic immunosorbants. It would indeed be fascinating would anti-allo-Ia reactive T cells turn out to also be selected for anti-idiotypic reactivity against anti-H-2 specific T cell receptors.

TABLE 1

C57BL/6-ANTI-CBA T BLASTS OF LYT-1^+2^- OR 1^-2^+ PHENOTYPE HAVE DIFFERENT IDIOTYPES AND FUNCTION

Serum	MLC response		CML activity	
	CBA	DBA/2	CBA	DBA/2
Normal	100%	100%	100%	100%
Anti-id	12.0%	112%	32.1%	88.6%
Anti-id abs Lyt-1^+2^-	78.4%	106%	38.2%	87.8%
Anti-id abs Lyt-1^-2^+	18.5%	100%	84.8%	81.8%

Anti-id = A C57BL/6 anti-C57BL/6-anti-DBA T blast serum known to contain anti-idiotypic antibodies (13). The serum was used in presence of rabbit complement to treat normal C57BL/6 T cells before MLC or already immune C57BL/6 T-MLC cells before CML tests.
MLC response in % of control response = 100%. Likewise for CML. Conditions as previously described (13). Absorption of anti-id serum carried out using C57BL/6-anti-CBA T blasts at 0°. Anti-Lyt-1 and -2 specific antisera for the corresponding Lyt-alloantigens were used in the presence of rabbit complement to selectively lyse the respective Lyt-positive cells before absorption of anti-id serum.

TABLE 2

INDUCTION OF CTL:S IN NORMAL T CELLS: A COMPARISON
BETWEEN ALLOGENEIC SPLEEN CELLS AND AUTOANTIIDIOTYPIC
ANTIBODIES WITH REGARD TO TRIGGERING ABILITY

Responder cells	Stimulating agent	CTL analyzed at day 6		
		$H-2^k$	$H-2^b$	$H-2^d$ targets
C57BL/6 T	CBA spleen cells	70.4%	-0.7%	4.5%
"	Anti-id serum	64.2%	0.6%	3.5%
C57BL/6 Lyt-1$^+$2$^-$	"	6.3%	-0.4%	0.9%
C57BL/6 Lyt-1$^-$2$^+$	CBA spleen cells	5.8%	2.3%	0.8%
"	Anti-id serum	64.0%	-0.8%	2.7%

CTL activity as % specific ^{51}Cr-release. Anti-id serum of
specificity = C57BL/6-anti-C57BL/6-anti-CBA T blasts.
Effector/target ratio = 12.5/1.

b. Preliminary evidence that a sizeable amount of the
helping ability of IgM-anti-SRBC antibodies may be of anti-
idiotypic nature. It has for long been known that IgM antibodies against antigens, particularly erythrocytes, may help
the humoral response against sub-optimal concentrations of
immunogen whilst IgG antibodies mostly act in the opposite,
inhibitory manner (14,15,16). In table 3 are summarized some
of the observations obtained by earlier workers when studying
this phenomenon.

TABLE 3

IgM-ANTI-SRBC ANTIBODIES ENHANCING IgM-ANTI-SRBC
SYNTHESIS: EARLIER FINDINGS

A) Antigen-specific enhancement
B) IgM is the active factor as shown by euglobulin
   preparations, gel filtration, sucrose gradient
   centrifugation or purification of anti-IgM immunosorbants
C) The enhancement requires presence of T cells
   (= does not replace T cells)
D) Is only functioning in certain dose intervals of
   antibody versus antigen
E) Antibody must be given before antigen to exert any
   sizeable impact
F) "Species and strain-specific properties of IgM seem
   to be of some consequence but not desicive for its
   enhancing property"

(see 14-16)

We have repeated and confirmed essential parts of the results of the earlier workers. Attempts were then made to compare the helping ability of IgM-anti-SRBC antibodies obtained
from early bleeds of mice identical as to MHC but differring
among other things with regard to heavy chain Ig genes. Purified IgM antibodies were tested in the same or the allogeneic
strain for ability to help the humoral antibody response
against suboptimal amounts of SRBC using a criss-cross approach.
Table 4 shows in a summary form one such experiment (out of 3
similar) demonstrating a quite clearcut strain specificity when
carrying out the "help"; that is help was always superior in
the autologous situation.

TABLE 4

STRAIN RESTRICTED HELP OF IgM-ANTI-SRBC ANTIBODIES FOR
IgM ANTI-SRBC ANTIBODY SYNTHESIS

Recipient	Origin of anti-SRBC	$PFC/10^6$ spleen	Relative* mean
CBA	CBA	1208	100%
"	AKR	468	38%
"	---	36	3%
AKR	CBA	280	36%
"	AKR	785	100%
"	---	2	0.3%

$4 \cdot 10^5$ SRBC given i.v. day 0. One hour later 0.1 ml IgM-
anti-SRBC hemolytic titer 1:4096 i.v. Day 6 test for
PFC in spleen.

   *100% = $PFC/10^6$ achieved when administered IgM-anti-
   SRBC was syngeneic

These experiments are preliminary. Yet, they suggest that
a sizeable part of the earlier observed helping activity of
IgM antibodies may occur because of idiotypic (anti-idiotypic)
rather than antigen-binding abilities of the administered antibodies. The use of mice congenic as to heavy chain Ig loci should
confirm or abrogate this present claim (one experiment carried
out is in support of this). It should be realized, however, that
it is quite clear from many earlier studies that class and antigen-binding specificity of antibodies may also be highly decisive as to specific regulation of the immune response (17).

ELIMINATION OF ANTIGEN-SPECIFIC IMMUNE REACTIONS
VIA AUTO-ANTI-IDIOTYPIC REACTIONS

Auto-anti-idiotypic immunity induced by the administration of antigen-specific T blasts generated in MLC reactions
using adjuvant can cause significant, specific depletion of
allo-reactivity in adult mice (9), rats (18) and primates (19).
Evidence that such specific unresponsiveness is caused by auto-
anti-idiotypic immune reactions at both the humoral and cellular levels is summarized in table 5. Likewise,. in the same
table are listed various adjuvants used when attempting to
achieve such specific unresponsiveness and problems encountered
when trying to induce specific transplantation tolerance in
this system. Here reproducibility (= only a fraction of the
auto-blast immunized individuals become suppressed to close to
complete levels) and variability in suppression (= when testing
for immune unresponsiveness in vivo beyond the MLC assay) con-
sistute areas which must be improved if this approach should
reach clinical trials.Examples of the impact of variability
between in vitro and in vivo assays are given in table 6 where
in a group of 10 Lewis rats which were close to 100 % MLC
suppressed in a specific manner against DA only 5 turned out
to be specifically tolerant when grafted with heart grafts of
DA compared to third party BN type. However, on the positive
side it should be recalled that so far no negative side effects
(i.e. kidney damage etc) have been noted subsequent to a successful and long-lasting immunosuppression induced by the auto-
blast procedures.

It is likely that further improvement using this approach
will come when antisera against constant regions of IgT chains
become readily available. This would allow the purification of
antigen-specific, idiotypic molecules from in vitro lymphocyte
cultures followed by the use of such autologous molecules in a
polymerized form to induce specific reductions or eliminations
of immune reactivity against allo-MHC structures in a way already found feasible (7).

EVIDENCE AT THE MOLECULAR LEVEL THAT ALLO-MHC REACTIVE
PURIFIED T CELL RECEPTORS CAN EXPRESS AUTO-IMMUNE, SELF-
MHC REACTIVITY

It has for long been known that a sizeable fraction of
normal T lymphocytes can express specific immune reactivity
when tested against a foreign MHC haplotype. This has been
shown using MLC (20), GvH (21) or idiotypic markers (22).Like-
wise, it is now well established that helper and killer T
cells within the individual can be shown to express clonally
derived receptors for self-MHC determinants (23,24) having

TABLE 5

ELIMINATION OF ALLO-MHC SPECIFIC RESPONSIVENESS VIA
AUTO-ANTI-IDIOTYPIC REACTIONS: EVIDENCE, CONDITIONS
AND PROBLEMS

A. Evidence of anti-idiotypic immunity as a cause of
   unresponsiveness
   1) Unresponsiveness can be induced by polymerized,
      syngeneic idiotypic molecules (IgG alloantibodies,
      heavy chains from these molecules, T cell derived
      chains) or MLC activated, purified T blasts.
   2) Unresponsiveness can be shown to be accompanied
      by active signs of auto-anti-idiotypic immunity
      (production of anti-idiotypic antibodies, induc-
      tion of anti-idiotypic killer and suppressor T
      cells).
   3) These induced anti-idiotypic agents can by them-
      selves also induce the same specific unresponsive-
      ness as the initial treatment.
B. Requirement for certain adjuvants to induce efficient
   unresponsiveness
   1) In the syngeneic situation efficient induction of
      specific unresponsiveness requires the use of ad-
      juvants.
   2) Successful adjuvants in this regard has been Freund´s
      complete adjuvant and some dimuramylpeptide rea-
      gents. Unsuccessful adjuvants include Freund´s
      incomplete adjuvant, Bordetella pertussis alum and
      LPS.
C. Problems in relation to possible clinical trials
   1) Variability with regard to efficiency of induction
      of unresponsiveness. Many auto-immunized animals
      fail to become suppressed. Reasons unknown.
   2) Variability with regard to correlating in vitro MLC
      suppression data with in vivo immune reactivity:
      Sometimes comparatively normal in vivo reactions
      may occur despite a close to complete suppression
      in MLC (see table 6).

been selected for such reactivity via passage over the thymic
epithelium (25,26). It is also suggested from several sets
of data that allo-reactive T cells may contain cells with
detectable activity against modified syngeneic cells (27,28,
29). It is still, however, debated whether allo-reactive T
cells are heteroclitic (= inclined to react against hetero
(30)) cells with their "proper" specificity being directed
against self-MHC (or self-MHC plus some additional determinant

or change) or if they constitute a population of cells clearly distinct from the anti-self-MHC reactive T cells (for the latter opinion see 31).

We have recently been able to demonstrate that allo-reactive T cells receptor can express significant selective affinity for self-MHC structures in addition to their relevant allo-MHC binding ability (32). The following system was used: Immunosorbants were made up of IgG Lewis-anti-DA allo-anbibodies or Lewis T cell receptors idiotypic for anti-DA reactivity and purified from normal Lewis serum using anti-Lewis-anti-DA idiotype-specific immunosorbants (33). Such immunosorbants were tested for ability to retain single, internally labelled chains of allo- or self-MHC nature (these chains were purified using alloantibody immunosorbants followed by reduction and purification via recycling using PAGE methodology). The results are summarized in table 7 and represent the results obtained in three large experiments yielding virtually identical profiles of separation. As seen, the Lewis-anti-DA alloantibody immunosorbant displayed selective ability to bind in a strong, retaining manner each of the three DA MHC chains analyzed (= the Ag-B heavy plus the two "Ia" chains). As this retention was selective (the columns failed to display any significant binding ability to Lewis or third party BN MHC chains) this would mean that MHC chains have enough renaturing ability to express alloantigenic determinants even after the comparatively rough purification procedures. Likewise, the results mean that alloantigenic variability can be detected at the serological level at all three groups of MHC chains (now disregarding that we do not know if the "Ia" molecules are only representative of part of the Ia-like determining region in rats). When the T cell receptor immunosorbant columns were tested, they expressed strong binding ability for only two of the DA MHC chains, namely the Ag-B heavy and the heavy "Ia" chains. Similar binding properties have been observed at the level of MLC activated rat T blasts (34). This may thus mean that T cells may only be "seeing" antigenic determinants coded for by these two MHC chains (or arising as an interaction between these chains and other structures). It should be realized, however, that this restricted ability may not be of general validity with regard to anti-MHC reactive T cells but may be confined to certain combinations.

When the T receptor columns were analyzed for binding ability to self-MHC chains a significant binding was noted with regard to one chain, the syngeneic Lewis heavy "Ia" chain, whereas no binding was detected when screening BN MHC chains. Thus, the Lewis-anti-DA T cell-derived molecules which can be shown to bind to DA spleen cells to close to 100% (32) do also

TABLE 6

SPECIFIC MLC UNRESPONSIVENESS IN LEWIS RATS IMMUNIZED
WITH LEWIS-ANTI-DA T BLASTS MAY NOT CORRELATE OF IN
VIVO REJECTION RESPONSE

Reduction in MLC reactivity against DA alloMHC antigens

Responder cells	Stimulator cells	Thymidine incorporation
Auto-anti-DA T	DA spleen	2.155 ± 146
-"-	BN "	17.984 ± 1.175
Normal Lewis T	DA "	24.484 ± 1.709
-"-	BN "	15.197 ± 817

Selective increase in survival of LewisxDA F_1 heart grafts

Recipients	LewisxDA F_1 grafts	LewisxBN F_1 grafts (days)
Auto-anti-DA Lewis	9,10,10,11,12,42, >180,>180,>180, >180	9,9,9,9,10,10, 10,10,11,11
Normal Lewis rats	8,9,9,9,10	9,10,10,10,11

display a weak but selective affinity towards Lewis self-MHC
determinants. We thus consider that these results show that
allo-reactive T cells indeed can also express clonally derived receptors binding to self-MHC using the very same
receptor for these two interactions. Furthermore, the results demonstrate at the molecular level that indeed normal
T cells have been skewed towards self-MHC reactivity when
undergoing maturation in the absence of deliberate immun-
zations. The fact that only the heavy Ia and not also the
self-Ag-B chain was retarded on the T cell receptor columns
we deem at present to quite likely be a technical artefact
(= the majority of the soluble T cell receptors isolated from
serum are most likely anti-Ia rather than anti-Ig-B in the
specificity). Experiments using purified anti-allo-Ag-B
reactive T cell molecules would be necessary to solve this
latter question.

The present results should also mean that the elimination of allo-MHC reactive T cells of a particular specificity
would cause a simultaneous depletion of cells with anti-self-
MHC reactivity (= normal helper or killer T cells). However,
this would only result in the "normal" elimination occurring
in the present idiotypic constellation in a (LewisxDA)F_1
hybrid. No evidence exist that F_1 hybrids in general are less
immunocompetent than their corresponding parents.

TABLE 7

FINE ANTIGEN-BINDING SPECIFICITY OF IgG LEWIS-ANTI-DA
ALLO-ANTIBODIES AND LEWIS-ANTI-DA T CELL RECEPTOR
MOLECULES

| Antigens** | Immunosorbants* | | |
	Lewis normal IgG	Lewis-anti-DA IgG	Lewis-anti-DA T
DA,Ag-B	−	+++	+++
DA,H-Ia	−	+++	+++
DA,L-Ia	−	+++	−
Lewis,Ag-B	−	−	−
Lewis,H-Ia	−	−	+
Lewis,L-Ia	−	−	−
BN,Ag-B	−	−	−
BN,H-Ia	−	−	−
BN,L-Ia	−	−	−

*   Immunosorbants = CNBR-Sepharose columns to which had
    been coupled the above reagents. Lewis-anti-DA IgG
    was obtained from Lewis rats immunized thrice with
    DA cells. Lewis-anti-DA T cell derived material was
    isolated as previously described (32) from normal
    Lewis serum using an anti-Lewis-anti-DA idiotypic
    immunosorbant.
** Antigens = Single polypeptide chains of MHC nature
    obtained from internally labelled LPS blasts of
    corresponding genotype using detergent lysates,
    Lewis-anti-DA IgG immunosorbants, reduction and
    PAGE techniques to obtain the single chains.
+++ = strong binding of virtually all chains applied =
    complete retention.
+   = weak binding of virtually all chains as indicated
    by significant retardation of passage.

ACKNOWLEDGEMENTS

This work was supported by Swedish Cancer Society, by
Swiss Cancer Society 135-AK-79, by Swiss National Science
Foundation grants 3.688-0.76 and 3.194-0.77, and by NIH grant
AI 13485-03.

REFERENCES

1. Wigzell, H. (1977). In "Autoimmunity" (Talal, ed.),
   pp, 693-707. Academic Press, New York, San Francisco,
   London.
2. Annales d'Immunologie, (1979). 130C, no. 2.
3. Cozensa, H. (1976). Eur.J.Immunol. 6, 114.
4. Urbain, J., Wikler, M., Franssen, J.D., and Collignon, C.
   (1977). Proc.Nat.Acad.Sci., U.S. 74, 5126.
5. Eichmann, K., Coutinho, A., and Melchers, F.(1977).
   J.Exp.Med. 146, 1436.
6. Jerne, N.K. (1974-5). Harvey Lect. 70, 93.
7. Binz, H., and Wigzell, H. (1977). Progress in Allergy
   23, 154.
8. Frischknecht, H., Binz, H., and Wigzell, H. (1978).
   J.Exp.Med. 147, 500.
9. Andersson, L., Binz, H., and Wigzell, H. (1976). Nature
   264, 778.
10. Binz, H., and Askonas, B. (1975). Eur.J.Immunol. 5, 618.
11. Auget, M., Andersson, L.C., Andersson, R., Wight, E.,
    Binz, H., and Wigzell, H. (1978). J.Exp.Med. 147, 51.
12. Cantor, H., and Boyse, E.A. (1977). Cold Spring Harb.
    Symp.Quant.Biol. 41, 23.
13. Binz, H., Frischknecht, H., Shen, F.W., and Wigzell, H.
    J.Exp.Med. in press.
14. Möller, G., Wigzell, H. (1965). J.Exp.Med. 121, 969.
15. Henry, C., and Jerne, N.K. (1968). J.Exp.Med. 128, 133.
16. Dennert, G. (1971). J.Immunol. 106, 951.
17. Uhr, J.W.,and Möller, G. (1967). Adv.Immunol. 19, 201.
18. Andersson, L., Aguet, M., Wight, E., Andersson, R.,
    Binz, H., and Wigzell, H. (1977). J.Exp.Med. 146, 1124.
19. Ahmed, A. Personal communication.
20. Wilson, D.B., Blyth, J.L., and Nowell, P.C. (1968).
    J.Exp.Med. 128, 1157.
21. Ford, W.L., Simmonds, S.J., and Atkins, R.C. (1975).
    J.Exp.Med. 141, 681.
22. Binz, H., Bächi, T., Wigzell,H., Ramseier, H., and
    Lindenmann, J. (1975). Proc.Nat.Acad.Sci., (U.S.) 72, 3210.
23. Paul, W.E., Shevach, E.M., Thomas, D.W., Pickeral, S.F.,
    and Rosenthal, A.S. (1976). Cold Spring Harb.Symp.Quant.
    Biol. 41, 571.
24. Zinkernagel, R.M., and Doherty, P.C. (1975). J.Exp.Med.
    141, 1427.
25. Fink, P.J., and Bevan, M. (1978). J.Exp.Med. 148, 766.
26. Zinkernagel, R.M., Callahan, G.N., Althage, A., Cooper, S.,
    Klein, P.A., and Klein, J. (1978). J.Exp.Med. 147, 882.
27. Shearer, G.M., and Schmitt-Verhulst, A.M. (1977).
    Adv.Immunol. 25, 55.

28. Bevan, M. (1977). Proc.Nat.Acad.Sci., U.S. 74, 2494.
29. Finberg, R., Burakoff, S.J., Cantor, H., and Benacerraf, B. (1978). Proc.Nat.Acad.Sci., U.S. 75, 5145.
30. Mäkelä, O. (1965). J.Immunol. 95, 378.
31. von Bockmer, H., Haas, W., and Jerne, N.K. (1978). Proc.Nat.Acad.Sci., U.S. 75, 2439.
32. Binz, H., Frischknecht, H., and Wigzell, H. J.Exp.Med., submitted.
33. Binz, H., and Wigzell, H. (1975). Scand.J.Immunol. 4, 591.
34. Fenner, M., Frischknecht, H., Binz, H., Lindenmann, J., and Wigzell, H. Scand.J.Immunol., in press.

ISOLATION AND PRELIMINARY CHARACTERIZATION OF HAPTEN REACTIVE MOLECULES FROM AFFINITY-ENRICHED AZOBENZENEARSONATE-SPECIFIC T CELLS[1]

George K. Lewis, Peter V. Hornbeck, and Joel W. Goodman

Department of Microbiology and Immunology, University of California School of Medicine, San Francisco, California 94143

ABSTRACT   Azobenzenearsonate-specific T cells were enriched from the spleens of A/J mice, primed 2 to 3 weeks earlier with ABA-conjugated mouse IgG, by adsorption of a T cell-enriched fraction onto ABA-coated plastic surfaces. Subsequent to release from the antigen-coated plates by cooling to 0°C, cell proteins were endogenously labelled by a 4 hour pulse with ^{35}S-methionine. The cells were lysed with Tris-buffered 0.5% NP-40 in the presence of protease inhibitors and the lysates were passed over ABA affinity columns. ABA-specific molecules were eluted by free hapten and analyzed by sodium dodecyl sulfate-polyacrylamide gel electrophoresis, which revealed a major specific band at 90,000 to 95,000 daltons. Additional minor bands were observed in the range of 30-45,000 daltons. Immunoprecipitation studies failed to reveal the presence of classical Ig determinants on the 90,000-95,000 dalton protein.

INTRODUCTION

Several recent investigations of the specificity of T cell regulation have resulted in the paradoxical conclusion that some T cells have receptors expressing idiotypes (1), while other T cells have receptors which recognize idiotypes (2). Although it is possible that different Lyt subsets express either idiotype or anti-idiotype recognition structures, it is perhaps equally likely that both types of recognition structures occur within a single Lyt subset. Thus, idiotype-anti-idiotype recognition may occur between Lyt subsets or within a single Lyt subset. While it is possible to obtain indirect evidence for one or the other of the above hypotheses by functional studies with idiotype-bearing and idiotype-recognizing T cells, a formal decision between the two alternatives requires the direct molecular analysis of the T cell recognition structures themselves. Such an analysis could also shed light on the third possibility that both types of

[1]This work was supported by NIH grant AI 05664-16 and NCI contract NO1 CB 74178.

461

recognition are normal T cell regulatory network elements.

If it is assumed that T cell recognition structures function at the cell surface, then several criteria should be established before a molecule is correctly called a recognition structure:

(1) The molecule should be demonstrable at the cell surface by either antigen-binding or idiotype-binding; (2) The functional activity of the cell should be affected by either antigen or anti-idiotype; (3) The putative receptor molecule should be in exact geometric association with the appropriate ligand as shown by procedures such as co-capping; (4) The putative receptor should be isolated by affinity chromatography from cell population which shows an identical specificity; (5) The recognition structure must be synthesized by the T cell in question.

Using the criteria outlined above, we will describe our most recent attempts to establish procedures which may permit the direct molecular analysis of T cell recognition structures.

METHODS

Immunizations and Cell Fractionation. The details of antigen preparation, immunization, and cell fractionation have been published elsewhere (3). Briefly, A/J mice were immunized ip with 100 μg of azobenzenearsonate-mouse-γ-globulin (ABA-MGG) in CFA. Two to three weeks later, single spleen cell suspensions were prepared and the B cells removed by passage over anti-Ig-coated plastic plates (3). This procedure generally gives preparations with B cell contamination of 5% or less. The T cell-enriched fraction was then allowed to settle onto plastic plates precoated with ABA-autologous mouse serum albumin (ABA-MSA). After 1 hour at room temperature, the non-adherent cells were removed and the plates washed and transferred to a melting ice bath. The adherent cells were recovered after 30 minutes by gentle pipetting. Generally, 1-2% of the total immune spleen cells adhere to ABA-MSA-coated plates.

Biosynthetic Labelling of Cell Proteins with ^{35}S-Methionine. Affinity enriched, ABA-primed T cells were cultured at 2×10^7 cells/ml in methionine-free Dulbecco's modified Eagle's medium (DME) containing 2.5% fetal calf serum. ^{35}S-methionine (>1000 Ci/mM) was added to a final concentration of 1mCi/ml at the beginning of culture. After 4 hours, the cells were diluted with cold PBS containing 2mM methionine to stop incorporation. The cells were then washed three times with cold PBS/methionine and lysed in Tris buffered NP-40 (0.05M Tris, 0.5% NP-40, 0.01M EDTA, 2mM

methionine, 20 units/ml trayslol, and 1mM PMSF). In some
experiments, the lysis buffer also contained 2 mM dithiothreitol and/or 0.15M NaCl. During lysis, the cell concentration was 5×10^7 to 10^8 cells/ml. After 15 minutes on ice
the lysates were spun at 10,000 X g for 10 minutes and stored
at -70C.

ABA-Specific Affinity Chromatography. Both ABA-BGG-
Sepharose-4B and ABA-tyraminyl-Affigel-10 were used with comparable success to purify ABA-binding molecules from T cell
lysates. Controls included both BGG-Sepharose-4B and tyra-
minyl-Affigel-10. Generally, 30 µl of lysate was loaded onto
30 µl of affinity or control matrix using a plastic 1 ml
tuberculin syringe as a column. The gel was held in place
by a piece of filter paper and the column flow regulated by
a three-way stopcock. After a 2 hour incubation at room T°,
the column was washed with 9 ml of lysis buffer and allowed
to run dry. For hapten elution, 30 µl of 10^{-3}M bis-2,4-
azobenzene-arsonyl-histidine (bis-RAH) was loaded onto the
column, followed by an additional 2 hour incubation period
at room T°. After incubation, the orange free hapten band
was allowed to pass through the column followed by a 400 µl
wash. During elution, fractions of three drops were collected. Subsequent to hapten elution, the column was washed with
3 ml of lysis buffer and allowed to run dry. Non-specifical-
ly binding material was eluted with 9M urea/0.5% NP-40.
Again, three drop fractions were collected.

After affinity chromatography, the samples were analyzed
by SDS-PAGE as described by Laemelli (4). Reduction and
alkylation were performed as described by Lane (5). In preliminary experiments, it was found that reduction and alkylation in the presence of hapten caused ^{35}S-proteins to precipitate; therefore, these experiments were performed only
on molecules purified by urea elution from ABA-BGG Sepharose.

RESULTS

Characteristics of Affinity-Enriched ABA-Specific T Cell
Populations. The serological and biological characteristics
of the affinity-enriched ABA-specific T cell populations used
in this study are listed in Table 1.

Although the preparations were clearly enriched for most
of the markers assayed, the cell populations were not abso-
lutely pure. Therefore, in the experiments to be cited
below, it should be remembered that the precise phenotype of
the cells from which the molecules were extracted remains
unknown.

TABLE 1

CHARACTERISTICS OF AFFINITY ENRICHED
ABA-SPECIFIC T CELLS

Serological or Biological Characteristics	Fraction of Positive Cells
Thy-1	~95%
Ig	2-6%
Ia^k (A.TH α A.TL)	60-80%
I-J^k [B10.A(3R) α B10.A(5R)]	20%
Antigen-binding by immunofluorescence	50-90%
Antigen-binding by rosetting	20%
Cross-reactive idiotype	54%
ABA-specific suppression	enriched 25-250 fold

ABA-Specific Micro-Affinity Chromatography.   Both ABA-BGG-Sepharose-4B and ABA-tyraminyl-Affigel-10 were used as affinity matrices with comparable success.   The results of an experiment using ABA-BGG-Sepharose and BGG-Sepharose are shown in Figure 1.   When free hapten was used as the eluant, approximately 10 times as much radioactivity was eluted from the ABA-BGG-Sepharose column as from the control BGG-Sepharose column.   In contrast, subsequent elution with 9M urea/0.5% NP-40 brought comparable amounts of radioactivity off both the ABA-BGG-Sepharose and the control BGG-Sepharose columns.   Additionally, irrelevant antigens (e.g., BSA) failed to selectively elute counts off the ABA-BGG-Sepharose column.   Therefore, these results document the specificity of the microimmunosorbent technique and demonstrate the feasibility of enriching T cell-derived ABA-binding molecules by micro-affinity chromatography.

Molecular Weight Analysis of T Cell-Derived ABA-Binding Molecules.   After enrichment on affinity columns, T cell-derived ABA-binding molecules were analyzed by SDS-PAGE.   The results of a single experiment are shown in Figure 2.   In this experiment, a ^{35}S-labelled lysate was passed over an ABA-tyraminyl-Affigel-10 column, the unbound material was washed off and the bound material was sequentially eluted with 10^{-3}M bis-RAH followed by 9M urea/0.5% NP-40.   Several bands of radioactivity having molecular weights ranging from approximately 55,000 to 120,000 were eluted by hapten (track H, Fig. 2).   In contrast, urea brought off only one major band at 45,000 m.w. (track U, Fig. 2).   Although several bands were eluted by free hapten in this particular experiment, only the

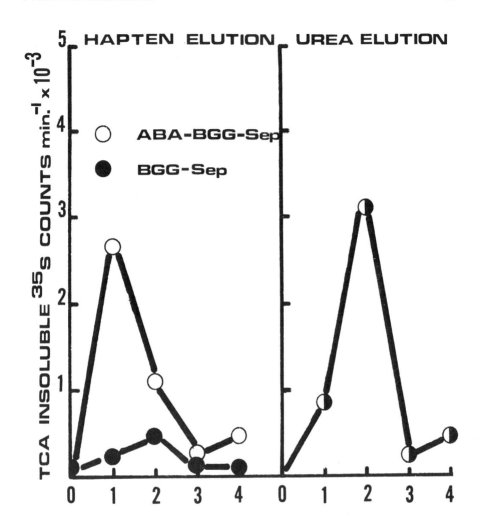

FRACTION NUMBER

FIGURE 1. Sequential elution by hapten and urea of a
^{35}S-methionine labelled, ABA-specific T cell lysate from
either ABA-BGG Sepharose or BGG-Sepharose columns.

protein migrating at 95,000 daltons has invariably shown
specificity. This protein binds only to ABA-columns and not
to control columns, and is always eluted by free ABA. In
contrast, as judged by both binding to control columns and
hapten elutions, the specificity of the smaller proteins has

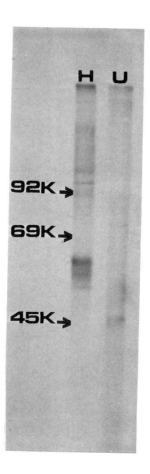

FIGURE 2. SDS-PAGE analysis of T cellderived ABA-
specific and non-specific molecules sequentially eluted from
ABA-tyraminyl-Affigel-10 by hapten and urea,respectively.

been variable. Since the reason for this is unknown, the
present report will focus on the 95K (p95) band. In our
earliest studies, p95 was not seen, but there was a corresponding increase of proteins having molecular weights in the
range of 50-60,000 and 30-40,000. Protease inhibitors in the
lysis buffer diminished these bands while p95 became more
apparent. These results suggest that p95 is degraded by
intracellular proteases released during lysis. Another interesting feature of p95 is that it often exists as a doublet

(Figure 2), which may be due to differences in glycosylation. Of particular significance, it should be noted that p95 is not found in lysates of an A/J anti-ABA producing B-cell hybridoma (31C3.2), where classical heavy (IgG$_1$) and light (κ) chains are apparent, thus providing an indirect argument for the T cell origin of p95.

Since the azo-linkage is reduced by sulfhydryls, we have been unable to perform satisfactory reduction and alkylation experiments on hapten-eluted material. On the other hand, reduction and alkylation of (1) whole cell lysates, (2) 95K material eluted by urea from ABA columns, and (3) SRBC-specific 95K material isolated from suppressive Con A-induced supernatants, have failed to reduce the apparent molecular weights of these 95K bands. Therefore, it is probable that p95 is monomeric. Since most of our lysates (including the one in Fig. 2) had 2mM dithiothreitol as a component of the lysis buffer, it is possible that p95 exists <u>in vivo</u> as a disulfide linked dimer. Recent preliminary findings, based on an experiment in which lysis was performed in the absence of a reducing agent, suggest that this may be the case. However, further experimentation is required to clarify this point.

T Cell-Derived p95 Molecules Lack Classical Immuno-
<u>globulin Determinants</u>. The presence of Ig and I-J^k deter-
minants on p95 was investigated by reacting ^{35}S labelled lysates from affinity enriched ABA-specific T cells with various anti-Ig and anti-I-J^k reagents, followed by immuno-precipitation with protein-A-bearing <u>Staphylococcus aureus</u> (6; Opperman, personal communication). After washing with Tris-saline (0.2M Tris, 1M NaCl), precipitated material was eluted with TUS (0.02M Tris, 6M Urea, 2% SDS) and analyzed under reducing conditions by SDS-PAGE. Using these proce-dures, we failed to precipitate p95 from any of our lysates using several anti-μ, anti-γ, anti-α, anti-κ and anti-λ reagents. These reagents readily precipitated classical heavy and light chains from control lysates as well as from highly labelled T cell lysates in which B cell contamination was 2% or greater. These findings suggest that p95 lacks conventional Ig determinants.

Similar experiments have been done using anti-I-J^k and rabbit anti-CRI. Although the anti-CRI had a titer of 40 μg/ml and the anti-I-J^k readily killed suppressor T cells, these antisera failed to precipitate p95. It is possible that the titers were not high enough for this immunoprecipitation technique. Clearly, positive controls are needed before the expression of these determinants can be definitively resol-ved.

DISCUSSION

Perhaps the most striking feature of p95, in comparison to T cell-derived antigen-binding molecules described by others, is its size. Most other reports cite monomer sizes of approximately 70-75,000 m.w., while p95 is approximately 20,000 daltons heavier. Although these differences may be partially attributable to such factors as cell sources and variation in degree of glycosylation, the most probable cause may be variable degradation by endogenous proteases. In the present investigation, the presence of protease inhibitors during lysis was essential for the recovery of p95. Interestingly, Taussig et al. (7) have recently reported an 85K dalton antigen-specific suppressor molecule. In collaboration with Dr. Daniele Primi, we have isolated a similar molecule which co-migrates with p95. Although these findings are highly suggestive, formal proof of identity awaits peptide mapping and sequencing of the two molecules.

The absence of classical Ig determinants on p95 is in excellent agreement with the findings of most other investigators. On the basis of these studies, it seems that T cells synthesize antigen-specific molecules having a unique heavy chain. Since we have consistently failed to find light chains in association with p95, our data support other investigations which point to the absence of conventional light chains on T cell-derived molecules.

Although our preliminary findings suggest that it is possible to chemically characterize T cell-derived antigen-binding molecules, the degree to which these molecules can be analyzed is limited by the number and purity of available cells. In a large series of experiments, we have found it difficult to obtain more than 4×10^7 affinity-enriched T cells, and such preparations are invariably contaminated with small numbers of B cells. While the B cell contamination appears to be non-specific, their products may interfere with the sensitive microchemical techniques required for receptor analysis. An obvious solution to these difficulties would be to make ABA-specific T cell hybridomas. Such efforts are currently in progress.

In summary, the present investigation clearly demonstrates the feasibility of isolating hapten-specific molecules from affinity-enriched, determinant-specific T cells. These preliminary observations should facilitate more detailed studies when ABA-specific T cell lines are available.

ACKNOWLEDGEMENTS

The authors wish to thank Drs. H. Opperman, R. Steinberg

and D. Primi for advice and discussions during the course of this work.

REFERENCES

1. Julius, M.H., Augustin, A., and Cosenza, H. (1977). "ICN-UCLA Symposium on Immune System: Genetics and Regulation" (E.E. Sercarz, L.A. Herzenberg and C.F. Fox, eds.), Vol. 6, p. 179. Academic Press, New York.
2. Owen, F.L., Ju, S.-T., and Nisonoff, A. (1977). Proc. Natl. Acad. Sci. USA 74, 2084.
3. Lewis, G.K., and Goodman, J.W. (1978). J. Exp. Med. 148, 915.
4. Laemmli, U.K. (1970). Nature 227:680.
5. Lane, L.C. (1978). Anal. Biochem. 86, 655.
6. Kessler, S.W. (1975). J. Immunol. 115, 1617.
7. Taussig, M.J., and Holliman, A. (1979). Nature 277, 308.

SPECIFIC TARGET CELL LYSIS BY SUPERNATANTS DERIVED
FROM ALLOIMMUNE MURINE CYTOTOXIC T LYMPHOCYTES:
POSSIBLE ROLE OF A LYMPHOTOXIN-T
CELL RECEPTOR COMPLEX

John C. Hiserodt, Gale A. Granger, and Benjamin Bonavida

Department of Microbiology and Immunology
UCLA School of Medicine
Los Angeles, California 90024

ABSTRACT   Lymphocytes or purified T cells obtained from
spleens or peritoneal exudate (PEL) of alloimmune
C57Bl/6 or BALB/c mice, when placed on monolayers of
lectin (PHA) coated allogeneic fibroblasts, rapidly
release (6-8 hr) into the supernatant antigen specific
cell lytic material(s). These supernatants could induce
rapid (10 hr) and *specific* lysis of the sensitizing
allogeneic target cells during *in vitro* [51]Cr release
assays. Analysis of the lytic supernatant revealed the
following properties: a) antisera which could neutralize murine lymphotoxin (LT) activity *in vitro* could
inhibit this effect; b) absorption of supernatants on
the specific target cells at 4°C removed both the specific lytic activity and nonspecific LT activity detectable on L-929 cells *in vitro;* c) polyspecific goat anti
mouse Ig sera had no effect on this lytic activity, and
removal of T cells by anti θ serum + C' removed the
capacity of the remaining cells to release these materials; and d) this material(s) was highly unstable.
Furthermore, biochemical fractionation of lytic supernatants by molecular sieving revealed the specific cell
lytic activity eluted in the void volume or in the
region of the high MW LT complex. Because the lytic
effects could not be shown to be due to classical Ab +
C', and since purified alloimmune T lymphocytes yielded
the most active supernatants, we feel the data is consistent with the concept that the short-lived specific
cell lytic material in these supernatants is a high MW
complex containing LT or LT-like molecules in functional
association with specific T cell antigen binding recep-
tor(s) molecules.

INTRODUCTION

Thymus derived cell-mediated cytotoxicity has been shown to require direct contact between the effector and target cell prior to the lytic step (1, 2, 3). However, the biochemical processes involved in cell lysis are largely unknown. Several unsuccessful attempts have been made to demonstrate the involvement of a soluble cytotoxic mediator(s) in T cell mediated cytotoxicity (4). Lymphotoxins are cell lytic proteins released *in vitro* by activated lymphoid cells from experimental animals and man. The most commonly detected and studied MW forms ($\leq$70,000 MW) can cause lysis or growth inhibition of certain target cell types *in vitro,* depending upon their concentration and the type of indicator cell·employed (5). However, because LT molecules are released into the soluble phase, appear to be nonspecific, and are slow acting, it has been difficult to envision their role as general effectors in cytotoxic reactions which require aggressor-target cell contact and in which cell lysis is unidirectional and highly specific. The present studies were designed to examine if alloimmune murine T lymphocytes could be activated to release lymphotoxin-like molecules that cause specific target cell lysis *in vitro.*

MATERIALS AND METHODS

Spleen cells were obtained from normal or alloimmune C3H, C57Bl/6, or DBA/2 mice immunized 11 days prior by IP injection of 10^7 allogeneic tumor cells (P815 or EL4). The adherent cells were removed by incubation in T flasks for 1 to 2 hours at 37°C. The nonadherent lymphocyte rich population was then activated by placing the lymphocytes (2.5 X 10^6/ml) on monolayers of PHA coated L929 cells (PHA/929) at a 40:1 ratio in serum free RPMI-1640 plus antibiotics. The lymphocytes and PHA/L cells were allowed to interact at 37°C for 6-8 hrs after which the supernatants were collected, concentrated 10-20 X by ultrafiltration and immediately tested for toxic (LT) activity on mitomycin C treated L-929 cells (6), or for lysis of ^{51}Cr labeled allogeneic target cells in a 10 hr ^{51}Cr release microplate assay. Two different rabbit antisera were also developed which will neutralize the capacity of murine LT molecules to destroy L-929 cells *in vitro:* a) polyspecific antisera made against protein-free fresh whole supernatant from activated normal C57Bl/6 splenic lymphocytes; and b) sera from an animal immunized with the (140,000-160,000 d) α_H MW LT class. The production and characteristics of these sera have been described in detail elsewhere (7).

RESULTS

Initial experiments were designed to test whether LT activity present in supernatants of nonspecifically activated alloimmune spleen cells could be functionally associated with target cell specific antigen binding receptor(s). Normal or alloimmune lymphocytes or nylon wool enriched (95% to 98% Ig negative) T cells were activated on monolayers of PHA/L cells for 8 hr, and the supernatants collected and incubated with various numbers of specific or unrelated target cells for 30 min at 4°C. The absorbed or control supernatants were then tested for LT activity on L-929 cells. Shown in Table 1 are representative experiments which indicate that absorption of alloimmune (C57 anti-P815 or DBA/2 anti-EL4) supernatants on the specific sensitizing target cell removes nonspecific LT activity detectable on L-929 cells *in vitro*. Up to 48% of the total LT activity could be removed when "immune" supernatants were incubated with the specific target cells, but little effect was observed when these same supernatants were absorbed on syngeneic or nonrelated allogeneic target cells. Furthermore, similar levels of LT activity were removed (46%) when supernatants collected from nylon wool enriched alloimmune T lymphocytes were absorbed on the specific sensitizing target cell (Table 1, Exp. 2).

Experiments were also designed to determine if soluble mediators released by alloimmune spleen or purified T cells were lytically active. Supernatants from alloimmune cells were produced as previously described, rapidly concentrated and tested for lytic activity on various target cells in a 6-10 hr ^{51}Cr release assay, and simultaneously tested for nonspecific LT activity on L-929 cells. Supernatants from enriched T cell populations or populations depleted of T cells by treatment with anti θ serum + C' were also tested. Shown in Table 2 are the results of several such experiments. In general, murine lymphoid cells (immune or nonimmune) released high levels of LT activity, detectable on L-929 cells, when activated on PHA/L cells *in vitro*. A lower but significant level of LT activity was also obtained on L cells in the absence of PHA. Furthermore, fresh supernatants collected from activated alloimmune lymphoid cells or alloimmune T cells caused significant levels of ^{51}Cr release when tested on the specific sensitizing target cell in 10 hr assays. In contrast, when the same supernatants were tested on syngeneic target cells, very low levels of ^{51}Cr release were observed. Finally, while nonimmune lymphoid cells did release high levels of LT activity detected on L-929 cells, these supernatants were not effective in causing ^{51}Cr release from P815 or EL4 target cells in the 10 hr assay. However, when

TABLE 1

SPECIFIC REMOVAL OF NONSPECIFIC LT ACTIVITY
BY INCUBATION OF IMMUNE SUPERNATANTS WITH
SPECIFIC TARGET CELLS *IN VITRO*

Exp.	Responder lymphocytes	No. of absorbing cells used/ml	% Neutralization of LT activity after absorption on:		
			P815	EL4	L929
1	C57 anti P815	2×10^6	19	0	1
		10×10^6	39	1	3
		40×10^6	45	5	4
2	C57 anti P815 (T lymphocytes)	10×10^6	37	2	0
		40×10^6	46	5	0
3	Normal C57	40×10^6	4	6	3
4	DBA/2 anti EL4	40×10^6	6	48	4

supernatants collected from nonimmune cells were assayed over
longer periods (i.e., 15-20 hr), a low but significant degree
of nonspecific lysis (5-10%) was observed (data not shown).
Furthermore, the results in Table 3 indicate these specific
cell-lytic effects are due to products released by activated
T cells, for nylon wool purified T cell populations (<4%
surface Ig[+] by immunofluorescence criteria) yielded very
active supernatants and treatment of unseparated alloimmune
spleen cells with anti-θ serum plus C' removed the capacity of
the remaining cells to release specific cell-lytic materials.
However, these supernatant effects were found to be highly
stable (half-life 30 min) at 37°C, and in experiments not
shown, polyspecific rabbit anti-mouse Ig serum had no effect
on this lytic activity, nor could fresh supernatants allowed
to lose activity by incubation for 2 hr at 37°C be reconstituted with fresh sources of mouse or guinea pig C'. These
data strongly indicate these effects are *not* due to cytotoxic
or cytophilic antibody plus C' components.
     To assess the biochemical nature of the labile materi-
al(s) having specific cell-lytic activity, supernatants were
subjected to rapid gel filtration chromatography employing AcA
44 and anti-LT neutralization studies. However, because of
the extreme instability of this activity, only minimal time
delay occurred between collection of supernatants,

TABLE 2

SPECIFIC TARGET CELL LYSIS BY SUPERNATANTS DERIVED FROM
ALLOIMMUNE MURINE CYTOTOXIC LYMPHOCYTES *IN VITRO*

Exp.	Effector cell	Units LT activity/ml (L929 cells)	Direct CML	% ^{51}Cr Release Supernatant killing on:	
				P815	EL4
1	C57 anti P815	600	42.5	24.6	3.3
	Normal C57Bl/6	510	2.3	0.4	1.2
2	C57 anti P815 (T cells)	410	69.8	33.6	4.2
	Normal C57 T cells	350	3.3	0.7	0.6
3	C3H anti P815	440	49.6	37.1	3.9
	C3H anti EL4	360	38.2	4.6	29.9
	Normal C3H	–	–	2.2	0.8
4	BALB/c anti EL4 (PEL)	–	53.6	6.1	41.2

TABLE 3

IDENTIFICATION OF EFFECTOR CELLS RELEASING SPECIFIC
CELL LYTIC MATERIALS AS T LYMPHOCYTES

Separation Technique	% ^{51}Cr release Supernatant killing on:		
	Direct CML	P815	EL4
Unseparated spleen[a]	36.7	13.9	2.4
Non adherent spleen cells	48.8	19.4	1.6
Nylon wool purified cells (T cells)	72.4	27.6	3.5
Spleen cells + (anti θ + C')	4.1	1.6	2.6
Nylon wool purified PEL	79.1	21.7	3.1

[a]Spleen cells were C57Bl/6 anti P815.

concentrattion, column chromatography, and assay on target
cells. Supernatants collected from activated C57 anti-P815
alloimmune spleen cells were concentrated 50 X and 2.0 ml was
chromatographed over a 2.5 X 55 cm Aca 44 column. Fractions
were collected in three pools corresponding to a) Pool 1 (Cx)

(the void volume) (>200,000 d); b) Pool 2 (α_H) (100-150,000 d); and c) Pool 3 (α_L + rest of column) (≤90,000 d). Each pool was then concentrated to 1 ml and assayed on ^{51}Cr labeled specific allogeneic targets, syngeneic targets, or LT sensitive L-929 cells. In addition, two different types of rabbit anti-LT sera recently developed were also tested. As can be seen in Table 4, significant ^{51}Cr release was induced from the P815 target cells by materials present in the void volume (or in the region of the high MW LT complex (8). Materials present in Pool 2 or Pool 3 only induced low levels of ^{51}Cr release during a 10 hr microplate assay. It should be noted that the normal distribution of various nonspecific LT MW classes were detected on L-929 cells. Finally the two anti-LT sera effectively neutralized the cell-lytic activity observed in these supernatants or MW pools.

TABLE 4

EFFECT OF HETEROLOGOUS RABBIT ANTI-LT SERUM ON THE SPECIFIC *IN VITRO* LYSIS OF ^{51}Cr LABELED P815 TARGET CELLS MEDIATED BY HIGH MW SUPERNATANT COMPONENTS RELEASED BY ACTIVATED ALLOIMMUNE MURINE LYMPHOID CELLS

Fraction tested	% ^{51}Cr release in the presence of:				
	NRS (100 μl)	Anti-WS (25 μl)	% Inh.	Anti-α_H (100 μl)	% Inh.
C57 anti-P815 whole supernatant (50 X conc.) (25 μl)	40 ± 2	12 ± 1	(65)	19 ± 3	(50)
Pool 1 (Cx) (100 μl)	11 ± 1	2 ± 1	(85)	3 ± 1	(75)
Pool 2 (α_H) (100 μl)	2 ± 1	0	(100)	0	(100)
Pool 3 (α_L + Rest) (100 μl)	0	0		0	

DISCUSSION

These experiments indicate that nonspecific LT activity, measured on L-929 cells, was removed when fresh supernatants

from activated immune cells were absorbed on specific target
cells and not removed by non-related targets. Moreover, no
target cell binding materials were evident in supernatants
from nonimmunized donors. Removal of LT activity was due to
binding to target cell surface structures, for all absorptions
were conducted rapidly (30 min) at 4°C. It is hypothesized
that the soluble cytotoxic material is a complex formed by LT
and the putative antigen specific T cell receptor (termed LT
C_x-R). However, it is not yet evident if the LT complexes and
T receptor molecules are released together as a single unit by
the activated lymphocyte or associate after the receptor has
reacted with antigen. Data not presented here supports the
former situation.

These findings confirm previous studies which revealed LT
molecules from lectin activated alloimmune human lymphoid
cells can associate with target cell specific antigen binding
receptor(s). While the physical-chemical nature of the
receptor materials in LT C_x-R forms is not known, certain of
these complexes are of T cell origin. That LT molecules are
associated with T cell receptor molecules is suggested by the
finding that specific target cell lytic forms were detected in
supernatants from activated purified T cell populations and
were not found in supernatants from T cell depleted cell populations. Additional studies, not shown here, reveal specific
P815 cell-lytic activity from alloimmune C57Bl/6 supernatants
was unaffected by polyspecific xenogeneic anti-murine Ig sera,
but totally inhibited by anti-α_H sera. These observations
suggest that the R material is not a traditional Ig molecule.
However, it is possible LT molecules could mask Fc region Ag
determinant sites. Similar and concurrent studies with LT
C_x-R forms from alloimmune human lymphocytes reveal reactivity
with anti-Fab$_2'$ (IgG) sera, but no reactivity with antisera
directed at human Ig heavy chain determinants (μ, γ, α). It
is significant that reactivity with anti-Fab$_2'$ may reflect
presence of V_H regions, which may be part of T cell recep-
tor(s), as suggested by Janeway et al. (9).

Supernatants from activated alloimmune or normal murine
lymphocytes possess different in vitro cell-lytic capacity.
These supernatants were rapidly concentrated and tested on
[51]Cr labeled P815 and EL4 targets in a 6-10 hr microplate
assay, and the standard 16 to 20 hr LT assay employing L-929
cells. Supernatants from both alloimmune or nonimmune cells
contained high levels of LT activity as measured on L-929
cells (up to 240 units of activity). While not shown here,
these supernatants are also capable of low level nonspecific
lysis (^{51}Cr release) of EL4 or P815 cells in a 16 hr assay
(0-10%). However, supernatants from alloimmune murine lymphocytes caused from 25 to 50% of the lysis of the specific

target cells *in vitro* in 6 to 10 hr assay. That this was
specific lysis was evident for: a) C57Bl/6 anti-P815 supernatants caused lysis of P815 cells and not EL-4; b) DBA/2
anti-EL-4 supernatants caused lysis of EL-4, and not P815; and
c) C3H alloimmune supernatants caused lysis of either EL-4
(C57Bl/6) or P815 (DBA/2) target cells, depending upon which
donor cell type the recipient C3H animals had been sensitized
against. The material(s) responsible for these "specific"
cell lytic effects was shown to be high MW (>200,000 d),
released by alloimmune T cells, highly unstable, and completely neutralized by rabbit anti-murine α_H-LT sera. In addition,
extensive experiments not shown in this manuscript revealed
these supernatant cell lytic effects are not due to classical
antibody and C'.

The present studies further support the concept that
lymphotoxins must be viewed in a new perspective, for they
appear to be part of an interrelated "system" of cell lytic
molecules. Based on these findings, a model was constructed
to explain the data and is described in a separate report (10).

The model suggests that upon receiving the appropriate
activating signals, the various MW LT subunits could be
assembled and focused as complexes around or with specific
receptor(s) on a target cell surface where they become, as a
result of collective action, highly cell-lytic. If Cx forms
are released into the soluble phase, they rapidly dissociated
into nonactive or weakly active subunits, so as not to affect
self tissues. The identification of similar physical and
functional forms of these molecules in several animal species
suggests this may be a common cell-lytic system, which has
been conserved through evolution.

ACKNOWLEDGMENTS

The authors wish to acknowledge R. S. Yamamato and G. J.
Tiangco for their excellent technical assistance.
This work was supported by NIH CA-12800 and in part by
CICR and the UCLA Cancer Center.

REFERENCES

1. Martz, E. (1977). In "Contemporary Topics in Immunobiology" (Osias Studman, ed.), 7, 301. Plenum Press, New York.
2. Goldstein, P., and Smith, E. T. (1977). In "Contemporary
   Topics in Immunobiology" (Osias Studman, ed.), 7, 273.
   Plenum Press, New York.
3. Berke, G., and Amos, D. B. (1973). Transplant. Rev. 17,
   71.

4. Henney, C. S. (1975). J. Reticuloendothelial Soc. 17, 231.
5. Granger, G. A., Daynes, R. A., Runge, P. E., Jeffes, E. W.
   B., and Priem, A. M. (1975). In "Contemporary Topics in
   Molecular Immunology" (F. P. Inman and W. J. Mandy,
   eds.), Vol. 4. Plenum Press, New York.
6. Spoffard, B. T., Daynes, R. A., and Granger, G. A. (1974).
   J. Immunol. 112, 2111.
7. Hiserodt, J. C., Tiangco, G. T., and Granger, G. A. (1979).
   J. Immunol. (in press).
8. Hiserodt, J. C., Yamamoto, R. S., and Granger, G. A.
   (1978). Cell. Immunol. 41, 380.
9. Janeway, C., Wigzell, H., and Binz, H. (1976). Scand. J.
   Immunol. 5, 993.
10. Hiserodt, J. C., Yamamoto, R. S., Tiangco, G. J., and
    Granger, G. A. (1979). Proc. Nat. Acad. Sci. (in press).

WORKSHOP SUMMARY: Molecular and Cellular Characterization of Antigen-binding Receptors

Workshop Conveners: John J. Marchalonis, NCI Frederick Cancer Research Center, Frederick, Maryland 21701; Darcy Wilson, Department of Pathology, University of Pennsylvania School of Medicine, Philadelphia, Pennsylvania; David Givol, Department of Chemical Immunology, Weizmann Institute, Rehovot, Israel

This workshop focused on the functional, serological and molecular properties of T-cell surface receptors and factors that exhibit specificity for foreign antigens. Although diverse experimental models were considered, a common theme emerged that antigen-specific T cells and factors express antigenic determinants associated with Ig V-regions and that these determinants are carried chiefly by a polypeptide of approximate mass 65,000-70,000 daltons.

Wilson introduced the problem of antigen recognition by T cells. This process is markedly specific, but has the striking property of responding to foreign antigen in association with products of the MHC. This is manifest in functional association of T_H cells with I region products and T_C cells with K and D end markers. Ir gene function is probably most stringent in presentation of antigen by macrophages, but a T-cell component might also be required. Furthermore, antigen-specific factors are now being described in systems showing genetic restriction. Are these factors related to T-cell surface receptors? Does study of them shed further light on the association of functional T-cell recognition with the MHC?

Givol introduced the structural and serological aspects of T-cell receptors for antigen. Recent evidence indicates that T-cell receptors can share V_H regions with serum antibodies and B-cell receptors (IgM, IgD) of similar specificity but that constant region determinants typical of serum or B-cell Ig isotypes probably do not occur on T cells. What new evidence could be considered regarding the following issues pertinent to expression of Ig V-regions by T cells: (1) Do T cells express V_H framework determinants as well as idiotypes? (2) Do T cell receptors express V_L determinants, including framework? (3) Are T-cell receptors of the form V_H/V_L (like antibodies), or V_H/V_H or V_L/V_L? (4) How do these interactions affect the relative affinities of T-cell receptors? (5) What kinds of constant region do T-cell receptors express?

The data and discussion were directed primarily to the nature of Ig V-region determinants occurring in antigen-

specific T-cell surface receptors and in specific suppressor
factors. Little new material was educed to explain the propensity of T cells to recognize antigen in association with
MHC products.

Several workers reported studies with anti-idiotype sera
which demonstrated the presence of idiotype-bearing receptors
on antigen-specific T cells. The response of strain A/J
mice to the arsonate hapten (ARS), originally reported by A.
Nisonoff et al., was a popular model system. The presence of
peripheral T cells (approx. 3%) reacting specifically with
ARS (G. Warr, J. Goodman) and bearing the anti-ARS idiotype
were reported. M. Greene and B. Bach described an ARS-
specific suppressor factor, which, likewise, carried the
anti-ARS idiotype and was produced by suppressor T cells.
Warr presented data showing the binding of the ARS-hapten by
both idiotype-bearing antibody in solution and idiotype-
bearing T-cell receptors in situ was blocked by anti-idiotype
antibodies. Also, specific binding of ARS by antibodies and
T cells was inhibited by chicken antibodies produced against
the Fab-fragment of normal serum IgG. The chicken antibodies
react with an interaction determinant formed by combination
of κ-chain and heavy chain Fd-region determinants. These
results suggest that the ARS-specific T-cell receptor contains
V_H-determinants, and might express V_L-determinants because
the anti-Id and chicken anti-Fab react with interaction
(V_H/V_L) determinants. Moreover, involvement of V_H framework
and other Fd-determinants (Warr), including allotypes (Greene),
was suggested. The latter possibilities require direct
serological or biochemical confirmation, particularly because
some workers were unable to detect V_H (a) allotypes on T cells
(rabbit; J. Jensenius).

H. Callahan and P. Maurer described the isolation of an
antigen-binding fragment from the plasma membranes of T cells
of BALB/c mice immunized with the random sequence synthetic
polypeptide L-GA (Glu ^{60}Ala^{40}). The immune-affinity purified
material had an apparent MW. of approx. 66,000 (PAGE) and
bound specifically to GA, but not to D-GLA or D-GAT (D-Glu^{60}-
D-Ala^{30}-D-Tyr^{10}) or L-GAT. R. Germain reported that antibodies to L-GAT express a widely cross-reactive idiotype
(found in all strains tested) and that T-cell-derived GAT-
specific suppressor factors bear this idiotype. It was of
considerable interest that the GAT-specific suppressor factor
could be bound by both anti-Id and by antibodies to I-J region
determinants. This result suggests that V_H and I-J determinants are either covalently or noncovalently associated in the
GAT-specific suppressor factor.

Specific antigen binding by murine T cells was described by D. DeLuca for normal T cells and fluorescent protein antigens, keyhole limpet hemocyanin, myoglobin and ferritin and by N. Ruddle for a T cell hybridoma that bound sheep erythrocytes. DeLuca found that about 0.5% of normal thymic T cells bound the protein antigens, and fluorescein-labeled chicken anti-mouse Fab allowed a critical test of the hypothesis that the Ig-like surface component on T cells is a primary receptor for antigen. In double-label experiments, anti-Fab and antigen were found to strictly coincide on both T and B cells, thereby suggesting that the Ig-like surface components carry out a receptor role. In control experiments, antigen did not codistribute with either Thy 1 or H-alloantigens. The T-cell hybridoma that bound SRBC biosynthetically incorporated ^{3}H-leucine into components of apparent mass (SDS-PAGE) of 68,000 and 45,000 daltons, which bound specifically to SRBC. Further antigenic and structural characterization of these components is eagerly awaited.

Cone described the production and specificity of rabbit antisera to Ig variable region framework determinants that react with a surface component of normal T cells and with an antigen (DNP or TNP)-specific factor produced by spleen T cells of tolerant mice. The specific suppressor factor is a single polypeptide chain of mass 68,000 daltons on SDS-PAGE. It does not bear known Ig constant region determinants, but is bound by antisera produced against Ig κ chains in association with variable region determinants.

There was much discussion of the properties of antigen-specific T-cell derived suppressor factors. It is not clear whether such factors are directly related to T-cell surface receptors for antigen, but they express idiotypic determinants (Germain, Greene) and possible V-region framework determinants (Cone) and have a major component of approx. 68,000 daltons (Greene, Cone), which is comparable in size to that of the heavy chain of the Ig-like T cell receptor (Marchalonis). An association with Ig allotype was also suggested (Greene, B. Rubin), and except for the GAT-specific suppressor (Germain) no association with the MHC was observed. Goodman isolated ARS-binding molecules from a T-cell population activated as suppressors. This factor had a major component on SDS-PAGE of approx. 90,000 daltons and lacked Ig constant region determinants, MHC determinants and Id. The ARS-specific cells, however, are Id[+]. Possibly the Id determinant might be labile under the conditions used to purify the factor. The 90,000 dalton factor might be a precursor of the 70,000 dalton fragments, which could arise via proteolysis.

Wigzell described the idiotype-bearing rat T-cell receptor. The molecule can occur as dimers or as monomers of a polypeptide chain of approx. 70,000 daltons. The molecule showed no association with MHC products. The chain was susceptible to proteolysis by chymotrypsin and papain with degradation products of approx. 50,000 and 25,000 daltons being produced.

Marchalonis presented serological and biochemical characterization data for the Ig-like T-cell receptor of normal mouse T cells and monoclonal T lymphoma cells. The molecule consists of a covalent dimer of heavy chains of mass 65,000-70,000 daltons. These heavy chains lack class-specific Ig determinants, but share Fd-region peptide determinants with heavy chains of serum Ig. Comparison of radioiodinated tyrosine-containing tryptic peptides of the T-cell heavy chain with serum Ig heavy chains by ion-exchange chromatography showed that the T-cell chain shared about 50% of its labeled peptides with μ and α chains. No similarity was found to the viral glycoprotein gp71, β_2 microglobulin or bovine serum albumin. The heavy chain was cleaved by limited tryptic proteolysis into fragments of approx. 50,000 and 35,000 daltons. Although the predominant component isolated was the heavy chain, small amounts of a component of approx. mass 25,000 daltons, which was not covalently bound to the heavy chain, was isolated. This material lacked κ chain constant region determinants, but showed some cross-reaction with myeloma κ chains, which was probably confined to the V-region. Ion exchange chromatographic comparisons of this chain with myeloma κ (MOPC 41) and λ (RPC 20) chains indicated that the T-cell product shared the two major labeled tyrosine-containing peptides with κ chain, but the two chains differed in other peptides. No clear similarity with λ chain was noted. The T-cell Ig heavy chain most probably represents a new isotype which shares V_H regions with serum and B cell surface Ig isotypes, but is restricted to the T-cell surface.

It is possible that T-cell-derived antigen-specific suppressor and helper factors are directly related to this surface component; but it is also possible that all of these components might share V_H-region structures but possess distinct constant region genes lying in the heavy chain gene cluster. The association of T-cell recognition with MHC products was not clarified in molecular terms during this workshop; but it is possible the V-regions are involved in primary recognition (binding of antigen), whereas MHC products are required for cell/cell interactions in activation and differentiation. We thank all of the participants for providing an informative and stimulating workshop.

MOLECULAR MODIFICATIONS IN VSV-INFECTED CELLS[1]

Paul L. Black, Ellen S. Vitetta, James Forman, Chil-Yong Kang
and Jonathan W. Uhr

Department of Microbiology, University of Texas Health Science
Center, Dallas, TX 75235

ABSTRACT   Three major observations have emerged from our
studies of molecular changes in P815 cells infected with
vesicular stomatitis virus (VSV). 1) Glycosylation of
H-2 and/or viral glycoprotein is a prerequisite for
lysis of infected cells by VSV-sensitized, H-2 identical
killer T cells. Treatment of P815 cells before and during VSV infection with the antibiotic Tunicamycin,
which specifically inhibited addition of sugars to polypeptides of glycoproteins, inhibited both glycosylation
of proteins and lysis of infected P815 cells by syngeneic, virus-immune killer cells. 2) VSV infection
caused a 50% decrease in the amount of H-2 on the surfaces of P815 cells 3 hr. after VSV infection. 3) Surface H-2 and viral proteins do not form a detergent-
stable association. P815 cells were surface-labeled,
then VSV-infected and lysed. The lysate was treated
with rabbit anti-VSV (or control) serum plus S. aureus.
Immunoprecipitation of VSV antigens failed to deplete
H-2 antigens.

INTRODUCTION

Infection of mice with a variety of viruses elicits the
development of cytotoxic T lymphocytes which can lyse syngeneic cells infected with the same virus. Lysis of infected
target cells requires expression of both viral determinants
and H-2K or H-2D antigens (1). However, the molecular nature
of the antigenic modification which cytotoxic T cells recognize on the surfaces of virus-infected target cells remains
unclear. Several possible mechanisms have been proposed (1).

[1]This work was supported by NIH Grants AI-11851,
AI-13448, AI-13111, and CA-20012.

Viral antigens may associate physically with surface H-2 molecules, and killer T cells could recognize such hybrid antigens. Alternatively, infected cells may express both viral and H-2 antigens as physically separate molecular entities on their surfaces, and cytotoxic T cells could recognize viral and H-2 antigens independently. An additional possibility not usually discussed is that viral infection may cause biosynthetic alterations in the cells' H-2K or H-2D antigens, and cytotoxic T cells could recognize such "altered-self" H-2 antigens. The aim of the present studies was to examine the molecular modifications which occur on the surfaces of virus-infected cells and which render such cells susceptible to lysis by syngeneic, virus-immune cytotoxic T cells.

METHODS

P815 cells (DBA/2 mastocytoma) were maintained by serial passage in vitro in Dulbecco's modified minimal essential medium containing 10% fetal calf serum and supplemented with glutamine and antibiotic-antimycotic mixture. Tunicamycin was used at a final concentration of 1 μg/ml; cells were pretreated with Tunicamycin for 18 hr. before labeling or virus infection. Vesicular stomatitis virus (VSV) of the Indiana serotype was used. VSV infection and cytotoxic assays were performed as described elsewhere (2). Cells were labeled by culturing for 6 hr. in the presence of ^{3}H-leucine (3), or were surface-labeled by lactoperoxidase-catalyzed radioiodination (4). Labeled cells were lysed in 0.5% Nonidet P40 (NP40) detergent, and the lysates chromatographed on Lens culinaris lectin-sepharose (LcH-sepharose). The lectin-adherent glycoprotein pool (GPP) eluted with 0.5 α-methyl mannoside, was treated with rabbit anti-mouse immunoglobulin serum plus Staphylococcus aureus (Cowan I strain bearing Protein A) to reduce non-specific binding. Supernatants were then immunoprecipitated with mouse alloantisera (plus goat anti-mouse serum) or rabbit anti-VSV serum (plus S. aureus). Anti-H-2^d serum was raised against BALB/c cells in C57.B16Ka mice; A.TH anti-A.TL was used as control. Specificity of the anti-H-2^d serum was established by immunoprecipitation of splenic lysates from B10.D2(H-2^d), B10(H-2^b), B10.A(4R) (H-2^{h4}), B10.M(H-2^f), B10.P(H-2^p), B10.Q(H-2^q), B10.RIII(H-2^r) and B10.S(H-2^s) mice. Rabbit anti-VSV serum was raised by immunization with detergent-lysed whole virions. The antiserum was adsorbed twice with an equal volume of uninfected P815 cells before use. Immune precipitates were washed, dissolved, and subjected to SDS-polyacrylamide gel electrophoresis (SDS-PAGE).

RESULTS

Role of Glycosylation in Susceptibility of Infected
Cells to Lysis by T Lymphocytes. As suggested earlier, viral
infection might induce an alteration in the carbohydrate
moiety of cell-surface H-2. In order to investigate the role
of the carbohydrate moeity, the glucosamine-containing antibiotic Tunicamycin (TM) was employed. Tunicamycin specifically inhibits addition of sugars to polypeptides of glycoproteins by preventing transfer of the core sugar N-acetyl
glucosamine to the dolichol-lipid carrier intermediate from
UDP-glucosamine (5, 6). P815 cells were treated for 16 hours
with TM (1 μg/ml) before VSV infection and/or labeling. Fig.
1 shows the inhibition of glycosylation of H-2 by TM. In the
top panel H-2 could not be detected in the GPP from lysates
of TM-treated cells. Untreated cells had a 45K H-2 peak in
the GPP, as shown in the bottom panel.

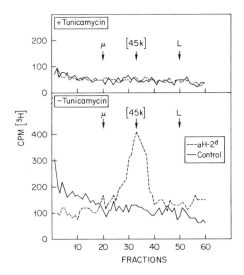

Fig. 1.   Effect of Tunicamycin on glycosylation of H-2.
P815 cells were incubated for 18 hr. in the presence or ab-
sence of TM (1 μg/ml), followed by labeling for 6 hr. with
^{3}H-Leu in the continued presence or absence of TM. Cells
were lysed, and the lysates chromatographed on LcH-Sepharose.
The adherent GPP were immunoprecipitated, the precipitates
dissolved and subjected to SDS-PAGE. Top panel + TM.
Bottom panel - TM.

Fig. 2 shows the effect of TM treatment on lysis of VSV-
infected P815 cells by syngeneic, VSV-immune effector cells.

TM treatment inhibited lysis. In contrast, TM treatment had no significant effect on lysis of P815 cells by alloimmune cytotoxic cells, as shown in Fig. 3.

VSV-IMMUNE SYNGENEIC KILLERS

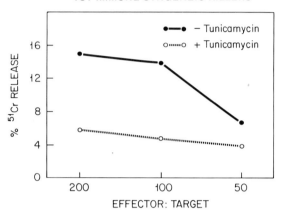

Fig. 2. Effect of TM treatment on lysis of VSV infected P815 cells by VSV-immune BALB/c spleen cells. P815 cells were treated with TM as described in Fig. 1, before and during VSV infection (2 hr.) and the cytolytic assay (4 hr.). Infection was done at a multiplicity of infection (MOI) of 50 plaque-forming units (PFU)/cell. MOI's of 500 and 5 were also tested, but not shown.

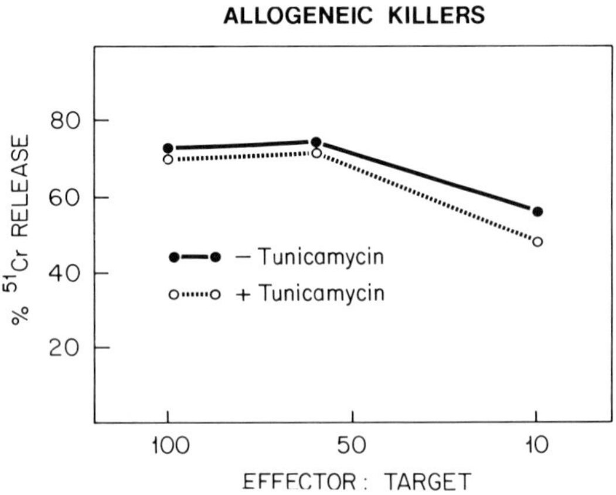

ALLOGENEIC KILLERS

Fig. 3. Effect of TM treatment on lysis of P815 cells by B10.PL spleen cells.

Effect of VSV Infection on the Expression of Cell Sur-
face H-2. Surface radioiodination of P815 cells following
VSV infection revealed a decrease in the amount of surface
H-2 on infected cells, compared with uninfected cells (Fig. 4).
The amount of H-2 in the GPP of VSV-infected cells was about
half that of uninfected cells. This finding suggests that

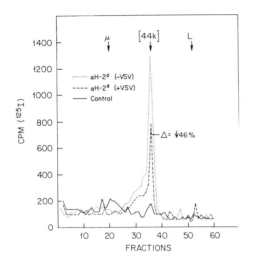

Fig. 4. Effect of VSV infection on expression of cell
surface H-2. P815 cells were surface radioiodinated 3 hr.
after VSV infection (or 3 hr. culture without VSV), lysed
and chromatographed on LcH-Sepharose. The adherent GPP were
immunoprecipitated, the precipitates dissolved and subjected
to SDS-PAGE.

surface H-2 is lost (internalized, shed or incorporated into
the viral envelope) during budding of the virus at the cell
surface. An alternative explanation is that virus infection
either sterically prevents radioiodination of surface H-2 or
alters the ability of surface H-2 to react with alloantibody.

Effect of Depleting VSV-Associated Antigens on the Recovery of H-2. One hypothesis to explain H-2 restricted
lysis of virus-infected cells proposes that H-2 and viral
antigens form a physical association on the cell surface. In
order to test this hypothesis, the effect of depleting VSV-
associated antigens on the recovery of H-2 was studied. P815
cells were surface radioiodinated, then infected with VSV,
lysed 3 hr. after infection, and chromatographed on LcH-
Sepharose. The adherent GPP was precleared and then depleted

of VSV-associated antigens by exhaustive treatment with
rabbit anti-VSV (or control hyperimmune) serum plus S. aureus.
The supernatants were then tested for H-2. If H-2 and viral
antigens form a detergent-stable physical association, then
depletion of VSV antigens should deplete H-2. As shown in
Fig. 5, depleting VSV antigens had no effect on the subsequent recovery of H-2. Thus, H-2 antigens do not form a
detergent-stable bond with viral antigens.

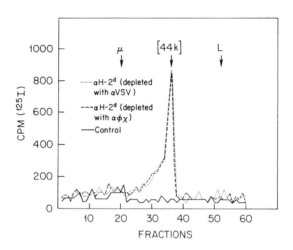

    Fig. 5. Effect of depleting VSV antigens on the recovery
of H-2. P815 cells were surface radioiodinated, infected with
VSV (MOI=50), lysed after 3 hr., and chromatographed on LcH-
Sepharose. The GPP was treated 2X with rabbit anti-VSV or
rabbit anti-ØX plus S. aureus and then with S. aureus alone.
Supernatants were immunoprecipitated, the precipitates dissolved and subjected to SDS-PAGE.

DISCUSSION

    The observations to emerge from our studies bear on the
hypotheses mentioned above to explain the modifications
occurring in H-2 restricted lysis of virus-infected cells.
    Thus, the antibiotic Tunicamycin, which prevents the
addition of sugars to polypeptides of glycoproteins (Fig. 1)
by inhibiting the N-acetyl glucosamine transferase (5, 6),
also inhibited the lysis of infected cells by VSV-immune,
syngeneic cytotoxic T cells (Fig. 2). Tunicamycin itself had
no effect on the lytic process as shown by the failure of
Tunicamycin treatment of target cells to inhibit allogeneic
lysis (Fig. 3). There are two possible explanations for the
inhibition of lysis by Tunicamycin. First, inhibition of

glycosylation blocks the surface expression of the glycoprotein (G) of VSV and thus prevents lysis. Second,
Tunicamycin causes the surface expression of a non-glycosylated H-2, which cannot be recognized by virus-immune
cytotoxic cells. Evidence from other laboratories favors the
first possibility. Thus, expression of VSV G protein is required for H-2 restricted lysis (2, 7, 8), and Tunicamycin
treatment inhibits the surface expression, but not the synthesis of VSV G protein (9). However, one cannot rule out
the other possibility that VSV infection causes an alteration
in the surface H-2 carbohydrate moiety, which is recognized
by virus-immune cytotoxic cells. Tunicamycin treatment would
prevent the expression of such an altered carbohydrate and
would thus inhibit lysis. We have no direct evidence to
exclude this intriguing hypothesis.

   Several different mechanisms could explain our observation of a decrease in surface H-2 antigen in VSV-infected
cells. VSV antigens may displace H-2 from the plasma membrane during the process of virus maturation and budding at
the cell surface with surface H-2 being either internalized
or shed from the cell. It is also possible that VSV
infection could block cell surface H-2 from radioiodination
or could alter the antigenicity of surface H-2 so that it no
longer reacts with alloantibody. In view of the short time
after VSV infection (3 hr.), it is unlikely that inhibition
or alteration in new H-2 synthesis could be responsible for
the major loss in H-2. Others (10) have shown decreases in
H-2 expression on VSV-infected cells by different techniques
and suggested that H-2 is displaced from the cell surface
during VSV budding by inclusion of H-2 in the virus envelope.
However, we have detected no decreases in H-2 when cells were
surface radioiodinated before VSV infection and their lysates
prepared and analyzed 3 hours after infection (data not
shown). This finding is consistent with internalization or
blocking of H-2 rather than its loss from the cell through
budding.

   Probably the most widely held hypothesis to explain H-2
restricted lysis of virus-infected cells is physical
association between viral antigens and H-2 on the cell surface. Evidence to support this view has come from studies
involving cocapping (11, 12), detection of H-2 in viruses
(10, 13), chemical crosslinking (14), and immunoprecipitation
and SDS-PAGE of transformed cell lines (15, 16). In particular, the last two studies (15, 16), which report detergent-
stable associations between histocompatibility antigens and
tumor-specific antigens, conflict with our findings. Our
studies failed to demonstrate association between H-2 and
viral antigens in detergent. Similarly, Fox and Weissman (17)

have failed to find a detergent-stable association between
H-2 and viral antigens.

In the early phases of this study (data not shown), we
found an apparent association between H-2 and a cellular
protein present on the cell surface before infection. When
P815 cells were surface labeled, then infected with VSV,
lysed and processed in the usual manner, immunoprecipitation
with rabbit anti-VSV and SDS-PAGE revealed a peak of >80K
mol. wt. However, uninfected cells showed the same peak, and
adsorption of the anti-VSV serum on uninfected cells removed
its capacity to precipitate this peak. This observation
emphasizes the problems in proving a molecular association
between H-2 and viral antigens using the above approaches.

ACKNOWLEDGEMENTS

We would like to thank Ms. J. Tsan and Ms. Y.M. Tseng
for technical assistance and Ms. J. Hahn for secretarial
assistance. Tunicamycin was the kind gift of Dr. Robert
Vandlen of Merck & Co. and of Dr. Robert Hamill of Lilly
Laboratories.

REFERENCES

1. Doherty, P.C., Blanden, R.V., and Zinkernagel, R.M.
     (1976). Transplant. Rev. 29, 89.
2. Forman, J., and Kang, C.-Y., submitted for publication.
3. Vitetta, E.S., Capra, J.D., Klapper, D.G., Klein, J.,
     and Uhr, J.W. (1976). Proc. Natl. Acad. Sci. USA 73, 905.
4. Baur, S., Vitetta, E.S., Sherr, C.J., Schenkein, I., and
     Uhr, J.W. (1971). J. Immunol. 106, 1133.
5. Takatsuki, A., Arima, K., and Tamura, G. (1971). J.
     Antibiot. 24, 215.
6. Tkacz, J.S., and Lampen, J.O. (1975). Biochem. Biophys.
     Res. Commun. 65, 248.
7. Hale, A., Witte, O.N., Baltimore, D., and Eisen, H.N.
     (1978). Proc. Natl. Acad. Sci. USA 75, 970.
8. Zinkernagal, R.M., Althage, A., and Holland, J. (1978).
     J. Immunol. 121, 744.
9. Leavitt, R., Schlesinger, S., and Kornfeld, S. (1977).
     J. Biol. Chem. 252, 9018.
10. Hecht, T.T. and Summers, D.F. (1972). J. Virol. 10, 578.
11. Schrader, J.W., Cunningham, B.A., and Edelman, G.M.
     (1975). Proc. Natl. Acad. Sci. USA 72, 5066.
12. Senik, A., and Neuport-Sautes, C. (1979). J. Immunol.
     122, 1461.
13. Bubbers, J.E., and Lilly, F. (1977). Nature 266, 458.

14. Zarling, D.A., Duke, R.E., Watson, A., and Bach, F.H. (1978). Fed. Proc. 37, 1570.
15. Kvist, S., Ostberg, L., Persson, H., Philipson, L., and Peterson, P.A. (1978). Proc. Natl. Acad. Sci. USA 75, 5674.
16. Callahan, G.N., Allison, J.P., Pellegrino, M.A., and Reisfeld, R.A. (1979). J. Immunol. 122, 70.
17. Fox, R.I., and Weissman, I. (1979). J. Supramolec. Struct. Supple 3, 327.

ALTERED EXPRESSION OF T-LYMPHOID CELL SURFACE ANTIGENS ASSOCIATED WITH VIRAL INFECTION[1]

Kim S. Wise, Susanne L. Henley, and Ronald T. Acton

Departments of Microbiology and Biology, and the Diabetes Research and Training Center, University of Alabama in Birmingham, Birmingham, Alabama 35294

ABSTRACT   Variants of a murine T-lymphoblastoid cell line (EL4) differing in their production of murine leukemia virus (MuLV) and in their expression of MuLV gene products at the cell surface, have similar morphological, growth and size characteristics, and express similar amounts of the normal T-cell surface differentiation alloantigen Thy-1. However, gene products of the $H-2K$ and $H-2D$ regions of the major histocompatibility complex (MHC) are present on the surface of the productively infected variant at a level approximately ten times that of the non-producing variant. Altering expression of $H-2$ products on the non-producing variant by infection with vesicular stomatitis virus (VSV), resulted in a concomitant and selective decrease in the expression of both $H-2K$ and $H-2D$ region products. VSV-infection of the MuLV producer line, however, resulted only in a modest decrease in $H-2K$ antigen expression, with no effect on $H-2D$ antigen expression. These results indicate possible differences between the two variant lines in cellular processing of $H-2$ antigens, and further suggest that $H-2K$ and $H-2D$ region products differ in their susceptibility to virus-induced alterations of surface expression in cells productively infected with MuLV.

INTRODUCTION

Virus replication and synthesis of viral products in T-lymphoid cells play a key role in numerous aspects of normal and neoplastic processes involving this cell population. Expression of MuLV-coded surface antigens on T-lymphoid cells of mice provides markers for normal events in differentiation (1,2,3) and signals the onset of neoplasia (4). In addition, expression of MHC $(H-2)$ antigens on thymocytes is markedly

[1]This work was supported by USPH grants CA18609, CA09128 and GM07561.

increased during early stages of infection with some oncogenic
viruses of mice (5), raising the possibility that control of
these antigens may be influenced in part by virus-induced
changes in the metabolic processes of T-cells. Recent studies
(6,7) suggest also that only certain functional subpopulations
of T-cells are capable of supporting replication of enveloped
viruses, such as the rhabdovirus, vesicular stomatitis virus
(VSV). Interestingly, infection of mouse lymphoblastoid tumor
cells with VSV and other enveloped viruses can also produce
marked changes in surface antigen expression, and can enhance
the potential of these cells (or cell membranes) to induce
anti-tumor responses *in vivo* (8,9,10). The expression of viruses and concomitant changes in surface membrane constituents
of lymphoid cells may then be fundamentally related to immunological phenomena associated with neoplastic diseases, and may
also reflect normal functional differences within lymphoid
cell populations. Clarification of these relationships would
be facilitated by a more detailed understanding of virus replication in lymphoid cells, and particularly, of virus induced
alterations of T-cell surface constituents.

A system is described in which selective increase of *H-2*
surface antigen expression is associated with MuLV production.
The effects of VSV infection on the expression of these antigens is also examined. This may provide a useful model for investigating possible virus-related control mechanisms regulating surface antigen expression on murine T-lymphoid cells.

MATERIALS AND METHODS

Cell Growth, Size Determinations and Phenotype. The
source and growth of EL4 murine T-lymphoblastoid cell lines
producing MuLV (EL4G+), or not expressing detectable amounts
of virus (EL4G-) have been described (8,11,12). Cell size was
measured in a Cytograf (Biophysics Systems, Inc., Mahopac,
N.Y.) as previously described (13). Results reported here
were obtained with cells taken from logarithmic growth phase,
and shown to be free of mycoplasmas by previously reported
methods (14).

Phenotypically, both lines express the Thy-1.2 differentiation alloantigen and $H-2^b$ histocompatibility antigens
(8,12). The EL4G+ variant line expresses the MuLV-related
Gross Cell Surface Antigen (GCSA,15,16) whereas this antigen
is not detectable on the EL4G- line (8,16). In addition to
GCSA, a marker of productive MuLV infection (15,17) the quantity of surface antigen related to the viral envelope glycoprotein gp70 is markedly elevated on the EL4G+ line compared to
the non-producing EL4G- line (8).

   Assays for Cell Surface Antigens. Quantitative absorption
of complement-dependent cytotoxic assays for lymphoid cell
surface antigens has been described in detail (8,13,18). Thy-
1 antigen was quantitated using goat antiserum to purified
Thy-1.1 (19), obtained from Dr. R.K. Zwerner of this department, diluted 1:60, and assayed against AKR/J mouse thymocytes
as target cells. $H-2^D$ specificities were measured in a similar assay system, using anti-$H-2D^b$ serum [(BALB/c x HTI)F_1
anti-EL4] (20), kindly provided by Dr. F. Lilly, Albert
Einstein College of Medicine, Bronx, N.Y., and used at a 1:8
dilution; or anti-$H-2K^b$ serum [antiserum D33: (B10.D2 x A)F_1
anti-B10.A (5R), from the Research Resources Branch, National
Institutes of Health], used at a 1:50 dilution. Both $H-2$
antisera were assayed on C57BL/6J splenocyte targets. Serum
dilutions represented approximately four times the concentration of antiserum needed to produce 50% cytotoxicity in the
respective assay system. Guinea pig serum (Flow Laboratories,
McLean, VA), diluted 1:3 in the appropriate medium, was added
to all cytotoxic reactions as a source of complement. Percent
inhibition and the absorption dose$_{50}$ (AD$_{50}$) were calculated as
previously described (13). Cell counts for all absorption assays were obtained directly from microplate wells following
the absorption step.
   A two-stage competition radioimmunoassay (RIA) was used
to assess quantitative differences in cell surface expression
of MuLV p30 determinants. Cultured cells were twice washed
and serially diluted with phosphate buffered saline (PBS). To
50 μl of each cell suspension, 50 μl of goat antiserum to AKR
MuLV p30 (No. 5S-333, obtained from the Office of Program Resources and Logistics of the National Cancer Institute and diluted 1:150 with PBS) was added in V-bottom 96-well Microtiter
plates (Dynatech Laboratories, Alexandria, VA). After thorough
mixing and incubation for 60 min at $0°C$, plates were centrifuged at 1000 x g for 10 min at $4°C$, and 50 μl of supernatant
transferred to empty wells. Fifty microliters of 0.5% sodium
deoxycholate in 0.01 M Tris hydroxymethylaminomethane, 0.5
mM phenylmethyl sulfonyl fluoride, pH 8.0 (DOC/Tris), containing approximately 3 x 10^5 trichloroacetic acid precipitable
counts per minute of ^{125}I-labeled p30 from Rauscher MuLV, was
then added to the wells. [Rauscher MuLV p30 was isolated from
preparative polyacrylamide gels by procedures previously described (21), using disrupted, fluorescamine labeled Rauscher
MuLV to mark the major p30 viral component. Purified p30 was
iodinated as described (21), resulting in a specific activity
of approximateley 10^7 CPM/μg protein]. After thorough mixing,
plates were incubated for approximately 18 hours at $5°C$.
Following incubation, 50 μl of formalin-fixed, DOC/Tris washed
Staphylococcus aureus (10% v/v) was added to each well to
precipitate immune complexes (22). After 4 rinses (1000 x g,

10 min, 4°C) with 0.15 ml DOC/Tris, radioactivity in final
pellets was determined in a Biogamma counter (Beckman Instru-
ments, Palo Alto, CA). Percent inhibition obtained for a given
number of absorbing cells was calculated as $[1-(CPM_n-CPM_o/CPM_c-CPM_o)]$ x 100, where CPM represents counts per minute in the
final pellet obtained with supernatants of absorption reactions
containing no antiserum (o), no cells (c), or cells at a given
concentration (n).

Infection of Cells with VSV. Infection of EL4 cells with
Indiana serotype VSV was performed by procedures described in
detail elsewhere (8,9), at a multiplicity of infection of
approximately 5 $TCID_{50}$ per cell. VSV-infected cultures were
used for absorption studies at 5.5 hours post infection (p.i.)
after maximal supernatant infectivity (typically $10^{7.5}$ $TCID_{50}$/
ml) was reached, but before the onset of viral cytopathogeni-
city (8).

RESULTS

Quantitative Comparison of EL4G- and EL4G+ Cell Surface
Antigens. Both EL4G+ and EL4G- cells shared size and certain
phenotypic characteristics. The two lines were indistinguishable by comparison of scatter/absorption histograms, indicating similar sizes, and hence surface areas (Figure 1A). In
addition, quantitative absorption assays for Thy-1 antigen
indicated that the amount of surface Thy-1 exposed per cell
was the same on both EL4G+ and EL4G- variant lines, as reflected in the identical AD_{50} values obtained from absorption data
(Figure 1B).
    In contrast, GCSA, a serologically defined set of anti-
genic specificities residing on MuLV *gag* gene products at the
cell surface (23,24,25,26) is expressed on the EL4G+ MuLV
producing line *in vitro*, but is not detectable on EL4G- cells
by standard cytotoxicity assays (8). Identification of a more
restricted set of *gag* gene products residing on the surface of
EL4G+ cells is illustrated in Figure 2, which depicts inhibition of a two-stage competition RIA for MuLV p30 by EL4G+ and
EL4G- cells. Lack of p30 determinants on the EL4G- line and
their presence on EL4G+ cells productively infected with MuLV
confirms the phenotypic difference in MuLV *gag* gene expression
between these variant cell lines, and demonstrates that p30-
containing portions of *gag* gene products are accessible to
antibody at the cell surface.

Increased *H-2* Antigen Expression Associated with MuLV
Production. Quantitative comparison of *H-2* antigen surface
expression on EL4G- and EL4G+ cells revealed a marked eleva-

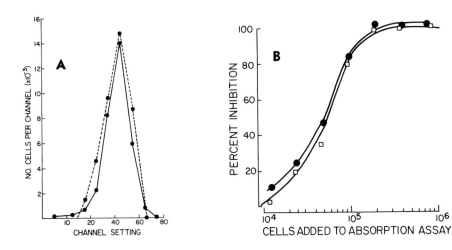

Figure 1. Size and antigenic similarities between EL4G+ and EL4G- cells. (A) Histogram comparing absorption/scatter properties of EL4G+ (———) and EL4G- (----) cells. (B) Analysis of Thy-1 antigen expression comparing EL4G+ (□———□) and EL4G- (●———●) cells by quantitative absorption of cytotoxic antiserum to Thy-1.

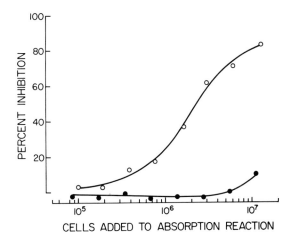

Figure 2. Expression of MuLV p30 on EL4G+ and EL4G- cells. Inhibition of antiserum binding to ^{125}I-labeled p30 by EL4G+ (0———0) and EL4G- (●———●) cells.

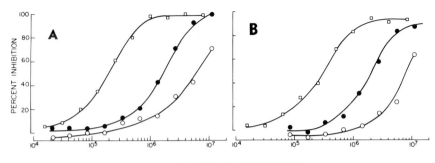

CELLS ADDED TO ABSORPTION ASSAY

Figure 3. Expression of H-2 antigens on EL4 cells.
Comparison of H-$2D^b$ (A) and H-$2K^b$ (B) expression by quantitative absorption of cytotoxic antiserum to these antigens by
EL4G+ (□——□) cells, EL4G- cells (●——●), or EL4G- cells
infected with VSV (0——0).

tion in the amount of both H-$2D$ and H-$2K$ region products per
cell on the MuLV-producing EL4G+ line (Figure 3). Absorption
of cytotoxic antiserum detecting H-$2K^b$ specificities resulted
in an AD_{50} (2.1 x 10^6 cells) for EL4G- cells, approximately
seven-fold higher than that for EL4G+ cells (3.2 x 10^5 cells),
indicating a much greater antigen activity per cell for the
EL4G+ line (Figure 3B). Similarly (Figure 3A) EL4G+ cells
showed a nine-fold greater amount of H-$2D^b$ surface antigen expression per cell (AD_{50} = 2.0 x 10^5 cells) compared to the
non-producing EL4G- line (AD_{50} = 1.8 x 10^6 cells). Thus, in
contrast to the similar levels of Thy-1 expressed on these
cell lines, a pronounced elevation in H-2 antigenic expression
was associated with MuLV production and expression of MuLV
gene products on the EL4G+ line.

     Altered H-2 Expression in VSV Infected EL4 Cells. To
investigate further effects of viral infection on H-2 antigen
expression at the surface of EL4 cells, and to evaluate the
possibility that replication of enveloped viruses in these
cells may generally produce increased levels of H-2 antigen
expression, quantitative absorption assays for H-2 antigens
were performed with EL4 cells following infection with VSV.
Comparison of VSV-infected and uninfected EL4G- cells revealed
a marked decrease in both H-$2K^b$ and H-$2D^b$ antigenic expression
occurring during VSV replication (Figure 3). By 5.5 hours
p.i., the amount of both H-$2K^b$ and H-$2D^b$ antigens per cell had
decreased in VSV infected EL4G- cells by a factor of approximately four. Increased H-2 antigen expression was not,
therefore, augmented in these cells by infection with VSV.
     Analysis of H-2 antigens on EL4G+ cells infected with

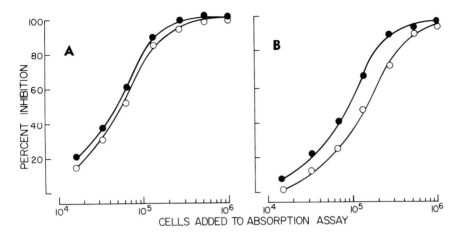

Figure 4. Effect of VSV infection on H-2 antigen expression in EL4G+ cells. Comparison of EL4G+ cells, either uninfected (●———●) or infected with VSV (O———O) by quantitative absorption of cytotoxic antiserum to H-$2D^b$ (A) or H-$2K^b$ (B) antigens.

VSV gave similar but not identical results (Figure 4). The specific activity of H-$2K^b$ antigens was also decreased on VSV infected EL4G+ cells, but only by a factor of two. However, no significant decrease in H-$2D^b$ expression was detected. Thus, the magnitude of VSV-induced changes in H-2 expression was less pronounced on the MuLV-producing EL4G+ line and, unlike VSV-induced changes in the surface expression of both K and D region products on EL4G- cells, a preferential decrease in H-$2K^b$ antigens was detected during infection of EL4G+ cells with this virus.

DISCUSSION

These findings describe an *in vitro* system which may be useful in examining mechanisms underlying changes in H-2 expression associated with productive infection of T-lymphoblastoid cells with MuLV. An association between increased MuLV production (and surface expression of MuLV gene products) and increased expression of both H-$2K^b$ and H-$2D^b$ products at the surface of these cells was established by comparison of variant cell lines differing in MuLV expression. The similarity of growth and size characteristics between these variant lines, and their nearly identical expression of the T-lymphoid surface antigen Thy-1, suggested that the concomitant elevation of MuLV and H-2 products is not merely a reflection of general-

ly increased expression of cell surface constituents or increased surface area of the MuLV-producing line.

Determining the effect of VSV infection on the surface
antigen expression in these two variants revealed further
interesting features of this model. While the non-producing
EL4G- line showed a marked and roughly similar decrease in
both $H-2K^b$ and $H-2D^b$ antigen expression during infection with
VSV, the EL4G+ line differed in its susceptibility to VSV-
induced alteration of $H-2$ surface expression. First, a significant but lesser decrease in $H-2K^b$ antigen expression was
observed during VSV infection of EL4G+ cells. Second, no
significant decrease in $H-2D^b$ expression was observed during
VSV infection of these cells. Thus the magnitude and selectivity of VSV-induced change differed between these variant
lines. Since VSV efficiently and rapidly inhibits protein
synthesis in both EL4G+ and EL4G- cells (K. S. Wise, unpublished observations), these results may reflect dissimilarities
in the metabolic fates of $H-2$ gene products in these two lines.
If the major effect of VSV infection is to terminate synthesis
of $H-2$ products, then there is an apparently slower "decay
rate" of $H-2$ surface antigens on EL4G+ cells; most notably the
disappearance of $H-2D^b$ antigens at the surface of these cells
is negligible during the time observed. These differences
could arise from greater initial synthesis rates, larger precursor pools, or decreased degradation of $H-2D^b$ gene products
in EL4G+ cells. These points may be clarified by ongoing
pulse-chase and metabolic inhibition experiments.

One possible mechanism by which MuLV production might
decrease $H-2$ degradation at the cell surface (which may normally occur by processes of enzymatic degradation or "shedding")
is the stabilization of $H-2$ products by direct interaction
with MuLV virions, a proposed phenomenon also invoked to explain a) $H-2$ associated restriction in the ability of immunocompetent cells to interact with virus antigens at the cell
surface (27), b) the apparent inclusion of $H-2$ antigens in
MuLV virions in the circulation (20) and c) the possible
attachment of MuLV to cells by interaction with $H-2$ "receptors"
(28). To assess in the present system any preferential association of $H-2$ gene products with MuLV particles, virions isolated from large scale cultures of EL4G+ cells (29) have been
measured to determine the specific activities of $H-2K^b$, $H-2D^b$
or Thy-1 (per protein) compared with a standard reference
preparation of membrane purified from the cells (29). These
studies (30) indicate that the relative proportions of $H-2D^b$
and $H-2K^b$ antigens in virus and membrane preparations are
indistinguishable by this technique, thus providing no evidence for preferential association of either $H-2D$ or $H-2K$ region specificities with MuLV isolated from EL4G+ cultures.
However, these studies have indicated a markedly increased

proportion of Thy-1 antigen (relative to *H-2* antigens) in virus preparations, compared with the proportion found in membranes. This result is compatible with (but does not prove) a preferential association of Thy-1 with MuLV virions, and raises the possibility that MuLV may interact with a number of cell surface glycoproteins not associated with products of the MHC. Our recent findings (14), that Thy-1 antigen is selectively associated with mycoplasmas in contact with lymphoblastoid cells, also underscores the interesting possibility that this membrane glycoprotein may have a particular propensity for interaction with membrane-bounded structures at the cell surface.

That MuLV production is associated with and may possibly regulate *H-2* antigen expression provides an impetus for further mechanistic analysis of these processes. In light of recent findings of markedly increased *H-2* expression on thymocytes during early stages of neoplasia induced by some oncogenic viruses of mice (5), and the apparent association between elevated *H-2* antigen expression and susceptibility to cell mediated lympholysis of virus infected cells (31), further investigations into the nature of possible interactions of MuLV with cell surface constituents may help elucidate these putative control processes.

ACKNOWLEDGEMENTS

We are grateful to Dr. Maurice Kemp for his help in preparing Rauscher MuLV p30, to Ms. Barbara Patterson and Mr. Jim Bradac for their helpful assistance in these experiments, and to Ms. Candy Gathings for preparation of this manuscript.

REFERENCES

1. Old, L. J., and Boyse, E. A. (1973). Harvey Lect. 67, 273.
2. Boyse, E. A. (1977). Immunol. Rev. 33, 125.
3. Del Villano, B. C., Nave, B., Croker, B. P., Lerner, R. A. and Dixon, F. J. (1975). J. Exp. Med. 141, 172.
4. Kawashima, K., Ikeda, H., Stockert, E., Takahashi, T. and Old, L. J. (1976). J. Exp. Med. 144, 193.
5. Meruelo, D., Nimelstein, S. H., Jones, P. P., Lieberman, M. and McDevitt, H. O. (1978). J. Exp. Med. 147, 470.
6. Bloom, B.R., Jimenez, L., and Marcus, P. I. (1970). J. Exp. Med. 131, 16.
7. Minato, N., and Katsura, Y. (1978). J. Exp. Med. 148, 837.
8. Wise, K. S., and Acton, R. T. (1978). In "Protides of the Biological Fluids" (H. Peeters, ed.), pp. 707-714. Pergamon Press, Oxford and New York.

9. Wise, K. S. (1977). J. Natl. Canc. Inst. 58, 83.
10. Lindenmann, J. (1974). Biochim. Biophys. Acta. 355, 49.
11. Acton, R. T., Barstad, P. A., and Zwerner, R. K. (1979). In "Methods in Enzymology" Vol. 48 (W.B. Jakoby and I.H. Pastan, eds.), pp. 211-221. Academic Press, New York.
12. Chesebro, B., Wehrly, K., Chesebro, K., and Portis, J. (1976). J. of Immunol. 117, 1267.
13. Zwerner, R. K., and Acton, R. T. (1976). J. Exp. Med. 142, 378.
14. Wise, K. S., Cassell, G. H., and Acton, R. T. (1978). Proc. Natl. Acad. Sci. USA. 75, 4479.
15. Old, L.J., Boyse, E. A. and Stockert, E. (1965). Canc. Res. 25, 813.
16. Aoki, T., Herberman, R. B., Hartley, J. W., Liu, M., Walling, M. J., Nunn, M. (1977). J. Natl. Cancer Inst. 58, 1069.
17. Boyse, E. A., Old, L. J., and Stockert, E. (1972). In "RNA Viruses and Host Genome in Oncogenesis" (P. Emmelot and P. Bentvelzen, eds.) p. 171. North Holland Publishing Co., Amsterdam, The Netherlands.
18. Barstad, P. A., Henley, S. L., Cox, R. M., Lynn, J. D. and Acton, R. T. (1977). Proc. Soc. Exp. Med. Biol. 155, 296.
19. Zwerner, R. K., Barstad, P. A., and Acton, R. T. (1977). J. Exp. Med. 146, 986.
20. Bubbers, J. E., Chen, S., and Lilly, F. (1978). J. Exp. Med. 147, 340.
21. Kemp, M. C., Wise, K. S., Edlund, L. E., Acton, R. T. and Compans, R. W. (1978). J. Virol. 28, 84.
22. Cullen, S. E., and Schwartz, B. D. (1976). J. Immunol. 117, 136.
23. Tung, J-S., Pinter, A. and Fleissner, E. (1977). J. Virol. 23, 430.
24. Snyder, H. W. Jr., Stockert, E., and Fleissner, E. (1977). J. Virol. 23, 302.
25. Ledbetter, J., and Nowinski, R. C. (1977). J. Virol. 23, 315.
26. Ledbetter, J. A., Nowinski, R. C., and Eisenman, R. N. (1978). Virology. 91, 116.
27. Zinkernagel, R. M., and Doherty, P. C. (1974). Nature (Lond.). 248, 701.
28. Schrader, J. W., Cunningham, B. A. and Edelman, G. M. (1975). Proc. Natl. Acad. Sci. USA. 72, 5066.
29. Zwerner, R. K., Wise, K. S., Acton, R. T. (1979). In "Methods in Enzymology" Vol. 48 (W. B. Jakoby and I. H. Pastan, eds.) Academic Press, New York.
30. Henley, S. L., Acton, R. T. and Wise, K. S. (1979). Fed. Proc. 38, 927 (Abstr. 3683).
31. Meruelo, D. (1979). J. Exp. Med. 149, 898.

MHC-RESTRICTION AND DIFFERENTIATION OF T CELLS[1]

Rolf M. Zinkernagel

Department of Immunopathology, Scripps Clinic
and Research Foundation
La Jolla, California 92037

Thymus-derived lymphocytes (T cells) are generally specific for a self determinant (self H) expressed on the target cell-surface and coded by the major histocompatibility gene complex (MHC) (Summarized in 1-3). T cells that mediate nonlytic functions such as T helper cells, proliferating T cells, and T cells involved in delayed-type hypersensitivity against contact allergens or intracellular bacteria are specific for H-2I determinants, whereas cytolytic T cells are specific for H-2K or D structures. Specificities both for self-H and for foreign antigen (X) are clonally expressed and highly specific. It is still unclear whether this dual specificity reflects that T cells express a single receptor for a neoantigenic determinant resulting when self-H complexes with X or that T cells express two independent receptor sites for self-H and for X (1-10).

How T cells acquire specificity for self-H during ontogeny has been the focus of several experiments with chimeras formed either by reconstituting lethally irradiated mice with lymphohemopoietic stem (bone marrow) cells from various sources or by reconstituting mice lacking a thymus and T cells with thymus grafts. These experiments have revealed the following: 1) Precursor T cells select the receptor-specificity for self-H independent of antigens in the thymus; radioresistant thymic cells seem to be responsible for this selection (11-15). Macrophage-like cells do not seem to be involved importantly since $F_1 \rightarrow$ parent irradiation bone marrow chimeras do not express substantial restriction to the non-host H-2 of reconstituting macrophages (11-13, 16). One must conclude that such cells are not involved or else do not repopulate the thymus in contrast to the exchange of Kupffer cells in liver, of lung macrophages and of all other lymphohemopoietic cells. Nor does suppressive activity explain the

[1]This work was supported by United States Public Health Service Grants A1-13779, A1-00273 and A1-07007 and is publication No. 1757 from the Department of Immunopathology of Scripps Clinic and Research Foundation, La Jolla, CA.

thymic influence on restriction, at least in the extensive
but unsuccessful search conducted so far (12, 17). 2) The
restriction specificity selected by T cells maturing in the
thymuses of chimeras is as specific or strict as that expressed by T cells from unmanipulated mice. Thus, T cells
from (H-2^k x H-2^b)F$_1$ → H-2^k irradiation chimeras lyse infected H-2^k cells at least 50 times better than infected H-2^b
cells (11-13). Similarly, spleen cells made tolerant to an
alloantigen by negative selection often lack the capacity to
become sensitized to lyse infected cells expressing the tolerated H-2 type (18). However, exceptions do exist and have
been used to argue that in a state of tolerance, restriction
specificity is relative (19-21). Indeed, all immunological
specificity is relative. Therefore, one should expect to
find rare "cross-reactivities" of T cell restriction that may
be boosted or selected under some extreme experimental protocols. Primary in vivo anti-viral responses exemplify the
relative frequency pattern of restriction specificities found
among precursor T cells under minimally selective conditions.
The general similarities in the response in chimeric and unmanipulated mice must therefore be considered real and more
relevant to any model devised to explain H-2 restriction of
effector T cells than the rare exceptions mentioned.
3) Apparently thymic selection alone is not sufficient for T
cells to mature to immunocompetence. For example, H-2^k mice
lacking thymuses and having T cells from a transplanted F$_1$
(H-2^k x H-2^d) thymus do not express H-2^d restriction specificity (13, 22). However, if the thymus graft is eliminated
and lymphohemopoietic cells of H-2^d type are transfused, such
animals may also express H-2^d-restricted T cells after some
time. Therefore, it seems that T cell maturation occurs in
at least two steps: thymic and post-thymic. Whether the
second step involves some I region-dependent amplification of
T cells that are relatively rare and "committed" or whether
it influences and/or promotes diversification of the T cell
repertoire for X is unknown (22). 4) Thymic selection of the
restriction specificity simultaneously includes selection of
the immune response (Ir) phenotype expressed by T cells.
Thus, selection of a restriction specificity for a nonresponder K, D or I-A allele that regulates the responsiveness of
their cytotoxic or nonlytic T cells, respectively, automati-
cally fixes the responder phenotype to high, low or nonre-
sponse. Apparently, then, Ir gene products and K, D or I-A
products are identical (26). Therefore, Ir-phenomena may
simply be a direct consequence of T cells being restricted.
That is, Ir phenomena arise because a T cell's function is
determined by that cell's restriction specificity, and because
this selection of a particular receptor for self-H that

mediates the T cell's effector function (lysis via K, D or further differentiation via I-A) influences the receptor repertoire available to recognize X (3, 13, 26, 27).

Several speculations have been proposed to explain this effect of anti-self-H recognition on the anti-X repertoire: a) In the altered self model self-H may or may not complex immunogenetically with X (5, 9, 10). b) With the Langman-Cohn preclusion rule expression of a particular receptor for self-H precluded the expression of some receptors for X by the same T lymphocyte (6, 7). c) von Boehmer, Haas and Jerne speculate that anti-self and anti-X start out identically and that anti-X, by somatic mutation, diversifies away from anti-self; this diversification from self-H cannot accomodate the generation of all possible anti-X receptors, thus Ir defects result (23). d) Certain anti-self-H receptors may be incapable of combining with certain anti-X receptors, much as immunoglobulin allotypes reflect framework sequences on specific hypervariable regions (13). e) In certain combinations tolerance may play some role in influencing responsiveness (13, 26, 27). All of these speculations may apply to Ir gene phenomena that are a consequence of T cells being restricted. However, still another possibility exists. f) If in addition to the restricting elements parts of the T cell receptor are coded within the MHC (e.g., in the I-J - I-C regions) (7, 28), then a completely different class of MHC-linked Ir gene regulation may occur. Thus, regulation resembles Ir genes with similar allotypes may be functioning in addition to the class of restriction specificity Ir genes discussed in the first five models (a-e). Neither of these models are fully satisfactory and supported by experimental data.

In summary, MHC restriction reflects the fact that T cells perform a particular effector function according to what kind of self-H they recognize along with foreign antigen. Apparently T cells kill in response to K and D, which are receptors for lytic signals, and participate antigen-specifically in cell differentiation in response to I determinants, which are receptors for cell differentiation signals. In vivo, MHC-restricted cytotoxic T cells are crucially involved in early anti-viral recovery, whereas nonlytic T cells act anti-virally or anti-bacterially via I-mediated macrophage activation. MHC products define the effector function and also influence the receptor repertoire that can be expressed by T cells. Therefore, we consider MHC polymorphism and gene duplication to have evolved together with T cells -- all under the selective pressure of intracellular parasites to expand the T cell receptor repertoire optimally at the level of the population and the individual (3, 5, 13). MHC polymorphism and MHC-associated diseases are consequences of the fact that T cell functions are determined by MHC-coded cell surface antigens, i.e., because T cells are restricted and because this limits responsiveness. Various ways of explaining MHC polymorphism and the association of certain disease susceptibilities with particular MHC haplotypes in this context have been discussed in detail elsewhere as have been some consequences for attempts at reconstituting immunodeficient patients with either stem cells or thymus transplants (13). However, to unravel the reciprocal regulation of restriction specificity and receptor repertoire for foreign antigens, ultimately it will be essential to understand the genetic organization and molecular nature of the genes and/or gene products that are involved.

ACKNOWLEDGMENTS

Part of this work has been supported by NIH-Public Health Service Grants Al-13779, Al-00273 and Al-07007. I thank Ms. Phyllis Minick, Andrea Rothman and Annette Parson for their excellent editorial and secretarial assistance in completing this manuscript. This is publication no. 1757 from the Department of Immunopathology of Scripps Clinic and Research Foundation, La Jolla, California.

REFERENCES

1. Transplantation Review. (1976). Volume 29.
2. Transplantation Review. (1978). Volume 42.
3. Zinkernagel, R. M., and Doherty, P. C. (1979). In "Advances in Immunology" (F. J. Dixon and H. G. Kunkel, eds.) Academic Press, New York. In press.
4. Zinkernagel, R. M., and Doherty, P. C. (1974). Nature 251, 547.
5. Doherty, P. C. and Zinkernagel, R. M. (1975). Lancet 1, 1406.
6. Langman, R. E. 1978). Rev. Phys. Bioch. Pharm. 81, 1.
7. Cohn, M., and Epstein, R. (1978). Cell. Immunol. In press.
8. Matzinger, P., and Bevan, M. J. (1977). Cell. Immunol. 29, 1.
9. Rosenthal, A. S. (1978). Immunol. Rev. 40, 136.
10. Benacerraf, B. (1978). J. Immunol. 120, 1809.
11. Zinkernagel, R. M., Callahan, G. N., Althage, A., Cooper, S., Klein, P. A., and Klein, J. (1978). J. Exp. Med. 147, 882.
12. Bevan, M. J., and Fink, P. J. (1978). Immunol. Rev. 42, 4.
13. Zinkernagel, R. M. (1978). Immunol. Rev. 42, 224.
14. Waldmann, H., Pope, H., Bettles, C., and Davies, A. J. S. (1979). Nature 277, 137.

15. Miller, J. F. A. P., Gamble, J., Mottram, P., and Smith, F. I. (1979). Scand. J. Immunol. 9, In press.
16. Bevan, M. J. (1977). Nature 269, 417.
17. Zinkernagel, R. M., and Althage, A. (1979). J. Immunol. In press.
18. Bennink, J. R., and Doherty, P. C. (1978). J. Exp. Med. 148, 128.
19. Matzinger, P. and Mirkwood, G. (1978). J. Exp. Med. 148, 84.
20. Doherty, P. C., and Bennink, J. R. (1979). J. Exp. Med. 149, 150.
21. Blanden, R. V., and Andrew, M. E. (1979). J. Exp. Med. In press.
22. Zinkernagel, R. M., Althage, A., Waterfield, E., Pincetl, P., and Klein, J. (1979). Nature. In press.
23. von Boehmer, H., Haas, W., and Jerne, N. K. (1978). Proc. Natl. Acad. Sci. U.S.A. 75, 2439.
24. Zinkernagel, R. M., Althage, A., Cooper, S., Callahan, G. N., and Klein, J. (1978). J. Exp. Med. 148, 805.
25. Billings, P., Burakoff, S. J., Dorf, M. E., and Benacerraf, B. (1978). J. Exp. Med. 148, 352.
26. Zinkernagel, R. M., Althage, A., Cooper, S., Kreeb, G., Klein, P. A., Sefton, B., Flaherty, L., Stimpfling, J., Shreffler, D., and Klein, J. (1978). J. Exp. Med. 148, 592.
27. Snell, G. (1978). The Harvey Lectures. In press.
28. Benacerraf, B., and Germain, R. (1978). Immunol. Rev. 38.

H-2 LINKED RESISTANCE TO SPONTANEOUS AKR LEUKEMIA: A MECHANISM[1]

D. Meruelo,[2] D. Smith, N. Flieger, and H.O. McDevitt[*]

Irvington House Institute, Department of Pathology,
N.Y.U. Medical Center, New York, N.Y. 10016;
[*]and Department of Medicine, Division of Immunology,
Stanford University School of Medicine,
Stanford, CA. 94305

ABSTRACT The role played by immune responses in resistance to virus-induced leukemogenesis has not been precisely defined. The present communication provides direct evidence for the involvement of genes in the B, J or E subregions of the H-2 complex in conferring humoral mediated resistance to the spontaneous AKR leukemia. Humoral immunity, but not cellular immunity, is effective in preventing the in vivo proliferation of AKR tumor cells. Furthermore, the development of effective humoral immunity depends on Lyl$^+$, 2$^-$, 3$^-$ helper T cells bearing the I-J^k phenotype.

INTRODUCTION

The involvement of the murine major histocompatibility complex, H-2, in virus-induced leukemogenesis was first demonstrated experimentally by Lilly et al. (1). To date the exact mechanisms of action of H-2 linked loci in disease associations are unknown. Some investigators (2, 3) have suggested that H-2 linked resistance to virus-induced leukemogenesis may result from genetically controlled variation in immune responses to virus-induced antigens. This hypothesis was put forth after several observations were made. One of these observations was that Rgv-1, a gene conferring resistance to Gross-virus induced tumorigenesis, was mapped near

[1]This work was supported by NIH Grants # CA22247 and AIO 7751, ACS Grant # IM-163, and a grant from The Irma T. Hirschl   Foundation.
[2]Leukemia Society of America   Scholar

or within the I region of the H-2 complex to which most immune response genes have been mapped (4). Support for this hypothesis was provided by studies of Aoki et al. (5) demonstrating that serum levels of anti-Gross virus antibodies were higher in mice homozygous or heterozygous for the resistant H-2 haplotype than in animals homozygous for the susceptible H-2 type.

Whether immune reactions to murine leukemia virus (MuLV) play a determining role in the development of naturally occurring leukemia in the mouse remains unknown. The question has become increasingly difficult to answer with the recognition that MuLV is not a single virus, but rather a complex family of viruses, making it uncertain which, if any, of the currently defined MuLV classes actually represents the etiological agent of spontaneous leukemia (6).

The present communication provides direct evidence for the involvement of immune mechanisms in conferring resistance to the spontaneous AKR leukemia and defines the humoral response involved, including the involvement of an $I-J^+$, $Ly-1^+$, $2^-,3^-$ T cell.

MATERIALS AND METHODS

Mice. All mice used in the present studies were bred at New York University Medical Center from animals derived from the Stanford University School of Medicine's colony.

Cells. BW5147 cells were originally obtained from the Salk Institute, San Diego, CA. and have been maintained independently since 1975. Their karyotype and growth conditions have been described previously (7).

Antisera. All antisera, with the exception of D-30 (anti-D^q) and rabbit anti-mouse IgG were prepared at Stanford University School of Medicine or New York University Medical Center. Antisera were produced as per published protocols (8-10). The following sera were utilized: α Thy 1.2 (AKR/J anti-AKR/Cum); α J^k ((BALB.BxB10.A(3R))F_1 anti-B10.A(5R));α A^k((B10.S(9R)x A.TFR5)F_1 anti-A.TL);$\alpha A^k B^k J^k E^k C^k S^k G^k$ (see ref. 13 regarding potential contaminants) (A.TH anti-A.TL); $\alpha A^S B^S J^S E^S C^S S^S G^S$ (A.TL anti-A.TH); $\alpha A^k B^k J^k$ ((B10.HTTxA.TH)F_1 anti-A.TL) ; αD^k ((A.TLxB10.A)F_1 anti-B10.BR) ; αK^k ((A.TLxC3H.OL)F_1 anti-C3H); $\alpha E^k C^k S^k G^k$ (B10.S(7R) anti-B10.HTT). Anti-D^{q}

(B10.AxLP.RIII)F$_1$ anti-B10.AKM) was kindly provided by
Dr. John G. Ray, Jr., of the Research Resources Branch, Na-
tional Institutes of Health, Bethesda, Md. Rabbit anti-mouse
IgG (RAMIG) was purchased from Antibodies, Inc., Davis,
CA.

Nylon Wool Purification; antiserum plus complement mediated cytotoxicity;cell binding radioimmunoassay; cell mediate cytotoxicity assay; absorption studies; irradiation of mice
and intravenous injections of alloantisera were done as described elsewhere (11).

RESULTS

Gene(s) in the B,J, or E Subregions of H-2I Confer
Resistance to Malignant AKR Cells. In previous studies (7)
AKR mice were crossed with animals of various H-2 congenic
strains on the C57BL/10 or C3H genetic background and the
hybrid mice injected intraperitoneally with AKR thymoma cells,
BW5147. Comparison of the cell-mediated immune response
of hybrid mice differing in their H-2 genotype showed a genetically controlled immune response difference. A continuing
study of the nature of this H-2 restriction on CML responsiveness indicates that hybrids unable to mount a vigorous CML
response to the injected tumor cells (namely H-2$^{k/q}$ mice
(B10.GxAKR)F$_1$ and (C3H.QxAKR)F$_1$) survive longer than hybrids capable of responding in a cell-mediated assay (primarily H-2$^{k/k}$ mice (CKBxAKR)F$_1$ and (B10.BRxAKR)F$_1$) . The results of four independent experiments in which various hybrid
mice received 5 x 10^6 BW5147 cells intraperitoneally and were
followed for at least 43 days are shown in Table I. Analysis
of the varying H-2 haplotypes of the F$_1$ hybrids demonstrates
that gene(s) mapping in the B,J, or E subregions of the I region
confer resistance or susceptibility to BW5147 cells. Thus,
only hybrids carrying at least one copy of the q or d allele in
these three subregions survive to any significant degree beyond 43 days. These studies were repeated numerous times
with the same results each time. The lack of additional recombinants does not permit more precise assignment of the
gene(s) involved to either B,J, or E.

The Importance of the Humoral Response and Effects of
Passive Antiserum Treatments. While a reciprocal correlation

Table I

MAPPING OF TUMOR RESISTANCE TO THE B,J OR E SUBREGION(S) OF H-2

	Strain	% Survival (day 43)	\-	H-2 haplotype of non AKR parent								
			K	A	B	J	E	C	S	G	D
Exp. 1	(B10.D2x AKR)F₁	67	d	d	d	d	d	d	d	d	d
	(B10.A(5R)x AKR)F₁	0	b	b	b	k	k	d	d	d	d
	(B10.A(3R)x AKR)F₁	0	b	b	b	b	k	d	d	d	d
	(B10.BRxAKR	0	k	k	k	k	k	k	k	k	k
	(B10xAKR	0	b	b	b	b	b	b	b	b	b
Exp. 2	(B10.GxAKR)F₁	90	q	q	q	q	q	q	q	q	q
	(B10.AQRxAKR)F₁	0	q	k	k	k	k	d	d	d	d
	(B10.AxAKR)F₁	0	k	k	k	k	k	d	d	d	d
	(B10.BRxAKR)F₁	0	k	k	k	k	k	k	k	k	k
Exp. 3	(C3H.QxAKR)F₁	80	q	q	q	q	q	q	q	q	q
	(CKBxAKR)F₁	0	k	k	k	k	k	k	k	k	k
	(B10.BRxAKR)F₁	0	k	k	k	k	k	k	k	k	k
Exp. 4	(D2GDxAKR)F₁	0	d	q	b	b	b	b	b	b	b
	(B10.D2xAKR)F₁	31*	d	d	d	d	d	d	d	d	d
	(B10.Gx AKR)F₁	73	q	q	q	q	q	q	q	q	q
	(B10.BRxAKR)F₁	0	k	k	k	k	k	k	k	k	k

*Repeats of this experiment indicate that (B10.D2xAKR)F₁ are consistently more resistant than all other F₁ mice, except (B10.GxAKR)F₁ and a significant number usually survive tumor inoculation.

was found between CML responsiveness and survival, a direct relationship was found between the latter and humoral responsiveness (Fig. 1A). (B10.GxAKR)F₁ mice (H-$2^{q/k}$) make a stronger response to an i.p. injection of BW5147 cells than do (B10.BRxAKR)F₁ mice (H-$2^{k/k}$). The humoral response is measurable equally well with BW5147 cells or AKR virus (Figs. 1A and B). Linkage of the humoral response to H-2 is readily demonstrable in a backcross segregation analysis of (AKRxB10.G)F₁xAKR progeny (Fig. 1C).

Gene(s) associated with survival map in the B,J, or E subregions and genes associated with the I-J subregion appear to code for antigenic determinants present on suppressor cells (12) and their soluble factors (13). Therefore, it is possible that mice unable to survive inoculation of BW5147 cells are prevented from mounting an effective humoral response by suppressor lymphocytes. To study this question experiments, patterned after Greene et al. (14) were carried out and are illustrated in Table II. In particular these authors have found that daily injection of a J^k serum results in retarded tumor

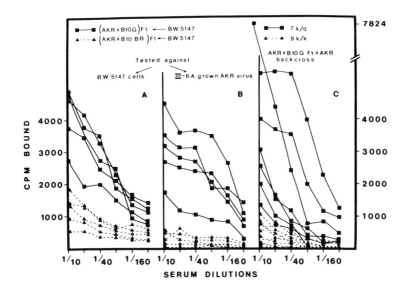

Figure 1. Humoral immune response of various mice injected 10 days prior with 5 x 10⁶ BW 5147 cells. Tested by radioimmunoassay against (A & C)BW5147 cells; (B)AKR-MuLV.

growth, presumably by abolishing tumor specific suppressor cells. Resistant ((AKRxB10.G)F_1) and susceptible ((AKRxB10.BR)F_1) mice were injected every other day with 10 μl of one of many different antisera (Table II-1).No effect of anti-I-J^k serum could be detected on survival by susceptible mice. In fact, a contrary result was obtained: resistant mice receiving injections of a J^k showed reduced resistance to the tumor suggesting that a I-J^k treatment eliminated a helper rather than a suppressor cell. This effect on resistant mice was examined in a second experiment (Table II-2) with similar results.

A more extensive analysis of the effect of antiserum treatment on resistant mice (AKRxB10.G) is shown in Table III. It can be seen from this experiment: (1) that treatment with $_aA^kB^kJ^k$, a Ly-1.2 or a Θ^{C3H} markedly reduced mean survival time and final survival incidence; (2) that absorption of $_aA^kB^kJ^k$ serum with BW5147 cells did not affect the serum's activity; and (3) that lowered resistance to the injected tumor cells was always associated with a reduction in the antiviral

Table II

EFFECT OF INTRAVENOUS INJECTION OF SEVERAL ANTISERUM SURVIVAL OF

$(AKR \times B10, G)F_1$ RECEIVING 5×10^6 BW5147 CELLS

Experiment #1

Antiserum potentially recognizes	Mean survival time (days)	% survival end of experiment
D^k	73.1 ± 12.2	50
$A^k B^k J^k E^k C^k S^k G^k$	87.1 ± 13.0	67
K^k	87.2 ± 12.1	58
A^k	114.8 ± 5.3	87.5
J^k	51.1 ± 13.2	0
None (PBS)	105.5 ± 8.9	75

Experiment #2

$A^k B^k J^k E^k C^k S^k G^k$	79.9 ± 20.3	57
A^k	97.8 ± 16.5	75
$A^k B^k J^k$	36.9 ± 12.3	0
$E^k C^k$	76.3 ± 16.8	63
$A^s B^s J^s E^s C^s$	81.3 ± 19.7	57
None (PBS)	89.5 ± 16.3	62

or antitumor humoral response.

Mouse alloantisera directed against H-2 determinants often contain antibodies to virus determinants (15). To insure against a role for these possible contaminants in the effects observed, the various sera used in these studies were tested for their reactivity with BW5147 cells. While significant

Table III

EFFECT OF INTRAVENOUS INJECTIONS OF VARIOUS ANTISERA ON SURVIVAL

AND HUMORAL IMMUNITY OF $(AKR \times B10, G)F_1$ INJECTED WITH 5×10^6

BW5147 CELLS

Potential determinants recognized by antiserum	Mean survival time (days)	% Survival end[b] of experiment (90 days)	% Reduction in[b] titer of a BW5147 serum
D^q	48.2 ± 6.3	67	5
D^k	54.0 ± 6.8	75	7
A^k	51.3 ± 6.5	67	8
J^k	30.9 ± 5.7	22	69
$A^k B^k J^k$	34.4 ± 6.1	25	50
$A^k B^k J^k{}^a$	37.7 ± 7.6	28	53
Ly-1.2	38.8 ± 4.6	36	69
Ly-2.1	52.8 ± 6.4	64	10
θ^{C3H}	37.0 ± 4.9	33	54
None (PBS)	56.4 ± 6.7	66	0

[a] Absorbed with BW5147 cells.

[b] Correlation analysis of % survival with % reduction in titer shows a coefficient of −0.94 which for n=10 is highly significant (> .01).

activity was detected in some sera, no correlation could be found between this activity and an effect on survival of (AKRxB10.G)F$_1$ mice (data not shown).

Effect of Various Antisera in Cell Transfer Experiments. To insure that effects seen with serum injections indeed reflected an effect on lymphocytes involved in the humoral response, a series of cell transfer experiments were carried out. These experiments demonstrated: (1) that transfer of non-immune (AKRxC3H.Q)F$_1$ (resistant) spleen cells to syngeneic, lethally irradiated recipients, did not reconstitute the humoral response (Fig. 2r); although, it resulted in a cellular immune response, not normally seen in H-2$^{k/q}$ mice (Fig. 3); and rendered the

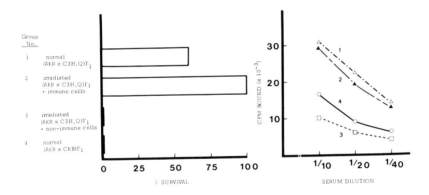

Figure 2. Transfer of survival and humoral immunity to BW5147 cells by syngeneic immune lymphocytes.

mice completely unable to resist tumor growth (Fig. 2l). (2) On the other hand, when reconstitution of irradiated (AKRxC3H.Q)F$_1$ mice was carried out with immune, syngeneic spleen cells, the humoral response was equal to that of normal hosts (Fig. 2A) and rendered the mice completely resistant to tumor growth (Fig. 2B). (3) The requirement that transferred

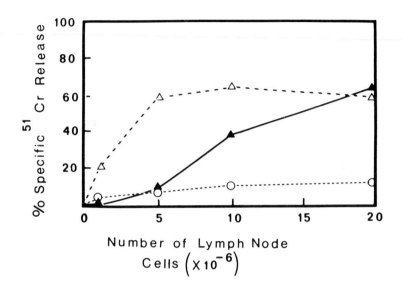

Figure 3. Cell mediated immune response of normal
responder (H-2$^{k/k}$) (▲——▲); nonresponder mice (H-2$^{q/k}$)
(o----o) as well as irradiated noresponder mice (△-----△)
10 days after injection of 5x10^6 BW 5147 cells.

cells be preimmune applied only to T cells (Fig. 4A). When
immune or normal T and/or B cells were transferred, it could
be shown that normal B cells would function to protect the
host in the presence of immune, but <u>not</u> non-immune, T cells
(Fig. 4<u>l</u>). A similar finding was obtained with respect to the
humoral response (Fig. 4<u>r</u>).

Further analysis of the characteristics of the transferred
immune T cells demonstrated that these cells were sensitive
to treatment with either a J^k or a Ly-1.2 antisera plus complement. When treated with either of these two sera plus complement prior to their transfer into irradiated syngeneic recipients, the capacity of the transferred immune T cells to reconstitute the host's humoral response (Fig. 5B) or its ability
to survive the tumor inoculation (Fig. 5A) were completely
abolished. On the other hand, treatment with a Ly-2.1 serum
plus complement in exactly the same fashion had no effect on
the transferred cells.

<u>Only J^k Positive Helper T Cells are Required for Effective</u>

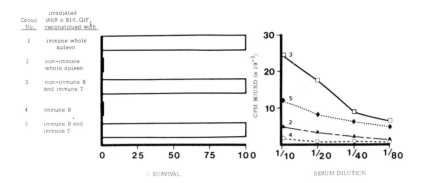

Figure 4. Role of immune T and/or B cells in transfer of survival and humoral immunity to a dose of 5×10^6 BW5147 cells.

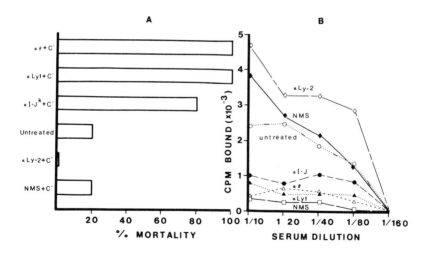

Figure 5. Effect of various antisera on the capacity of immune T cells to transfer (A) survival, and (B) humoral immunity to an inoculum of 5×10^6 BW5147 cells.

Humoral Anti-Tumor Immunity.   Because anti-$A^k B^k J^k$ was as effective as anti-I-J^k, one possibility that needed analysis was that two T cells, for example, one A^k positive and one J^k

Table IV

SURVIVAL OF VARIOUS MICE AFTER RECEIVING 10^7 SPONTANEOUS AKR LEUKEMIA CELLS (INTERPERITONEALLY			
Strain of Mice	Antiserum Treatment	Mean Survival Time	Mortality day 43
(AKRxB10.G)F$_1$	$_a A^k$	66 ± 10	17%
"	$_a A^k B^k J^k$	45 ± 7	75%
"	$_a J^k$	44 ± 3	67%

positive were required to help T dependent B cells make an effective humoral response.   Elimination of either one would be sufficient to abolish humoral immunity and resistance to BW5147 cells.   Under this assumption $_a J^k$ would work by abolishing I-J positive T cells, and $_a A^k B^k J^k$ by abolishing I-J^k positive and/or I-A^k positive cells.   This hypothesis was tested by absorption of $_a A^k B^k J^k$ with either B10.A(4R) (kkbbbbbbb), B10.A(3R) (bbbbkdddd), or B10.A(5R) (bbbkkdddd) cells (data not shown).   Absorption with B10.A(4R), which removed all anti-A^k activity, rendered the serum even more powerful in abolishing resistance to growth of BW5147 cells. In fact, this absorbed serum showed the strongest activity of any serum tested in the current experiments. Absorption with B10.A(5R), which removed anti-I-J^k reactivity, rendered the serum ineffective in abolishing resistance.   Absorption with B10.A(3R) did not alter the serum's behavior as would be expected.   Therefore, all the helper T cell(s) involved in resistance to the tumor must display the I-J^k phenotype.

Relevance of Finding to the Spontaneous AKR Leukemia. Malignant AKR cells were prepared from the thymus and spleen of an overtly (spontaneously) leukemic AKR mouse and injected into $(AKRxB10.G)F_1$ mice undergoing the injection protocol of 10 μl of serum every other day (Table IV). The observed effect on survival for each sera was similar to that obtained in mice receiving BW5147 cells.

DISCUSSION

The experiments reported here strongly indicate that a T cell, expressing the $I-J^k$, $Ly-1^+$, 2^-, 3^- phenotype, is crucial for the development of a humoral response capable of rendering mice resistant to the growth of spontaneously developing malignant cells of AKR origin.

The previously observed (7) genetic control of CML response may be understood in terms of the current findings. It would seem that the first line of defense against growth of BW5147 cells is an effective humoral response. $\underline{H-2^{q/k}}$ mice make such a response and usually eliminate the growing tumor cells. Therefore, the antigenic load may never become sufficient to trigger the second line of defensive responses: cell-mediate immunity. However, some $(AKRxB10.G)F_1$ mice do die from the tumor load. The growing tumor cells in these mice might still fail to elicit a cellular immune response because their surfaces may be covered by antibodies or the antigenic determinants may be immunomodulated. In contrast to $\underline{H-2^{q/k}}$ animals, $\underline{H-2^{k/k}}$ mice are unable to make a vigorous antibody response, possibly due to the action of suppressor lymphocytes, but can mobilize their secondary defense mechanism: cellular immunity. However, such immunity may arrive too late to achieve tumor regression, or may be too limited in extent, since, for example, effector cells in these mice cannot be found in the spleen (7).

In view of the effect of a J^k serum on spontaneous tumor proliferation in AKR mice, it would appear that AKR mice could overcome the disease if they could be brought to make the appropriate immune response. To achieve this experimentally it would be required that the antigen recognized by the humoral response be clearly identified, and the antigen be presented to unresponsive $\underline{H-2^{k/k}}$ mice in a manner which can elicit a response. Further studies are in progress to achieve this.

ACKNOWLEDGEMENT

We wish to thank Ms. Anna Paolino for her invaluable help in the breeding of mice, Ms. Diane Teece for production of antisera, and Ms. Beverly Coopersmith for her excellent secretarial assistance.

REFERENCES

1. Lilly, F., Boyse, E. A., and Old, L. J. (1964). Lancet 2, 1207.
2. McDevitt, H. O., and Bodmer, W. F. (1972). Am.J.Med. 52, 1.
3. Lilly, F., and Pincus, T. (1973). Adv.Cancer Res. 17, 231.
4. Lilly, F. (1970). Bibl. Haematol. 36, 213.
5. Aoki, T., Boyse, E. A., and Old, L. J. (1966). Cancer Res. 26, 1415.
6. Elder, J. H., Gautsch, J. W., Jensen, F. C., and Lerner, R. A. (1978). J.Natl. Cancer Inst. 61, 625.
7. Meruelo, D., Deak, B., and McDevitt, H.O. (1977). J.Exp.Med. 146, 1367.
8. Shen, F. W., Boyse, E. A., and Cantor, H. (1975). Immunogenetics 2, 591.
9. Reif, A. E., and Allen, J. M. V. (1963). Nature 200, 1332.
10. Murphy, D. B., and Shreffler, D. C. (1975). J.Exp.Med. 141, 374.
11. Meruelo, D., Flieger, N., Smith, D., and McDevitt, H.O. Submitted for publication.
12. Murphy, D. B., Herzenberg, L. A., Okumura, K., Herzenberg, L. A., and McDevitt, H. O. (1976). J.Exp. Med. 144, 699.
13. Tada, T., Taniguchi, M., and David, C.S. (1976). J.Exp. Med. 144, 713.
14. Greene, M.I., Dorf, M. E., Pierres, M., and Benacerraf, B. (1977). Proc.Natl.Acad.Sci. 74, 5118.
15. Nowinski, R. C., and Klein, P. A. (1975). J.Immunol. 115, 1261.

WORKSHOP SUMMARY: Learning of H-2 Restriction and Lymphocyte-
Virus Interactions, Peter C. Doherty, The Wistar Institute,
36th & Spruce Streets, Philadelphia, PA 19104, and Irving L.
Weissman, Department of Pathology, Stanford University School
of Medicine, Palo Alto, CA 94305.

The major theme of this workshop centered around the
question, "What do cytotoxic T cells see?" The workshop was
divided into four subsections, each defining a separate aspect
of T cell recognition. The first session dealt with thymic
maturation and the thymic microenvironment, especially with
respect to the eventual H-2 restriction of emerging T lymphocytes. The second subsection asked the question, "Does MHC
restriction exist, and are there any exceptions?" The third
section dealt with responder and nonresponder situations and
the MHC, while the fourth section centered around possible
association of virus and MHC components on the cell membranes
of target cells for H-2 restricted cytotoxic T cell action.

In the first session, R. Rouse presented evidence that
thymic cortical epithelial cells express I-A determinants, and
thymic medullary cells express I-A, K and D antigens, and perhaps other gene products of the H-2 region. The cortical I-A
positive dendritic epithelial cells were stable to irradiation
and/or transplantation, whereas some question about the origin
of medullary I-A antigens still remained to be resolved.
Waksal presented the hypothesis that prothymocytes are natural
killers, each of which is H-2 restricted in its cytotoxicity,
but is not yet selected for the self vs. nonself components of
H-2 restriction. He envisioned that these cells would enter
the thymus and be selected according to recognition of self
specificities.

We then approached the question of whether MHC restriction exists and whether MHC restriction is totally defined by
the environment encountered during differentiation in thymus.
The first presentation by J. Bennink concerned the use of T
cells that were filtered through semi-allogeneic irradiated
recipients, and then restimulated with virus in further sets
of recipients which shared at least some part of the H-2 gene
complex of the responder T cells. It seems that C57B1/6,
BALB/c, and B.10D2 T cells (which are H-2^b and H-2^d respectively) can be sensitized in an appropriate environment to
vaccinia virus and can recognize vaccinia virus presented in
the context of H-2K^k. However, it seems that the converse
does not apply, and that H-2^k T cells do not respond to vaccinia virus presented in association with H-2^d or H-2^b. We
thus have an apparent exception to the rule that T cells are
totally restricted to the MHC components encountered in
thymus. Further experiments indicate that this may not be a
widespread phenomenon and may, in effect, be the exception

which proves the rule. R. Korngold then followed with similar experiments, using negative selection protocols to look at the response to minor histocompatibility components. In this case there was no evidence that T cells of one H-2 type could, after negative selection, be induced to respond to minor H determinants in the context of H-2 antigens not encountered during differentiation.

H. Kreth then presented the first evidence to date that the primary response to virus in man is HLA restricted. Work from the group in Würzburg has shown that individuals with measles make a cytotoxic T cell response which is restricted by HLA determinants. It is important to recognize that these were primary infections, and that the usual dose of virus used for immunization does not lead to differentiation of detectable cytotoxic T cells. Furthermore, there are difficulties in restimulating measles immune memory T cells in vitro, a problem which has also been encountered by K. Lucas.

We then turned to the problem of the hamster in a presentation by M. Nelles from Dallas. The hamster has proven somewhat of an enigma, because what appeared to be a cytotoxic T cell response seemed not only to cross between different strains of hamsters, but also between Syrian and European hamsters, which are totally different species. It transpires, however, that this group has recently found that the phenomenon probably reflects the activity of antibody dependent cell mediated cytotoxicity; we will thus be able to dispose of this somewhat problematic set of findings in a rather relieved manner. The third question was concerned with responder and nonresponder situations with relation to the major histocompatibility complex. The two central papers in this area were from A. McMichael, S. Shaw and W. Biddison from Oxford and NIH, respectively. Both groups are working with the secondary in vitro T cell response to the influenza A viruses. The Washington group has documented responses to influenza A viruses and in the context of HLA-1, A2, B7, B8, and BW 44. There are some discrepancies with the Oxford group, but it probably is not wise to make a great point of this as only a limited number of individuals have been tested in each case. McMichael established that the human cytotoxic T cell response that can be stimulated in vitro is totally crossreactive for all influenza A viruses. This presumably reflects presensitization with other influenza A viruses, as it also is very difficult to stimulate T cells which are hemagglutinin specific in mice which have been previously primed with another influenza A virus. McMichael also showed that the HLA restricted response could be blocked with antibodies to HLA determinants, and not with antibodies to virus. This has been a common finding in the virus systems, but recent evidence from Doherty's group shows that virus-immune murine cytotoxic T cells can be blocked with monoclonal antibodies of high titer for particular influenza HA determinants.

We then left the virus systems for the moment and Mary Brenan, from London, summarized very interesting findings from the H-Y system, where there seems to be a hierarchy in responsiveness associated with particular H-2 alleles. Response to a strong combination will suppress that to a weaker combination, whereas if that (strong) response is not present, the weaker response will emerge.

The fourth section dealt with various approaches to determine whether virus and MHC components are either associated on cell membranes, or linked in a fashion which endures following detergent lysis and immunoprecipitation of either component. The first three presentations all demonstrated that H-2 and viral components appear not to be covalently or stably associated following detergent lysis and immunoprecipitation, using both VSV and oncornavirus systems. These studies were carried out by Black's group, Wise, and Fox and Weissman. The latter investigators also demonstrated that H-2 products appear not to be structurally altered to the extent that is detectable by isoelectric focusing and SDS-PAGE. Thus the attention of the group centered about demonstrating whether or not there are stable associations of these markers on the cell membrane, and if one can detect these associations by nearest neighbor crosslinker analysis or by utilizing artificial vesicle systems. A. Hapel used lipid vesicles containing H-2 antigens to demonstrate that he could create targets for cytotoxic T cells directed against Sendai virus by fusing in the appropriate H-2 type to a Sendai virus infected, H-2 different cell. This demonstrates the point that if any H-2 virus associations occur in the cell membrane, they must be sufficiently unstable to permit reassociation of viral components with the transferred H-2 determinants. S. Burakoff demonstrated that stimulation of secondary cytotoxic T cells to Sendai virus could be accomplished by incubating these cells with liposomes containing inserted H-2 and Sendai viral proteins only if a single liposome fraction contained both components; addition of liposomes containing H-2 determinants plus liposomes containing viral determinants did not lead to stimulation of restricted cytotoxic effectors. Thus the two components must be presented together to stimulate the secondary cytotoxic T cell and, if antigen processing is required for secondary stimulation, it evidently cannot function independently presented H-2 and viral components contained on and/or in liposomes. Finally, Takemoto and D. Zarling discussed the utility of bifunctional crosslinking reagents to study nearest neighbor associations of H-2 and viral components in oncornavirus infected cells which are subject to H-2 restricted cytotoxic T cell lysis. It appears that the technology is still in its infancy, and that the major congenors following crosslinking are oncornaviral glycoprotein dimers and trimers, or H-2 dimers and trimers. Some association of gp70 with molecules of 45,000 and 12,000 molecular weight was reported by Zarling in short term incubations, although he has not yet tested whether these represent the expected H-2 light and heavy chains, or some other cellular or viral products. Thus these studies have not yet provided us with an estimate of the frequency of association of viral and H-2 components on the cell membrane.

If we were to identify the most significant advances that have been made in this area since the last of these meetings two years ago, the most obvious one is the definition of the role of the thymus in restricting cytotoxic T cell responses to self. This seems to be a general rule, though there may be some exceptions. The second gratifying point is a clear demonstration of HLA restricted cytotoxic T cell responses to influenza A viruses in man, something that we had no information about two years previously. We have also been able to identify responder/nonresponder situations in various virus infections associated with H-2K, H-2D, or HLA-A and HLA-B. The final point is that very serious attempts are being made to evaluate the possibility that virus and MHC components associate on the cell membrane. The overall impression seems to be that if such associations do occur, they are rather tenuous.

T LYMPHOCYTE REACTIVITIES TO ALLO- AND ALTERED-SELF ANTIGENS[1]

Fritz H. Bach[2] and Barbara J. Alter[3]

Immunobiology Research Center
University of Wisconsin, Madison, Wisconsin 53706

ABSTRACT The diversity of T lymphocytes that play a role in the response to alloantigens and altered-self antigens is great. In addition to the classical Ly 1, helper T lymphocytes and Ly 2, cytotoxic T lymphocytes, it is now clear that one must consider participation by suppressor T lymphocytes that are separate from the cytotoxic T lymphocytes, and Ly 1,2 T lymphocytes that are involved at the precursor level in the response to K/D alloantigenic stimuli as well as in the response to "altered-self" antigens. It appears that there are two alternative pathways that T lymphocytes can use in their response to foreign antigens: first, a pathway consisting of collaboration between Ly 1, helper T lymphocytes and Ly 2, cytotoxic T lymphocytes and second, a pathway dependent on an Ly 1,2 cell at the precursor level. The factors that may influence the balance between these two pathways as well as consideration of the nature of the antigenic stimuli needed to elicit a secondary response, perhaps dependent on which pathway(s) is used in the primary, are discussed.

INTRODUCTION

T lymphocyte reactivities have been related in a most interesting and exciting manner to antigens encoded by genes of the major histocompatibility complex. An enormous

[1]Supported by NIH grants AI 08439, CA 16836, AI 15588, and National Foundation grants 6-78 and 1-246.
[2]Departments of Medical Genetics and Surgery and the Immunobiology Research Center, University of Wisconsin.
[3]Immunobiology Research Center, University of Wisconsin.
This is paper no. 191 from the Immunobiology Research Center and paper no. 2355 from the Laboratory of Medical Genetics.

literature has developed which is consistent with the concept that evolution has allowed adaptation between the "types" of stimulating antigenic determinants and their differential recognition by functionally disparate subpopulations of T lymphocytes. Support for this has emerged not only from studies of alloantigenic reactivities in which the pre-eminence of MHC encoded antigens in activating helper T lymphocytes (T_h), cytotoxic T lymphocytes (T_c) and suppressor T lymphocytes (T_s) has been extensively documented (1) but also from experiments in which recognition by these different T cells of antigens other than MHC encoded determinants is in turn restricted by the MHC encoded structures (2,3,4).

The realization that antigens associated with the MHC can be divided into different types of determinants on the basis of the T lymphocyte subpopulations that they activate has lead to the concept of LD-CD collaboration (1). LD (L determinant) antigens preferentially stimulate T_h cells whereas CD (C determinant) antigens interact with precursor and effector T_c. It is, of course, the joint activation of both LD responsive T_h and CD responsive T_c that leads to the strong generation of a cytotoxic response in vitro and probably also in vivo. Separation of T_h and T_c cells in terms of their reactivity to MHC encoded determinants was first accomplished by monolayer adsorption techniques (5) in which the T_c cells adhered to the monolayer in an antigen specific manner and the proliferating (presumed T_h) cells did not. Subsequently the use of anti-Lyt sera has permitted separation (6,7), as well as reconstitution (7,8), experiments to gain further insights into the cellular and corresponding antigenic dichotomy.

With respect to Lyt phenotypes of precursor responding T lymphocytes, the T_h cells are Ly 1+2- (Ly 1) whereas the cytotoxic T lymphocytes are Ly 1-2+ (Ly 2) at least when Ly 1+2+ (Ly 1,2) cells are removed from the precursor population and the stimulating cells differ from the responding cells by an entire H-2 complex. It is important to stress that the model that has emerged, i.e. collaboration between the Ly 1 T_h and Ly 2 T_c cells, is based on both of these factors: first, the presumed absence of Ly 1,2 cells in the population and second, stimulation of the responding cells by both the strong LD antigens encoded by H-2 I region genes and strong CD antigens encoded by the K and/or D regions. These are important considerations because in studies of precursor Ly phenotype of cells responsive in altered-self situations, including TNP modified cells and syngeneic tumors, it was noted that an Ly 1,2 cell appeared to play a critical role as a precursor (9,10,11) in allowing the generation of a cytotoxic response. All of these systems have indicated an

Ly 2 cytotoxic effector T cell. On the basis of these
findings it has been suggested there is a fundamental
difference between altered-self and alloantigen evoked
responses. Such a hypothesis would place the emphasis on a
difference at the level of the type of antigen recognized,
that is, the "altered-self" as opposed to alloantigens.

We have performed experiments to test whether generation
of cytotoxic T lymphocytes to alloantigens can, under some
circumstances, involve an Ly 1,2 cell in a manner similar to
the response evoked by altered-self antigens; further we
have tested whether effector T$_c$ are in all cases Ly 2 cells
even when an Ly 1,2 cell may function as a precursor.
Materials and methods used in the studies reported here have
been described in detail elsewhere (12).

Lyt Phenotype of Precursor Cells Responding to K/D
Alloantigen Differences. We have previously published data
showing the importance of an Ly 1,2 cell at the precursor
level for proliferative and cytotoxic responses to K/D
alloantigenic stimuli (12,13). Presented in Table I are
results of MLC proliferative responses of cell populations
pretreated with either normal mouse serum, anti-Lyt 1 or
anti-Lyt 2 sera and complement and subsequently stimulated
by cells differing for various regions of H-2. In addition,
results are presented when the anti-Lyt 1 treated and anti-
Lyt 2 treated populations are mixed. This type of reconstitution experiment is designed to ask whether the presence of
both Lyt 2 cells (present after treatment with anti-Lyt 1
serum) and Lyt 1 cells (present in the other population)
will synergize to produce a response. As previously demonstrated, the vast majority of the proliferating cells against
an entire H-2 difference are of the Lyt 1 phenotype; pretreatment of the responding cells with anti-Lyt 2 serum has
little effect on proliferation. On the other hand, precursor
cells proliferating against K/D alloantigenic differences
are eliminated with either anti-Lyt 1 or anti-Lyt 2 serum
and little if any reconstitution occurs when these two
populations are mixed. Thus, at the proliferating cell
level, an Ly 1,2 cell appears to play a crucial role in the
response to K/D alloantigenic differences, as also appears
to be the case for the response to the H-2 mutants (14).

As demonstrated in Table II, pretreatment of the cells
with either anti-Lyt 1 or anti-Lyt 2 serum fails to allow
the generation of a cytotoxic response against either K/D
alloantigens or complete H-2 differences on stimulating
cells. Admixture, however, of the two pretreated populations results in little if any response to K/D stimulation
whereas the response to an entire H-2 haplotype difference

TABLE I
MLC PROLIFERATIVE RESPONSE OF LY SUBPOPULATIONS AGAINST
SELECTED MHC REGION DIFFERENCES ON STIMULATING CELLS

AQR responding cells treated with[*]	MHC region difference of stimulator[†] net cpm[°]		
	K	I+S	K+I+S+D
C (5)[**]	2,565	14,885	14,207
αLy 1.2 + C (5)	-4	4,695	1,118
αLy 2.2 + C (5)	-178	20,773	15,903
αLy 1.2 + C (2.6) + αLy 2.2 + C (2.6)	317	13,183	12,153
αLy 1.2 + C (4.0) + αLy 2.2 + C (3.6)	312	10,423	11,733

[*]Prior to culture AQR spleen cell aliquots are treated
separately with each antiserum plus complement (C) or C
alone after which they are stimulated with 5 x 10^5 irradiated
spleen cells for 4 days.

[**]Number of responding cells x 10^5 per well.

[†]K region difference = B10.A; I+S = B10.T(6R); K+I+S+D
= B10.M.

[°]Net cpm refers to cpm remaining after background cpm
of responding cells incubated with syngeneic irradiated
cells has been subtracted. Background cpm are as follows:
C(5) = 2725; αLy 1.2 (5) = 1155; αLy 2.2 (5) = 1868; αLy 1.2
(2.6) + αLy 2.2 (2.6) = 1660; αLy 1.2 (4.0) + αLy 2.2 (3.6)
= 2608.

is reconstituted to a very major degree. These results
argue strongly for participation by Ly 1,2 cells at the
precursor stage in the generation of the cytotoxic response
to K/D stimuli and thus, at least at this level, there is no
fundamental difference in response to allo- and altered-self
antigens.

Lyt Phenotype of Effector T_c. As mentioned earlier,
the data presented in the literature to date suggests that
effector T_c are of the Ly 2 phenotype even in those
situations where an Ly 1,2 cell plays a role as a precursor.
We have examined this question not only with respect to
effector T_c following activation to K/D alloantigenic
differences but also in situations where stimulating and
responding cells differ by an entire H-2 haplotype or by
"mutant" H-2 encoded differences. Our results suggest that
in all of these situations there are some effector T_c that
are of the Ly 1,2 phenotype (12,15,16) although our

TABLE II

LY PHENOTYPE OF CELLS REQUIRED FOR CTL DEVELOPMENT TO H-2
VS D-REGION DISPARATE CELLS

| | | % CML ± SD | | |
| | | | Targets | |
B10.T(6R) responding cells*	E:T†	B10.T(6R)	B10.M	B10.G
I. H-2 Disparate Stimulating Cells; B10.T(6R) Responding Cells				
C treated	40:1	-3.2 ± 4.1	49.2 ± 3.3	
αLy 2.2 + C	40:1	-6.0 ± 3.8	9.2 ± 2.5	
αLy 1.2 + C	6:1	NT	2.6 ± 1.4	
αLy 1.2 + C + αLy 2.2 + C	40:1	-3.4 ± 3.5	44.9 ± 4.5	
II. D-Region Disparate Stimulating Cells; B10.T(6R) Responding Cells				
Untreated	50:1	-3.2 ± 5.0		38.4 ± 4.8
αLy 1.2 + C	50:1	NT		2.6 ± 5.2
αLy 2.2 + C	50:1	0.7 ± 5.8		12.8 ± 6.3
αLy 1.2 + C + αLy 2.2 + C	50:1	-2.3 ± 4.1		8.1 ± 4.3

* B10.T(6R) cell aliquots are treated separately with either antiserum plus
complement or complement alone after which they are stimulated with (I) B10.M_x or
(II) B10.G_x spleen cells.
†Effector:target cell ratio.
For further details, see reference 12.

impression is that the percentage of these cells as compared with Ly 2 effector T_c is greater when the stimulating cells used differ from the responding cells by only K/D allo-antigens. Recent data published by Nakayama et al (17), also indicate that effector Tc can express an Ly 1 pheno-type.

Presented in Table III are results of an experiment in which effector cell populations on day 5 of a primary MLC are treated with anti-Ly sera and complement immediately prior to their use as effector cells in the CML assay. Treatment with anti-Ly 2 serum plus C' essentially eliminates cytotoxicity both when the stimulating cells differ from the responding cells by an entire H-2 difference and when only a D region difference is present. Treatment of the effectors with anti-Lyt 1 serum plus C' very markedly reduces the cytotoxic activity of the cells following D region stimula-tion; treatment of the effectors that have been stimulated by an entire H-2 difference also significantly reduces cytotoxic activity although not as much as in the case when the stimulating cells differ by only the D region. In all of these experiments the effectors after treatment with either normal mouse serum or either of the anti-Ly sera were readjusted to the same effector/target cell ratio after

TABLE III

SUSCEPTIBILITY OF D-END VS K+I+S ACTIVATED

T_c TO LYT ANTISERA PLUS COMPLEMENT

Effector cells†	Lytic Units/10^6 cells on:
B10.T(6R) + B10.A$_x$ treated with:	B10.A Target
Complement (c) (2x)	27.5
αLy 1.2 + c (2x)	6.5
αLy 2.2 + c (2x)	0
B10.T(6R) + B10.G$_x$ treated with:	B10.G Target
Complement (2x)	7.5
αLy 1.2 + c (2x)	<0.25
αLy 2.2 + c (2x)	0

†Effector cells generated in vitro were treated twice on day 5 either with complement alone or with antisera plus complement, sequentially, and then allowed to interact with ^{51}Cr labeled target cells for 3.5 hours.

counting viable cells remaining after antiserum treatment.
Thus, any decrease in cytotoxic activity following treatment
with an antiserum as compared with normal mouse serum must
reflect the presence of effector T_c that are sensitive to
lysis with that antiserum.   The results from this, and
similar experiments, clearly indicate the presence of Ly 1,2
effector T_c.   This general problem, with a detailed presentation of the experimental data, is discussed elsewhere
(16).

   A Model for Alternative Pathways of T Lymphocyte
Activation.   Presented in Figure 1 is a theoretical schema
for T lymphocytes that respond to foreign antigens, presumably in altered-self or in alloantigenic situations.   The
pathway first described is depicted at the bottom of that
figure in which Ly 1 precursor T_h collaborate with Ly 2
precursor T_c.   This is the pathway in which the Ly 1 precursor T_h is presumably preferentially activated when the
stimulating cells carry the LD stimulus encoded by genes in
the H-2 I region.   This response can occur in the presence
or absence of Ly 1,2 cells.   The alternative pathway, which
is activated under situations where the stimulating cells
present only those antigens encoded in the K or D region to

PRIMARY RESPONSE

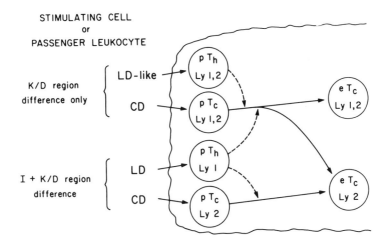

FIGURE 1.   A schematic representative of possible
pathways by which T lymphocytes can respond to allo- or
altered-self antigens.

the responding cells, involves participation by an Ly 1,2
precursor cell. We would hypothesize based on the data of
Swain et al (18) that there may be two Ly 1,2 cells involved:
first, an Ly 1,2 T_h that can respond to the uv-light or heat
sensitive component encoded in the K or D region (1) which
we have referred to as LD-like and second, an Ly 1,2 precursor
T_c. We would further hypothesize, as we have detailed
elsewhere (15), that in most responses there is a balance
between the two pathways which may depend on the presence of
the type of LD stimulus encoded in the I region in mouse or
the HLA-D region in man. Whether a threshold level exists
for the amount of LD stimulus needed to provide access to
the Ly 1 plus Ly 2 pathway (as compared with the Ly 1,2
dependent pathway) will need to be established in the future.
It appears that Ly 1,2 precursor cells can differentiate to
Ly 2 effector cells (19). At the same time, based on our
previously published data and the data included in Table
III, it seems likely that Ly 1,2 precursor T_c can also
differentiate into active cytotoxic T lymphocytes that still
carry the Ly 1,2 phenotype. Other evidence has been presented also suggesting that Ly 1,2 precursor T_c cells can
respond to alloantigens (20,21).
    The data presented and discussed above thus indicates
that at least with respect to the parameters enumerated, T
lymphocyte responses to altered-self are not fundamentally
different than those to alloantigens. In addition, the
findings raise the possibility that "memory" or "secondary-
type" lymphocytes generated by one or the other of the two
pathways of T lymphocyte activation may differ. Such a
difference could, in turn, lead to differential antigenic
requirements for activation of progeny cells derived from
the pathway dependent on collaboration between the Ly 1 and
Ly 2 cells as opposed to the antigenic requirements required
for activation of progeny cells derived from the Ly 1,2
dependent pathway.

SECONDARY RESPONSES

    Whereas a fair amount of information has been gained
regarding the antigens responsible for elicitation of
secondary responses to alloantigens, the situation with
altered-self has been more difficult to analyze. It is our
purpose in this section of the paper to review, with certain
points of emphasis, findings regarding secondary responses
to alloantigens and then pose questions based on data using
the Sendai virus system concerning possible parallelisms
between alloantigenic and altered-self recognition in the
secondary response. The possibility that we would want to

consider is that the antigenic requirements for restimulation following in vitro sensitization may differ depending on the genetic disparities present in the primary, sensitizing MLC. In turn, the differences in antigenic requirements may relate to the pathway that predominates during the primary, sensitizing culture.

Presented in Table IV are results obtained following in vitro sensitization to an entire H-2 haplotype in a primary MLC and evaluation of antigens encoded by various regions of the H-2 complex which are most effective in eliciting a secondary response on day 14 following primary sensitization. Restimulation with uv-light treated cells carrying the CD determinants initially used for sensitization elicits essentially no, or only a very weak, antigen specific cytotoxic response. Yet, the CD determinants on those uv-light treated cells elicit a strong, and highly specific, cytotoxic response in a primary MLC-CML in the presence of an additional LD stimulus in a three-cell protocol (22,23). On the other hand, restimulation on day 14 with cells carrying an I region difference leads to the production of a secondary-type cytotoxic response aimed at the K/D encoded CD antigens present on the initial sensitizing cells. The combined addition of the I region different restimulating cell and uv-light treated cell carrying the initial sensitizing CD antigens leads to a significantly, but only slightly, stronger cytotoxic response than does the I region different restimulating cell itself. This additive effect of the presence of the K/D encoded CD antigens on the restimulating cell mixture is antigen specific.

In further support of the findings shown in Table IV, Kuperman et al (24) have observed that animals sensitized in vivo to either normal cells or uv-light treated cells which differ by a K or D region show differential response patterns when restimulated in vitro with normal cells or uv-light treated cells. Results are summarized in Figure 2. If animals are sensitized on day 0 with normal cells differing by the D region, then spleen cells taken from the sensitized animals on day 7 and restimulated with x-irradiated cells show a marked memory type response, i.e. a stronger response (which is also detectable on an earlier day) than the response seen with spleen cells from an unprimed animal. Spleen cells taken from such an animal do not show a significant response against uv-light treated restimulating cells.

In contrast, if the animals are primed in vivo with uv-light treated cells then a marked secondary-type, memory response is elicited not only by x-irradiated cells but also by uv-light treated cells where both types of restimulating

TABLE IV

RESPECTIVE ROLE OF LD, CD AND LD + CD IN
GENERATION OF A SECONDARY CYTOTOXIC RESPONSE

Sensitization	Day of assay[a]	MLC (cpm ± S.D.)	Effector/Target	6R	D2
Primary					
6R + D2$_x$	5	51,769 ± 616	70/1	-2.8	57.4
	12	NT	70/1	-0.1	24.6
Secondary [6R + D2$_x$]					
+ 6R$_x$[b] (5 x 10^6)	3	2,335 ± 80	30/1	-2.7	5.8
+ D2$_x$ (5 x 10^6)	3	15,532 ± 751	30/1	-0.3	59.5
+ D2$_{uv}$ (5 x 10^6)	3	1,717 ± 126	30/1	-2.1	9.3
+ AQR$_x$ (5 x 10^6)	3	19,735 ± 265	30/1	1.4	35.3
+ D2$_{uv}$ (2.5 x 10^6) / AQR$_x$ (5 x 10^6)	3	26,815 ± 445	30/1	0.1	51.5
+ B10$_{uv}$ (2.5 x 10^6)	3	1,589 ± 140	30/1	-1.9	6.5
+ B10$_{uv}$ (2.5 x 10^6) / AQR$_x$ (2.5 x 10^6)	3	10,867 ± 463	30/1	-0.4	20.3

[a]Day of assay: day following primary sensitization or secondary
sensitization on day 14.
[b]5 x 10^6 primed responding spleen cells are restimulated in flasks with
the number of x-irradiated or uv-treated stimulating cells given in parentheses.
[c]Standard deviations on all targets <6.7%.
Reproduced from Grillot-Courvalin et al. (1977).

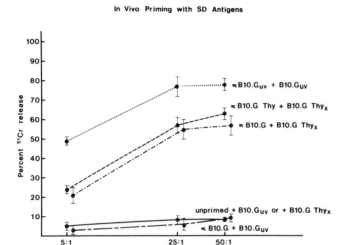

FIGURE 2. The response of in vivo sensitized cells to antigens presented in different combinations and after treatment of the restimulating cells in various manners.

cells are syngeneic with the priming cells. Although there are several interpretations of these findings, one possibility is that in vivo the animal has used different pathways of T lymphocyte activation in the generation of the response to alloantigens as presented on normal cells versus those presented on uv-light treated cells. These results, then, at least raise the possibility of a difference in antigenic requirement(s) for the elicitation of a secondary response depending on the pathway used in the primary sensitization. Thus, in analyzing the antigenic requirements for elicitation of secondary responses following sensitization to altered-self antigens, these considerations must be kept in mind to the extent that the rules governing the responses to allo-antigens will be paralleled in the altered-self systems.

We and others have studied the basis of the cytotoxic T response to Sendai virus with respect to the nature of the antigens that elicit the response (25,26,27,28). Our previous work has shown the importance of the fusion (F) glycoprotein and more specifically its fusion activity for target cell formation. Recently, results presented in detail elsewhere (29) and in preparation, we have made two further observations that may be relevent to parallelisms between alloantigenic and altered-self responses. First, it appears that whereas the primary response to Sendai virus is markedly dependent on the presence in the responding cell population of adherent cells, the secondary response seems relatively independent of or at the very least much less dependent on, the presence of adherent cells. Second, in possible direct analogy with the experiments just discussed fusion glycoprotein isolated from virions on a fetuin column and then coupled covalently to chicken red blood cells appears to be able, by itself, and presumably without the concurrent presence of H-2 antigens, to stimulate a highly significant secondary response. Although certain caveats must be considered in the interpretation of these data, it seems possible that following activation at least under some circumstances the CD antigen can, without the concurrent presence of the H-2 molecule which restricts recognition, activate a secondary response, not unlike the ability of uv-light treated restimulating cells to elicit a secondary response after sensitization with similar cells. This finding may relate directly to the apparent lack of a need for adherent cells in the secondary response which may be needed in a primary to "present" the CD antigen in the right context.

DISCUSSION

We would suggest from the data presented and reviewed in this paper that, at least with regard to the parameters that we have discussed, the basis for different T lymphocyte responses is not stimulation by altered-self vs alloantigens, but rather, that T lymphocyte responses may use one or the other of the two pathways depicted in Figure 1 depending, perhaps in large measure, on the presence of an LD stimulus as encoded in the I region, or a similar stimulus, with perhaps a quantitative requirement for the strength of that stimulus to reach a necessary activation level. The LD stimulus may give "access" to the Ly 1 T_h which would play a major role in the activation and expansion of the responding precursor Ly 2 T_c. To what extent the problem of dual recognition (given that as the explanation of MHC restriction) will apply not only to the altered-self situation but to the allogeneic response remains an open question at the present time with regard to the strong H-2 K and H-2 D encoded CD antigens.

The finding that effector T_c can carry the Ly 1,2 phenotype not only following activation against K/D allo-antigenic differences but also when stimulation has occurred with an entire H-2 haplotype or the H-2 mutants (12,16,17), not only supports the possible existence of mature precursor Ly 1,2 T_c, but also leads to the question whether effector T_c that carry the Ly 1,2 phenotype recognize the same determinant(s) as effector T_c that are of the Ly 2 phenotype. Could it be, for instance, that restricted responses use one of these two types of populations whereas non-restricted use the other?

With respect to the secondary response, a great deal more work is needed before tests of parallelism and difference between allo- and altered-self antigen induced responses can be adequately evaluted. We recognize, for instance, that our findings on the ability of fusion glycoprotein linked covalently to chicken red blood cells to elicit a secondary cytotoxic response contrast with the data published (30) studying the antigenic requirements of the elicitation of an anti-Sendai cytotoxic response using molecules incorporated into artificial membranes. It would appear to us that these differences might not only be explained by the method of sensitization of the animals but also by the method of presentation of the Sendai related glycoproteins in the two systems. We have attempted in this paper to draw some possible parallelisms but recognize that other interpretations exist for the data we have presented. Finally, as the complexity of T lymphocyte responses leading to the effector arm of that immunological system is recognized, it would seem likely to us that the selection of which system is used in any given situation or, even more probable, what balance there is between the different arms of the response would be determined by the types of antigens that are presented to the responding cells.

ACKNOWLEDGMENTS

We thank Dr. Kazuo Sugamura whose work, as yet unpublished, is referenced in this article; also our colleagues at the Immunobiology Research Center for discussion of these topics. The expert secretarial assistance of Ms. Michelle Howard and Ms. Cindy Smith is gratefully acknowledged.

REFERENCES

1. Bach, F.H., Bach, M.L., and Sondel, P.M. (1976). Nature 259, 273.

2.   Zinkernagel, R.M., and Doherty, P.C. (1974). Nature 248, 701.

3.   Bevan, M.J. (1975). J. Exp. Med. 142, 1349.

4.   Shearer, G.M. (1974). Eur. J. Immunol. 4, 527.

5.   Bach, F.H., Segall, M., Zier, K.S., Sondel, P.M., Alter, B.J., and Bach, M.L. (1973). Science 180, 403.

6.   Kisielow, P., Hirst, J.A., Shiku, H., Beverly, P.C.L., Hoffmann, M.K., Boyse, E.A. and Oettgen, H.F. (1975) Nature (London) 253, 219.

7.   Cantor, H., and Boyse, E.A. (1975). J. Exp. Med. 141, 1376.

8.   Cantor, H., and Boyse, E.A. (1975). J. Exp. Med. 141, 1390.

9.   Cantor, H., and Boyse, E.A. (1977) Cold Spring Harbor Symp. Quant. Biol. 41, 23.

10. Shiku, H., Takahashi, T., Bean, M.A., Old, L.J., and Oettgen, H.F. (1976). J. Exp. Med. 144, 1116.

11. Stutman, O., Shen, F.-W., and Boyse, E.A. (1977). Proc. Natl. Acad. Sci. USA 74, 5667.

12. Bach, F.H., and Alter, B.J. (1978). J. Exp. Med. 148, 829.

13. Bach, F.H., and Alter, B.J. (1977). In "Immune System: Genetics and Regulation" (E.E. Sercarz, L.A. Herzenberg, and C.F. Fox, eds.), pp. 631-637, Academic Press, New York.

14. Wettstein, P.J., Bailey, D.W., Mobraaten, L.E., Klein, J., and Frelinger, J.A. (1978). J. Exp. Med. 147, 1395.

15. Alter, B.J. and Bach, F.H. (1979). Speculations on Alternative Pathways of T Lymphocyte Response. Scand. J. Immunol., submitted.

16. Bach, F.H., Roehm, N., and Alter, B.J. (1979). Lyt Phenotype of Effector Cytotoxic T Lymphocytes Generated in Response to Alloantigens. In preparation.

17. Nakayama, E., Shiku, H., Stockert, E., Oettgen, H.F.,
     and Old, L.J. (1979). Proc. Natl. Acad. Sci. 76,
     1977.

18. Swain, S.L., and Panfili, P.R. (1979). J. Immunol.
     122, 383.

19. Stutman, O., and Shen, F.W. (1979). Transpl. Proc.,
     in press.

20. Wu, S., Bach, F.H. and Auerbach, R. (1975). J. Exp.
     Med. 142, 1301.

21. Burakoff, S.J., Finberg, Robert, Glimcher, L.,
     Lemonnier, F., Benacerraf, B., and Cantor, H. (1978).
     J. Exp. Med. 148, 1414.

22. Alter, B.J., Grillot-Courvalin, C., Bach, M.L., Zier,
     K.S., Sondel, P.M. and Bach, F.H. (1976). J. Exp.
     Med. 143, 1005.

23. Grillot-Courvalin, C., Alter, B.J., and Bach, F.H.
     (1977). J. Immunol. 119, 1253.

24. Kuperman, O.J., and Bach, F.H. (1977). Scand. J.
     Immunol. 6, 161.

25. Sugamura, K., Shimizu, K., Zarling, D.A., and Bach,
     F.H. (1977). Nature 270, 251.

26. Sugamura, K., Shimizu, K., and Bach, F.H. (1978).
     J. Exp. Med. 148, 276.

27. Schrader, J.W., and Edelman, G.M. (1977). J. Exp.
     Med. 145, 523.

28. Koszinowski, U., Gething, M.J., and Waterfield, M.
     (1977). Nature (London) 267, 160.

29. Sugamura, K., Shimizu, K., and Bach, F.H. (1978). J.
     Exp. Med. 148, 276.

30. Finberg, R., Weiner, H.L., Fields, B.N., Benacerraf,
     B., and Burakoff, S.J. (1979). Proc. Natl. Acad. Sci.
     76, 442.

T CELL CYTOTOXICITY IN MICE ELICITED BY IMMUNIZATION WITH SYNGENEIC TUMOR CELLS INDUCED BY DIFFERENT STRAINS OF MOUSE LEUKEMIA VIRUSES[1]

Fernando Plata[2] and Frank Lilly

Department of Genetics, Albert Einstein College of Medicine
Bronx, New York 10461

ABSTRACT   Mice of the BALB/c strain or its congenic partner strains differing in H-2 type produced cytotoxic T lymphocytes (CTL) when immunized with cells of syngeneic lines derived from tumors induced *in vivo* by Gross (GV) or Friend (FV) viruses. The cytotoxic activity of these lymphocytes depended on the presence on target cells of two immunologically distinct specificities: a viral specificity and an H-2 specificity. Little or no crossreactivity was seen on target cells that were either induced by different strains of virus or of a different H-2 haplotype, although extensive crossreactivity was seen among H-2-identical tumor target cells induced by the serologically crossreactive Friend, Moloney and Rauscher viruses. In the FV system, CTL activity elicited by immunizing with H-2^b cells depended exclusively on the presence on target cells of H-$2D^b$, H-$2K^b$ being irrelevant. By contrast, in the GV system, CTL activity elicited by immunizing with H-2^b cells depended on either H-$2D^b$ or H-$2K^b$.

INTRODUCTION

Mice immunized with viruses of diverse types often produce both an antibody response and a cell-mediated immune response. One component of this cellular response which has received particular attention is that of thymus-derived lymphocytes, or T cells. In several viral systems it has been possible to demonstrate the occurrence in immunized mice of cytotoxic T lymphocytes (CTL) capable of destroying virus-infected target cells (1,2).

Our own studies in this area have concentrated on two strains of murine leukemia virus (MuLV): Gross lymphatic

[1]This work was supported by a grant (NO1 CP 71017) from the National Cancer Institute, Bethesda, Maryland.

[2]Supported by a fellowship from Cancer Research Institute, Inc., New York, New York.

leukemia virus (GV) and Friend erythroleukemia virus (FV).
This paper summarizes our recent work, which demonstrates
that the activities of CTL generated in response to the two
different virus strains do not crossreact with each other,
and that the patterns of H-2 restriction of these CTL activities is also not identical in the two viral systems.

MATERIALS AND METHODS

For our studies of the CTL response to syngeneic MuLV-
induced tumor cells, we have taken advantage of the existence
of a series of mouse strains which differ from each other
with respect to the H-2 chromosomal region but share >99.9%
of the rest of their BALB/cAnLi-derived genetic material, so
that differences seen from one strain to another are attributable with a high degree of confidence to a gene of the H-2
region itself. In addition to the unrelated $H-2^b$, $H-2^d$ and
$H-2^k$ haplotypes, we have also used certain haplotypes representing recombination events occurring within H-2 itself. The
H-2K and H-2D region genotypes of these haplotypes are summarized in Table I.

TABLE I
MOUSE STRAINS AND H-2 HAPLOTYPES

Mouse strain	H-2 haplotype	Origin of	
		H-2K region	H-2D region
BALB/cAnLi	$H-2^d$	d	d
BALB.B	$H-2^b$	b	b
BALB.K	$H-2^k$	k	k
BALB.G	$H-2^g$	d	b
BALB.5R	$H-2i^5$	b	d
(BALB.B × BALB/c)F$_1$	$H-2^b/H-2^d$	b,d	b,d

Tumors were induced *in vivo* in mice of these strains with
both FV (3,4) and GV, and cells from these tumors were adapted for growth in culture as continuous cell lines. In the
FV tumor series, cell lines were designated generically as HFL
lines and individually with a letter identifying the H-2 haplotype of the strain of origin, e.g., HFL/b, of BALB.B ($H-2^b$)
origin. In the GV system cell lines were designated according to the strain and sex of the primary tumor-bearing donor,
e.g., CδGV from a BALB/c male.

Cells of each of these tumor lines have been used to
study the T cell response of the host. Primary immunization
was performed *in vivo*. Cells of the GV lines were heavily
X-irradiated (5000 r), and cells of the FV lines were fixed

by a 15 second exposure to 0.15% glutaraldehyde solution before use as immunogen. Twenty to thirty days later the spleens of the immunized mice were removed, and lymphocytes from them were restimulated by cultivation in the presence of X-irradiated cells of the same tumor line used for primary immunization. Six days later these lymphocytes were used as effector cells in cell-mediated cytolysis (CMC) assays in order to determine their capacity to lyse various ^{51}Cr-labeled target cells over a range of lymphocyte-to-target cell ratios.

RESULTS

The immunization procedure employed was uniformly sucessful in generating CTL in all mouse strains tested. In all cases but one the activity of the CTL was readily demonstrable on target cells of the same line used for immunization of the CTL donor. This exception was noted in the case of CTL from BALB/c mice immunized with CδGV cells, and the anomaly appeared to be due to a property of the tumor cell line rather than to the CTL population, since cells of B/CF$_1$δGV, a line derived from a (BALB.B × BALB/c)F$_1$ tumor, were highly susceptible to lysis by these CTL. In all experiments reported here the identity of the effector lymphocytes as T cells was confirmed by showing that their activities were abolished by pretreatment with anti-Thy-1.2 and complement.

The viral specificity of the CTL population was investigated in tests of lymphocytes of BALB.B mice immunized with either BδGV or HFL/b, using as targets various tumor cells derived from $H-2^b$ mice. Anti-BδGV CTL were strongly active on both BδGV and EδG2, the latter a GV-induced tumor line of C57BL/6 origin; no significant activity was detected on RBL-5 (C57BL Rauscher virus-induced leukemia), HFL/b or EL4 (C57BL chemically induced leukemia) target cells. Anti-HFL/b CTL showed marked activity on HFL/b and RBL-5, but none on BδGV, EδG2 or EL4 target cells. The crossreactivity of anti-HFL/b CTL on HFL/b and RBL-5 targets confirms previous indications that the Friend and Rauscher viruses, which induce markedly crossreactive cellular antigens detectable in serological assays (FMR antigen), also belong in the same category with respect to induction of the antigens recognized in the CMC assay (5,6). The failure to detect crossreactivity between these viruses, on the one hand, and GV, on the other hand, also establishes a parallel between the tumor cell antigens demonstrated in serological and T cell assay systems.

Previous studies from our laboratory have demonstrated that CTL activity in the FV system is $H-2$-restricted, i.e., that their activity depends upon at least partial $H-2$ identity

TABLE II

H-2 RESTRICTION OF CTL ACTIVITY ELICITED BY IMMUNIZATION
WITH SYNGENEIC, GV-INDUCED TUMOR CELLS[a]

^{51}Cr-labeled target cells	% ^{51}Cr release with CTL from:		
	BALB.B α-B♂GV	BALB/c α-C♂GV	BALB.K α-K♀GV
B♂GV	54	5	3
C♂GV	0	2	4
B/CF$_1$♂GV	33	48	5
K♀GV	8	11	26
G♂GV	23	53	5
5R♀GV	48	6	0

[a]CMC assay performed at a 30:1 ratio of CTL restimulated
in vitro and labeled tumor target cells.

between the target cell and the cell used for immunizing the
CTL donor (7). We now report that CTL activity in the GV
system is also strongly H-2-restricted, as demonstrated both
by direct CMC assays and by tests of the capacity of GV-
induced tumor cells of various H-2 types to inhibit the
specific activity of the CTL. CTL derived from BALB/c anti-
C♂GV, BALB.B anti-B♂GV and BALB.K anti-K♀GV immunizations
showed marked activity on the homologous tumor target but
little or no activity on the other two tumor targets (Table II).
In both the BALB/c anti-C♂GV and the BALB.B anti-B♂GV systems,
the capacity of the CTL to lyse B/CF$_1$♂GV target cells was
markedly inhibited by addition into the reaction mixture of
unlabeled cells of other GV-induced tumor lines, but only if
the added tumor cells were homozygous or heterozygous for the
same H-2 haplotype as the labeled target cell. (Although CTL
from BALB/c mice immunized with C♂GV cells were anomalously
ineffective in killing the homologous C♂GV target cells, as
noted above, the activity of these same CTL on B/CF$_1$♂GV target
cells was strongly inhibited by addition of C♂GV cells into
the reaction mixture.)

Extensive studies in other viral systems have indicated
that the requirement for at least partial H-2 identity, in
addition to viral antigen identity, between potential targets
for a given CTL population can be mapped within the complex
H-2 region, and that the relevant portions of the complex are
the H-2K and H-2D genes (8). In our previous work in the FV
system, we have studied the fine mapping of the H-2 restriction of BALB.B anti-HFL/b CTL and shown that crossreactivity

of the lytic effect of these cells depends on the presence of the $H-2D^b$ gene in potential target cells, $H-2K^b$ being apparently irrelevant (9). We have now performed a similar set of experiments regarding the $H-2$ restriction of BALB.B anti-BδGV and BALB/c anti-CδGV CTL. For this purpose we have developed and used as target cells for these two CTL populations two tumor lines from mice bearing intra-$H-2$ recombinant haplotypes: GδGV ($H-2^g$) and 5R$_Q$GV ($H-2^{i5}$). Table I shows the $H-2K$ and $H-2D$ constitution of these haplotypes. Table II indicates that BALB.B anti-BδGV CTL were effective not only against BoGV targets but also against both GδGV and 5R$_Q$GV targets, showing that possession of either $H-2K^b$ or $H-2D^b$ by a target cell permits expression of lytic activity in the GV/$H-2^b$ system. BALB/c anti-CδGV CTL, on the other hand, were effective only against GδGV and not 5R$_Q$GV targets, suggesting that only $H-2K^d$ and not $H-2D^d$ could serve as the basis for CTL crossreactivity.

DISCUSSION

Leukemogenic retroviruses of the mouse have been classified into two groups according to the cell surface antigens (CSA) induced by them on membranes of infected cells. These antigens have been extensively studied with serological techniques, but it has only recently been possible to investigate these or other CSA with techniques of cell-mediated immunity. Serologically, the CSA induced by a number of MuLV, including the Friend, Moloney and Rauscher prototype strains, crossreact broadly, permitting their classification into a category called FMR viruses (10). The FMR category of CSA has never been identified in tissues of uninfected mice, and recently it has been proposed that these viruses represent a purely contagious entity in mice that is transmitted horizontally but not within the germ line cells (11). The CSA induced by Gross MuLV shows no serological crossreactivity with FMR CSA, but crossreacts extensively with those of other strains of MuLV which share the property of being in some sense endogenous virus transmitted mainly as mendelian genetic units within the species.

The results summarized here are the first from detailed studies of the cellular immune response to GV-induced tumors of mice, although studies in the rat, where GV is markedly more immunogenic than in the mouse, have been reported (12). The methods used in our studies permitted the demonstration of high levels of GV-specific CTL generated in mice immunized with GV-induced, syngeneic tumors. From an analysis of the target cell specificities of these anti-GV CTL by comparison with anti-FV CTL prepared in an analogous manner, it appears that the virus-induced CSA recognized on target cells by the CTL lead to a classification of MuLV strains similar to the classification resulting from serological studies. We have also demonstrated that the cytolytic activity of the anti-GV CTL is strongly *H-2*-restricted, as had been the case in previous studies of anti-FV CTL (7). However, a detailed analysis was performed in order to determine the contributions to this *H-2* restriction phenomenon of different subregions of the *H-2* complex in the two viral systems. Whereas in the FV system BALB.B anti-HFL/b CTL were effective only if the prospective target cells possessed *H-2D^b* antigen specificities (9), we found that BALB.B anti-B̃GV CTL were effective on target cells possessing either *H-2D^b* or *H-2K^b* specificities. Thus, the CSA recognized by anti-GV and anti-FV CTL populations differ not only in their immunological specificities but also in their capacity to function as targets in the presence of *H-2K^b* gene product.

It has been postulated that the phenomenon which we call *H-2* restriction might be based upon the recognition by CTL of a self *H-2D* or *H-2K* molecule which has been modified by physical association with a virus-encoded molecule in such a way that it has become a specific type of non-self (13). If this hypothesis is true, it follows that GV and FV molecules show different patterns of affinity for various *H-2D* and *H-2K* molecules and form different types of non-self even when associated with the same *H-2D^b* molecule.

REFERENCES

1. Zinkernagel, R.M., and P.C. Doherty (1973). J. Exp. Med. *138,* 1266.
2. Koszinowski, U., and H. Ertl (1975). Nature *255,* 552.
3. Freedman, H.A., and F. Lilly (1975). J. Exp. Med. *142,* 212.
4. Freedman, H.A., F. Lilly and R.A. Steeves (1975). J. Exp. Med. *142,* 1365.
5. Herberman, R.B., T. Aoki, M. Nunn, D.H. Lavrin, N. Soares, A. Gazdar, H.T. Holden and K.K.S. Chang (1974). J. Nat. Cancer Inst. *53,* 1103.
6. Plata, F., J.C. Cerottini and K.T. Brunner (1975). Europ. J. Immunol. *5,* 227.
7. Blank, K.J., H.A. Freedman and F. Lilly (1976). Nature *260,* 250.
8. Blanden, R.V., P.C. Doherty, M.B.C. Dunlop, I.D. Gardner and R.M. Zinkernagel (1975). Nature *254,* 270.
9. Blank, K.J., and F. Lilly (1977). Nature *269,* 808.
10. Old, L.J., and E.A. Boyse (1965). Federation Proc. *24,* 1009.

11. Barbacid, M., K.C. Robbins and S.A. Aaronson (1979).
    J. Exp. Med. *149*, 254.
12. Bruce, J., N.A. Mitchison and G.R. Shellam (1976). Int.
    J. Cancer *17*, 342.
13. Zinkernagel, R.M., and P.C. Doherty (1974). Nature *251*,
    547.

DICHOTOMY OF MHC CONTROL OVER
ANTI H-Y CYTOTOXIC T CELL RESPONSES

Takeshi Matsunaga[1], Mary Brenan,
David Benjamin[2], and Elizabeth Simpson

Transplantation Biology Unit, Clinical Research Centre,
Watford Road, Harrow, Middlesex HA1 3UJ, England

ABSTRACT Anti H-Y cytotoxic T cell (Tc) responses in
mice are not only H-2 K/D restricted, but also under the
control of I-region Ir genes. We propose that such Ir
gene products are Ia antigens and function in the same
way as K/D antigens, i.e. Ia antigens are associative,
restrictive elements for helper T cells (Th) and such a
Th subset is required for the generation of anti H-Y Tc
responses. A non-responder situation may arise from a
failure of such associative recognition at either the Th
or the Tc subset level.

INTRODUCTION

T cells cannot recognize foreign antigens alone. Rather,
they "see" them in association with self major histocompatibility complex (MHC) antigens which T cells encounter and
learn in the thymus (1). This mode of cell recognition seems
to be the rule with at least three T cell subsets, i.e. cytotoxic T cells (Tc) in association with H-2 K/D in mice (2),
helper T cells (3,4) and cells for delayed-type responses (5)
in association with I-region antigens.

Our studies on H-2 gene control of Tc responses against
male specific antigens (s), H-Y, have shown that two different sets of H-2 genes (K/D and I) must somehow co-ordinate
properly in order to generate anti H-Y Tc responses and have
suggested collaborative interaction among different T cells
and antigen presenting macrophages (6).

[1]Present address: Department of Biology, City of Hope
National Medical Center, Duarte, CA 91010

[2]Present address: Department of Microbiology, School of
Medicine, University of Virginia, Charlottesville, VA

There are three points to be mentioned about the H-2 control in this system. (1) Anti H-Y Tc are K/D restricted in the analogous manner to the K/D restriction of anti virus Tc responses (7). (2) I-region Ir genes are critically involved in anti H-Y Tc responses (8). A particular I-region haplotype determines whether an animal can make anti H-Y Tc or not. Genetic studies revealed that two types of Ir genes can operate. The first is a dominant type of gene(s) which when present in appropriate F_1 hybrids makes such an F_1 female a responder to male antigens present on the parental cells of a non-responder haplotype. One of these dominant genes has been mapped at IA^b subregion (8). The second are complementary type Ir genes which can be recognized in appropriate F_1 hybrids. In these cases, two non-responder parental strains give F_1 hybrids which are responders and anti H-Y Tc can be elicited in association with K/D antigens of either parent. One of these complementary genes has been mapped to IC^k in the $H-2^k$ x $H-2^s$ combination (8). (3) There are several K/D antigens which we call "non-associative" in the sense that no anti H-Y Tc could be elicited in association with these antigens under any circumstances. Examples are K^b, D^d, K^q, K^s (6).

In order to shed more light on the underlying cellular mechanism of H-2 control, we studied anti H-Y responses in chimeric mice. Two kinds of chimeras were used: Allophenic mouse chimeras which can be produced by aggregating two 8-cell stage embryos, and irradiation bone marrow chimeras (double $P1 + P2 \rightarrow F_1$, single $P \rightarrow F_1$). The strain combination we were interested in for the chimeric studies was BALB/c and C3H (or CBA) for the following reasons.

BALB/c ($K^d I^d D^d$) and C3H/He ($K^k I^k D^k$) are both anti H-Y non-responders. Yet, their F_1 hybrids are responders although the response is found only with $H-2^k$ (K^k, D^k) of C3H male cells. This "one-way" type F_1 complementation was generally observed in F_1 animals between BALB/c and other non-responder parents (9). C3H.OH recombinant mice ($K^d I^d D^k$) are also responders with D^k association (8). We speculated that BALB/c must already possess dominant-type Ir gene(s) in the I region but that they lack appropriate associative K/D antigens for H-Y. In F_1 hybrids or C3H.OH, associative K^k or D^k are available.

The results from chimeric experiments led us to construct an "association model" (10) in which (1) the dichotomous nature of H-2 gene control on Tc response was emphasized, i.e. K/D and I gene products are associative, restrictive antigens for Tc and Th respectively implying that a specific Th subset is required to generate anti H-Y Tc responses. (2) Non-responders may arise from a failure of such associative recognition.

MATERIALS AND METHODS

Chimeras

Allophenic chimeras (BALB/c $\leftrightarrow$ C3H/He) were produced by aggregating a pair of 8-cell stage embryos in vitro and transferring them into uterii of a "incubator" mother (13,14). Mice born females, considered to be XX/XX karyotype, were selected for anti H-Y experiments.

Irradiation bone marrow chimeras [BALB/c + C3H/He $\rightarrow$ (BALB/c x C3H/He) F_1, BALB/c $\rightarrow$ (BALB/c x CBA) F_1] were produced by i.v. injection of bone marrow cells which had been treated with anti Thyl. 2 antiserum and complement into lethally irradiated F_1 mice (15).

In vitro Generation and Assay
of Anti H-Y Tc Responses

The method used to elicit and assay anti H-Y Tc responses have been described (7,8). In order to disect anti H-Y Tc responses in allophenic and double irradiation chimeras, anti H-2 serum plus complement treatment was employed to remove one or the other cellular genotype in the chimeric lymphoid population before sensitization in vitro (10).

RESULTS

Anti H-Y Responses in Allophenic and
(BALB/c + C3H/He) $\rightarrow F_1$ Irradiation Chimeras

Examples of anti Tc responses by an allophenic and a double irradiation chimera (d + k $\rightarrow F_1$) are represented in Table 1. It was found that, in both kinds of chimeras, the actual genotype of anti H-Y ($H-2^k$) Tc was of BALB/c origin. Chimeric spleen cells treated with anti $H-2^k$ plus complement before the in vitro boosting step generated anti H-Y Tc, whereas anti $H-2^d$ plus complement treatment abolished the responses completely. These anti $H-2^d$ treated cells gave anti third party H-2 responses indicating unresponsiveness to H-Y is specific. Five chimeras (3 allophenic, 2 irradiation) gave similar results but, in one allophenic chimera, there was evidence that $H-2^k$ cells may have produced anti H-Y Tc as well.

Anti H-Y Response in "Single"
BALB/c $\rightarrow F_1$ Irradiation Chimeras

As shown in Table 1, BALB/c $\rightarrow F_1$ chimeras responded to CBA ($H-2^k$) male cells.

TABLE 1

	Target Cells		
	H-2^k ♂	H-2^k ♀	Third party
Allophenic chimera #88 □			
(BALB/c ↔ C3H/He)			H-2^b (B10)*
anti H-2^k + C'	9.3 ± 1.7	1.1 ± 0.3	44.2 ± 1.0
anti H-2^d + C'	3.6 ± 1.3	-1.2 ± 2.0	43.8 ± 1.7
Irradiation double chimera ○			
H.W. # 1(BALB/c + C3H/He→F$_1$)			H-2^s (B10.S)*
unseparated	27.4 ± 0.8	0.4 ± 0.5	34.3 ± 1.8
anti H-2^k + C'	25.2 ± 1.6	1.0 ± 0.2	20.8 ± 0.4
anti H-2^d + C'	1.7 ± 1.3	0.7 ± 0.1	16.4 ± 0.8
Irradiation single chimera △			TNP-CBA*
(BALB/c→F$_1$)	32.8 ± 1.5	1.4 ± 2.0	45.6 ± 2.0

□ Allophenic chimera. lymphoid chimerism, H-2^d 20%, H-2^k 80%, primed in vivo with C3H/He male cells twice, 21 and 2 weeks before in vitro stimulation. Percent corrected lysis at attacker: target ratio = 8:1 (see reference 7). The r^2 value from regression analysis from four different points laid between 0.9 and 1.0. ○ Irradiation double chimera, H-2^d 27%, H-2^k 73%, primed in vivo 8 weeks before. △ irradiation single chimera, H-2^d cells more than 95%, primed in vivo 6 and 2 weeks before in vitro boosting. *Third party cells used as in vitro stimulator and target cells as positive control. Spontaneous release was between 10 and 20% except C3H female cells used for allophenic experiment (27%).

DISCUSSION

Our association model simply proposes that I-region Ir gene products are Ia antigens and that they participate in Tc responses as associative antigens responsible for the induction of Th as well as for the collaboration between Th and Tc precursors.

Chimeric Experiments

The experimental facts are that both allophenic chimeras (BALB/c $\leftrightarrow$ C3H/He) and irradiation chimeras (BALB/c + C3H/He $\rightarrow$ F_1) generated anti H-Y Tc in association with H-2^k and that in most cases (4/5) anti H-Y Tc were found to be BALB/c genotype. The latter point convinced us that indeed I-region restricted Th subsets are operative in anti H-Y Tc responses.

When C3H male cells are introduced into chimeras in priming, there are two cellular sites of antigen presentation to T cells (see Figure 1). Direct interaction occurs between Tc precursors and immunizing male C3H cells carrying H-Y and K/D antigens (H-2^k). Presentation of H-Y antigens to Th is executed by host macrophages which process H-Y antigens from degraded male antigen cells. However, it is only BALB/c macrophages, not C3H macrophages, that can offer associative Ia antigens to H-Y, such that both BALB/c and C3H Th cells can interact only with BALB/c macrophages. This is because only BALB/c cells possess dominant-type Ir gene(s) expressed on the macrophages (3,4). Consequently, the anti H-Y Th subset induced in these chimeras are restricted to I^d-coded Ia antigens and collaborate preferentially with Tc precursors bearing the same I^d antigens (i.e. BALB/c cells) in analogy to I-restricted Th for B cells (12). This explanation is based on the concept that Ir gene products = Ia antigens, and that these are restrictive entities.

The reason why we assumed direct interaction of Tc with antigen male cells was prompted by the observation that anti H-Y Tc generated in F_1 females after priming with male cells of one parent are always associated with K/D of the same parent used for priming (6). However, this might be a mere quantitative matter and, under certain immunization conditions, host macrophage-Tc interaction might become predominant.

On one occasion (in an allophenic chimera) there was some evidence for the presence of anti H-Y Tc of C3H type. This could be due to cross-reactivity between I^d and I^k antigens in that Th recognizing such cross-reactive determinants might have been induced.

It might be noted that, in these chimeras, both H-2^d and H-2^k antigens are present in the thymic epithelium (Figure 1).

FIGURE 1

Cellular Pathway of Anti H-Y Tc Response
in BALB/c (ddddd) ⟷ C3H/He (kkkkk) chimeric mice

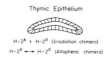

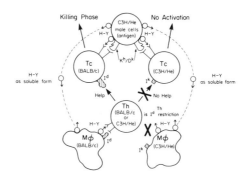

Thus, BALB/c precursors of Tc cells learned K^k and D^k antigens in the thymus such that they could react or recognize H-2^k determinants on C3H male cells. We favor the idea that thymus MHC learning represents clonal selection for anti MHC low affinity receptors (20).

     According to our explanation for the chimeric results outlined so far, BALB/c cells are crucial in that (1) BALB/c offers antigen presenting macrophages that express associative I^d-coded antigens (products of dominant Ir gene) (2) BALB/c Tc precursors learn H-2^k on the thymic epithelium.

     For this reason, there is no need for the presence of C3H cells (Tc, Th, macrophage) in this chimeric combination. The experimental results to support this point were obtained from the experiments using P→F$_1$ irradiation chimeras (Table 1),i.e. BALB/c→F$_1$ gave anti H-Y Tc (CBA H-2^k associated) responses. Analogous results were reported by von Boehmer et al. (15) using B10.A. (5R)→(B6 x CBA) F$_1$ chimeras in which B10.A. (5R) offer associative IA^b antigens for Th.

     Implicit with our association model is an emphasis that both K/D and Ia antigens of associative type are minimum requirement for eliciting anti H-Y Tc responses. Thus, H-2^b (e.g. B6 mice) are only responder strains, since H-2^b possess both associative D^b and IA^b antigens. A cellular pathway in

FIGURE 2

Cellular Pathway of Anti H-Y Tc Response
in C57 BL6 (bbbbb) Mice

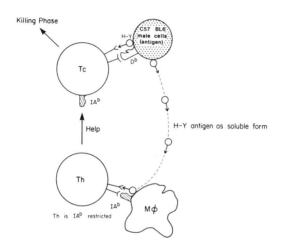

$H-2^b$ mice for anti H-Y response is depicted in Figure 2.

F_1 Complementation

Our association model can also explain the complicated pattern of F_1 complementary responses (9). In short, we see only two types of H-2 complementation in anti H-Y Tc responses observed in F_1 hybrids. The first type is a complementation between <u>associative K/D and associative Ia antigens</u> (associative Ia = products of dominant Ir gene). For example, BALB/c x C3H/He, a combination used for our chimeric studies, belongs to this class. Associative Ia antigens come from I^d of BALB/c and associative K/D are from C3H/He, $(H-2^k)$. Therefore, anti H-Y Tc are associated only with $H-2^k$ antigens (in vivo priming and in vitro boosting with BALB/c male cells gave no anti H-Y Tc). Since most strains of independent H-2 have associative K/D but lack associative (= dominant Ir) Ia for H-Y, F_1 hybrids with BALB/c are invariably "one-way" type responder. Apart from BALB/c and B10.A. (5R), $H-2^r$ (B10 R III.71NS) was found to have associative Ia but not K/D (9). In the case of F_1 animals with $H-2^b$ responder parent, anti H-Y response is "two-way", since these F_1 have associative IA^b and associative K/D from both parents $(D^b$ of $H-2^b$, associative K/D of other parent).

The second type is the complementation between at least two different I-region Ir genes. It has been suggested that complementary Ir genes may consist of the modification of Ia antigens of one haplotype by the presence, in F_1 hybrids, of I-region genes of another haplotype (16). Another possibility is that two Ia antigens form hybrid molecules. In either case, such newly formed Ia antigens become "associative", i.e. they will be presented to Th together with H-Y on macrophage surface. We believe that two complementary gene products must be localized within the same cells for the response to occur. F_1 hybrids that belong to this category of complementation usually give "two-way" anti H-Y Tc responses in spite of the fact that both parents are non-responders (e.g. $H-2^k$ x $H-2^s$, $H-2^k$ x $H-2^q$).

H-Y Antigen May Physically Associate With MHC

The terms "associative" and "association" have been used in a functional sense in the above section. We mean by these that H-Y antigens do actually associate physically with either K/D or Ia antigens on the plasma membrane of cells. Recently, it has been shown that spike proteins of Semliki forest virus (17) and bacterial particles (18) can indeed bind purified K/D or human HLA A, B and D antigens. There is some indirect evidence for H-Y-HLA association (19). Although MHC molecules may have broad specificity for binding many antigens, it is conceivable that some MHC products may bind less efficiently or may not bind at all. We favor the idea that such non-associative (non-binding) K/D or Ia antigens cause the non-responder condition (Figure 3). A corollary to this postulate would be that Th or Tc cannot be activated unless H-Y and MHC are jointly recognized. If T cells use two V_h receptors (20), one for H-Y and the other for MHC, both polypeptide chains must come close to each other to send an "on signal" to the cells. Alternatively, one V_h receptor with wide combining site is also compatible with the notion of joint recognition. In any case, these possibilities suggest evolutionary kinship between specificities of T cell V_h receptors and MHC molecules(21).

In an F_1 or H-2 recombinant female mouse which has two possible associative K/D antigens, the anti H-Y Tc response is directed predominantly at the "stronger" of the two antigens, i.e. of two possible clones of Tc cells, only one is activated. Quite clearly therefore the relative strength of the associative K/D antigens can control the response. Amongst associative K/D antigens, there is apparently a hierarchy of association: $D^k > D^b > K^k > K^d$ (6). Thus, K^d in BALB/c is the most weakly associative antigen and K^d associated anti H-Y Tc can only be demonstrated in (BALB/c x B10) F_1 hybrids where I^b as well as I^d induce abundance of Th help. This parental preference phenomena may be due to the relative difference in binding force of K/D molecules for H-Y antigen.

The presence of H-Y non-associative I-region alleles (non-responder Ir genes) widely spread among many inbred mouse strains is in contrast to the situation in H-2 restricted anti virus Tc responses. Although non-associative K/D have been reported with a group of alpha viruses (22), no I-region non-responder Ir gene has been identified. It might well be that such non-responder alleles for viruses have been eliminated by natural selection. In addition, the number of epitopes on H-Y antigens might be small, thus decreasing the chance of interacting with MHC antigens. According to Nagai et al. (23), human H-Y antigens are proteins with molecular weight being around 18,000.

If Tc responses generally require participation of both K/D and I antigens of associative type, selective forces might act on the particular combination of K/D and I alleles rather than on each of them separately. Thus, linkage disequilibrium observed between HLA A, B and D alleles (24) could be explained on this basis, as individuals with the capacity to generate Tc against some harmful viruses or other antigens should enjoy selective advantage. Although the Th subset alone may have some protective role against viruses (25), significance of Th participation in Tc responses remains to be elucidated.

FIGURE 3

Schematic Illustration of Association Model

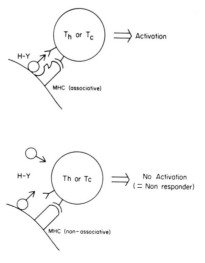

ACKNOWLEDGEMENTS

We are grateful to Dr. A. McLaren (Medical Research Council, Mammalian Development Unit) for kindly offering T.M. facilities to produce allophenic chimeras, Dr. H. Waldmann (Department of Pathology, Cambridge) for his kind gift of some irradiation chimeras used for our experiments.

REFERENCES

1. Zinkernagel, R.M., Callaghan, G.N., Althage, A., Cooper, S., Streilein, J.W., Klein, J. (1978) J. Exp. Med. 147, 897.
2. Doherty, P.C., Blanden, R.V., Zinkernagel, R.M. (1976) Transplant. Rev. 29, 89.
3. Rosenthal, A.S., Shevach, E.M. (1973) J. Exp. Med. 138, 1194.
4. Erb, P., Feldmann, M. (1975) J. Exp. Med. 142, 460.
5. Miller, J.F.A.P., Vadas, M.A., Whitelaw, A., Gamble, J. (1975) Proc. Natl. Acad. Sci. USA 72, 5093.
6. Simpson, E., Gordon, R.D. (1977) Immunol. Rev. 35, 59.
7. Gordon, R.D., Simpson, R., Samuelson, L.E. (1975) J. Exp. Med. 142, 1108.
8. Hurme, M., Hertherington, C.M., Chandler, P.R., Simpson, E. (1978) J. Exp. Med. 147, 758.
9. Brenan, M., Brunner, C., Matsunaga, T., Hetherington, C.M., Benjamin, D., Simpson, E. (submitted).
10. Matsunaga, T., Simpson, E. (1978) Proc. Natl. Acad. Sci. USA 75, 6207.
11. von Boehmer, H., Sprent, J., Nabholz, M. (1975) J. Exp. Med. 141, 322.
12. Sprent, J. (1978) J. Exp. Med. 147, 1142.
13. Mintz, B. (1971) IN: Methods in Mammalian Embryology, ed. Daniel, J.C. (Freeman, San Francisco), p. 186.
14. McLaren, A. (1976) IN: Mammalian Chimeras (Cambridge University Press, Cambridge), p.10.
15. von Boehmer, H., Haas, W., Jerne, N.K. (1978) Proc. Natl. Acad. Sci. USA 75, 2439.
16. Jones, P.P., Murphy, D.B., McDevitt, H.O. (1978) J. Exp. Med. 148, 925.
17. Helenius, A., Morein, B., Fries, E., Simons, K., Robinson, P., Schirrmacher, V., Terhorst, C., Strominger, J.L. (1978) Proc. Natl. Acad. Sci. USA 75, 3846.
18. Klareskog, L., Bank, G., Forsgren, A., Peterson, P.A. (1978) Proc. Natl. Acad. Sci. USA 75, 6197.

19. Beutler, B., Nagai, Y., Ohno, S., Klein, G., Shapiro, I.M.
    (1978) Cell 13, 509.
20. Janeway, C.A., Wigzell, H., Binz, H. (1976) Scand. J.
    Immunol. 5, 993.
21. Jerne, N.K. (1971) Eur. J. Immunol. 1, 1.
22. Mullbacher, A., Blanden, R.V. (1979) J. Exp. Med. 149,
    786.
23. Nagai, Y., Ciccarese, S., Ohno, S. (1979) Differentia-
    tion (in press).
24. Terasaki, P.I., Bernoco, D., Park, M.S., Ozturk, G.,
    Iwaki, Y. (1978) Amer. J. Clin. Path. 69, 103.
25. Howes, E.L., Taylor, W., Mitchison, N.A., Simpson, E.
    (1979) Nature 227, 67.

MOUSE ALLOANTIBODIES WHICH BLOCK
CML BY REACTING WITH KILLER CELLS

Nobukata Shinohara and David H. Sachs

Transplantation Biology Section, Immunology Branch,
National Cancer Institute, National Institutes of Health,
Bethesda, Maryland   20205

ABSTRACT   In an attempt to produce alloantibodies to
T cell receptors, hyperimmune anti-lymphocyte sera
raised in mice of various strain combinations have
been tested for their ability to block allogeneic CML
in the absence of complement at the T killer cell
level.   Although most of the sera failed to show
significant inhibitory effects, some C3H anti-B10.BR
antisera were found to be capable of significantly
inhibiting CML.   This effect was attributable to
antibodies reacting with the killer population rather
than the target cells, since the sera inhibited B10
anti-C3H CML but not C3H anti-B10 CML.   Among mouse
strains tested, sensitivity of killer cells to the
inhibitory effect correlated well with the strain
distribution of the Lyt-2.2 antigen.   In order to
study the relationship between the antigen(s) responsible for the blocking effect and Lyt-2-linked genes
as well as Igh-C-linked genes, killer cells from
Lyt-2 congenic and Ig congenic strains were tested.
Among B6, B6.Ly2.1, C3H.SW and CWB strains, only the
B6 strain was significantly sensitive despite the
fact that in the presence of complement the same sera
were toxic to >98% of 5 day in vitro sensitized cells
of B6 and B6.Ly2.1 strains with comparable titers.
These results indicate that the target molecules
reactive with the blocking antibodies are encoded by
genes linked to or identical with Lyt-2, and that
coating killer cells with antibodies of other specificities does not affect the killer cell functions.

INTRODUCTION

Available information on the nature of antigen recognition structures on T cells has been sparse and controversial.   Nevertheless, evidence obtained primarily by idiotypic

ISBN 0-12-069850-1

analyses suggests that at least a part of antigen combining
site of a T cell receptor is encoded by Ig heavy chain-linked
Igh-V genes (1, 2). However, conventional Ig constant region
determinants have not been detected on the molecules. If
T cell receptors have constant regions, antibodies to such
determinants might interfere with achievement of T cell
effector functions by blocking receptor-antigen interactions.
      Allogeneic CML reactions can be inhibited by anti-H-2
antibodies reactive with the relevant antigens of target
cells (3). Such inhibitory effects probably reflect
blocking of interaction between antigen molecules on target
cells and antigen-specific receptors on killer T cells. On
the other hand, the effector functions of cytotoxic T cells
in allogeneic CML reactions have been shown to be insensitive to treatment with a variety of mouse alloantibodies in
the absence of complement (4, 5). If alloantibodies with
such inhibitory activity could be raised, they would provide
a useful tool for analysis of the nature and genetics of
molecules involved in cytotoxic T cell effector functions.
Therefore we have made attempts to raise mouse alloantibodies
capable of inhibiting allogeneic CML by reacting with killer
cells in the absence of complement. Although most of our
attempts were unsuccessful, we could obtain mouse alloantisera with the requisite properties in one strain combination.
The properties of these sera as well as the linkage relationships of genes coding for the antigens on the cytotoxic T
cells reactive with the inhibitory antibodies have been
analyzed.

MATERIALS AND METHODS

      Mice. Adult mice, 8 to 10 weeks old, of both sexes were
used.

      Immunization. Recipient mice were immunized with i.p.
injections of 2 to 5 x 10^7 cells of a mixture of thymus,
spleen and lymph node cells of normal donor mice at 1- to
2-week intervals. For the first immunization, the cell
suspension was emulsified in CFA, and following immunizations were administered without adjuvant. Seven to eight
days after each immunization, mice were bled and pooled
sera were decomplemented (56°C, 30 min).

      Target Cells. Normal spleen cells and tumor cells were
used as target cells for CML assays. K46 BALB/c tumor cell
line (6) was kindly provided by Dr. J. Kim and maintained

in culture. Target cells were labeled by incubation with ^{51}Cr.

CML Assay. Methods for in vitro sensitization of
lymphocytes to alloantigens and CML assay have been described elsewhere (7). To study inhibitory activities of
alloantisera, 20 microliters of decomplemented serum was
placed in microtiter wells in triplicate and 100 µl of cell
suspension containing 1.6×10^5 attackers were added. After
shaking the plate, 2×10^4 ^{51}Cr-labeled target cells in 100
µl were added and the CML assay was performed. Fetal calf
serum used in all experiments was decomplemented (56°C for
30 min).

Complement-mediated Cytotoxicity Assay. Trypan blue
cytotoxicity tests were performed as previously described
(8).

RESULTS

Screening of Mouse Alloantisera for CML-blocking
Activity. Hyperimmune mouse alloantisera were raised in
various strain combinations including H-2 and non-H-2
incompatible pairs. Mice were immunized with mixtures of
normal spleen, lymph node and thymus cells up to 8 to 18
times, and they were bled 7 to 8 days after each immunization. Decomplemented sera were tested for their ability
to inhibit allogeneic CML when added to CML assay culture in
the absence of complement, using strain combinations chosen
to assess effects on the killer cells. Killer cell functions
were remarkably insensitive to such a treatment. Most of
these sera failed to show any significant and reproducible
inhibitory effect, although many of them had high-titered
antibodies reactive with 100% of donor spleen cells (Table
1). However, among the C3H anti-B10.BR (non-H-2) antisera
tested, some were found to have significant inhibitory
effects on CML.

Specificity of CML-inhibiting Activity of C3H Anti-
B10.BR Sera. In order to study whether or not the observed
inhibitory effect of these sera was attributable to alloantibodies reactive with the killer population, the effects of
the serum on killer cells of the donor and recipient strains
were examined. Since this serum (C3H anti-B10.BR) should
not contain anti-MHC antibodies, all H-2 congenic strains on
the B10 background would be expected to show reactivity to
this serum similar to that observed for B10.BR. Therefore,
C3H and B10 cells were sensitized to each other in vitro and

TABLE 1

SCREENING OF VARIOUS MOUSE ALLOANTISERA FOR
INHIBITORY EFFECT ON ALLOGENEIC KILLER CELLS[a]

Strain combination	Maximal cytotoxicity[b]		Inhibition of CML
	%		
BALB/cαB6	>90	1:2042	-, +[c]
A/JαB10.D2	>90	1:256	-, +
CBA/JαB10	>90	1:8000	-
B10.D2αB10.BR	>90	1:128	-
C3H/HeJαC3H.SW	>90	1:5120	-, +
BALB/cαB10.D2	>90	1:128	-
DBA/2αBALB/c	50	1:512	-
DBA/2αB10.D2	40	1:256	-
A/JαB10.A	>90	1:64	-
C3H/HeJαCBA/J	60	1:128	-
CBA/JαC3H/HeJ	70	1:64	-
CBA/JαB10.BR	>90	1:512	-, +
C3H/HeNαB10.BR	>90	1:1024	-, ++[d]
C3H/HeJαB10.BR	>90	1:512	-, ++
CB-20αBALB/c	<10		-
BALB/cαCB-20	<10		-
(PL/JxB6.PL-Thy1[a])F$_1$αB6	>90	1:256	-

[a]Animals of each group received 8 to 18 immunizations. Decomplemented pooled sera collected after each immunization were tested for their ability to inhibit CML in the absence of complement. Killer-target combinations were chosen so that the antisera should react only with the killer population.

[b]Complement-dependent cytotoxicity of the serum on donor spleen cells which showed the highest cytotoxic activity among the sera obtained within the immunization group. The left column shows the maximum percent of spleen cells killed by the serum. The right column indicates the maximal dilution of the serum required to kill more than half of the maximum killing.

[c]Inhibition with marginal significance or with poor reproducibility.

[d]Some sera showed significant and reproducible inhibition.

TABLE 2
SPECIFICITY OF CML-INHIBITORY ANTIBODIES IN
THE C3H ANTI-B10.BR SERUM

Inhibitor	Killer/target combination			
	B10αC3H on C3H	C3HαB10 on B10	B10αBALB/c on K46	C3HαBALB/c on K46
none	17.3 + 1.1[a]	36.2 + 1.3	47.1 + 2.0	51.9 + 1.7
NMS[b]	19.1 + 5.0	35.3 + 7.3	44.9 + 1.4	52.4 + 0.7
C3H B10.BR	8.9 + 1.0	38.9 + 7.2	16.2 + 0.1	40.9 + 0.2

[a]Precent specific release + standard deviation, in the presence of the indicated serum.
[b]Normal mouse serum.

the inhibitory effect of this serum was assessed on CML of the two reciprocal combinations of killers and targets (Table 2). In the combination of B10 killers and C3H targets, this serum caused significant reduction of specific lysis of target cells, whereas it did not show a significant effect on C3H anti-B10 CML. When B10 and C3H killers directed to a third strain (BALB/c, $\underline{H-2}^d$) were tested on the same target cell preparation, only B10 killers showed significant sensitivity to the inhibitory effect. These results indicated that the inhibitory activity of this serum on CML was achieved by antibodies reacting with the killer population rather than with target cells. Furthermore, specificity of killer cells, i.e., H-2 type of target cells recognized by the killers, did not seem to affect sensitivity to the inhibitory effect of this serum.

Correlation Between Sensitivity of Killer Cells to the Inhibitory Effect and the Lyt-2 Phenotype. In order to study the genetic relationship of the molecules reactive with the inhibitory antibodies present in these complex sera, sensitivity of CML effector cells of various mouse strains to the inhibitory effect of these antisera was examined. As shown in Table 3, killer functions of A/J, BALB/c, B10 and B6 strains were significantly inhibitable by these sera while those of AKR, CBA, C3H, and DBA/2 strains were insensitive. This pattern of strain distribution was found to be very well correlated with that of the Lyt-2 allele.

Linkage Analysis Using Congenic Strains. In order to examine the possible relationship between the antigen reactive with the inhibitory antibody and Lyt-2-linked genes

TABLE 3

EFFECT OF C3H ANTI-B10.BR SERA ON KILLER
CELLS OF VARIOUS STRAINS

| Killer | Inhibitor | | | Sensi- | |
strain	None	NMS	C3H B10.BR	tivity[a]	Lyt-2
AKR/N*	7.0[b]	9.2	9.9	−	1
A/J†	8.9	10.1	0.4	+	2
BALB/c†	13.0	10.8	2.3	+	2
B10*	18.0	16.2	−1.5	+	2
B6*	20.8	21.3	8.2	+	2
CBA/J*	17.9	18.2	19.3	−	1
C3H/HeJ*	13.7	12.8	13.1	−	1
DBA/2†	10.5	13.0	9.6	−	1

Normal splenic lymphocyes of indicated strains were
sensitized in vitro to C3H.SW cells (marked with †) or to
BALB/c cells (marked with *) and tested on C3H.SW spleen
cells (†) or K46 tumor cells (*).

[a]Sensitivity of killer cells to the inhibitory effect
of the C3H anti-B10.BR serum.

[b]Percent specific release in the presence of the
indicated serum.

as well as Igh-C-linked genes, killer cells from Lyt-2
congenic and Ig congenic strains were studied. Among B6
(Lyt-2[b], Igh-C[b]), B6.Ly2.1 (Lyt-2[a], Igh-C[b]), C3H.SW (Lyt-2[a],
Igh-C[a]), CWB (Lyt-2[a], Igh-C[b]), B10.BR (Lyt-2[b], Igh-C[b]) and
C3H (Lyt-2[a], Igh-C[a]) strains, only B6 and B10.BR strains
showed a significant sensitivity to the inhibitory effect
of C3H anti-B10.BR sera (Table 4). Killer cells of the
B6.Ly2.1 strain, which differs from the B6 strain at a
single chromosomal segment including the Lyt-2 locus, were
totally insensitive to the CML-inhibiting effect of these
sera. Complement-dependent cytotoxicity of the C3H/HeJ
anti-B10.BR serum was tested on Ficoll-Hypaque-separated
killer populations used in this experiment. As shown in
Fig. 1, this serum killed more than 98% of in vitro
sensitized killer cells of B6, B6.Ly2.1 and B10.BR strains
with almost identical titers. These results suggest that
the CML-inhibiting activities of these complex sera are
almost exclusively attributable to antibodies specific for
molecules encoded by a single genetic locus linked to or
identical with Lyt-2.

TABLE 4
EFFECT OF C3H ANTI-B10.BR SERA ON KILLER
CELLS OF CONGENIC STRAINS

Killer strain	Inhibitor			
	None	NMS	C3H/HeNα B10.BR	C3H/HeJα B10.BR
B6	26.3 + 1.3	25.5 + 0.8	11.7 + 0.7	14.8 + 1.2
B6-Ly2.1	20.6 + 0.5	18.1 + 0.7	22.1 + 0.1	21.8 + 1.9
C3H.SW	45.9 + 1.7	41.9 + 1.1	43.3 + 5.1	42.7 + 2.2
CWB	24.4 + 0.5	23.6 + 2.3	30.7 + 0.4	25.0 + 0.3
B10.BR	20.6 + 1.0	20.1 + 2.8	8.5 + 0.7	10.3 + 1.1
C3H	22.7 + 1.3	19.7 + 1.4	24.1 + 0.9	20.5 + 1.7

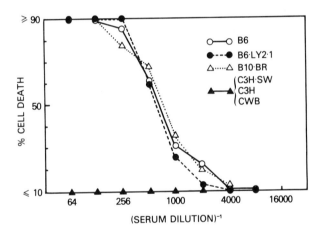

FIGURE 1. Complement-dependent cytotoxicity of the C3H anti-B10.BR serum on day five in vitro sensitized cells.

DISCUSSION

The observations made in this paper can be summarized as follows:
1) Some C3H anti-B10.BR sera are capable of inhibiting effector functions of allogeneic CML in the absence of complement.
2) This effect is attributable to antibodies reactive with killer cells rather than with target cells.

3) The target molecules reactive with the blocking anti-bodies are encoded by genes closely linked to or identical with the Lyt-2 locus.

4) Treating killer cells with antibodies of other specificities does not cause significant inhibition.

The identity of the molecules responsible for the anti-body-mediated inhibition of CML still remains to be studied. Lyt-2 molecules have been shown to be expressed on certain subpopulations of T cells including H-2D and K specific killer cells (5). However, earlier reports by other investigators have suggested that anti-Lyt-2 antibodies do not inhibit CML (4, 5). The discrepancy between the present observation and those observations might imply that the molecules reactive with the inhibitory antibodies are not Lyt-2 molecules but rather distinct molecules encoded by Lyt-2-linked genes. The discrepancy could also be due to differences in amounts and titers of antisera used for inhibition experiments.

At present we can only speculate on the possible mechanisms of the antibody-mediated inhibition of CML we have observed. The possibility of non-specific inhibitory mechanisms due to high-titered antibodies, such as massive agglutination of killer cells, has not been ruled out. However, it does not seem likely since the inhibitory anti-serum C3H anti-B10.BR did not affect the function of B6.Ly2.1 killer cells despite the fact that the reactivity of the serum as judged by complement-dependent cytotoxicity was indistinguishable from that on B6 killer cells. Further-more, treating killer cells with high-titered antibodies of other specificities did not cause significant inhibition (Table 1).

A second possibility is alteration of the cell surface by antibodies which somehow results in the inability of killer cells to achieve normal function. Since many other antibodies reactive with T cells failed to cause inhibition, this model requires a certain peculiar nature of the mole-cules reactive with the inhibitory antibodies. Such a relationship could be a close physical association of the Lyt-2 related determinants with some functional molecule necessary for killing. Even without physical association of the two kinds of molecules, such specific interference might occur.

A third possibility is that the inhibitory antibodies react with functional molecules other than antigen recep-tors. After interacting with the antigen on target cells, killer cells may deliver a killing message to the target cells through mediators either expressed on their surfaces or released locally. If the antibodies reacted with such molecules, killing might not take place.

Perhaps the most attractive possibility is that the observed inhibition reflects interaction of anti-receptor antibodies and antigen-recognition structures of killer T cells. In this model, the anti-receptor antibodies would be directed to the constant region of the receptor, since they inhibited the function of killer cells with various different specificities, i.e., anti-H-2^d, anti-H-2^k and anti-H-2^b.

Although the Lyt-2 antigen has been shown to be a marker for a subpopulation of T cells with certain functions including H-2K, D specific killer cells and suppressor cells (5, 9, 10), the function of this molecule is unknown. The present study may suggest a possibility that the Lyt-2 molecules play an essential role in effector functions of allogeneic killer T cells.

REFERENCES

1. Binz, H., and Wigzell, H. (1977). Contemp. Top. Immunobiol. 7, 113.
2. Rajewsky, K., and Eichmann, K. (1977). Contemp. Top. Immunobiol. 7, 69.
3. Nabholz, M., Vives, J., Young, H. M., Meo, T., Miggiano, V., Rijnbeck, A., and Shreffler, D. C. (1974). Eur. J. Immunol. 4, 378.
4. Kimura, A. K., and Wigzell, H. (1977). Contemp. Top. Mol. Immunol. 6, 209.
5. Shiku, H., Kisielow, P., Bean, M. A., Takahashi, T., Boyse, E. A., Oettgen, H. F., and Old, L. J. (1975). J. Exp. Med. 141, 227.
6. Kim, K. J., Kanellopoulos-Langevin, C., Merwin, R. M., Sachs, D. H., and Asofsky, R. A. (1979). J. Immunol. 122, 549.
7. Neefe, J. R., and Sachs, D. H. (1976). J. Exp. Med. 144, 996.
8. Sachs, D. H., Winn, J., and Russel, P. S. (1971). J. Immunol. 107, 481.
9. Cantor, H., Shen, F. W., and Boyse, E. A. (1976). J. Exp. Med. 143, 1391.
10. Huber, B., Devinsky, O., Gershon, R. K., and Cantor, H. (1976). J. Exp. Med. 143, 1534.

WORKSHOP SUMMARY: Genetics and Cell Interactions in Cell-Mediated Lympholysis. Gene Shearer, Immunology Branch, National Cancer Institute, Bethesda, MD 20205 and Benjamin Bonavida, Department of Microbiology and Immunology, UCLA School of Medicine, Los Angeles, CA 90024.

The workshop discussion was divided into four broad categories which addressed questions dealing with:
1) Specificity in cell-mediated lympholysis
2) Regulatory cells involved in cytotoxic T-lymphocyte generation
3) Mechanism of cytotoxic T-lymphocyte generation and cytotoxic lysis
4) Ir gene control of cytotoxic T-lymphocyte responses

Many of the questions raised during the workshop were related to the results presented in the poster session of the panel topic.

1) Specificity in cell-mediated lympholysis: The question was raised whether antigenic structures other than MHC gene products have been recently identified which are recognized by cytotoxic T-lymphocytes (CTL) and whether such responses would be major histocompatibility complex (MHC) restricted. It was reported that a secondary in vitro T-cell mediated lympholysis (CML) response could be generated against products of the Qa-1 region. Qa-1-directed cytotoxicity was not H-2 restricted, and therefore, appeared to behave like other major alloantigenic systems.

The function of the L antigen (a second D region product) was compared to that of the K and D antigens in various CTL responses. The results indicated that: a) CTL responses against products of the D region included reactivity against L as well as D alloantigens; b) CTL against TNP-modified syngeneic cells (TNP-self) did not include reactivity against L-TNP; and c) CTL against influenza infected syngeneic cells included recognition of influenza in association with L antigens. These results indicate that L antigens can function analogously to K and D antigens in some but not all CTL responses.

Another aspect of CTL specificity was concerned with inhibition of the lytic phase of an allogeneic CML reaction by mouse alloantibodies. In contrast to other effector phase blocking studies, these antibodies interacted with determinants on the effector rather than on the target cells. A careful analysis of the phenomenon in a number of inbred mouse strains indicated that the target molecules responsible for blocking was encoded by a gene linked to or identical with Lyt-2.

The cytotoxic activity of H-2-restricted influenza specific

CTL was shown to be inhibited by pre-incubating infected
target cells with monoclonal anti-influenza antibodies.
Although the hybridomas used were all directed against the
hemagglutinin antigen, they differed in their ability to
inhibit CTL. Spleen cells and TDL from immunized mice
appeared to be differentially inhibited by these hybridomas.

Effector cell activity generated by F_1 hybrid anti-parent
CTL responses were found to specifically lyse only parental
and not F_1 target cells. However, cold target cell inhibition
of lysis could be achieved by F_1 as well as parental blockers.
These observations raise the possibility that the antigenic
requirements for lysis and inhibition of cytolysis may be
different.

2) Regulatory cells involved in cytotoxic T-lymphocyte
generation: The questions of whether direct evidence exist
for helper and suppressor cells in CML was considered.
Subcutaneous immunization of mice with trinitrophenyl-modified
syngeneic cells (TNP-self) resulted in enhanced secondary in
vitro CTL responses. The increment of enhanced CTL due to
priming was abolished by antigen-specific suppressor T cells.

The generation of CTL against alloantigens was shown to
be regulated by radioresistant helper cells which were Ly6(-),
Ly7(+), but their precursors were Ly6(+), Ly7(-), and their
precursors were also Ly6(+), Ly7(-). Such Ly studies may be
useful in characterizing helper and suppressor functions for
regulation of cytotoxicity.

3) Mechanism of CTL generation and cytotoxic lysis: The
question was raised regarding the precursor frequency analysis
of cytotoxic T cells. Using a battery of H-2 mutant strains
sensitized against the strains of origin, it was shown that
the number of CTL precursors against allogeneic H-2 molecules
does not increase as serological and structural similarities
diverge. These results suggest that the T cell receptor repertoire recognizes those H-2 molecules or determinants closest
to self. The repertoire of cytotoxic precursors to TNP-
modified self and TNP-modified allogeneic cells was examined.
It was shown that a high degree of cross-reaction exists
between allodeterminants and TNP-modified self determinants
and consistent with the hypothesis that cytotoxic responses
to TNP-modified self antigens may be similar to responses to
alloantigens. The allodeterminants are being created as a
result of modification of H-2 antigens with TNP. An analysis
was made of the mechanism of recognition by cytotoxic T cells.
It was shown that there was a dissociation between recognition
and binding using various metabolic inhibitors and requirements. Consequently, it was suggested that the step of antigen specific recognition which is sufficient for subsequent
cytolysis may be of weak affinity with the T cell receptor and

the receptor having more of a reading than a binding role.
In another study, the role of $^{++}$Ca in killing was examined.
Since the lytic hit is calcium dependent, it was questioned
whether killing of target cells by CTL is due to a selective
incorporation of lethal amount of calcium into the target
cell. Using P815 mastocytoma cells, allowing measurement of
secretion in addition to lysis, it was found that a high concentration of calcium ionophore A23187 induced calcium dependent lysis and this was preceded by a secretion of ^{14}C serotonin. However, when CTL were directed against mast cells,
^{14}C serotonin was not released from the target until after
^{51}Cr. These results argued against selective calcium influx
being the sole primary event effected by the killer T lymphocytes. The issue as to whether cytotoxic T lymphocytes mediate killing by a soluble mediator was reexamined. Supernatants derived from allosensitized lymphocytes following
incubation with L929 cells was primarily cytotoxic to the
original sensitizing target cell. It was hypothesized that
the supernatant may consist of a short-lived lymphotoxin in
association with antigen specific receptor. Finally, it was
proposed that antigen recognition and binding by single CTL
can be used to measure directly the frequency of cytotoxic T
lymphocytes. Effector target cell conjugates were prepared
and lysis of individual target cells measured. Using this
assay, it was proposed that a single rate-binding step is
operational in CMC, and that measurement of target lysis is
best represented as an exponential function.

    4) Ir gene control of cytotoxic responses: Certain
similarities have been observed for immunoregulation among
H-2 restricted CTL responses. For example, some unrelated
CTL respond to antigens in association with D-coded self
structures, but not in association with K-self. In contrast,
a number of (but not all) H-2 restricted CTL responses including that to trinitrophenyl-modified syngeneic cells show the
similar pattern of reduced or absent CTL to antigens in
association with D region self products when that antigen was
recognized in association with $\underline{K^k}$. Regulation of the D restricted response of F_1 mice to TNP-self was shown to be
dependent on an active response to TNP-self in association
with $\underline{K^k}$.

    Genetic regulation of CTL to syngeneic cells modified with
low concentrations of TNBS (low dose TNP-self) was found to
be H-2 linked. $\underline{H-2^{k,a}}$ mouse strains were responders, whereas
$\underline{H-2^{b,d}}$ strains were low responders to low dose TNP-self.
(Responder x non-responder) F_1 responded when recognizing TNP
in association with responder self structures, but did not
respond when recognizing TNP in association with non-responder
self structures.

Genetic control of specificity of human cytotoxic T-cells to influenza infected autologous cells was investigated in a large family. Influenza specific CTL were generated by all family members and the specificity of the effectors was shown to be HLA-linked. Leukocytes from siblings consistently generated CTL activity which was predominately in association with only one HLA haplotype. These preferential patterns of responses were similar among HLA-identical siblings, indicating that HLA-linked genes were responsible for this haplotype preference in T-cell recognition of influenza-infected cells.

HYBRID I REGION ANTIGENS AND I REGION
RESTRICTION OF RECOGNITION IN MLR

C. G. Fathman and H. Hengartner

Department of Immunology, Mayo Clinic, Rochester, MN.
Basel Institute of Immunology, Basel, Switzerland

Recent studies from this laboratory have demonstrated the existence of a unique murine hybrid MLR
stimulating determinant(s) on stimulator cells from
(C57 Bl 6 x A/J)F$_1$ (B6A) mice. This determinant(s) has
been demonstrated to be encoded by genes residing within
the I region of the murine major histocompatibility
complex (H-2) and the recognition of this product has
likewise been demonstrated to be controlled by products
of the I region of the H-2 complex. Using appropriate
recombinant mice it has been possible to further
localize the site of interaction which leads to the
production and recognition of this hybrid MLR stimulating determinant(s). Additionally, it has been
possible to derive clones of alloreactive T cells using
techniques of soft agar cloning which have specificity
for the unique MLR stimulating determinant(s) on B6A
stimulator cells.

INTRODUCTION

The studies of Irvin in the mid-sixties suggested that
non-allelic genes could form "interaction" products recognized as hybrid cellular antigens in eukaryotic species (1).
Additional reports of the interaction of non-allelic genes
have appeared (2,3). Until recently, however, hybrid histocompatibility antigens had not been described. Using techniques of in vitro secondary mixed lymphocyte cultures, we
have been able to demonstrate hybrid histocompatibility
determinants (4,5,6). The results obtained in our studies
suggest that in vitro primed populations of alloreactive
cells (primed responder cell = PRC) can recognize determinants
on hybrid cells which are not present on either parental cell
type. Furthermore, using techniques of soft agar cloning, it
has been possible to derive clones of alloreactive T cells
which recognize the unique hybrid histocompatibility deter-
minant(s) on B6A stimulator cells (7,8,9).

577

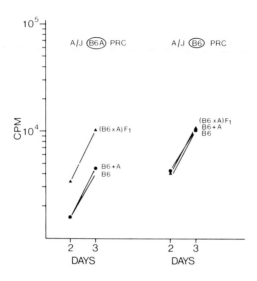

FIG.1   The response expressed as cpm of incorporated
$[^3H]$dThd, of 50×10^3 A(B6A)PRC and A(B6)PRC to restimulation
with allogeneic (B6), semi-allogeneic (B6xA)F_1, or a mixture
of syngeneic and allogeneic (B6+A) stimulator cells. The
$[^3H]$dThd incorporation in the syngeneic control culture has
been subtracted from each experimental group.   Reprinted by
permission (4).

1. <u>Hybrid Histocompatibility Determinants</u>. Figure 1
demonstrates the phenomena of enhanced MLR reactivity of F_1
primed responder cells.   A/J (A) responder lymph node cells
were cultured <u>in vitro</u> with either allogeneic C57BL/6 (B6) or
semi-allogeneic (B6xA)F_1 B6A irradiated stimulator spleen
cells.   Two weeks later these cultures were harvested and the
surviving viable cells (PRC) were tested in secondary MLR
against allogeneic B6, semi-allogeneic B6A or 1:1 mixtures of
A and B6 stimulator cells. A(B6A)PRC (cells from strain A
primed with B6A stimulator cells) recognized F_1 stimulator
cells about twice as well as they recognized allogeneic cells
or the mixture of A and B6 cells. A(B6)PRC recognized all
three stimulator populations equally well. The genes controlling the expression of this F_1 MLR stimulating determi-
nant(s) were mapped to the H-2 complex. Table 1 demonstrates
the H-2 linkage of expression of the F_1 MLR determinant(s).
When the mapping of the genes controlling expression of the
F_1 MLR determinant(s) was extended using recombinant congenic
mice, the genetic control of the hybrid determinant(s) became
more complex. Table 2 presents the data obtained using hybrids
derived from crosses of recombinant mice with the allogeneic
parent, B10, as a source of stimulator cells for A(B6A)PRC.

Table 1. H-2 linkage of F_1 MLR determinants[a]

Stimulator strain	H-2 haplotype	A(B6A)PRC	A(B6)PRC
		(cpm ± SE)	
A/J	a/a	2 632 ± 137	3 980 ± 276
(B6 x A)F$_1$	a/b	39 608 ± 2317	36 329 ± 4124
B6 + A	a/a + b/b	21 094 ± 1206	35 071 ± 524
B6	b/b	19 921 ± 732	33 770 ± 1274
(A.BY x B6)F$_1$	b/b	20 374 ± 978	37 324 ± 5176
(A.BY x A/J)F$_1$	a/b	41 913 ± 142	35 245 ± 1076
(B10.A x A)F$_1$	a/a	2 570 ± 240	2 984 ± 360
(B10.A x B10)F$_1$	a/b	40 176 ± 2274	34 773 ± 332

a) The response on day 2 of 50x10^3 A(B6A)PRC and A(B6)PRC expressed as cpm ± SE of incorporated [^{3}H]dThd to a variety of stimulator cell types bearing MHC haplotypes of strain A and/or B6 is given. Reprinted by permission (4).

Table 2. Mapping of genes controlling F_1-MLR determinants[a]

Stimulator strain	H-2 haplotype		A(B6A)PRC	A(B6)PRC
			(cpm ± SE)	
A	a	(kkkkkddd)	4 376 ± 11	3 742 ± 173
B6 + A	b + a	(bbbbbbbb + kkkkkddd)	25 522 ± 76	21 148 ± 950
B6	b	(bbbbbbbb)	22 260 ± 2260	18 999 ± 1110
(B6 x A)F$_1$	b/a	(bbbbbbbb/kkkkkddd)	46 804 ± 2492	23 552 ± 834
(B10 x B10.A(5R))F$_1$	b/i5	(bbbbbbbb/bbbkkddd)	20 545 ± 759	18 578 ± 1490
(B10 x B10.A(4R))F$_1$	b/h4	(bbbbbbbb/kkbbbbbb)	18 693 ± 1387	19 324 ± 1258
(B10.A(4R) x B10.A(5R))F$_1$	h4/i5	(kkbbbbbb/bbbkkddd)	49 646 ± 416	21 536 ± 1948

a) The response on day 2 (as cpm ± SE) of 50x10^3 A(B6A)PRC and A(B6)PRC to a variety of stimulator cells including cells from certain hybrid mice, sharing regions of the MHC with both strain A and B6. For presentation purposes the MHC regions shared between the stimulator cells and strain A are underlined. Reprinted by permission (4).

These results clearly demonstrate that expression of the F$_1$ MLR stimulating determinant(s) on B6A cells requires the presence (in cis- or in trans-position) of at least two loci within the MHC.

Using selected recombinant mice, it has been possible to further localize the site of interaction which leads to the production and recognition of this hybrid MLR stimulating determinant(s). Prerequisites for expression of the hybrid MLR stimulating determinant(s) between strains A and B6 include an I-E region of the k haplotype and an I-A of both

b and k haplotypes. F_1 mice derived from recombinant strains
which lack any of these subregions fail to express the F_1 MLR
stimulating determinant(s). Table 3 presents data which
support the hypothesis that the product(s) recognized by
strain A present on B6A stimulator cells is an altered form
of I-A^b resulting from genes residing within the I-E region
of haplotype k and that the recognition of this altered form(s)
of I-A^b is restricted by I-A^k region products. This hypothesis
is based in part upon recent studies by Dr. P. Jones and
collaborators who have demonstrated using two-dimensional gel
electrophoresis that the cell surface expression of some I-A
antigens appears to be controlled by two genes (10). One
locus maps in the I-A subregion and is probably the structural
gene for an I-A encoded polypeptide, whereas the second locus
which maps between the I-J and the H-2D regions, controls the
cell surface expression of this I-A molecule. Furthermore,
complementation between these two loci allowing cell surface
expression can occur in cis- or trans- chromosomal position.
Mice of haplotype H-2^b generate a cytoplasmic precursor for
an I-A^b molecule which can be expressed in recombinant or
hybrid animals who have "permissive haplotypes" in the region
of H-2 between I-J and D. It is possible that the hybrid
determinant(s) recognized on B6A stimulator cells is the same
molecule that has been detected by two-dimensional gel electrophoresis; (i.e., the cell surface expression of the cytoplasmic precursor of I-A^b which is allowed, in combination
with the permissive haplotype of strain A.) However, if this
alone were enough for expression of the hybrid MLR stimulating
determinant(s) on B6A stimulator cells, then recombinant
strains B10.A(5R) and B10.A(3R) should be able to express the
hybrid stimulating determinant(s). As demonstrated in Table
3A, A(B6A)PRC do not recognize B10.A(5R) nor B10.A(3R) stimulator cells any better than they recognize B6 or B10 stimulator cells. Thus, it is apparent that the simple expression
of the altered form of the I-A^b antigen recognized by two-
dimensional gel electrophoresis is insufficient to generate
the augmented responsiveness of A(B6A)PRC seen when they are
restimulated with B6A stimulator cells. Furthermore, if the
hybrid MLR stimulating determinant(s) were simply an interaction of allelic products of either I-A or some other region
of the mouse H-2 complex between haplotypes a and b, then
recombinant F_1 hybrids [B10.A(5R)xB6]F_1 and/or [B10.A(4R)xB6]F_1
should be capable of reconstituting a response similar to the
augmented responsiveness seen when A(B6A)PRC are stimulated
with B6A stimulator cells. As demonstrated previously (4)
(and in Table 3B) neither of these F_1 stimulator cells is
capable of reconstituting the responsiveness of A(B6A)PRC for
the F_1 hybrid determinant(s). Not only can [B10.A(4R)xB10.A
(5R)]F_1 mice reconstitute the augmented responsiveness of

TABLE 3-A

Mapping of genes which allow expression and/or recognition
of F_1 "hybrid MLR determinant"

Strain	K	A	B	J	E	C	S	D	A(B6A) PRC	A(B6) PRC
									CPM ± SD	
A	k	k	k	k	k	d	d	d	546 ± 25	349 ± 21
B6	b	b	b	b	b	b	b	b	16,577 ± 1,538	21,901 ± 1,494
B6A	k	k	k	k	k	d	d	d	29,677 ± 3,388	21,629 ± 1,363
	b	b	b	b	b	b	b	b		
B10	b	b	b	b	b	b	b	b	17,013 ± 138	23,017 ± 1,714
B10.A(5R)	b	b	b	k	k	d	d	d	16,986 ± 531	21,776 ± 911
B10.A(3R)	b	b	b	b	k	d	d	d	15,524 ± 337	20,177 ± 1,706

TABLE 3-B

	K	A	B	J	E	C	S	D	A(B6A) PRC	A(B6) PRC
[B10.A(4R)xB10]F_1	k	k	b	b	b	b	b	b	14,028 ± 288	10,150 ± 1,322
	b	b	b	b	b	b	b	b		
[B10.A(5R)xB10]F_1	b	b	b	k	k	d	d	d	18,598 ± 2,694	21,068 ± 474
	b	b	b	b	b	b	b	b		
[B10.A(5R)xB10.A]F_1	k	k	b	b	b	b	b	b	7,132 ± 973	6,139 ± 104
	k	k	k	k	k	d	d	d		
[B10.A(5R)xB10.A]F_1	b	b	b	k	k	d	d	d	31,306 ± 653	19,634 ± 617
	k	k	k	k	k	d	d	d		
[B10.A(4R)xB10.A(5R)]F_1	k	k	b	b	b	b	b	b	30,911 ± 1,077	20,017 ± 391
	b	b	b	k	k	d	d	d		

TABLE 3-C

	K	A	B	J	E	C	S	D	A(B6A) PRC	A(B6) PRC
[A.TFRIxB10.A(5R)]F_1	s	k	k	k	k	k	k	f	32,805 ± 1,398	18,828 ± 3,504
	b	b	b	k	k	d	d	d		
[A.TFRIxB10.A(4R)]F_1	s	k	k	k	k	k	k	f	6,832 ± 1,006	8,911 ± 397
	k	k	b	b	b	b	b	b		
[B10.A(3R)xB10.A(4R)]F_1	b	b	b	b	k	d	d	d	28,667 ± 1,161	19,695 ± 1,934
	k	k	b	b	b	b	b	b		

Table 3A, 3B & 3C. The results of one of several experiments in which 25×10^3 A(B6A) or A(B6)PRC are restimulated in secondary MLR with 1×10^6 irradiated (3300R) cells from a variety of mice. At the termination of a 72 hour culture, proliferation is assayed as counts per minute (CPM) plus or minus standard deviation (± SD) of standard scintillation counting following a 16 hour pulse with 2 mci of ^{3}HTdr(5). The responses of A(B6A)PRC to restimulation with B6A have been underlined as have similar responses against other stimulator cells. Subregions of H-2 shared among the genotypes of the cells generating this amount of response in A(B6A)PRC have been underlined.

A(B6A)PRC but [B10.A(5R)xB10.A]F_1 mice can reconstitute this
responsiveness. This confirms our initial observations which
suggest that we are looking at an interaction of genes or
gene products of haplotypes a and b which can interact in
cis- or in trans-configuration. Data presented in Table 3C
further localizes the areas of interaction which allow
expression of the F_1 MLR stimulating determinant(s) by
examining responsiveness of A(B6A)PRC to stimulator cells
from hybrid mice derived between crosses of A.TFR1 and
B10.A(5R) and A.TFR1 by B10 A(4R). The augmented responsiveness of A(B6A)PRC for [A.TFR1xB10.A(5R)]F_1 stimulator cells
excludes the need for sharing at the k of K and any a haplotype products to the right of the I-E region and by examining
the responsiveness of A(B6A)PRC to stimulation by cells from
the recombinant F_1 hybrid B10.A(3R)xB10.A(4R) it is possible
to exclude the I-J of k as a prerequisite for expression of
the F_1 MLR stimulating determinant(s). Thus these data suggest
as one possible explanation that the hybrid determinant(s)
recognized by A(B6A)PRC on B6A stimulator cells is indeed the
altered form of I-A^b allowed by the permissive haplotype H-2^a
and that recognition of this altered form of I-A^b is
restricted by the I-A^k gene product.

2. Clones of Alloreactive T Cells. The results above
suggest that not only is there a unique hybrid determinant(s)
but that clones of cells must exist in the A(B6A)PRC population which recognize this unique F_1 determinant(s). We therefore attempted to derive clones of cells which would recognize this unique F_1 MLR determinant(s). Previous studies
demonstrated that colonies of mouse T cells could be obtained
in vitro in soft agar following mitogen stimulation (11).
Additionally, transformed cells could be cloned in soft agar
(12). We therefore attempted to obtain clones of alloreactive
T cells from soft agar which would recognize the unique F_1
MLR stimulating determinant(s). Figure 2 depicts earlier
results obtained from such experiments. Not only did we
obtain clones of the uniquely F_1 reactive cells [A(B6A)1-1]
but we were able to derive clones of cells which recognized
homozygous B6 stimulator cells better than heterozygous B6A
cells (7). It is apparent from these data that although clone
A(B6)1-1 seems to uniquely see the F_1 determinant(s) on B6A
stimulator cells, clone A(B6)1-13, in addition to seeing the
homozygous B6 stimulator cells, is weakly stimulated by B6A
and, at least initially after cloning, is also stimulated by
DBA/2 stimulator cells. Two simple explanations for these
data are that,(a) there are indeed crossreactive determinants
expressed on B6 cells, some of which are also expressed on
B6A and on DBA/2 stimulator cells, or (b) that we have not

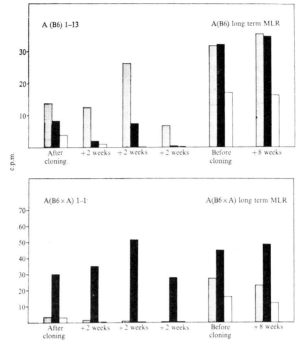

Fig. 2 Serial proliferative responses of 'cloned' PRC. Cells from selected PRC colonies (obtained as outlined in Table 1) were re-stimulated at 14-d intervals with stimulator cells from strain A (as control), B6 (stippled columns), DBA/2 (open) or (B6 × A) F_1 hybrid mice (solid). 10×10^3 PRC were re-stimulated with 1×10^6 irradiated (3300R) stimulator cells and collected at day 3 (ref. 4). The results of two such serial re-stimulations are presented as c.p.m. $\times 10^{-3}$ of incorporated ^{3}H-thymidine at each 14-d interval (control counts have been subtracted). Parallel cultures of both parental PRC populations were re-stimulated as controls, and the results of assays carried out at the beginning and end of the time course are included for comparison.

Reprinted by permission (7).

truly cloned these cells and that although the majority of cells are derived from a clone which uniquely sees B6 stimulator cells, there are contaminant cells derived from either a clone or several clones which recognize other stimulator cell types. In order to examine these two possibilities, we subcloned a selected clone which exhibited more than single reactivities for the stimulator cells we assayed. Our initial results were unsuccessful. However, following the reports by Gillis and Smith (13) on the use of ConA activated supernatant to enhance the growth of colonies (clones) of cytotoxic murine T lymphocytes, we attempted to subclone in the presence of such activated ConA supernatant. We were successful with this procedure in obtaining subclones, and a typical example is presented in Table 4 in which we show the

TABLE 4

SUB-CLONES OF A(B6)3-6
Results of MLR as CPM

CLONES		STIMULATORS			
		A/J	B6	$(B6xA)F_1$	DBA/2
A(B6)II°		1,500	38,100	37,717	24,603
A(B6)3-6		1,742	18,931	4,713	6,214
A(B6)3-6	2	1,064	38,907	3,926	576
	3	927	34,184	1,895	140
	5	1,230	14,291	6,527	1,114
	8	1,578	71,584	4,910	91
	14	215	41,048	1,163	584
	18	2,318	28,010	2,604	372
	22	829	24,427	253	176
	25	483	81,322	4,178	311
	31	5,076	32,038	1,996	2,058

reactivities of a parental culture A(B6)11°, the putitive
clone A(B6)3-6 and subclones derived from A(B6)3-6 numbered
serially A(B6)3-6,-1,-2, etc.

3. Cross-Reactive MLR Determinants Recognized by
Cloned Alloreactive T Cells. It is apparent from these data
that one of our original hypotheses is seemingly correct--
that there are, in fact, contaminant cells in our "clone
A(B6)3-6" but that a majority of the cells uniquely recognize
"homozygous" stimulating determinants on B6, as exemplified
by subclones A(B6)3-6,14,18,22,31, etc. Although this answered
our question concerning the clones of A(B6) and A(B6A)
reactive T cells, we were still left with no explanation for
possible cross-reactivities which we recognized in bulk
cultures in which A primed to B6 seemed also to generate
cells reactive with, for instance, DBA/2 stimulator cells.
Therefore, we attempted another cloning in which we used long-
term primed responder cells which were either primed with B6
or B6A for six or seven generations in vitro. Then we primed
these prior to the cloning with either B6, B6A or DBA/2
stimulator cells. Once we observed colonies in soft agar
following this stimulation, we picked the colonies and restimulated them serially with any one of three stimulator
cell types. Thus, it might be possible to derive a colony
from A(B6) parental cells which were cloned in the presence
of DBA/2 stimulator cells, harvested and carried with serial
challenges in the presence of B6A stimulator cells. This
allowed us to examine what was happening in the "black box"
following harvesting of the colonies prior to expansion of
the clones to the point where we would question their
reactivities. It was possible that by stimulating them only
with one stimulator cell type we were picking the colonies

out of soft agar and cloning them, in effect, by limiting
dilution. In an attempt to examine this problem, we devised
the experiments outlined above using the checkerboard pattern
of priming and restimulation for clone selection. Results
presented in Table 5 suggest that this is one possible interpretation of our data. If in the parental cultures there are

TABLE 5

3HTdr incorporation of selected clones of A(B6A) PRC

A(B6A) IV Parental Culture

A/J	3,914	±	507
B6	52,321	±	4,277
B6A	81,844	±	4,908
DBA/2	38,651	±	2,602

	Clone 5 D´-AB1			Clone 4-AB-AB 7		
A	594	±	139	294	±	44
B6	628	±	151	19,485	±	930
B6A	26,794	±	1,929	19,165	±	2,793
DBA/2	28,536	±	3,044	22,248	±	2,491

	Clone 4-AB-AB´ 6			Clone 4-AB-B´ 5		
A	943	±	290	462	±	128
B6	938	±	292	39,722	±	2,966
B6A	10,250	±	595	27,235	±	1,501
DBA/2	722	±	296	1,764	±	494

a variety of clones, each of which has specificities either
unique for the priming stimulator cell or for cross-reactive
determinants shared between the priming stimulator cell and
third party cells, we should derive clones of cells which
either uniquely see the priming stimulator cell or see some
combination of priming stimulator cell and a third party.
As demonstrated in Table 5, these are exactly the results we
obtained. We derived several different types of clones
recognizing all possible combinations of priming stimulator
cell and third party cells used to push or retrieve the
colonies from agar. Studies are now in progress to subclone
these "clones" to see if there are, in fact, truly crossreactive determinants recognized by clones such as 4D´AB1,
etc., or whether this "clone" contains mixtures of clones,
some of which recognize B6A stimulator cells and others which
recognize DBA/2 stimulator cells.

DISCUSSION

The studies outlined above have demonstrated several new
observations. First, it has been possible to demonstrate
hybrid histocompatibility determinants recognized in secondary
mixed lymphocyte reactions; second, it has been possible to

derive clones of alloreactive T cells; third, it has been possible to demonstrate crossreactive determinants recognized by these cloned alloreactive T cells; and finally, it has been possible to suggest that recognition in mixed lymphocyte reactions leading to proliferation is restricted by I region gene products on the stimulator cell. The data outlined above and the fact that it has not yet been possible to demonstrate these determinants serologically support the concept that T cell recognition is distinct from B cell recognition.

From these isolated observations it is possible to derive a generalized hypothesis concerning recognition and proliferation in mixed lymphocyte reactions. First, the problem alluded to many times in the literature concerning the numbers of cells that seemingly react against single allotype disparities in mixed lymphocyte reaction (14) can perhaps now be answered by the observation that there are multiple clones of allo- reactive cells, many of which see crossreactive determinants on totally dissimilar haplotype stimulator cells. Thus, the sum of reactivity in a bulk culture mixed lymphocyte reaction is simply the total of many individual clonal responses, many of which would be primarily stimulated by other haplotype stimulator cells. Additionally, if (as suggested by the data) the response in mixed lymphocyte reaction is restricted by I region determinants, this would suggest that the reason alloreactivity, as measured by proliferation in mixed lympho- cyte reactions, seems to be directed toward I region disparity may simply be the result of restriction of the recognition of numerous cell surface antigens by an I region determinant on the stimulator cell. This would suggest that the I region determinant, itself, was the stimulus in mixed lymphocyte reaction, but, in fact, the reactivity would be due to the I region restriction imposed upon many separate clones re- sponding against a variety of different antigens, all of which would be restricted by I region determinants on the stimulator cell. This would fit very nicely with the observa- tions that conservation of I region recognition has been preserved, even through speciation (15) and would support the concept that the I region is of critical importance in immuno- regulation. As to the question of the nature of T cell receptors for determinants which give rise to proliferative responses in mixed lymphocyte reaction, nothing new can be added to current conjecture. It is, however, now possible, using clones of alloreactive T cells, to attempt to chemically characterize the receptors which recognize the determinant or determinants which give rise to alloreactive mixed lymphocyte reactions.

ACKNOWLEDGEMENTS

We acknowledge the expert technical assistance of Ms. Phyllis D. Infante.

REFERENCES

1. Irwin,M.R.(1966). Proc.Natl.Acad.Sci. 56, 93.
2. Silvers,W.K. and Wachtel,S.S.(1977). Science 195, 956.
3. Melvold,R.W. and Kohn,H.I.(1977). Immunogenetics 5, 351.
4. Fathman,C.G. and Nabholz,M.(1977). Eur.J.Immunol. 7, 370.
5. Fathman,C.G. (1978). (in) Ir Genes and Ia Antigens, ed. H.O.McDevitt, Academic Press, New York, 97-103.
6. Fathman,C.G., Watanabe,T. and Augustin,A.(1978). J. Immunol. 121, 259-264.
7. Fathman,C.G. and Hengartner,H.(1978). Nature 272,617-618.
8. Hengartner,H. and Fathman,C.G. Manuscript submitted.
9. Fathman,C.G. and Hengartner,H. Manuscript submitted.
10. Jones,P.P.(1977) J.Exp.Med. 146,1261.
11. Sredni,B.,Kalechman,Y.,Michlin,H. and Rozenszajn,L.A. (1976). Nature 259, 130.
12. Cotton,R.G.H., Secher,D.S. and Milstein,C.(1973) Eur. J. Immunol. 3, 135.
13. Gillis,S. and Smith,K.A.(1977) Nature 268, 154-156.
14. Matzinger,P. and Bevan,M.J.(1977) Cell.Immunol. 29, 1.
15. Sachs,D.H., et al. (this symposium).

SPECIFIC KILLER AND SPECIFIC AND NONSPECIFIC SUPPRESSOR ACTIVITIES INDUCED IN A PRIMARY MLC ARE MEDIATED BY DISTINCT T CELL SETS[1]

Anthony Schwartz, Charles A. Janeway and Richard K. Gershon[2]

Section of Comparative Medicine and Department of
Pathology, Yale University, and Cellular Immunology Laboratory,
Howard Hughes Medical Institute, New Haven, Connecticut 06510

ABSTRACT T cells derived from mixed leukocyte cultures
(MLC's) make accelerated responses to the original stimulating antigen and little or no response to other alloantigens. The present experiments examine this finding
to determine if it reflects positive selection of responding clones, suppression of nonresponding clones, or
both. We found evidence for generation of at least four
distinct types of T cells in a primary MLC: primed CTL
precursors; cytotoxic T lymphocytes (CTL's); specific
suppressor T cells; and non-specific suppressor T cells.
Interestingly, primed CTL precursors were insensitive to
suppressor T cells under the current experimental conditions, a finding which differentiated them from naive
CTL precursors. An important outgrowth of this study
was the discovery that the addition of pyrilamine, a
histamine$_1$ receptor antagonist and local anesthetic, to a
primary MLC permitted selective in vitro induction of
specific suppressor T cells.

INTRODUCTION

The specificity of alloreactive T cells has been examined
by a number of investigators by taking cells from a primary
MLC and restimulating them. When exposed to the primary stimulating antigen, such cells show highly specific secondary
proliferative and cytotoxic responses (memory), but in general
they do not respond to other alloantigens (reviewed in ref 1).

[1]This work was supported by U.S.P.H.S. Grant AI-10497
and The Howard Hughes Medical Institute.
[2]Director, Cellular Immunology Laboratory, Howard
Hughes Medical Institute.

This could be due to a pure positive selection of specific clones of alloreactive T cells, or it could reflect the activity of suppressor T cells. In primary MLC's, in addition to CTL memory cells and CTL effectors, specific and nonspecific suppressor T cells are generated (2-7). While others have shown that nonspecific and specific suppressors belong to different cell sets (5, 8), it has not been clear whether specific suppressive and cytotoxic activities are mediated by different cells. The present experiments have examined these questions by adding cells from primary MLC's to fresh MLC's. By using Thy 1 congenic responding T cells, it has been possible to determine the origin of CTL's found after the second MLC, and thus, to accurately estimate suppression of the fresh culture. We have also taken advantage of the inhibitory effect of pyrilamine (a histamine$_1$ receptor antagonist and local anesthetic) on the induction of CTL's and of nonspecific suppressor T cells, to examine the importance of these cell types in suppression of the MLC. Thereby, we have succeeded in defining a T cell set which in the absence of CTL effectors, specifically suppresses CTL responses. We have also detected nonspecific suppressors which may account for the specificity of secondary MLC cultures. Finally, we have been able to demonstrate that the specific suppressor T cell will not suppress primed CTL precursors, but will suppress normal spleen cell precursors of the same specificity.

MATERIALS AND METHODS

Mice. Male C57BL/6 (B6)($H-2^b$, Thy 1.2$^+$), DBA/2($H-2^d$), B6 x $\overline{DBA/2}$ (B6D2F$_1$) C3H/He ($H-2^k$, Thy 1.2+), AKR/J ($H-2^k$, Thy 1.1+) and B10.BR ($H-2^k$) mice, 6 to 8 weeks of age, were obtained from the Jackson Laboratories, Bar Harbour, Maine. B6.PLThy1^a mice ($H-2^b$, Thy 1.1+)(B6 1.1) were bred at Yale Medical School by Dr. Donal Murphy.

Mixed Leukocyte Cultures (MLC's). Spleens from normal mice were prepared in phosphate buffered balanced salt solution containing 5% fetal bovine serum (BSS-FBS). Cells were suspended in Mishell-Dutton culture medium (9) containing 10% FBS (plating medium). To prepare suppressors, 5 x 10^6 viable B6 responding spleen cells (responders) were mixed with 5 x 10^5 mitomycin C treated DBA/2 or B6D2F$_1$ stimulating spleen cells (stimulators) in a total volume of 2 ml in 24 well Linbro tissue culture trays(#76-033-05, Linbro Scientific, New Haven, CT). At least triplicate cultures per group were incubated for 4 or 5 days in an atmosphere of 5% CO$_2$ in humidified air at 37°C. Cells recovered from replicate cultures were pooled and were washed 3X in BSS-FBS.

Cells, counted for viability by trypan blue exclusion, were
then transferred to fresh second cultures and/or were assayed
for cytotoxicity. Following 5 days incubation, viable cell
yields were from 50 to 70% unless 10^{-4}M pyrilamine (Sigma
Chemical Co., St. Louis, MO) had been added at the start of
culture when yields were 20%. In some cases, second culture
responders were B6.PLThy1[a]; stimulators were either DBA/2 or
B6D2F$_1$, to assess specific suppression, or C3H or B10.BR to
assess nonspecific suppression.

Assay of CTL's. MLC cells were suspended in BSS-FBS and
were added to 2 x 10^4 erythrocyte-depleted, ^{51}Cr labelled
DBA/2 mastocytoma P815 cells, or 3-4 day thioglycolate in-
duced peritoneal exudate cells (PEC) from C3H, DBA/2 or
B10.BR mice. Cytotoxicity tests were done in quadruplicate
in Falcon #3040 96 well culture trays (Falcon Plastics,
Oxnard, Calif.). Following centrifugation, trays were incubated for 4 hrs at 37°C. Release into the supernatant of
^{51}Cr was compared with release from target cells incubated
with either medium (0% or spontaneous release) or 2% Triton
X-100 (Amersham-Searle, Arlington Heights, Ill) (100% release).
Spontaneous release usually varied from 10 to 25% of Triton-
X-100 controls. When significant cytotoxicity (i.e., 20%
release or greater) was detected, the standard deviation (SD)
generally was 10% or less of the mean release.

Anti-Thy 1.2 Serum Treatment of Cell Suspensions. In
certain experiments, prior to transfer or assay for cytotoxic
potential, MLC-derived cells were treated with either Anti-
Thy 1.2 (AKR-anti-C3H thymocyte) or Anti-Thy 1.1(C3H-anti-AKR
thymocyte) serum or with normal mouse serum (NMS), followed
by low cytotoxicity rabbit serum as a source of complement
(C). The cells were washed 3X, diluted to equal volumes
(yield equivalents) in the appropriate medium and either
tested for cytotoxicity or for suppression.

                           RESULTS

     Early in our investigations we noted that cells trans-
ferred from 4 or 5 day primary allogeneic MLC's suppressed
CTL generation in a fresh MLC of homologous responder cells
and third party stimulator cells. This demonstrated the generation of nonspecific suppressor cells in the primary MLC.
However, these cells did not decrease CTL's produced in a
fresh MLC in which both stimulators and responders were identical to those in the first culture. In the experiment represented in Table I, 2.5 x 10^5 B6-anti-DBA/2 MLC cells
(1 suppressor/20 responders) were able to decrease generation

TABLE I

COMPARISON OF SUPPRESSION OF KILLING EFFECTED
By B6-ANTI-DBA MLC CELLS TRANSFERRED TO HOMOLOGOUS
OR THIRD PARTY -STIMULATED MLC's

Suppressors Transferred	Second Culture Cytotoxicity[a]	
	Fresh Cells	Suppression
B6-Anti-DBA/2	B6-Anti-DBA/2	-13%
B6-Anti-DBA/2	B6-Anti-C3H	56%

[a]Stimulators and PEC targets from same strain

of CTL's when transferred to a B6-anti-C3H MLC but did not affect the CTL response of a fresh B6-anti-DBA/2 MLC.

In contrast to these results, specific suppressor T cells have been detected by others in similar systems (2, 3, 5-7). It was possible that specific suppression was masked by cytotoxic activity transferred from the first culture. Were this the case, the actual level of suppression only could be measured if CTL's derived from the first culture were removed prior to assay. To test this we used B6(Thy 1.2+) responder spleen cells in the first MLC. These cells were transferred to a second MLC in which responders came from the Thy 1 congenic strain, B6PLThy1[a] (Thy 1.1+) (see Fig. 1). After harvest from the second culture the cells were treated with NMS or with Anti-Thy 1.2 serum + C. Therefore, all CTL's derived from the first or second culture could be assessed.

'The experiment summarized in Table II demonstrates the feasibility of this approach. Thy 1.2+ CTL derived from the first or second MLC were eliminated by anti-Thy 1.2 serum + C treatment, while Thy 1.1+ CTL were unaffected, and vice versa. The results confirmed our hypothesis that suppression of the second MLC had occurred, but that suppression was obscured by CTL precursors or effectors transferred from the first culture. In control studies (not shown) Anti-Thy 1.1 serum + C treatment depleted Thy 1.1+, but not Thy 1.2+ CTL.

While the experiment in Table II suggests that specific suppressor cells are generated in primary MLC's, two other types of cells may have similar effects: nonspecific suppressor cells or CTL effector cells derived from the first culture. It was necessary to eliminate the possible effects of these other cell types. To block the induction of CTL's,

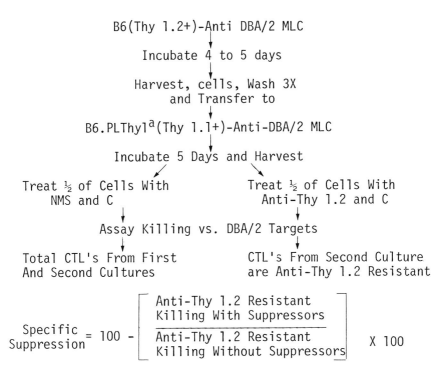

FIGURE 1.   Sample protocol for use of Thy 1 congenic B6
            responders cells and anti-Thy 1.2 serum to
            define specific suppression.

we used pyrilamine, a histamine$_1$ receptor antagonist with
local anesthetic effects. As can be seen in Table III,
pyrilamine, when present at 10^{-4}M from the time of initiation
of a primary MLC totally inhibits CTL induction. This inhibition is complete through at least 5 days of MLC. We also
asked whether the addition of 10^{-4}M pyrilamine to MLC's would
     prevent induction of suppressor cells.

     In our system, nonspecific suppressors are first detect-
able by day 4 of culture of responding cells with or without
stimulator cells. We have found that pyrilamine inhibits the
induction of non-specific suppressor cells both in non-allo-
antigen stimulated cultures (not shown) and in MLC's. Table
IV summarizes an experiment in which the effects of pyrilamine
on specific and nonspecific suppression were tested simultaneously. Using the protocol in Fig. 1, B6-anti-DBA/2
suppressors, incubated in the presence or absence of 10^{-4}M
pyrilamine, were transferred to a second MLC in which B6(1.1)
responders were incubated with either DBA/2 stimulators and

TABLE II
USE OF A THY.1 CONGENIC MOUSE SYSTEM AND ANTI-THY-1.2 SERUM
TREATMENT AFTER THE SECOND CULTURE TO DETERMINE THE SOURCE OF
CTL's DETECTED FOLLOWING TRANSFER OF MLC-DERIVED CELLS TO A
FRESH MLC

Cells Transferred From First Culture[a]	Second Culture	Treatment Before Assay	Killing of DBA/2 PEC Target Cells[b]
None	B6(1.1) α DBA	NMS + C	++++
		αThy 1.2 + C	++++
None	B6 α DBA	NMS + C	++++
		αThy 1.2 + C	-
B6(1.1) α DBA	B6 α DBA	NMS + C	++++
		αThy 1.2 + C	++++
B6 α DBA	B6 α DBA	NMS + C	++
		αThy 1.2 + C	-
B6 α DBA	B6(1.1) α DBA	NMS + C	++
		αThy 1.2 + C	-

[a]After 5 days 5 x 10^5 cells were transferred

[b]45:1 Killer to target cell ratio; ++++ is 40-49%; +++is 30-39%; ++ is 20-29%; + is 10-19%; ± is 5-9%; - is <5%.

TABLE III
PYRILAMINE INHIBITS ALLOGENEIC CTL GENERATION

Cells in Culture[a]	Drug Added	% ^{51}Cr Release (±SD)[b]		
		Killer to Target (K:T) Cell Ratio		
		10:1	30:1	90:1
B6	-	0(2)	0(1)	1(1)
B6 α DBA	-	23(2)	44(2)	49(2)
B6 α DBA	10^{-4}M Pyrilamine	1(0)	0(1)	1(0)

[a]Harvested after 4 days

[b]P815 target cells

tested against DBA/2 PEC target cells (specific) or with B10.
BR stimulators and tested against B10.BR PEC target cells
(nonspecific). The results show that pyrilamine strongly
inhibits nonspecific suppressor cell generation. It also can

TABLE IV
EFFECT OF PYRILAMINE ON FIRST CULTURE DERIVED CTLS's AND
NONSPECIFIC AND SPECIFIC SUPPRESSOR CELLS

Treatment of B6 α DBA/2 Suppressors	Killing From First Culture[a]	Killing From Second Culture[b]
	B6(1.1) α B10.BR Second Culture[c]	
No Suppressors	−	++++
Medium	+	+
Pyrilamine, 10^{-4}M	±	+++
	B6(1.1) α DBA/2 Second Culture[d]	
No suppressors	−	++
Medium	+++	−
Pyrilamine, 10^{-4}M	+	−

[a] 20:1 K:T ratio; see legend, Table II for estimates
of % cytotoxicity. Killing from first culture
determined by formula: (killing by cells treated
pre-assay with NMS + C)-(killing by anti-Thy 1.2
treated cells).

[b] Anti-Thy 1.2 serum + C-resistant killing.

[c] B10.BR PEC Target Cells.

[d] DBA/2 PEC Target Cells.

be seen in Table IV that pyrilamine does not inhibit induction
of specific suppression; a conclusion supported by cell titration studies which showed that pyrilamine - treated specific
suppressors were somewhat more potent than medium treated
suppressors on a cell/cell basis (data not shown). Furthermore, while no CTL effectors are present in pyrilamine-treated
MLC's at the time of transfer, CTL activity derived from the
first, pyrilamine-treated MLC, was demonstrable after the
second MLC. Therefore, pyrilamine prevents the development of
CTL effectors in the primary culture and decreases either the
number of CTL precursors or their ability to develop into effectors in the second culture, while apparently not affecting
specific suppressor cell activation. Similar studies performed with B6 responders in both the first and second cultures
showed that use of pyrilamine also allowed demonstration of
specific suppression in a non-Thy 1 congenic system by partially decreasing total CTL's in the second culture (data not
shown). These results support the notion that specific suppression is not due to transferred CTL effectors and indicate
that specific and nonspecific suppressors belong to different
cell sets. In addition, the results in Table IV demonstrate

TABLE V

EFFECT ON SUPPRESSION AND SECONDARY CTL
ACTIVATION OF INCREASING STIMULATORS IN THE SECOND MLC

Treatment of Suppressors[a]	Second Culture[b] Stimulators x 10^{-5}	Cytotoxicity[c] Pre-Assay Treatment	
		NMS + C	α Thy 1.2+C
No suppressors	0.	$-$	Not Done
"	5.	+++	++++
Medium	0.	$-$	$-$
"	1.25	+++	$-$
"	5.	+++	$-$
"	20.	++++	$-$
"	80.	++++	$-$
Pyrilamine 10^{-4}M	0.	$-$	$-$
"	1.25	+	$-$
"	5.	+	$-$
"	20.	++	$-$
"	80.	+++	$-$

[a]2 x 10^5 B6-anti-DBA/2 suppressors were transferred after 5 days culture in the presence or absence of pyrilamine .

[b]5 x 10^6 B6(1.1) responders, 5 day culture.

[c]P815 target cells; 37:1 K:T ratio; See legend, Table II, for estimates of % cytotoxicity.

transfer of cross-reactive CTL precursors from the first culture. That is, cells transferred from primary B6-anti-DBA/2 MLC's provided precursors for B6-anti-B10.BR CTL's. This has not been found following transfer of nonspecific suppressors generated in the absence of stimulators in the first culture (not shown). From this it follows that cross-reactive CTL precursor activity is not necessary for nonspecific suppression.

Even though no detectable CTL's are present in 10^{-4}M pyrilamine-treated MLC's it could be argued that CTL precursors might be activated early after transfer to the second culture and prematurely deplete stimulator cells. This could then lead to inhibition of the induction of CTL's by fresh cells in the second culture. If this were the case, suppression should be overcome by adding large numbers of stimulators to the second culture. The results of an experiment to test this possibility, presented in Table V, indicate that this did not occur. Adding as many as 640×10^5 stimulators (320:1 stimulator:suppressor ratio) has failed to decrease suppression (data not shown). Therefore, premature removal of stimulator cells in the second culture probably is not the mechanism of specific suppression. Results of preliminary studies of the kinetics of the secondary CTL response described in this system have detected no first culture derived CTL's 2 days following transfer of pyrilamine treated MLC cells, which further supports this conclusion (data not shown). The data in Table V also show that restimulation with antigen is necessary for first culture derived CTL precursors to become optimal effectors. This is particularly evident in the case of pyrilamine treated cells. These findings indicate that our system detects a form of CTL memory. It is evident that the response to secondary stimulation contrasts with the primary response in its lack of sensitivity to suppression.

We should note that all activities (specific and nonspecific suppression, CTL effector function and CTL memory) were mediated by T cells since they could be generated using nylon passaged spleen cells and they could be depleted completely by treatment with anti-Thy 1 serum + C (not shown).

DISCUSSION

We have detected four distinct activities present in cells derived from primary MLC's. Nonspecific suppressor cells, which could ablate primary MLC responses to third party alloantigen, were sensitive to the addition of 10^{-4}M pyrilamine to the primary MLC in which they were generated. CTL precursors, also generated in primary MLC, were largely sensitive to pyrilamine as well, while the development of CTL effector function was totally inhibited by pyrilamine. Finally, specific suppressor T cells induced in primary MLC's were detected by their ability to inhibit a second completely homologous MLC. This activity could not be accounted for by either nonspecific suppressor cells, or by removal of stimulating antigen by CTL's transferred from the primary culture, since development of specific suppression was not sensitive to pyrilamine. One interesting feature of such cells, clearly revealed by use of Thy 1 congenic spleen cell responders, was that they could suppress naive but not antigen primed CTL precursors. Whether resistance to suppression represents an increase in the number of precursors, or a differentiative event, is not yet known.

Our system also permitted simultaneous study of primary

and secondary CTL responses. Others have shown that cells harvested from allogeneic MLC's can be restimulated for proliferative and cytotoxic responses by specific antigen but not by a third party alloantigen (reviewed in ref 1). This could be explained in one of two ways. 1. Specific proliferation of T cells occurs during an MLC "at the expense" of proliferation of other T cells, thereby leading to positive selection of specific responders; or 2. Inhibition of all other responders occurs due to the activity of suppressor cells. Our data are consistent with both mechanisms since specific and nonspecific suppressor cells are generated in a primary MLC, and since precursor cells derived from the first culture are not susceptible to this suppression, (positive-selection) while naive cells are.

Investigations are continuing to determine the surface antigenic phenotypes of the various T cells involved in this system and the mechanism of action of pyrilamine. In addition we will further define the cell interactions required for both the generation and effector function of allo-specific and nonspecific suppressor T cells.

ACKNOWLEDGMENTS

The authors sincerely thank Ms. Sandra Sutton, Mr. Keith Rasmussen and Mr. Thomas Whitney for their excellent technical assistance, and Ms. Gloria Ramos for typing the manuscript.

REFERENCES

1. Bach, F.H., Grillot-Courvalin, C., Kuperman, O.J. Sollinger, H.W., Hayes, C., Sondel, P.M., Alter, B.J., and Bach, M. (1977). Immunological Rev. 35, 76.
2. Fitch, F.W., Engers, H.D., Cerottini, J.-C., and Bruner, K.T. (1976). J. Immunol. 116, 716.
3. Sinclair, N.R. Stc., Lees, R.K., Fagan, G., and Birnbaum, A. (1975). Cell. Immunol. 16, 330.
4. Hirano, T., and Nordin, A.A. (1976). J. Immunol. 116,1115.
5. Hodes, R.J., Nadler, L.M., and Hathcock, K.S. (1977). J. Immunol. 119, 961.
6. Eisenthal, A., Nachtigal, D. and Feldman, M. (1977). Cell. Immunol. 34, 112.
7. Ferguson, R.M., Anderson, B.A., and Simmons, R.L. (1978). Transplantation. 26, 331.
8. Ferguson, R.M., Anderson, S.M., and Simmons, R.L. (1977). Transplant. Proc. 9, 919.
9. Mishell, R.I., and Dutton, R.W. (1967). J. Exp. Med. 126, 126, 423.
10. Gey, G.O., and Gey, M.K. (1936). Am. J. Cancer. 27, 45.

WORKSHOP ON MIXED LYMPHOCYTE REACTIONS

Hilliard Festenstein*, Kirsten Fischer Lindahl**, Sid Golub***

*Department of Immunology, London Hospital Medical College, Turner Street, London E1 2AD, England. **Basel Institute for Immunology, Grenzacherstrasse 487, Basel, Switzerland. ***Department of Bacteriology, UCLA, Los Angeles, California 90024, USA.

Two main topics were identified as foci for discussion: lymphocyte activating determinants (Lads) on stimulating cell populations — genetics and biological function; and H-2 restriction of Mls mixed lymphocyte reactions (MLR).

AHMED (Navy) presented his view that there are at least two different independently segregating genetic regions which code for lymphocyte activating determinants (Lads) for primary, and one for secondary MLR on mouse lymphoid cells. These include the Lads of the H-2 locus, the Mls locus and a new locus defined by secondary MLR which appears to be linked to the IgC_H. In all three cases the responding cell is Thy-1 positive. Splenic adherent cells (SAC) seem also to be required for an MLR. Purified T cells when cultured with purified Ig^+ cells (with the use of fluorescent anti μ and the use of the fluorescence activated cell sorter (FACS)) gave only a weak MLR. In the primary response, the SAC could be either from the responder or stimulator population. The SACs used during the primary MLR and secondary MLR had to be of the same H-2, e.g. B10.D2 ($H-2^d$) primed T cells in the presence of B10.D2 SACs and B10.BR ($H-2^k$) B cells. These data strongly suggest that the phenotype of the antigen presenting cell, SAC, seems to restrict secondary responsiveness in MLR. This was also found to be true for secondary Mls responses.

In the mouse model, AHMANN (NIH) studied six different spleen cell populations or combinations of populations as stimulators in mouse MLR and unfractionated responders. The stimulator populations consisted of T cells (nylon non-adherent); B and macrophage (rabbit anti-mouse brain (RAMB) and complement treated); T and B (G10 passed); B cells (G10 passed, RAMB, and complement treated); and splenic adherent cells (SAC). Only the SAC and unfractionated cells stimulated an MLR, and the SAC were 50 fold more effective. Stimulation was abrogated by treating the SAC with anti-I-A or anti-I-E/C antisera. Thus, SAC and not B cells appear to bear the key Lads, although the possibility of a highly selected B cell subset retained on G10 and contaminating the SACs cannot be ruled out.

BACH (Wisconsin) emphasised the importance of determining which functions (cytotoxic, suppressor, helper) are activated by Lads on any particular cell type.

The discussion then turned to human studies. GOLUB (UCLA) pointed out that while B cell lines are the most potent known activators of T cells, MANN (NIH) found that isolated T cells nevertheless stimulate in MLR and therefore investigated the presence of DRw antigens on T lymphocytes using the fluorescence activated cell sorter (FACS). Isolated T cells were positive with anti DRw sera which had been found to be cytotoxic to B cells from the particular donor and stained with a fluorescinated anti Ig reagent.

Control sera, normal human sera, NHS as well as DRw sera, not reacting with the B cells from the donor were negative. The result demonstrates the presence of DRw antigens on peripheral blood T lymphocytes. The T cells were found to express the DRw antigens of the donor; however, the amount was only 1/50th that of B cells.

STEEL (Edinburgh) described a heteroantiserum which he showed to have anti DR activity as well as strong MLC inhibitory activity. He could differentially remove the cytotoxic activity without affecting the blocking activity.

GATTI (Cedars—Sinai, Los Angeles) then described the extensive cross—reactivity found in the D region when one types by PLT using lymphoblastoid cell lines from homozygous donors as the priming cells. For example, Dw1, 3, 6, 8 and maybe 2 fall into one cross—reactive group while Dw4, 5, 7, 11 fall into another. FESTENSTEIN (London) suggested that this method is probably the most sensitive cellular method and picks up Lad differences not seen by homozygous typing cells and conventional PLT tests.

SHAW (NIH) studied a family with a member with B/D recombination. By primary MLR and by PLT, his data suggest two regions, presumably within HLA, that can stimulate.

FESTENSTEIN (London) showed that Ia (DR) antigens are normally expressed on B but not on T cells, and these sub—populations are believed to be stable.

Activation with sperm (and allogeneic lymphocytes) produced transformation with 20—30% blast cells after six days.

Typing of these T blasts produced positive results with anti—DRw sera, indicating either derepression of silent genes or cloning up of DR positive T cell sub—populations.

H—2 restrictions for Mls MLR responses were then discussed in the mouse model. MOLNAR (Philadelphia) questioned whether Mls^a and Mls^d were different on the basis of negative selection by acute blood to lymph recirculation, and direct MLC tests between AKR/Cum and CBA/J, (C3H/HeJ x DBA/2)$_{F_1}$ and CBA/J.

Secondary MLC tests were also used, i.e. T cells were specifically restimulated and Mls^a was found to be highly cross—reactive with Mls^d. In answer to this, FESTENSTEIN (London) cited original double F1 experiments in which Mls^a was defined separately from Mls^d using the F1 combination CBA/H.T6 x AKR/J and CBA/H x CBA/J, while BALB/c x AKR and CBA/H.T6 x DBA/2 failed to stimulate. The difference in these reactions may be attributed to the different AKR sublines. For example, it is not known for sure that AKR/Cum is Mls^a. It could be Mls^d. FESTENSTEIN (London) confirmed from data of his own laboratory and of others that Mls^a and Mls^d are highly cross—reactive.

MOLNAR (Philadelphia) also discussed whether the T cell responses to the strong Mls alleles are not MHC—restricted:

1.   T cells negatively selected to H—2 determinants by passage through allogeneic irradiated mice respond well to an Mls incompatible Lad on H—2 stimulator cells syngeneic to the irradiated mice.

2.   T cells fail to react against a "self" strong Mls allele on H—2 disparate cells. In support of the contention that Mls responses are not restricted, FESTENSTEIN (London) quoted the experiments in which much greater stimulation was found with H—2 plus Mls disparity compared with H—2 disparity alone.

In contrast, JANEWAY (Yale) described primary MLC experiments in which reactions to Mls^a or Mls^d determinants by Mls^b mice were examined for MHC restriction. Evidence favouring MHC restriction was obtained by: blocking with anti—Ia antisera reacting to stimulator determinants; BUdR and light suicide; and F1 ⟶ parent radiation chimaeras. Whether an unrestricted component exists is not known. He also cited his original experiments with secondary MLR.

FATHMAN (Mayo Clinic) suggested that lymphocyte proliferative responses to Ia alloantigens might be restricted by syngeneic I—A determinants. These data are described elsewhere in this volume.

MODULATION OF TUMOR CELL MEMBRANES WITH LIPOPHILIC HAPTENS: AN APPROACH TO MODIFYING TUMOR IMMUNOGENICITY[1]

V.S. Byers[2] and R.W. Baldwin[3]

Department of Dermatology, School of Medicine
University of California, San Francisco, California 94143
and
Cancer Research Campaign Laboratories
University of Nottingham, England

ABSTRACT Modification of tumor immunogenicity by insertion of lipophilic molecules into the lipid phase of tumor cells has been investigated. A series of alkylcatechols including pentadecylcatechol and the natural plant oil urushiol have been selected for these studies since they are lipophilic and are highly potent hypersensitizing agents. The lipophilic properties of these compounds was demonstrated by the high uptake of ^{3}H-labeled pentadecylcatechol and the heptadecyl derivative heptadecylcatechol into erythrocyte membranes as well as normal and neoplastic cells. Furthermore model membrane studies indicated that incorporation of pentadecylcatechol or urushiol led to changes in membrane fluidity as determined by polarization of fluorescence from a fluorescence probe, 1,6-diphenyl-1,3,5 hexatriene. These membrane changes were also reflected in alterations in the antibody induced redistribution of β-2-microglobulin on pentadecylcatechol or urushiol treated lymphocytes.

The influence of alkylcatechols on tumor immunogenicity has been approached firstly by demonstrating that treatment enhances the capacity of a weakly immunogenic rat hepatoma to induce immunity against transplanted tumor cells. Secondly, since these compounds are potent inducers of delayed hypersensitivity in humans and guinea pigs, experiments have been carried out to show that intralesional injection of pentadecylcatechol into intra-

[1]This work was supported by NIH grant 501 AI-12947 and by a block grant from the Cancer Research Campaign (UK).

[2]Present address: Department of Dermatology, School of Medicine, University of California, San Francisco, California 94143.

[3]Present address: Cancer Research Campaign Laboratories, The University of Nottingham, England NG7 2RD

dermal grafts of the Line 10 hepatoma in sensitized
guinea pigs suppresses growth of the local tumor and
markedly restricts the development of regional lymph
node metastases.

INTRODUCTION

Tumors induced with chemical carcinogens or oncogenic
viruses may express neoantigens capable of eliciting immunological rejection of transplanted tumor in syngeneic recipients (1). This led to the widespread acceptance that human
tumors also exhibit this type of neoantigen and so immunotherapy is being evaluated in the treatment of many types of
human cancer (2). But, insufficient attention has been given
to studies on naturally occurring (spontaneous) animal tumors,
these being defined as tumors arising without deliberate in-
ducement in animal strains not selected for a high natural
tumor incidence. Within this definition there are only a few
reports on the induction of immunity to transplanted tumor
cells, and by and large, these have been equivocal. For
example in an early report, Prehn and Main (3) showed that
naturally arising murine sarcomas were not immunogenic,
whereas those induced by 3-methylcholanthrene (MCA) were able
to induce immunity to transplanted cells from the autologous
tumor. More recently, Hewitt and his colleagues (4) presenting results of a long term study in which the transplantation
characteristics of 27 spontaneous murine tumors including
leukemias, carcinomas and sarcomas, were evaluated, came to
the conclusion that none displayed immunogenicity. The immunogenicity of spontaneous tumors arising in inbred WAB/Not
rats has been the subject of study in our laboratory for some ·
years alongside extensive studies with carcinogen-induced
tumors (5). The earliest report (6) showed that rats immunized with cells from a squamous cell carcinoma exhibited
weak resistance, but immunity could not be induced to a reti-
culum cell sarcoma. In a later study (7) 6 of 9 spontaneous
mammary carcinomas were found to be non-immunogenic and it
has now been shown that spontaneous sarcomas have a similar
incidence of immunogenicity (8). Since 1976 more than 50 new
spontaneous tumors have been transplanted into syngeneic WAB/
Not rats and in tests with 33 tumors by challenge protection
procedures, none have so far provided clear cut evidence of
tumor immunogenicity.
      It must be concluded from these studies as well as the
published investigations, that a high proportion of naturally
occurring tumors do not express tumor rejection antigens, at
least in a manner such that they are able to elicit significant tumor immune responses. It may be argued that these

tumors in fact do not express tumor antigens at all, in which
case any form of specific immunological defense will be ruled
out. Alternatively, it may be that they do express neoantigens, but these are inadequately, or inappropriately expressed
with the result that only low levels of immunity are induced,
these being insufficient to provide protection against a
developing tumor. This latter hypothesis is preferred since
most studies showed that at least some of the naturally
arising tumors did induce immunity, albeit at low levels. But
this implies that alternative approaches have to be sought to
increase recognition of 'weak' neoantigens.
     One approach has been to modify cell surface determinants
by chemical coupling (9). This has included methylation of
tumor cell surface components by treatment with dimethylsul-
phate (10) or the introduction of haptenic determinants such
as trinitrophenyl. For example, mice injected with trinitrophenylated Moloney virus induced YAC tumor cells rejected
viable YAC cells more effectively than those immunized with
unmodified YAC cells (11). A further variant of this approach recently developed involves attachment of PPD to tumor
cells by the addition of PPD cross-linked concanavalin A, the
suggestion here being that the insertion of helper determinants may enhance the response to tumor associated antigens
(12). In the original study, a positive but weak response
was obtained against MCA-induced murine sarcomas in mice pre-
sensitized to Bacillus Calmette Guerin (BCG). But this approach has not materially altered the immune response to a
weakly immunogenic rat hepatoma, D23, nor has it induced any
detectable resistance to a rat mammary carcinoma which has
not demonstrated any immunogenicity (13). Virally-induced
antigen modification has also been considered as a means for
increasing tumor cell immunogenicity (14-17). Here the precise combination of tumor, virus and host seems to be crucial
in determining whether viral xenogenization leads to enhanced
immunogenicity. For example, infection of MCA-induced murine
sarcomas with Moloney sarcoma or leukemia virus did not lead
to increased tumor immunogenicity (15), whereas rat tumors
infected with endogenous mouse C-type virus induced tumor
resistance (17).

RESULTS

Modulation of Tumor Cell Membranes by Lipophilic
Compounds. An alternative approach to modifying cell antigen
expression by the insertion of lipophilic compounds into the
lipid phase of the cell membrane has been suggested by
studies indicating that manipulation of the lipid composition
of mammalian cells, including tumor cells, can profoundly
alter their properties (18-20). Changes in membrane fluidity

would be expected to modify lateral mobility of cell surface receptors. This is exemplified by studies showing that conversion of a murine thymic leukemia to an ascitic form was associated with a decrease in membrane microviscosity, and correlated with this change, these cells showed a markedly lower ability to form caps with respect to virus related and H-2 antigens (21). Also, changes in cell membrane phospholipids may have an influence on transmembrane exchange processes which may lead to quantitative changes in cell surface receptor expression (22).

A series of alkylcatechols including 3n-pentadecylcatechol (PDC), 3n-heptadecylcatechol (HDC) as well as analogs with unsaturated hydrocarbon side chains have been selected for these studies.

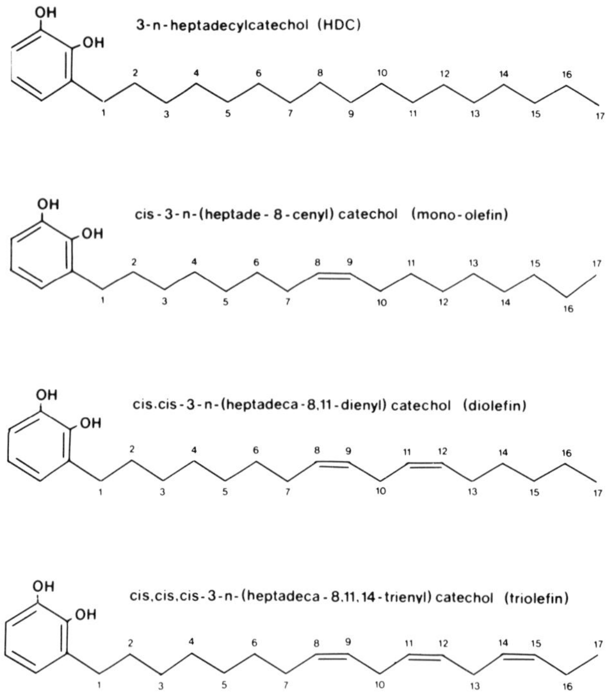

FIGURE 1. Alkylcatechols in poison oak urushiol

These are amphipathic molecules which on account of their hydrocarbon side chains would be expected to possess considerable lipophilicity. Furthermore, these compounds are highly potent hypersensitizing agents and are components of the natural plant oil urushiol which causes poison ivy, and poison oak dermatitis (23,24). This second functional activity was considered to be potentially important since immunotherapy with bacterial immunostimulants such as BCG is most effective when they are administered into the site of a tumor deposit so eliciting local host responses (25,26). It was considered, therefore, that incorporation of alkylcatechols into tumor cell membranes may also elicit local delayed hypersensitivity responses which may produce anti-tumor effects.

Although the relationship between chemical structure of the alkylcatechols and the capacity to induce delayed type hypersensitivity remains to be completely elucidated, in vivo studies emphasize a requirement for both the catechol ring and the hydrocarbon side chain for activity. For example, 3-n-pentadecylcatechol (PDC) but not 3-n-pentadecylresorcinol or 3-methylcatechol elicit delayed type hypersensitivity following epicutaneous application to guinea pigs (23). In order to explore further the function of these compounds, they have been tested for their capacity to induce a blastogenesis response in vitro when added to peripheral blood lymphocytes from naturally sensitized donors (27). In view of the highly lipophilic properties of these compounds, they cannot be added directly to lymphocyte cultures, but advantage was taken of their uptake into erythrocyte membranes to use these preparations as carriers for the alkylcatechols. This is illustrated in Figure 2 which shows that addition of 3-n-heptadecylcatechol

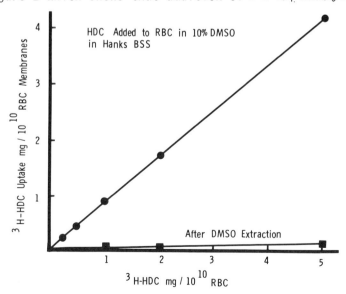

FIGURE 2.   3H-Heptadecylcatechol uptake into human RBCs

(HDC) to human erythrocytes in amounts up to 5mg/10^{10} cells
led to approximately 80% of the compound being taken up. But
most of this was present in an unbound form (DMSO-extractable)
and so available for transfer from membrane preparations.
The blastogenesis responses elicited when urushiol and PDC are
added on erythrocyte membrane carriers to sensitized peripheral blood lymphocytes indicate that the natural product is
most active (Fig. 3).

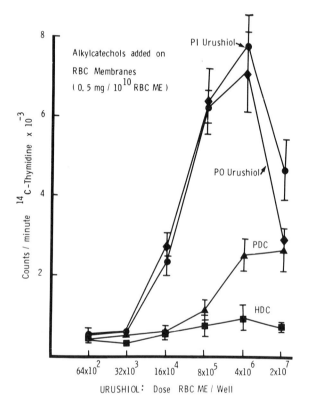

FIGURE 3. Blastogenesis response of human peripheral
blood lymphocytes from a sensitized donor to urushiols and
3-n-pentadecylcatechol.

But from the comparative tests summarized in Figure 4, the
resorcinol compound (PDR) as well as 3-n-heptadecylveratrole
(HDV) in which the hydroxyl groups of the catechol ring are
methylated were essentially inactive. Comparably, methylation
of urushiol rendered the compound inactive and simple compounds such as 3-methylcatechol and linoleic acid were also
unable to generate blastogenesis responses. These findings
indicate that a catechol ring with free hydroxyl groups as

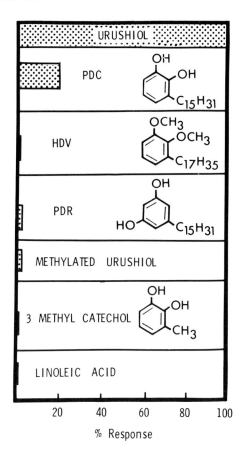

FIGURE 4. Blastogenesis response of urushiol-sensitized peripheral blood lymphocytes to urushiol analogs: response expressed as a % of the urushiol response.

well as the hydrocarbon side chains are essential structural components for reactivity. One proposal is that oxidation of the catechol to its quinone leads to covalent protein binding of urushiol and its analogs (23). In this context, conjugates prepared by interaction of ovalbumin with PDC-quinone can generate a delayed hypersensitivity skin response in PDC-sensitized guinea pigs and these preparations are being evaluated for their capacity to generate blastogenesis responses with sensitized lymphocytes. The function of the hydrocarbon side chain in alkylcatechols is less clear. As already discussed, lipophilic properties of the compound depend upon the hydrocarbon side chain and this may be important in cell uptake. Here it should be noted that the urushiol is more active than PDC in eliciting blastogenesis responses with sensitized lymphocytes (Fig. 3). Since urushiol consists of a mixture

of alkylcatechols with mono, di- and tri-unsaturated hydrocarbon side chains, this suggests that this structural feature
is necessary for maximal reactivity.

Alkylcatechol Uptake into Cells: The incorporation of
alkylcatechols into cells is illustrated by the uptake of HDC
into human erythrocyte membranes (Fig. 2) and as already indicated this is one of the vehicles used to present compounds to
sensitized lymphocytes (27). Comparably PDC was readily taken
up into both normal and neoplastic rat and guinea pig cells.
This is illustrated in Figures 5 and 6 which show the essentially linear uptake of ^{3}H-PDC as well as freshly prepared
quinone derivatives (^{3}H-PDQ) by guinea pig Line 10 hepatoma
cells and peritoneal exudate cells. Furthermore within two
hours, some 13% of the compound added to guinea pig PE cells
(100µg/10^7 cells) is covalently bound to protein.

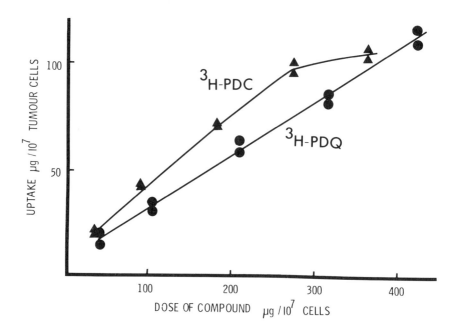

FIGURE 5. Alkylcatechol binding to guinea pig Line 10
hepatoma cells
     3H - PDC   3-n-pentadecylcatechol
     3H - PDQ   3-n-pentadecylcatechol-quinone

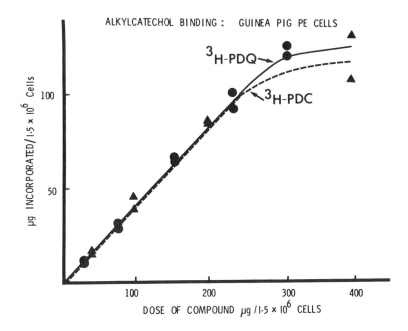

FIGURE 6.   3H-PDC binding to guinea pig peritoneal exudate cells.

Response to Cell Membrane Uptake of Alkylcatechols.
From the cell binding studies, it was concluded that compounds such as PDC were taken up by cell membranes.   An examination of the interaction of these compounds with some bilayer lipid membranes was undertaken, therefore, to see if such an association could be detected and, if so, whether these compounds were able to modify the structural parameters of the membrane. The fluorescent probe 1, 6-diphenyl -1,3,5-hexatriene (DPH) was chosen for these studies since it is sensitive to structural modifications of membranes (28) and it has been used to measure membrane "microviscosity" (29).
The polarization of fluorescence from DPH embedded into the membranes of dipalmitoylphosphatidylcholine (DPPC) vesicles is shown in Figure 7 as a function of temperature. The well-established transition at ∿40°C is apparent, above which the membrane exists in the fluid liquid-crystalline state in which DPH exhibits low polarization of fluorescence. Incorporation of PDC into the DPPC membranes at a 2:1 (DPPC:PDC) molar ratio had no detectable effect on the rigid phase below the transition temperature, but increased the microviscosity of the fluid phase (T >40°C):   in this respect, PDC acts similarly to cholesterol (30).

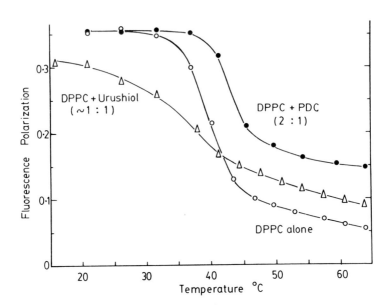

FIGURE 7.   Effect of urushiol and pentadecylcatechol on
the fluidity of dipalmitoylphosphatidylcholine vesicles.

    PDC also modifies the fluidity of erythrocyte ghost
membranes, but the effect is opposite to that observed with
lecithin membranes (Fig. 8). In the ghost membranes, PDC
causes an approximate 25% decrease in fluorescence polarization when present at a concentration of 40 μg/ml. This difference might be accounted for by the high concentration of
cholesterol in erythrocyte membranes (31). Such substantial
quantities of cholesterol have been shown to reverse the
effects of modulators on membrane fluidity (32).
    In comparison to the effects of PDC, addition of uru-
shiol to DPPC vesicles had a more marked effect upon membrane
fluidity as determined with DPH (Fig. 7). Above the phase
transition temperature of DPPC urushiol had a similar effect
to PDC in decreasing fluidity. But, unlike PDC, urushiol
increased the fluidity of DPPC vesicle membranes below the
transition temperature. Urushiol therefore broadens and
tends to obscure the phase transition of DPPC. The effect
upon the rigid crystalline phase is probably due to unsaturation in the hydrocarbon side chains of urushiol which will
prevent packing of the fatty acyl chains of membranes into a
crystalline array. Unsaturation in the urushiol molecule,
therefore, provides disorder in the membrane which results in
increased fluidity below 40°C.

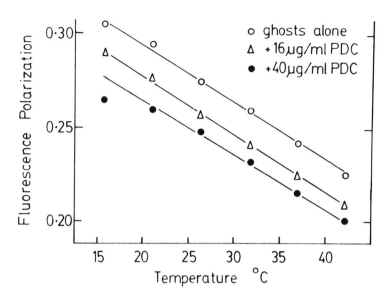

FIGURE 8.   Effect of 3-n-pentadecylcatechol on the
fluidity of human erythrocyte ghost membranes.

Mobility of Receptors on Cells Treated with Alkylcatechols.   In order to evaluate the influence of alkylcatechols
on cell membrane components, their effect was studied on the
antibody-induced redistribution of β-2-microglobulin associated with the surface of human peripheral blood lymphocytes.
Lymphocytes isolated by Ficoll-Hypaque separation were treated
at 0°C with either urushiol, PDC or, in controls, 10% DMSO in
HBSS. β-2-microglobulin moieties were then reacted with goat
anti-human β-2-microglobulin serum antibodies which after
washing were revealed by reaction with fluorescein labeled
rabbit anti-goat IgG.   All procedures up to this stage were
performed at 0°C to ensure random distribution of cell surface
associated β-2-microglobulin.   The data summarized in Figure
9 indicate that there is a decrease in the percentage of cells
treated with either PDC or urushiol, showing caps and patches
after incubation of samples for various intervals at 37°C
followed by addition of paraformaldehyde to prevent further
redistribution.

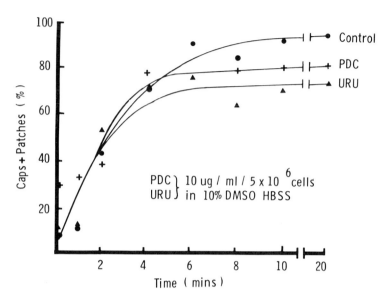

FIGURE 9.   Antibody induced β-2-microglobulin redistribution on peripheral blood lymphocytes and its modification
by treatment of cells with urushiol or PDC.

Immunogenicity of Alkylcatechol-Treated Tumor Cells.
Urushiol and related compounds can be incorporated into tumor
cells and model membrane studies previously discussed indicate that this leads to changes in membrane fluidity. Studies
have been undertaken, therefore, to determine whether this
treatment modifies the immunogenicity of tumor cells. This
has been approached with the following objectives:

    1. Modification of tumor cells so as to enhance re-
sponses to 'weakly' immunogenic tumors.
    2. Induction within tumors of delayed type hypersensi-
tivity responses to urushiol and analogs for regional immunotherapy.

Induction of Immunity to Hepatoma D23 with DPC - Treated
Tumor Cells. The first objective has been to determine
whether treatment of tumor cells with PDC modifies immunogenicity and these studies were carried out with an ascitic
variant of a carcinogen-induced hepatoma D23 AS which is maintained by intraperitoneal transfer in syngeneic WAB/Not rats
(33). This tumor is weakly immunogenic, rats immunized by
various means rejecting challenge with up to 10^5 tumor cells.
As with the guinea pig Line 10 hepatoma, D23 cells also
readily incorporate PDC. For example, treatment with up to

500 µg ^{3}H-PDC/10^7 D23 cells resulted in an essentially linear uptake of compound at both 0°C and 37°C (Fig. 10).

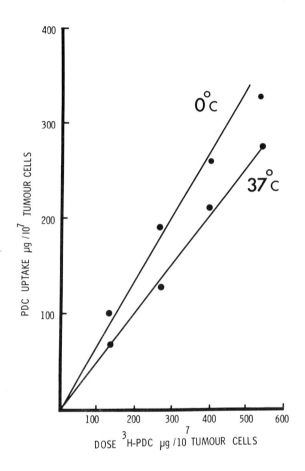

FIGURE 10. ^{3}H-Pentadecylcatechol uptake into rat hepatoma D23 cells.

Cells treated with 100 µg PDC/10^7 cells/ml were more than 90% viable as defined by trypan blue exclusion, although there was some loss of viability with increasing concentration of PDC. Nevertheless the cell survival under the conditions selected for tumor cell treatment (1 mg PDC/10^7 cells/ml) was more than adequate to produce tumor growth since the threshold dose of hepatoma D23 is of the order of 10^3 cells. Accordingly after PDC treatment, D23 cells were attenuated by γ-irradiation (15000R). Experiments in which immunity to

intraperitoneal challenge with hepatoma D23 AS cells (10^4) was
assessed following a single or multiple immunizations with
either irradiated D23 cells (Irr. D23) or irradiated PDC-
treated D23 cells (Irr-PDC-D23) are summarized in Figure 11.
Following a single immunization, none of the rats receiving
irradiated D23 cells showed any immunity, but in comparison
3/5 rats treated with irradiated PDC-treated tumor cells rejected the tumor challenge. As expected, the rejection response induced following multiple immunizations was more
effective and under these conditions, 4/8 rats receiving irradiated D23 cells rejected tumor challenge. However all of
the rats given PDC-treated D23 cells were immune.

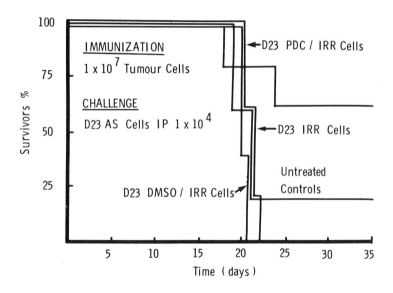

FIGURE 11a. Induction of immunity to rat hepatoma D23
with PDC-treated tumor cells. Immunization 1 x 10^7 tumor
cells.

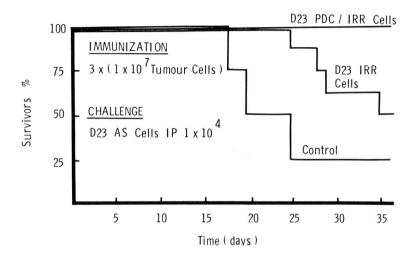

FIGURE 11B.   Induction of immunity to rat hepatoma
D23 with PDC-treated tumor cells.   Immunization 3 x (1 x 10^7
tumor cells).

These studies indicate that the immune response to the
weakly immunogenic hepatoma D23 can be enhanced by PDC treatment of the immunizing tumor cells.   But the conditions so
far used have invariably led to some loss of tumor cell viability and further studies are in progress to evaluate the
immune response to D23 cells treated with less toxic doses of
PDC.   In addition comparative studies with urushiol as well as
non-sensitizing analogs including 3-n-pentadecylresorcinol
(PDR) which also became incorporated into membranes will establish whether the effects on D23 cells correlate with the
haptenic function of the compounds or their lipophilicity.
Naturally arising rat tumors such as mammary adenocarcinomas
are also being tested for the response to alkylcatechols since
it has not been possible previously to reveal tumor immunogenicity using several immunization protocols.   These include
immunization with viable or radiation attenuated tumor cells
sometime with the incorporation of BCG or C. parvum in the
vaccines (34).   Also some of these tumors have been tested for
immunogenicity, without success, following neuraminidase
treatment (35).   These tests will indicate whether cell membrane modification can induce exposure of 'covert' neoantigens.

Intralesional Therapy.   Whilst bacterial agents like
BCG and C. parvum have been administered systemically for
tumor immunotherapy, infiltration into tumor deposits usually
has a more marked therapeutic effect (25).   For example, in-

jection of BCG into intradermal implants of the guinea pig
Line 10 hepatoma causes regression of the local tumor and
regional lymph node metastases are eliminated (36). Although
the mechanism of tumor rejection is not adequately understood, the local granulomatous response is recognized to be
important (26).   These observations suggest that urushiol or
its analogs may provide an alternative to BCG for intralesional (regional) immunotherapy, since these compounds are
potent inducers of delayed type hypersensitivity responses
in humans (27) and guinea pigs (23).   This has only been examined so far in pilot experiments, but the findings summarized in Figure 12 indicate the potential of this approach.

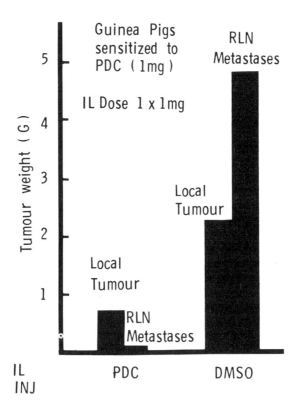

FIGURE 12.   Effect of intralesional injection of PDC
on growth of Line 10 hepatoma and the development of regional lymph node metastases.

Here, Line 10 hepatoma (10^6 cells) were injected intradermally into strain two guinea pigs sensitized epicutaneously to PDC. The intradermal tumors were then injected intralesionally either with PDC (1 mg) or its solvent (DMSO), and observed for 40 days when the development of regional lymph node metastases necessitated termination of the test. Growth of the intradermal tumor was suppressed by PDC treatment, although they were not completely rejected. However, the most pronounced effect was on the regional lymph node metastases which were almost completely controlled by intralesional injection of PDC into the primary tumor.

DISCUSSION

Alkylcatechols related to the natural plant oil urushiol were chosen as agents for insertion into the lipid phase of tumor cell membranes since they would be expected to possess considerable lipophilicity on account of their C 15 -C17 .hydrocarbon side chains. Secondly these compounds are highly potent hypersensitizing agents and it was considered that insertion of a haptenic moiety into the tumor cell membrane would provide a second approach for modifying tumor cell immunogenicity. In fact urushiol oil which is composed of mixtures of 3-n alk (en) ylcatechols with saturated and mono, di and triene forms (Fig. 1) is one of the most potent hypersensitizing agents known and it has been estimated that 80% of the United states population is naturally sensitized. This is further emphasized by comparative studies on the delayed type hypersensitivity response in guinea pigs which showed that PDC was some 20 times more potent than other chemical hypersensitizers including DNCB and DNFB (37).

Although the relationships between the chemical structure of the alkylcatechols and their capacity to elicit DHR remains to be fully elucidated, there is a requirement for free hydroxyl groups in the catechol ring and a hydrocarbon side chain. The hydroxyl groups in the catechol ring are considered to be involved in binding to tissue proteins following oxidation to a quinone intermediate (23). The function of the hydrocarbon side chain is less clear, but may indicate that an element of lipophilicity is required for haptenic activity. This may allow the compounds to be taken up into cell membrane lipids prior to their binding to membrane protein through the catechol ring. In this context, the natural oil urushiol is a much more potent hypersensitizing agent than compounds in which the hydrocarbon side chain is fully saturated. Here it may be suggested that the unsaturated bonds in the hydrocarbon side chains of the

urushiol compounds increases the degree of membrane modulation. This is emphasized by the studies showing that urushiol but not PDC increased the fluidity of DPPC vesicle
membranes below the transition temperature (Fig. 7).

A basic concept in these studies was that incorporation of the alkylcatechols into the lipid phase of tumor
cell membranes would lead to a degree of membrane distortion,
so possibly resulting in changes in membrane antigen expression. As already discussed, PDC, or more effectively
urushiol modifies the fluidity of artificial membranes and
similar effects were obtained with human erythrocyte membranes. The effect of alkylcatechols on the mobility of receptors in the plasma membrane is further illustrated by the
studies showing that antibody-induced redistribution of β2-
microglobulin on human lymphocytes was decreased in cells
treated with PDC or urushiol (Fig. 9).

Since alkylcatechols are avidly taken up into membranes of neoplastic cells, this provides several potential
possibilities for manipulating immune rejection responses.
Firstly, modulation of the lipid phase of tumor membranes
may increase the expression of neoantigens or even result in
the appearance of membrane components which are normally
'silent'. This is illustrated by the experiments showing
that there is an enhanced tumor rejection response in rats
immunized with PDC-treated hepatoma D23 cells (Fig. 11).
This approach is being extended to determine whether PDC
treatment enhances immune responses to naturally occurring
mammary carcinomas and sarcomas. These tumors generally do
not elicit significant immune rejection responses (5,34,35)
and so this will establish whether alkylcatechol treatment
of tumor cells leads to qualitative changes in neoantigen
expression.

Urushiol and analogs are also potent hypersensitizing
agents (23) and so it has to be considered that the enhanced
tumor rejection response elicited by PDC-treated hepatoma
D23 cells might be due to the compounds acting as helper determinants. This would be akin to other studies where the
immune response to a murine MCA-induced sarcoma was improved
using tumor cells coupled with the PPD derivative of tuberculin (12). This interpretation is considered less likely
with rat hepatoma D23 in view of the weak DHR response elicited in rats by alkylcatechols. However, the haptenic
function of these compounds does represent an important component which can be manipulated for tumor rejection. This
is illustrated by the tests on the Line 10 hepatoma in guinea
pigs since this species can be readily sensitized to urushiol
into intradermal tumor challenges inhibited growth of the
local tumor and essentially prevented the development of

regional lymph node metastases. These effects are similar to those obtained following intralesional injection of BCG organisms into Line 10 hepatoma (36). But the advantages of the alkylcatechols include the availability of well defined products which can be administered in several ways, e.g. in liposomes, so as to provide a regulated release of the compound into the tumor environment.

ACKNOWLEDGEMENTS

The assistance of Dr. M.V. Pimm with the tumor studies and Drs. R. Bisby and R.G. Dennick with membrane binding studies is gratefully acknowledged. Work is supported in part by NIH grant AI 14752, RO1 A1 12947 and FDA grant 223-77-1201.

REFERENCES

1. Herberman, R.B. (1977). Biochim. Biophys. Acta. 473,93.
2. Goodnight, J.E., and Morton, D.L. (1978). Annu. Rev. Med. 29,231.
3. Prehn, R.T., and Main, J.M. (1957). J. Nat. Cancer Inst. 18,769.
4. Hewitt, H.B. (1978). Advan. Cancer Res. 27,149.
5. Baldwin, R.W., Embleton, M.J., and Pimm, M.V. (1979). In "Antiviral Mechanisms in Control of Neoplasia" (P. Chandra, ed.), p. 333. Plenum Press, New York.
6. Baldwin, R.W. (1966). Int. J. Cancer 1,57.
7. Baldwin, R.W., and Embleton, M.J. (1969). Int. J. Cancer 4, 430.
8. Baldwin, R.W., Embleton, M.J., and Pimm, M.V. (1979). In "Carcinogens: Identification and Mechanisms of Action" (A. Clark Griffin and C.R. Shaw, eds), pp. 365-379. Raven Press, New York.
9. Naor, D., and Galili, N. (1977). Progr. Allergy 22,107.
10. Staab, H-J., and Anderer, F.A. (1978). Brit. J. Cancer 34,496.
11. Galili, N., Naor, D., Åsjo, B., and Klein, G. (1976). Eur. J. Immunol. 6,473.
12. Lachmann, P.J., and Sikora, K. (1978). Nature 271,463.
13. Baldwin, R.W., and Basley, W. (unpublished findings).
14. Kobayashi, H., Kodamu, T., and Gotuhda, E. (1977). Xenogenization of tumor cells Hokkaido University Medical Library Series, Vol. 9.
15. Kuzumaki, N., Fenyo, EM., Klein E., and Klein, G. (1978). Transplantation 26,304.
16. Takeichi, N., Austin, F.C., Oikawa, T., and Boone, C.W. (1978). Cancer Res. 38,4580.

17. Kuzumaki, N., Fenyo, E.M., Giovanella, B.C., and Klein G. (1978). Int. J. Cancer 21,62.
18. Inbar, M., and Shinitzky, M. (1974). Proc. Nat. Acad. Sci. USA 71,2128.
19. Horwitz, A.F. (1977). In "Dynamic Aspects of Cell Surface Organization" (G. Poste, and G.L. Nicolson, eds.), pp. 295-305. Elsevier/North Holland Biomedical Press, Amsterdam.
20. Kimelberg, H.K. (1977). In "Dynamic Aspects of Cell Surface Organization" (G. Poste, and G.L. Nicolson, eds.), pp. 205-293. Elsevier/North Holland Biomedical Press, Amsterdam.
21. Hilgers, J., Van Der Sluis, P.J., Van Blitterswijk, W.J. and Emmelot P. (1978). Brit. J. Cancer 37,329.
22. Kader, J.C. (1977). In "Dynamic Aspects of Cell Surface Organization. (G. Poste, and G.L. Nicolson, eds.), pp. 127-204. Elsevier/North Holland Biomedical Press, Amsterdam.
23. Baer, H., Watkins, R.C., and Bowser, R.T. (1966). Immunochemistry 3,479.
24. Gross, M., and Baer, H. (1975). Phytochemistry 14,2263.
25. Baldwin, R.W., and Pimm, M.V. (1978). Advan Cancer Res. 28,91.
26. Baldwin, R.W., and Byers, V.S. (1978). Seminars in Immunopathology, (in press). Springer-Verlag, Heidelberg.
27. Byers, V.S., Epstein, W.L., Castagnoli, N., and Baer, H. (Submitted for publication).
28. Andrich, M.P., and Vanderkooi, J.M. (1976). Biochem. 15,1257.
29. Shinitzky, M., and Inbar, M. (1976). Biochim. Biophys. Acta. 433,133.
30. Cogan, U., Shinitzky, M., Weber, G., and Nishida, T. (1977). Biochemistry 12,115.
31. Cooper, R.A., Duroches, J.R., and Leslie, M.H. (1977). J. Clin. Invest. 60,115.
32. Pang, K-YY., and Miller, K.W. (1978). Biochim. Biophys. Acta. 511,1.
33. Pimm, M.V., Hopper, D.G., and Baldwin, R.W. (1976). Brit. J. Cancer 34,368.
34. Pimm, M.V., Cook, A.J., Hopper, D.G., Dickinson, A.M., and Baldwin, R.W. (1978). Int. J. Cancer 22,426.
35. Pimm, M.V., Cook, A.J., and Baldwin, R.W. (1978). Eur. J. Cancer 14,359.
36. Zbar, B., and Tanaka, T. (1971). Science 172,271.
37. Friedlaender, M.H., and Baer, H. (1972). J. Immunol. 109,1122.

INDUCTION OF VIRUS-SPECIFIC H-2 RESTRICTED MURINE CTL BY LIPOSOMES[1]

Matthew F. Mescher, Robert Finberg,
Linda Sherman,[2] and Steven Burakoff

Department of Pathology, Harvard Medical School,
Boston, MA 02115

ABSTRACT   Reconstituted membranes and liposomes have
been used to study the requirements for the induction
of *in vitro* secondary CTL responses to allogeneic and
virus-infected, syngeneic cells. Evidence is presented
that partially purified H-2 antigens are able to induce
CTL activity from primed allogeneic spleen cells.
These partially purified H-2 antigens when incorporated
into reconstituted membranes or liposomes with Sendai
virus antigen are able to induce virally primed
syngeneic spleen cells to give a virus specific, H-2
restricted CTL response. Furthermore, when the hemag-
glutinin/neuraminidase (HN) protein of Sendai virus
was isolated and incorporated into liposomes with
partially purified H-2 antigens, virus specific CTL
are induced.

INTRODUCTION

Joint recognition of antigen and cell surface proteins
encoded by the major histocompatibility complex (MHC) is
involved in many of the humoral and cell mediated immune
responses. Genetic and serological evidence has provided
extensive information regarding the types of MHC molecules
involved in these phenomena and the requirements for effective interaction but the nature of the molecular events
occurring at the cell surface remains largely unknown.
Murine cytolytic T lymphocytes (CTL) have provided an
excellent system for studying MHC restricted recognition of
foreign antigens in that recognition can be assessed at three

[1]This work was supported by U.S. Public Health Service
grant CA-14723.
[2]Present address: Department of Cellular and Developmental Immunology, Scripps Clinic and Research Foundation,
La Jolla, California 92037.

different stages; induction of the primary response, induction
of the secondary response and interaction of the CTL and
target in the effector stage. While each of these stages may
have somewhat different requirements (e.g., accessory cells),
it is clear that all three require recognition of antigen and
H-2 gene products. The recent demonstration that purified
plasma membranes are able to induce a primary and secondary
CTL response (1) and that the activity for induction of a
secondary response is retained following detergent solubilization (2,3) has allowed us to begin to investigate the
recognition process at the molecular level. This report
describes the use of reconstituted membranes and liposomes to
study allogeneic and virus-specific CTL induction.

METHODS

     Induction of secondary CTL was measured by culturing
spleen cells from previously immunized animals together with
preparations being tested for activity. After 5 days of *in
vitro* culturing (1), CTL activity was assessed in a 4 hr
chromium release assay. P815 (H-2^d) and EL-4 (H-2^b) tumor
cells were used for *in vivo* immunization and as targets for
allogeneic CTL. These same cells, coated with β propiolac-
tone inactivated Sendai virus (Connaught Laboratories,
Willowdale, Ontario), were used as targets for virus-specific
CTL (4).
     Tumor cell membrane isolation (1), solubilization (2)
and reconstitution (5) have been previously described. H-2
antigens from solubilized P815 membranes were partially
purified by affinity chromatography on a *Lens culinaris*
(lentil) lectin column (6). Lipids were extracted from P815
membranes with chloroform:methanol (2:1, vol:vol), the
extract was washed with water (0.3 vol) and dried under a
stream of nitrogen. Dried lipids were dissolved in 0.5%
deoxycholate (DOC) in TBS at a concentration of 1 μmole
phosphate/ml.
     Sendai virus was solubilized in DOC as previously
described for reconstitution experiments (4). Purification
of the Sendai virus glycoproteins, hemagglutinin/neuramini-
dase (HN) and fusion (F) protein, will be described in detail
elsewhere (M. Lepreau-Jose and M. Mescher, in preparation).
Briefly, virus was solublized in Triton X-100 (TX-100), 1M KCl
and centrifuged to remove insoluble material. The supernatant was dialyzed to remove KCl and the insoluble matrix
protein removed by centrifugation. This supernatant was
chromatographed on DEAE-cellulose to separate HN and F and
the separated proteins further purified by affinity chromatography on a lentil lectin column. The purified proteins

were also exchanged from TX-100 into DOC at this stage. This procedure resulted in approximately 4.5 fold purification of the HN protein (as determined by specific neuraminidase activity) and the final preparation gave a single band on sodium dodecyl sulfate (SDS) polyacrylamide gel electrophoresis. The F protein was approximately 97% pure. The final preparation contained approximately 3% HN and gave a major band on SDS gels in the position expected for F protein and a faint band corresponding to HN.

Liposomes were prepared by mixing proteins and lipids, dissolved in 0.5% DOC in Tris-buffered saline (TBS), pH 8, and dialyzing for 24 hr against TBS followed by 24 hr dialysis against TBS, 5 mM $CaCl_2$. The resulting liposomes were sedimented by centrifugation at 100,000 xg for 45 min. and resuspended in TBS for use. Analytical analyses were done as previously described (4,5).

RESULTS AND DISCUSSION

Induction of Secondary Allogeneic CTL by Reconstituted Membranes and Liposomes. Deoxycholate solubilized tumor cell membrane proteins are able to stimulate the generation of an *in vitro* secondary allogeneic CTL response and the stimulation is dependent on the H-2 antigens present in the preparation (2). Detergent containing preparations are of limited usefulness in investigating antigen recognition and we therefore examined the ability of reconstituted membranes to stimulate the response. As seen in Table I, the reconstituted membranes formed upon removing the detergent by dialysis are able to stimulate a secondary response and the response is specific. Similar results have been reported by Fast and Fan (3).

Detergent solubilized H-2 antigens can be partially purified by affinity chromatography on a *Lens culinaris* (lentil) lectin column (5,7). This procedure results in approximately twenty-fold purification and separates the membrane lipids from the antigen containing fraction. The partially purified protein stimulates an allogeneic CTL response following removal of detergent by dialysis but better activity is obtained if the antigens are incorporated into liposomes. Table II shows the stimulation obtained by liposomes prepared by mixing lectin purified antigen and lipids in the presence of DOC, dialyzing in the presence of calcium to remove detergent and sedimenting the liposomes by centrifugation at 100,000 xg. The best activity was obtained with liposomes prepared using lipids obtained by chloroform:methanol extraction of P815 tumor cells.

TABLE I

CTL INDUCTION BY RECONSTITUTED MEMBRANES[a]

| Responder | Stimulator | Target | |
		P815 (H-2[d])	EL-4 (H-2[b])
C57BL/6 (H-2[b])	Reconstituted P815 (H-2[d]) [b]	67%	3%
	Reconstituted EL-4 (H-2[b]) [b]	1%	0%
CD2F$_1$ (H-2[d])	Reconstituted P815 (H-2[d])	0%	0%
	Reconstituted EL-4 (H-2[b])	1%	44%

[a]CTL activity was measured after 5 days of *in vitro* culture. Lysis is shown at an E/T ratio of 25:1 and values are corrected by subtracting lysis by responder cells incubated without stimulator cells. (2% for CD2F$_1$ responders and 20% for B6 responders.) Spontaneous release was 17% for P815 and 19% for EL-4.

[b]Reconstituted membranes were prepared from solubilized high speed pellet membrane fraction in the case of P815 (51 µg) and solubilized plasma membrane in the case of EL-4 (14 µg) (5).

TABLE II

CTL INDUCTION BY LIPOSOMES[a]

| Lipid[b] | % Specific release | |
	12.5:1	6.25:1
None	24	12
P815 membrane lipid	53	24
Lecithin + Cholesterol[c]	25	15
Lecithin	5	2

[a]CTL activity of B6 immune spleen cells was measured on P815 targets after 5 days of *in vitro* culture. Specific release values were corrected by subtracting lysis by responder cells cultured alone (13% at an effector to target ratio of 12.5:1, 9% at 6.25:1).

[b]Liposomes were prepared using lectin-purified H-2[d] (obtained from 115 µg of membrane) and 0.2 µmole of the indicated lipid.

[c]Mixture of 4:1 lecithin:cholesterol.

The greater activity obtained using antigen incorporated into liposomes indicates that recognition is critically dependent upon the physical presentation of the antigen. This is further suggested by several additional observations. It was previously found that DOC solubilized membrane proteins would induce a CTL response when added directly to cultures, as long as the final detergent concentration was sufficiently low (2). Nonidet P-40 (NP-40) solubilized antigen, however, was inactive even though this procedure yields serologically active H-2 antigens and the NP-40 itself did not interfere with the cultures at the levels added. One possible explanation for these findings is that the dilution of detergent occurring upon addition of the soluble protein to the culture medium results in formation of protein aggregates and that these aggregates form differently depending upon the detergent used. It was found that antigens solubilized in NP-40 become active if exchanged into DOC on a lectin column (5). Physical presentation has also been found to play an important role in determining the xenogeneic CTL inducing activity of liposomes containing pure HLA-A and HLA-B (8). The activity is dependent on the ratio of HLA to phospholipid in the liposomes. Additional evidence of the critical role of presentation is seen in the experiments described below using Sendai virus antigens.

The lectin purified preparations used in the experiments described above contain a number of membrane glycoproteins. In fact, H-2 antigens are a minor component of the mixture (5). It thus remains an open question whether allogeneic recognition involves recognition of the H-2 molecules alone or of H-2 molecules together with other cell surface proteins. It has recently become possible to isolate highly purified, detergent solubilized H-2 (S. Herrmann and M. Mescher, in preparation) and this question is currently being investigated.

Induction of Sendai Virus Specific CTL by Reconstituted Membranes and Liposomes. Recognition of syngeneic, virus-infected cells by CTL requires both viral antigen and H-2 molecules (9). It is not known whether these proteins are recognized independently on the cell surface or if recognition requires molecular interaction between the H-2 and virus protein(s). The use of isolated antigens incorporated into liposomes should provide a means of approaching this question and we have begun to examine the feasibility of using the approach described above for allogeneic CTL. Sendai virus specific CTL were chosen for investigation as it was known that formation of the cell surface antigen(s) necessary for recognition does not require viral infection of the cell (10, 11).

Initial experiments showed that mixing DOC solubilized tumor membranes with solubilized virus and forming reconstituted membranes by dialysis resulted in material active in induction of a secondary Sendai virus specific CTL response. Similar experiments were then done using B6D2F$_1$ (H-2$^{b/d}$) spleen cells in order to determine if the activity was dependent on the H-2 antigens present in the reconstituted membranes. Stimulation of spleen cells from these mice with reconstituted membranes containing P815 (H-2^d) and virus proteins should result in CTL able to lyse P815-Sendai targets and not EL-4 (H-2^b)-Sendai targets if the induction is dependent on the H-2 antigens present in the reconstituted membranes. Alternatively, if the reconstituted membranes fuse with the responder cells in culture or are taken up by macrophages and the viral proteins presented on responder cell membranes, then both types of target will be lysed. The results of such experiments demonstrate that the CTL induced by reconstituted membranes containing H-2^d antigens lyse H-2^d and not H-2^b targets (Fig. 1, M). Reciprocal results are obtained using reconstituted membranes containing H-2^b antigens. These results strongly suggest that both the H-2 antigens and viral proteins in the reconstituted membranes are recognized and determine the specificity of the response.

The requirements for recognition were further examined (Fig. 1) using reconstituted membranes containing only P815 antigens (P), only Sendai proteins (S) or a mixture of both (M). The results demonstrated that stimulation was obtained only if the reconstituted membranes contained both H-2 and virus proteins, thus confirming the above conclusion. Furthermore, no activity resulted if equivalent amounts of H-2 antigen and viral proteins were added to the same culture in separately reconstituted membranes (P + S, Fig. 1). It thus appears that not only must both types of antigen be added to the culture, but the H-2 and virus proteins must be present in the same lipid bilayer for effective recognition to occur. While this observation indicates that the antigens must be in relatively close physical proximity, it does not prove that a molecular interaction between H-2 antigens and viral proteins is necessary.

Sendai virus specific CTL have also been induced with liposomes containing viral proteins and lectin-purified H-2 antigens (4). As in the experiments described above, the H-2 antigens and viral proteins had to be present in the same membranes to obtain activity. Eliminating a large amount of the irrelevant membrane protein by lectin chromatography allowed us to examine the liposomes by SDS gel electrophoresis to determine which viral proteins were present. The major proteins present were the viral membrane glycoproteins, the fusion (F) protein and the hemagglutinin/neuraminidase (HN), along with some matrix and nucleoprotein. The viral protein composition of the liposomes was the same whether H-2 antigens were present or not (4).

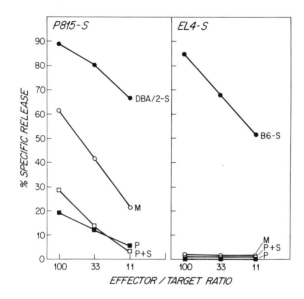

FIGURE 1. Stimulation of a secondary Sendai virus-specific syngeneic CTL response by whole cells and reconstituted membranes. Reconstituted membranes or virus-coated whole cells were placed in *in vitro* culture with spleen cells from B6D2F$_1$ mice immunized 1 week previously with Sendai virus. CTL activity was assayed 5 days later on Sendai virus-coated P815 H-2^d cells (A) or EL-4 H-2^b cells (B). Whole cells or reconstituted membranes were used: Sendai-coated DBA/2 spleen cells (closed circles, A); Sendai-coated B6 spleen cells (closed circles, B); reconstituted membranes (4 μg total protein) formed from a mixture containing both P815 membrane proteins and virus proteins (M), (open circles); reconstituted P815 membranes (P) (2 μg total protein) and reconstituted Sendai membranes (S) (2 μg total protein) added to the same culture (open squares); reconstituted P815 membranes (P), (2 μg total protein) (closed squares) (Ref.4).

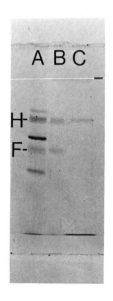

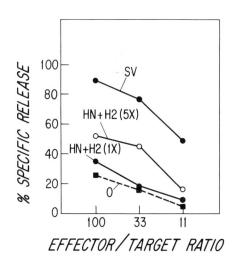

FIGURE 2.   Left. SDS gel electrophoresis of Sendai virus
proteins. A, whole virus (H = hemagglutinin/neuraminidase;
F = fusion protein). B, virus glycoproteins. C, purified HN
glycoprotein. The faint band indicated by the bar at the
right is an HN dimer.
Right. CTL induction by liposomes containing lectin purified
$H-2^d$ and purified HN. Responder spleen cells were from DBA/2
mice and targets were P815 tumor cells coated with Sendai
virus. HN + H-2(5X), liposomes made from .042 units of HN
and lectin purified protein from 400 µg of tumor cell membrane. HN + H-2(1X), liposomes made from .047 units of HN
and lectin-purified protein from 80 µg of tumor cell membranes. 0, CTL activity of responder cells cultured alone.
SV, response obtained when intact, inactivated Sendai virus
was added to the cultures.

     The use of liposomes for induction makes it possible to
determine which of the viral proteins are recognized by the
CTL. Purified HN glycoprotein (Fig. 2A) stimulates a response
when incorporated into liposomes along with lectin purified
$H-2^d$ (Fig. 2B) indicating that at least some of the CTL are
specific for this protein. The magnitude of the CTL response

is dependent on the amount of H-2 antigen present in the HN
liposomes (Fig. 2B), again indicating that recognition
requires the presence of both antigens. Preliminary experiments indicate that CTL can be induced with liposomes containing H-2 antigens and F protein. The F protein preparation
being used has about 3% HN in it, but the magnitude of the
CTL response obtained to these liposomes indicates that the
response cannot be attributed to the small amount of HN
present. These preliminary results suggest that there are
CTL populations specific for each of the two viral glycoproteins.

It has previously been shown that treatments of Sendai
virus which inactivate the F protein (12,13) or the HN protein (13) result in viral particles which can no longer
interact with tumor cells to form targets for CTL. These
treatments prevent fusion of the viral and cell membranes,
suggesting that insertion of the viral glycoproteins into the
cell membrane is required for recognition. This conclusion
is consistent with our results demonstrating that both the
H-2 and virus glycoproteins must be present in the same lipid
bilayer to stimulate induction of CTL. The results obtained
using purified F and HN further indicate that either glycoprotein alone, once inserted into a membrane along with H-2,
results in antigens able to induce a CTL response.

The use of reconstituted membranes and liposomes to
stimulate induction of secondary CTL responses provides a
valuable means of investigating the joint recognition of
foreign antigen and MHC products at the molecular level.
Using this functional assay, it should now be possible to
begin to investigate the nature of the interaction, if any,
between H-2 and foreign antigen in the membrane, *i.e.*, to
determine whether association of the molecules is necessary
for recognition or if physical proximity in the lipid bilayer
is sufficient.

There is also much that remains to be understood about
the interaction of liposomes and cells. While subcellular
materials are able to induce secondary CTL responses, plasma
membranes induce only a very weak primary response (1) and no
activity has been obtained using reconstituted membranes and
liposomes (unpublished results). We have also been unsuccessful in attempting to specifically block the CTL-target interaction using membranes or liposomes. Even in the case of
secondary CTL induction, subcellular materials are less
efficient that whole cells in inducing the response (1,2,4,5
8). Preliminary experiments comparing secondary CTL induced
with whole stimulator cells or purified plasma membranes
indicate that stimulation with membranes results in a smaller
number of CTL but that these cells have a higher average
affinity for targets than the CTL responding to whole cells

(S. Balk and M. Mescher, unpublished). Further studies of
these aspects of CTL recognition are in progress.

Liposomes containing pure or partially purified antigens
have been used in studies of allogeneic (5), xenogeneic (8)
and Sendai-virus specific (4) secondary CTL response. Membranes from TNP-modified cells (14) and influenza virus
infected cells (C. Reiss and S. Burakoff, unpublished) induce
specific CTL and Alaba and Low (15) have recently demonstrated
that detergent solubilized tumor cell membranes stimulate a
tumor-specific, syngeneic CTL response. Thus it appears that
in vitro secondary induction will provide a means of studying
the molecular requirements for recognition of most, if not
all, of the foreign antigens able to induce CTL responses.

REFERENCES

1. Lemonnier, F., Mescher, M., Sherman, L., and Burakoff, S.
   (1978). J. Immunol. 120, 1114.
2. Mescher, M., Sherman, L., Lemonnier, F., and Burakoff, S.
   (1978). J. Exp. Med. 147, 946.
3. Fast, L.D., and Fan, D.P. (1978). J. Immunol. 120, 1092.
4. Finberg, R., Mescher, M., and Burakoff, S.J. (1978).
   J. Exp. Med. 148, 1620.
5. Sherman, L., Burakoff, S.J., and Mescher, M.F. (1979).
   Submitted for publication.
6. Hayman, M.J., and Crumpton, M.J. (1972). Biochem. Biophys.
   Res. Comm. 47, 923.
7. Kvist, S., Sandberg-Trägårdh, L., Östberg, L., and
   Peterson, P.A. (1977). Biochem. 16, 4415.
8. Engelhard, V.H., Strominger, J.L., Mescher, M., and
   Burakoff, S. (1978). Proc. Natl. Acad. Sci. USA 75, 5688.
9. Doherty, P.C., Blanden, R.V., and Zinkernagel, R.M.
   (1976). Transplant. Rev. 29, 89.
10. Schrader, J.W., and Edelman, G.M. (1977). J. Exp. Med.
    145, 523.
11. Koszinowski, U., Gething, M.-J., and Waterfield, M.
    (1977). Nature 267, 160.
12. Sugamura, K., Shimizu, K., Zarling, D.A., and Bach, F.G.
    (1977). Nature 270, 251.
13. Gething, M.-J., Koszinowski, U., and Waterfield, M.
    (1978). Nature 274, 689.
14. Sherman, L., Mescher, M., and Burakoff, S. (1979).
    Submitted for publication.
15. Alaba, O., and Low, L.W. (1978). J. Exp. Med. 148, 1435.

INTERACTION OF LIPID VESICLES CONTAINING H-2 ANTIGENS WITH ALLOANTIBODY AND WITH ALLOIMMUNE CYTOTOXIC T LYMPHOCYTES [1]

Carol C. Whisnant and D. Bernard Amos

Division of Immunology, Duke University Medical Center
Durham, North Carolina 27710

ABSTRACT   Detergent solubilized, partially purified mouse H-2 antigens have been reconstituted in phosphatidylcholine and phosphatidylcholine/cholesterol lipid vesicles. These lipid vesicles inhibit lysis by alloantibody and complement and inhibit specific conjugate formation between alloimmune cytotoxic T lymphocytes and target cells. With this system the influence of antigen density and lipid composition on immune recognition can be studied.

INTRODUCTION

The importance of cell-cell interactions in the generation and regulation of immune responses and in the expression of certain immunologic effector functions is well established. The initial event in cell-cell interaction, "recognition," is based on the complementarity of cell surface components. Recognition may result in activation of one or both interacting cells and initiate a complex requence of events, some of which are designated the "function" of the activated cell(s).

The goal of the studies we describe here is to define molecular events in cell-cell interaction by studying the influence of membrane composition on interaction. Our experimental approach is to replace one of a pair of interacting cells with a lipid vesicle of defined chemical composition and to study the influence of bilayer composition on cell-vesicle interaction.

The importance of membrane composition in immune recognition and activation is demonstrated by the elegant experiments of McConnell and colleagues. By incorporating lipid antigens or lipid haptens in lipid bilayers of known composition, Humphries and McConnell (1) and Brulet and McConnell (2, 3) studied the importance of the physical state of the bilayer ("solid" or "fluid") for antibody binding and complement activation. At low hapten density the degree of

[1]This work was supported by USPHS grant AI-08897 and USPHS TG T32 GM-07003.

complement activation was greater if the bilayer were in a
fluid rather than solid state. The initial interpretation of
these results was that the reduced lateral mobility of hapten
(and therefore of hapten-antibody complexes) in the solid membrane decreased the probability of IgG molecules coming sufficiently close together to bind C1q. Diffusion constants for
lipids in the solid state were later measured by Smith and
McConnell (4) and were, in fact, lower than diffusion constants for fluid lipids, but the differences seemed insufficient to account for the observed differences in complement
activation. Parce et al. (5) subsequently showed that C1q
bound equally well to the solid and fluid bilayers. These
results indicate that the physical state of the bilayer influences a step or steps in complement activation subsequent
to C1q binding, such as activation of C1s or interaction of
nascent hydrophobic regions of complement components with
lipids.

The mole fraction (X) of cholesterol in phosphatidylcholine lipid bilayers was shown to have a marked effect on
recognition of hapten by antibody (2) and on complement activation by sensitized vesicles (1, 3). Cholesterol enhances
exposure of certain haptens at $X > 0.3$. The effects of lower
concentrations of cholesterol ($X = 0.2$) on antibody binding may
be related to the influence of cholesterol on lateral diffusion of lipids (6). The precise nature of the interactions
between phosphatidylcholine and cholesterol and how these
interactions affect antibody binding are not known.

Despite these complexities we are attempting to study the
influence of antigen density and lipid composition on recognition and activation in cell-cell interaction.

Gene products of the murine major histocompatibility
complex (H-2) have been shown to play key roles in immunologically relevant cell-cell interaction (7, 8). We have chosen
as a model system the recognition and lysis of murine target
cells by murine alloimmune cytotoxic T lymphocytes (CTL). In
this system immune recognition involves cell surface components determined by the H-2K and H-2D regions of the H-2
complex. Although the generation and expression of alloreactivity represents a somewhat artificial function of the immune
system, we believe that this model system offers several
important advantages:

1) while homogeneous populations of CTL are not
available, immune peritoneal exudate lymphocytes (IPEL)
contain a relatively high percentage of CTL (9);

2) the cell surface antigens recognized by alloimmune CTL have been identified (see below);

3) recognition can be studied directly without
relying on secondary or tertiary manifestations of immune
recognition; this is particularly important since events

subsequent to recognition (activation, lysis) may also be influenced by membrane composition.

Several lines of evidence strongly suggest that the cell surface components recognized by alloimmune CTL are the serologically detectable gene products of the H-2K and H-2D regions (10, 11). These gene products are integral membrane glycoproteins of molecular weight 45,000 daltons (12) which are noncovalently associated with B_2 microglobulin. It is not known whether determinants recognized by alloantibody are the same as those recognized by alloimmune CTL.

RESULTS AND DISCUSSION

To produce lipid vesicle "targets" for CTL we have used H-2 antigens solubilized in detergent (deoxycholate--DOC) from crude plasma membranes of the murine T-cell tumors EL4 (H-2^b) and RL♂1 (H-2^d) and partially purified by affinity chromatography on <u>Lens culinaris</u> hemagglutinin (LcH). On the average, crude plasma membranes from 10^{10} tumor cells yield 37 mg of DOC-soluble protein, and we recover 3.7 mg LcH adherent glycoprotein per 100 mg DOC-soluble protein applied to the affinity column. Serologically defined H-2 activity is demonstrated by the ability of these preparations to specifically inhibit lysis by alloantibody and complement. Inhibition of alloantibody and complement by LcH "purified" H-2 preparations is shown in Figure 1. LcH purification increases

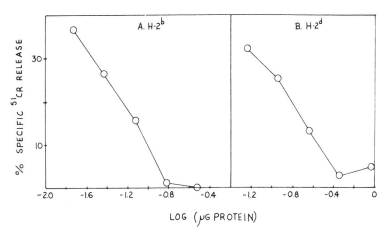

FIGURE 1. Inhibition of alloantibody and complement mediated lysis by LcH purified H-2 preparations. A. Effect of LcH purified H-2^b on lysis of EL4 by (BALB/c anti-EL4) + C'. B. Effect of LcH purified H-2^d on lysis of RL1 by (C57BL/6 anti-RL1) + C'. At these protein concentrations H-2^b does not inhibit lysis by (C57BL/6 anti-RL1) and H-2^d does not inhibit lysis by (BALB/c anti-EL4).

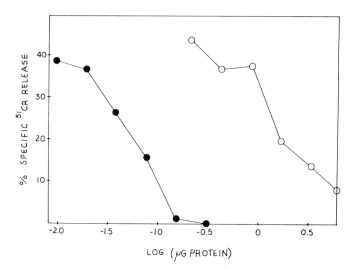

FIGURE 2.   Effect of DOC-sol H-2^b (O——O) and DOC-sol
LcH purified H-2^b (●——●) on lysis of EL4 by (BALB/c anti-
EL4) and C'. No inhibition of lysis by (C57BL/6 anti-RL1) is
observed at these protein concentrations.

inhibitory activity per weight of protein by approximately
30-fold (Figure 2), which is consistent with yield of glycoprotein in the LcH purification step.
     In interaction between CTL and target cells the formation
of stable conjugates or aggregates is a manifestation of
immune recognition and a prerequisite to lysis (13, 14). We
have measured conjugate formation between IPEL, a population
rich in CTL, and target cells as described in (15); the combined results of many experiments are given in Table 1. We
consistently observe binding of IPEL to "irrelevant" targets
(i.e., targets which are not lysed by the IPEL in ^{51}Cr release
assays), but this binding is always less than binding to
relevant targets. We define specific conjugate formation, a
parameter of immune recognition, as (A - B) where A = per cent
of cells in conjugates or aggregates with relevant targets and
B = per cent of cells in conjugates or aggregates with irrelevant targets.
     The effects of LcH purified H-2 preparations on specific
conjugate formation are shown in Figure 3. H-2^b preparations
inhibit specific conjugate formation by (IPEL anti-EL4) but
have no effect on specific conjugate formation by (IPEL anti-
RL1), while H-2^d preparations inhibit specific conjugate formation by (IPEL anti-RL1) without significantly affecting
specific conjugate formation by (IPEL anti-EL4). We attribute
these effects to binding of detergent-solubilized H-2 to

TABLE 1

CONJUGATE FORMATION

(IPEL anti-EL4) + EL4   36.9% (n=9)

(IPEL anti-EL4) + RL1   18.4% (n=12)

    specific conjugate   =   18.5%
      formation

(IPEL anti-RL1) + RL1   33.9% (n=9)

(IPEL anti-RL1) + EL4   19.1% (n=9)

    specific conjugate   =   14.8%
      formation

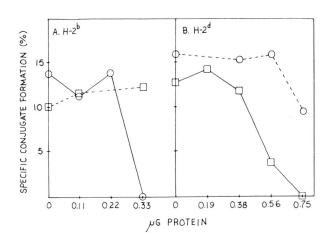

FIGURE 3. Effect of LcH purified H-2 preparations on specific conjugate formation. A. Specific conjugate formation by (IPEL anti-EL4) (O——O) and (IPEL anti-RL1) (□---□) in the presence of H-2^b. B. Specific conjugate formation by (IPEL anti-RL1) (□——□) and (IPEL anti-EL4) (O---O) in the presence of H-2^d.

antigen receptors on CTL, with concomitant loss of binding of
CTL to target cell H-2 antigens.

We have reconstituted these LcH purified H-2 preparations
in egg phosphatidylcholine (PC) and phosphatidylcholine/cho-
lesterol (PC/CHOL) lipid vesicles using the procedure of
Brunner et al. (16) with slight modifications. Lipid, protein
and detergent are dispersed in buffered saline, applied to a
Sephadex G-50 column and eluted with buffered saline. Large
vesicles consisting of lipid and protein are eluted in the
void volume, while smaller detergent micelles are eluted much
later. Preliminary studies indicate these are large unila-
mellar vesicles of average size 0.5-1.0 μ.

In Figure 4 inhibition of lysis by alloantibody and
complement is compared for a LcH purified H-2^b preparation and
the same preparation reconstituted in PC lipid vesicles
(estimated molar ratio lipid:protein = 80:1). The lipid
vesicle reconstituted H-2^b has about 40% inhibitory activity/
weight protein as the detergent-solubilized material. This
suggests that inside-outside orientation of proteins is random
in these lipid vesicles.

Inhibition of specific conjugate formation by H-2 preparations reconstituted in PC and in PC/CHOL lipid vesicles is
shown in Figure 5. H-2 containing lipid vesicles bind to CTL
and thereby inhibit specific conjugate formation between IPEL
and target cells.

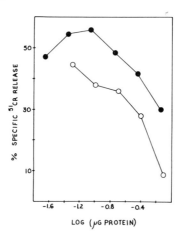

FIGURE 4. Effect of LcH purified H-2^b (O———O) and
LcH purified H-2^b reconstituted in phosphatidylcholine lipid
vesicles (●———●) on lysis of EL4 by (BALB/c anti-EL4) + C'.
Estimated molar ratio PC:protein = 80:1. No inhibition of
lysis by (C57BL/6 anti-RL1) is observed at these protein
concentrations.

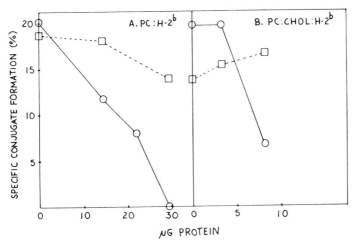

FIGURE 5. Effect of lipid vesicles containing H-2^D on specific conjugate formation by (IPEL anti-EL4) (O———O) and (IPEL anti-RL1) (□---□). A. Estimated molar ratio lipid:protein = 40:1. B. Estimated molar ratio lipid: protein = 200:1.

These results constitute a basis for studying the effects of antigen density and lipid composition on recognition of H-2 by alloimmune CTL. Currently we are attempting to quantitate binding of lipid vesicles loaded with 6-carboxy-fluorescein (17) to CTL and to demonstrate binding of CTL to black lipid membranes containing H-2 antigens. These may be more sensitive assays of antigen recognition by CTL than is inhibition of specific conjugate formation. Also we are attempting further purification of detergent-solubilized H-2K and H-2D gene products so that the term "antigen density" will be more meaningful.

In summary, we have shown that H-2 preparations reconstituted in phosphatidylcholine and in phosphatidylcholine/cholesterol lipid vesicles are recognized by alloantibody and by alloimmune CTL. The influence of antigen density and lipid composition on recognition can now be studied systematically.

ACKNOWLEDGMENTS

We have enjoyed many helpful discussions with Drs. P. Cresswell and K. Singer. Experiments demonstrating inhibition of alloantibody and complement mediated lysis were done by R. Zelman. We thank A. Cowles and K. Little for excellent technical assistance.

REFERENCES

1. Humphries, G. M. K., and McConnell, H. M. (1975). Proc. Natl. Acad. Sci. USA 72, 2483.
2. Brulet, P., and McConnell, H. M. (1976). Proc. Natl. Acad. Sci. USA 73, 2977.
3. Brulet, P., and McConnell, H. M. (1977). Biochemistry 16, 1209.
4. Smith, B. A., and McConnell, H. M. (1978). Proc. Natl. Acad. Sci. USA 75, 2759.
5. Parce, J. W., Henry, N., and McConnell, H. M. (1978). Proc. Natl. Acad. Sci. USA 75, 1515.
6. Rubenstein, J. L. R., Smith, B. A., and McConnell, H. M. (1979). Proc. Natl. Acad. Sci. USA 76, 15.
7. Katz, D. H., Hamaoka, T., and Benacerraf, B. (1973). J. Exp. Med. 137, 1405.
8. Doherty, P. C., Blanden, R. V., and Zinkernagel, R. M. (1976). Transplant. Rev. 29, 222.
9. Berke, G., Sullivan, K. A., and Amos, D. B. (1972). J. Exp. Med. 135, 1334.
10. Egorov, I. K. (1974). Immunogenetics 1, 97.
11. Todd, R. F., Stulting, R. D., and Berke, G. (1975). Cancer Res. 33, 3203.
12. Nathenson, S. G., and Cullen, S. E. (1974). Biochim. Biophys. Acta 344, 1.
13. Martz, E. (1975). J. Immunol. 115, 261.
14. Henney, C. S. (1977). In "Contemporary Topics in Immunobiology 7" (O. Stutman, ed.), pp. 245-272. Plenum Press, New York.
15. Whisnant, C. C., Singer, K. H., and Amos, D. B. (1978). J. Immunol. 121, 2253.
16. Brunner, J., Skrabal, P., and Hauser, H. (1976). Biochim. Biophys. Acta 455, 322.
17. Weinstein, J. N., Yoshikami, S., Henkart, P., Blumenthal, R., and Hagins, W. A. (1977). Science 195, 489.

T AND B LYMPHOCYTES

WORKSHOP SUMMARY: Synthetic Membranes as Markers for Immunological Recognition and Function. Pierre Henkart, Immunology Branch, National Cancer Institute, National Institutes of Health, Bethesda, MD 20205, and Harden McConnell, Department of Chemistry, Stanford University, Stanford, CA 94305

The workshop was comprised of a varied group of investigators who have used artificial membrane systems to shed light on a number of rather different biological problems. Although this area is still small, it is growing rapidly. The use of artificial membranes is a powerful tool to dissect many immunological processes involving membranes because it offers the opportunity to ask functional questions using chemically defined membrane components. Such artificial membranes are of course lacking many poorly understood "biological" activities of real cell membranes (e.g., capping, microvilli formation) and in well-defined systems any functional properties possessed by the artificial system can be assumed not to require such activities. More importantly, demonstration of biological functions by such biochemically defined membranes can provide a satisfying answer with regard to the role of MHC products which up until now has depended largely on inferences from genetics. While the latter has proved to be a powerful approach to analyzing the many functions of MHC molecules, the role of nonpolymorphic species may be underemphasized, and there always remains some doubt about the chemical identity of the molecules involved. It is only through the use of artificial membranes containing completely purified antigens and other species that a rigorous analysis of structure-function relationships of membrane components can be established.

The workshop attempted to assess the experience of the participants with regard to the optimal properties of artificial membranes required to give biological function in the different systems studied to see if any generalizations could be made at this early stage of experience.

Three laboratories presented results involving the afferent limb of the immune response. Engelhard, Burakoff, and Strominger prepared purified HLA-A and -B antigens from human lymphoblastoid cell line and incorporated these into phospholipid vesicles by detergent dialysis. Such vesicles stimulated the differentiation of mouse cytotoxic T lymphocytes previously primed with the intact human lymphoblastoid cells. The killer T lymphocytes selectively lysed human target cells bearing the appropriate alloantigens. Mescher, Finberg and Burakoff also studied the ability of artificial membranes to elicit secondary cytotoxic lymphocytes, but studied the Sendai virus specific H-2 restricted killer T cell

641

ISBN 0-12-069850-1

system in which much debate has been generated regarding the
molecular recognition mechanism. Lectin purified H-2 antigens
and purified Sendai membrane proteins were reconstituted into
phospholipid vesicles by detergent dialysis. Such artificial
membranes were able to stimulate secondary CTL responses in
vitro using Sendai primed mice. The resulting cells showed
appropriate virus and H-2 specificity. Both viral and H-2
antigens had to be in the same membrane; mixtures of liposomes
containing only H-2 and others containing only Sendai membrane
proteins did not stimulate the CTL response. Finally,
Humphries and McConnell showed that liposomes containing
phosphotidyl choline, chlosterol and DNP lipid would stimulate
the production of DNP-antibody forming cells during a 4-day
primary in vitro culture.

     Cytotoxic lymphocyte-target cell interactions were
studied by several groups beginning efforts to define the
molecular parameters for recognition and lysis. Hollander et
al. (Stanford) were able to demonstrate rapid (3 hr) specific
release of ^{51}Cr from vesicles formed from partially purified
H-2, eye muscle membrane proteins and exogenous lipids using
mouse cytotoxic T cells. The requirement for the eye muscle
protein for recognition or marker release was discussed, but
its role is unclear. This work shows that cytotoxic T cells
can cause permeability changes in artificial membranes.
Whisnant, Zelman and Amos have approached the molecular
requirements for killer T cell-target cell recognition by
inhibiting the formation of killer-target conjugates with
partially purified H-2 antigens which were detergent solubilized or reincorporated into liposomes. Specific inhibition
of conjugate formation by liposomes containing appropriate
H-2 was obtained. Eliott described the specific binding of
plasma membrane vesicles to allogeneically activated T cell
blasts, as detected by indirect immunofluorescence or by
radioacitively labeling the vesicles.

     It appears early at this stage to generalize as to the
optimal qualities of model membranes to interact functionally with lymphocytes, but current experience indicates that
variants of the cholate dialysis technique can give reconstituted liposomes containing H-2 and probably Ia which are
functional. In some cases such as CML stimulation and inhibition of killer-target conjugate formation, solubilized membrane antigens are active without reconstitution into
membranes, implying that lipid membrane carriers are not
required. If artificial membranes are used as immunogens,
the antigen/lipid ratio can affect the magnitude of the
response, as in the xenogeneic secondary CML with HLA or in
the in vitro induction of anti-hapten responses using liposomes. In the case of artificial membranes as targets for

killer T cells, an additional contribution from membrane protein seems required. In addition, cytotoxic cells may require
an optimal sized target; cytotoxic T cells released ^{51}Cr best
from ∿1-10μ vesicles, while ADCC effector cells released
marker from intact erythrocyte ghost targets but not from 0.2μ
vesicles derived from these ghosts (Simone and Henkart).
Little data is available at this point about the role of lipid
fluidity, phase transitions, and chlosterol requirements in
controling antigen presentation in these systems.

T-CELL GROWTH FACTOR DEPENDENT RESTORATION OF NUDE MOUSE T-CELL MITOGENESIS AND ALLOANTIGEN REACTIVITY[1]

Steven Gillis[2], Paul E. Baker[2], and Kendall Smith

Hematology Research Laboratory, Dept. of Medicine,
Dartmouth-Hitchcock Medical Center, Hanover, N.H.

ABSTRACT   We recently determined that T-cell growth factor (TCGF) in addition to promoting the sustained proliferation of antigen-specific cytotoxic T-cell lines, also
acted as the replication-inducing second signal in both
T-cell mitogen and antigen-driven proliferation. As such,
our hypothesis has been that TCGF functions as a key regulatory molecule in the development of T-cell immune reactivity.   In this communication we report the results of
experimentation detailing that TCGF is capable of restoring normal proliferative responses to T-cell mitogen
stimulated nude mouse spleen, lymph node, or bone marrow
cells.   Furthermore, addition of TCGF to either nude
mouse mixed lymphocyte cultures or allogeneic mixed tumor
lymphocyte cultures resulted in the generation of significant levels of T-cell mediated cytolytic reactivity.

INTRODUCTION

Due to our previous studies detailing the development of
culture methodologies allowing for the sustained in vitro proliferation of antigen-specific murine and human cytotoxic
T-cells (CTLL, 1,2), we have become increasingly interested in
how soluble factors regulate and control lymphocyte reactivity.   Recent investigations have determined that a particular
T-cell growth factor ((TCGF) responsible for the long-term exponential proliferation of CTLL) functions as the key prolif-
eration-inducing agent in both T-cell mitogen and antigen sen-
sization (3).   Further studies presented in this communication
have confirmed that (i) normal thymocytes produced little to
no TCGF and proliferated poorly in response to stimulation

1. Supported in part by NCI contract NO1-CB-74141, grant
CA-17643-04, and a grant from the National Leukemia Association, Inc.
2. Fellows of the Leukemia Society of America.

with Con A; (ii) cortisol-resistant thymocytes (predominantly mature T-cells) produced considerable quantities of TCGF and proliferated as well as peripheral splenocytes following stim- ulation with Con A and (iii) although incapable of producing TCGF or responding to purified TCGF, normal thymocytes were capable of proliferating to the same extent as Con A stimu- lated mature T-cells (peripheral splenocytes or cortisol- resistant thymocytes) provided exogenous TCGF was supplied to- gether with Con A.

The observation that TCGF was capable of promoting normal T-cell mitogenesis of immature thymocyte populations prompted an examination of the effects of TCGF on nude mouse lymphocyte reactivity. In experimentation reviewed in this report, we observed that addition of purified TCGF to nude mouse lympho- cyte populations resulted in the promotion of near-normal levels of proliferation in response to stimulation with Con A. Furthermore, addition of purified TCGF to both nude mouse mixed lymphocyte cultures (MLC) and allogeneic mixed tumor- lymphocyte cultures (MTLC) resulted in the generation of con- siderable T-cell mediated, alloantigen-directed cytotoxic re- activity. These results may have significant ramifications regarding the extent of T-lymphocyte reactivity in the nude mouse and the function of the thymus in programming the dif- ferentiation of effector cell reactivity.

MATERIALS AND METHODS

Animals.   Balb/c female, athymic nu/nu (nude) mice, 5-7 weeks of age were purchased from ARS Sprague-Dawley, Solon, Ohio. NIH female nude mice were purchased from Harlan Indus- tries, Indianapolis, Indiana. Normal female C57B1/6 mice (4-8 weeks of age) were purchased from the Jackson Laboratory, Bar Harbor, ME.

Purification of TCGF.   Mouse TCGF was prepared by the 18-20 hour Con A (2 ug/ml) stimulation of normal murine spleen cells (5×10^6 cells/ml) in serumless RPMI 1640 tissue culture medium supplemented with 5×10^{-5}M/ml 2-mercaptoethanol, 50 U/ml penicillin G, and 50 ug/ml streptomycin. Con A sensitized murine spleen cells were cultured in 300 ml volumes in roller bottles at 37^oC. Rat TCGF (Charles River Breeding Laborator- ies, Wilmington, MA) was produced under identical conditions in RPMI 1640 supplemented with 5% heat-inactivated (56^oC for 30 minutes) fetal calf serum (FCS, Grand Island Biologicals Co., Grand Island, NY). Both sources of crude TCGF (rat and mouse) were then subjected to sequential concentration (vacuum dialy- sis for mouse-conditioned medium; 85% ammonium sulfate preci- pitation for rat-conditioned medium), Sephadex G-100 gel ex-

clusion chromatography, ion exchange chromatography (diethyl-
aminoethyl cellulose, DEAE) and preparative flat-bed isoelectric focusing, using procedures previously detailed (4).

TCGF Microassay. TCGF activity contained in either culture supernates or in biochemically fractionated material was
assayed as previously described using either CTLL-1 or CTLL-2
(1) cells as the indicator cell populations (5). The results
were quantified by probit analysis and expressed as units of
activity based on a standard rat TCGF preparation. In experiments designed to test the ability of a particular lymphocyte
population to produce TCGF, lymphoid cells (10^7/ml) were cultured with Con A (5 ug/ml) in 10% FCS-supplemented RPMI 1640.
Supernates harvested from 24 hour cultures were then tested as
described above for TCGF activity. Splenocytes, thymocytes,
cortisol-resistant thymocytes, lymph node cells and bone marrow cell populations were prepared as detailed elsewhere (3,6).

Tritiated Thymidine (^{3}H-Tdr) Incorporation Assays For
Cellular Proliferation. Murine cells (100 ul, 10^6 cells/ml)
were seeded in triplicate in 96-well microtiter plates (#3596
Costar, Inc., Cambridge, MA) in Click's medium (Altick Associates, Hudson, WI) supplemented with 2% normal mouse serum.
Cells were stimulated by 100 ul addition of either purified
TCGF or purified TCGF plus Con A (5 ug/ml). After four days
of culture 0.5 uCi of ^{3}H-Tdr (Schwarz-Mann, Orangeburg, NJ,
specific activity 1.9 Ci/mM) was added to each well and the
incubation continued for 4 hours. Cultures were harvested onto glass fiber filter strips and ^{3}H-Tdr incorporation determined as previously described (5). Results were expressed as
the mean cpm ± 1 standard deviation of triplicate cultures.

Nude Mouse MLC, MTLC Stimulation. MLC/MTLC were conducted either as previously detailed (6,7) or in 200 ul volumes
in v-bottom 96 well microtiter plates (#1S-MVC-96-TC, Linbro
Chemical Co., New Haven, CT). For microplate stimulation, NIH
nude mosue splenocytes (1×10^6 cells/well) were cultured with
either an equal number of x-irradiated (1500 r) allogeneic
($H-2^d$) Balb/c spleen cells or with 1×10^5 x-irradiated (5000r)
allogeneic ($H-2^d$) P815 mastocytoma cells. After five days of
stimulation either in the presence or absence of purified TCGF,
effector cells were harvested and tested for cytolytic reactivity against an appropriate target cell in a standard four
hour ^{51}Cr-release assay.

Lymphocyte Mediated Cytolysis (LMC) Assays. Four hour
^{51}Cr-release assays were conducted in 96 well v-bottom microplates using methodology previously described (6). Percent
specific lysis was determined by using the following equation:

$$\% \text{ specific lysis} = \frac{\text{experimental cpm} - \text{medium control cpm}}{\text{maximum release cpm} - \text{medium control cpm}}$$

RESULTS

Ability of TCGF to Promote Thymocyte Mitogenesis.   The
data displayed below in Figure 1A summarizes results of experimentation conducted to ascertain the degree of TCGF production and cellular proliferation exhibited by both mature
and immature T-cell populations (10^7 cells/ml) stimulated with
a mitogenic concentration of Con A (5 ug/ml for 24 hours).

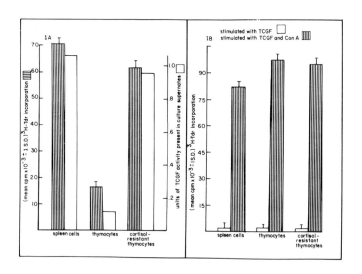

FIGURE 1. A. ^{3}H-Tdr incorporation and TCGF production
exhibited by 10^6, 24 hr. Con A-stimulated spleen, thymus, and
cortisol resistant thymus cells. B. ^{3}H-Tdr incorporation exihi-
bited by identical cell populations stimulated for 96 hrs with
either purified TCGF or TCGF plus Con A.

Normal thymocytes produced little to no TCGF and proliferated
poorly in response to Con A stimulation. Peripheral splenocytes as well as cortisol-resistant thymocytes (the mature
T-cell compartment of the thymus) produced similar high titer
TCGF-containing supernates and proliferated markedly in response to stimulation with Con A. The data in Fig. 1A further
supported our previous findings detailing the requirement for
mature T-cells to ensure TCGF production and once again
pointed out the strong correlation between TCGF production and
cellular proliferation exhibited by mitogen-activated T-cells
(3).
    Figure 1B details the ^{3}H-Tdr incorporation response of
identical lymphocyte populations (1x10^6 cells/ml) following
96 hour culture stimulation with either purified TCGF or puri-

fied TCGF to which a mitogenic concentration of Con A had been added. It is important to note that immature and mature (cortisol-resistant) thymocytes as well as peripheral splenocytes were incapable of responding to purified TCGF. However, immature thymocytes following dual stimulation with Con A and purified TCGF incorporated as much, if not greater amounts of ^{3}H-Tdr than did mature T-cell populations (spleen cells or cortisol-resistant thymocytes) stimulated with Con A alone (Fig. 1A). In addition to providing suggestive evidence that one possible function of the thymus may be to effect the maturation of T-cells capable of TCGF production, results of experimentation displayed in Fig. 1 supported our previous findings that TCGF was only capable of mediating the proliferation of activated lymphocyte populations (3). Furthermore it appeared that resting T-cells regardless of their state of maturation were incapable of responding to TCGF stimulation in the absence of concomittant mitogen triggering.

TCGF Dependent Nude Mouse Lymphocyte Mitogenesis. Based primarily on the data displayed in Fig. 1 we questioned whether TCGF supplementation might also prove effective in promoting T-cell mitogenesis in similar lymphocyte populations limiting for the presence of mature T-cells; namely, nude mouse lymphocytes. On the next page, Fig. 2A details the inability of BALB/c nude mouse spleen, lymph node, and bone marrow cells (10^7/ml) to produce TCGF or to incorporate high levels of ^{3}H-Tdr following stimulation with a mitogenic concentration of Con A for 24 hours (5 ug/ml). As was the case with other resting lymphocyte populations, nude mouse spleen, lymph node, or bone marrow cells exhibited little if any ^{3}H-Tdr incorporation, in response to culture stimulation with purified TCGF (Fig. 2B). However, stimulation with TCGF and Con A resulted in proliferation almost equal in magnitude to that mediated by normal thymocytes stimulated with purified TCGF and Con A, or for that matter, mature splenocytes stimulated with Con A alone (Fig. 1). Therefore, as was the case with normal thymus cells (predominantly an immature T-cell population) nude mouse lymphocytes could be induced to display near-normal T-cell mitogenesis provided Con A stimulation was conducted in the presence of exogenous purified TCGF.

TCGF-Dependent In Vitro Generation of Nude Mouse Cytolytic T-Cell Reactivity. The observation that TCGF supplementation could restore near-normal levels of T-cell mitogen-induced lymphocyte proliferation in nude mice, led us to question whether TCGF might be capable of provoking competent immune reactivity in response to antigen sensitization. Due to our previous studies establishing the obligatory role that TCGF plays in the in vitro generation of normal murine cytolytic reactivity (7), we felt that an appropriate model system to

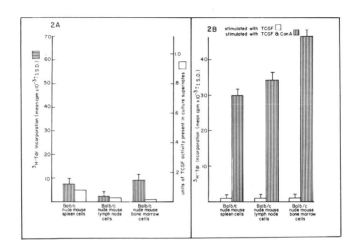

FIGURE 2. A. ^{3}H-Tdr incorporation and TCGF production exhibited by 10[6], 24 hr. Con A-stimulated nude mouse spleen,
lymph node, and bone marrow cells. B. ^{3}H-Tdr incorporation exhibited by identical cell populations stimulated for 96 hrs.
with either purified TCGF or TCGF plus Con A.

investigate would be the effect of TCGF supplementation on
nude mouse MLC responses. Spleen cells from both NIH and
BALB/c nude backgrounds were co-cultured in MLC with x-irradiated (1500r) allogeneic C57Bl/6 spleen cells. Cultures were
conducted in either 2% FCS-supplemented Click's medium or in
identical tissue culture media supplemented with purified
TCGF. Viable effector cells harvested from 5-day control and
TCGF supplemented cultures were then tested for cytolytic reactivity against radiolabeled C57Bl/6 tumor target cells
(FBL-3(Hn)) in a standard 4-hour ^{51}Cr-release assay. As shown
on the next page in Figure 3, only effector cells harvested
from TCGF-supplemented MLC mediated significant levels of
cytolysis. Further experimentation detailed in a separate report (8) confirmed that effector cells generated in TCGF-supplemented MLC were Thy-1 antigen positive in that pretreatment
of such cell populations with anti-Thy-1 serum and complement
resulted in the total abrogation of effector cell cytotoxicity.
Furthermore, nude mouse cytolytic lymphocytes (generated in
TCGF-supplemented MLC) have been maintained in TCGF-dependent
culture for more than 5 months, during which time they have
continued to demonstrate alloantigen-specific cytolytic reactivity along with Thy-1 antigen cell surface expression. (8)
    It is important to note that the TCGF used in the above-
detailed MLC supplementation experiments was obtained follow-

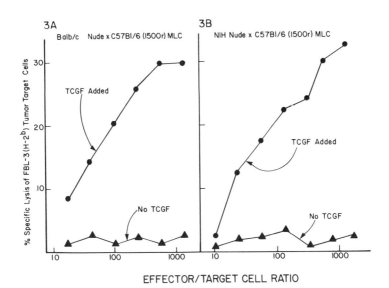

FIGURE 3. TCGF-dependent generation of nude mouse cytolytic effector cells in BALB/c nude x C57BL/6 (3A) and NIH nude
x C57Bl/6$_x$ (3B) MLC.

ing successive G-100 gel exclusion and DEAE ion exchange
chromatography of medium conditioned by Con A-stimulated rat
spleen cells. Therefore, the possibility remained that additional factors with molecular weight and charge mobility similar to that of TCGF might also have been involved in promoting
the in vitro generation of nude mouse splenic cytotoxic T-
lymphocytes. In an attempt to further establish that TCGF
alone was responsible for provoking nude mouse cytolytic reactivity, additional experiments were conducted in both MLC
and MTLC systems using purified TCGF preparations obtained
after a 3 step purification procedure. TCGF purified from
both mouse and rat sources, was subjected to successive gel
filtration chromatography, ion exchange chromatography, and
preparative flat-bed isoelectric focusing. Using such a
purfication system, mouse TCGF (30,000 mw) separated into two
distinct species with isoelectric points of 4.3 and 4.9.
Rat TCGF (15,000 mw) migrated with a single isoelectric point
of 5.5. The purification of both mouse and rat TCGF along with
data detailing the relationship of TCGF to previously detailed
T-cell regulatory factors (including T-cell replacing factor
(TRF,9) and thymocyte mitogenesis factor (TMF, 10) are the
subjects of separate communications (11,12). IEF pure mouse

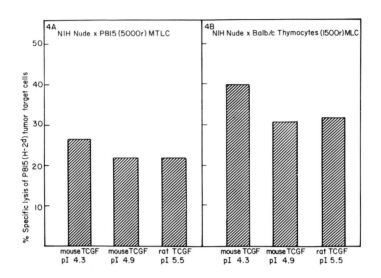

FIGURE 4. Ability of purified TCGF (mouse and rat) to sup-
port the in vitro generation of cytolytic effector cells in
NIH nude x P815$_x$ MTLC (4A) and NIH nude x BALB/c thymocyte$_x$
MLC (4B).

and rat TCGF (1/5 dilution) were tested for their ability to
promote the in vitro generation of NIH nude mouse cytotoxic
responses in 200 ul cultures following stimulation with either
(i) 1500r x-irradiated allogeneic BALB/c thymocytes (1/1,
stimulator/responder cell ratio) or (ii) 5000r x-irradiated
P815 (H-2^d) tumor cells (1/30 stimulator/responder cell ratio).
As detailed below in Fig. 4, both IEF pure rat and mouse TCGF
promoted the generation of significant cytolytic activity in
nude mouse MLC and MTLC. The data displayed in Fig. 4 provide
further evidence that exogenous TCGF in concert with antigen
stimulation constitutes sufficient sensitization to allow for
the proliferation of reactive nude mouse cytolytic pre-T-cells
to the point where meaningful in vitro reactivity can be observed.

                              DISCUSSION

     One implication of the studies detailed in this report
(Fig. 3 and 4) together with our previous findings regarding
the in vitro generation of cytolytic responses from nude mouse
spleen cells (8), is that antigen-specific pre-effector-T-cells

may exist in peripheral lymphoid organs of nude mice. The existence of antigen-specific pre-T-cells which are capable of mediating differentiated T-cell functions may call for a re-examination of previous studies detailing the mechanism of action of so-called T-cell replacing factors (9). TRF, harvested from either Con A-stimulation or MLC supernates has been shown to promote antibody production in cultures limiting from mature T-cells (either nude mouse splenocytes or in vitro manipulated T-cell deficient populations). The major hypothesis has been that TRF (by replacing T-helper cells) acts directly on antigen-activated B-cells to promote antibody production. However, in light of the observation that medium conditioned by either Con A or MLC-stimulation contains significant quantities of TCGF it is plausible to assume that TCGF present in "TRF-containing" supernates acts primarily by promoting nude mouse pre-helper T-cell proliferation to the point where newly differentiated helper cells are providing sufficient help to trigger antibody production.

The observation that nude mice are incapable of producing TCGF upon mitogen stimulation (Fig. 2) coupled with the demonstrated ability of exogenous purified TCGF to promote both T-cell mitogenesis (Fig. 2) and alloantigen reactivity (Fig. 3, 4) leads us to hypothesize that perhaps a major reason behind the well-documented immunodeficiency of the nude mouse may be its inability to produce TCGF. It should be pointed out, however, that the levels of cytotoxicity generated by TCGF-supplemented nude mouse MLC or allo-MTLC do not approach the efficiency of cytolysis that is demonstrated by normal mouse splenocytes following alloantigen stimulation (7). The observed difference in efficiency may simply be that far fewer numbers of alloantigen-reactive precursors are present in the spleens of nude mice than exist in normal mouse splenocyte populations. To answer this question, perhaps it will be possible to take advantage of the culture techniques detailed in this report (particularly the ability to generate positive cytolytic reactivity from TCGF-supplemented nude MLC conducted in 200 ul volumes) to conduct limiting dilution experiments to determine the frequency of alloantigen-specific cytotoxic precursors in nude mouse spleen cell populations.

Other investigators have previously reported the existence of cytotoxic cells in the nude mouse. However, the cytolytic reactivity mediated has most often been associated with the presence of natural cytotoxicity. Accordingly, the cells which mediate this reactivity have been termed "natural killer" or NK cells (see reference 13 for review). We feel assured that the cytolytic reactivity demonstrated by the nude mouse MLC or MTLC effector cells detailed in this report cannot be associated with NK activity. First, the NK cell has generally be

thought of as a non-T-cell. In studies using either conventional or nude mice, pretreatment of NK populations with
anti-Thy-1 serum and complement has resulted in only a partial
reduction of cytolytic reactivity (13,14). However, similar
pre-treatment of TCGF-supplemented nude mouse MLC effector
cells completely eliminated allo-antigen directed cytolysis (8).
Secondly, the cytolytic reactivity mediated by both nude mouse
MLC effector cells and nude CTLL cells has been shown to be
specifically directed against a particular allo-antigen (H-2^b)
(8). This is in direct contrast with NK activity which does
not appear to be specific for a particular cell surface antigen
whether or not of histocompatibility gene origin. Finally,
one characteristic of NK activity in mice has been the diminu-
tion of reactivity following prolonged culture (24 hours or
more) at 37°C (15). This was obviously not the case with the
nude mouse MLC effector cells detailed in this report in that
five day activation cultures and 4-hour LMC assays were all
conducted at 37°C.

The observation that purified TCGF is capable of restoring immune responsiveness to predominantly immature thymocytes
and nude mouse splenocytes, compounded with the finding that
neither lymphocyte population is capable of producing TCGF,
allows one to speculate that perhaps a major function of the
thymus is to program the differentiation of cells capable of
producing TCGF. Zinkernagel et al. recently found that upon
restoration of T-dependent function in B-mice (thymectomized,
lethally irradiated and reconstituted with anti-Thy-1 serum
and complement-treated bone marrow cells) by thymus grafting;
vaccinia virus directed cytolysis was H-2 restricted. However,
the restriction was conferred by the histocompatibility type
of the donor thymus (16). These results have been interpreted
to suggest that a major function of the thymus is to "teach"
precursor effector lymphocytes to recognize antigen in association with self H-2. The data presented in this report would
suggest that perhaps these same precursor populations are already capable of recognizing non-self without prior exposure
to thymic influence. Based on the methodology described herein,
it would be interesting whether in vitro treatment with purified
TCGF would be sufficient to allow for the generation of nude
mouse lymphocytes with cytolytic specificities directed against
antigens recognized in association with self H-2 (perhaps virus
encoded antigens (17) or TNP-modified cell membrane (18) structures).

Finally, it should be stressed that despite the sophisti-
cation of the purification processes used, it remains feasible
that TCGF itself is capable of mediating some differentiation-
inducing stimulus. Perhaps a more appealing hypothesis is that
the proliferation and differentiation of nude mouse splenocytes

(which results following co-stimulation with antigen and TCGF) may be inseparable biological pathways. It may even be plausible that the rate limiting step in the differentiation of effector T-lymphocytes may be the ability of ligand-stimulated cells to proliferate and in doing so, differentiate into cells capable of immune function. It is hoped that further studies of the effects of TCGF on the proliferation and function of T-cells isolated at different stages of maturity will provide greater understanding of the role that TCGF plays in the development of effector T-cell immune reactivity.

REFERENCES

1. Gillis, S. and Smith, K.A. (1977) Nature 268, 154.
2. Gillis, S., Baker, P.E., Ruscetti, F.W., and Smith, K.A. (1978) J. Exp. Med. 148, 1093.
3. Smith, K.A., Gillis, S., Baker, P.E., McKenzie, D., and Ruscetti, F.W. (1979) Ann. N.Y. Acad. Sci. in press.
4. Watson, J., Aarden, L., Shaw, J., and Paetkau, V. (1979) J. Immunol. in press.
5. Gillis, S., Ferm, M.M., Ou, W., and Smith, K.A. (1978) J. Immunol. 120, 2027.
6. Gillis, S., and Smith, K.A. (1977) J. Exp. Med. 146, 468.
7. Baker, P.E., Gillis, S., Ferm, M.M., and Smith, K.A. (1978) J. Immunol. 121, 2168.
8. Gillis, S., Union, N.A., Baker, P.E., and Smith, K.A. (1979) J. Exp. Med. in press.
9. Watson, J.D., Aarden, J., and Lefkovitz, I. (1979) J. Immunol. 122, 209.
10. Farrar, J.J., Simon, P.L., Koopman, W.J., Fuller-Bonar, J. (1978) J. Immunol. 121, 1353.
11. Watson, J.D., Gillis, S., Marbrook, J., Mochizuki, D., and Smith, K.A. (1979) submitted for publication.
12. Gillis, S., Watson, J., and Smith, K.A. (1979) submitted for publication.
13. Herberman, R.B. (1978) in: The Nude Mouse in Experimental and Clinical Research. Academic Press, New York, New York.
14. Paige, C.J., Figarella, E.F., Cittito, M.J., Cahan, M., and Stutman, O. (1978) J. Immunol. 121, 1827.
15. Herberman, R.B., Nunn, M.E., Holden, H.T., and Laurin, D.H. (1975). Int. J. Cancer 16, 230.
16. Zinkernagel, R.M., Callahan, G.N., Althage, A., Cooper, S., Klein, P.A., and Klein, J. (1978) J. Exp. Med. 147, 882.
17. Zinkernagel, R.M., Doherty, P.C. (1974) Nature 248, 701.
18. Schmitt-Verhulst, A.M., Pettinelli, C.B., Henkart, P.A., Lunney, J.K., and Shearer, G.M. (1978) J. Exp. Med. 147, 352.

FUNCTIONAL SPECIFICITY OF A PERMANENT T CELL LINE[1]

Gunther Dennert, and J. Douglas Waterfield[2]

Department of Cancer Biology
The Salk Institute for Biological Studies
San Diego, California and
Department of Biology, University of California
San Diego, California

ABSTRACT Mouse T cells selected in a one way mixed lymphocyte culture were maintained in tissue culture for three years by restimulation. These T cells proliferate only when stimulated with cells sharing H-2 antigens with the strain used for selection of the cell line. Intra H-2 mapping revealed that the IA^k subregion codes for the majority of stimulating determinants(s). Cytotoxic effector function could be induced by specific alloconfrontation and was directed against targets carrying IA^k coded antigens. This cell line was also able to induce a positive allogeneic effect by activating B cells in an in vitro primary humoral response to sheep erythrocytes. Helper activity was again specific for cells carrying IA subregion coded antigens. Supernatant factor(s) capable of substituting for the cell line could be generated by stimulation with cells expressing $H-2^k$ region coded determinants. Such supernatants, however, were not strain specific in their activation of an in vitro primary humoral response to sheep erythrocytes.

INTRODUCTION

Thymus derived lymphocytes (T cells) stimulated in a primary mixed lymphocyte culture can be propagated in tissue culture for several months or even years provided they are periodically stimulated with allogeneic spleen cells (1-4).

[1]This work was supported by grants CA 15581 and CA 19334 from National Institute of Health to G. D. and in part by grants AI 08795 and IM-1K (American Cancer Society) to Dr. R. W. Dutton.

[2]Recipient of a postdoctoral fellowship from the Anna Fuller Fund.

Many of these cell lines, although they retain their proliferative activity, tend to lose their cytotoxicity after several
months (2,3,5). This of course makes these cell lines less
useful for studying receptor specificities and function of
cytotoxic T cells. Here we report the successful establishment of a cell line in tissue culture which has retained not
only specific proliferative and cytotoxic activity but also
displays strong and specific helper activity in the in vitro
induction of a humoral response to sheep erythrocytes (SRBC).

RESULTS

Establishment in Culture of a BALB/c anti C3H Cytotoxic
T Cell Line. Mixed lymphocyte cultures containing 10^5/ml
responder BALB/c spleen cells and 10^5/ml 1000 r irradiated C3H
stimulator cells were set up in medium containing 5% fetal
calf serum and 5×10^{-5} M 2-mercaptoethanol in 20 ml Falcon
tissue culture bottles (2,3). Every two weeks the culture
supernatant was replaced with new medium containing 10^5/ml
irradiated C3H spleen cells. The cultures were routinely
split when the cell density reached 5×10^5 per ml. The established line was called C·C3·11·75 since it was a BALB/c ($H-2^d$)
anti C3H ($H-2^k$) T cell culture, originally set up in November,
1975 (3). After 5 months C·C3·11·75 showed strong proliferation (about tenfold over background) when challenged with
C3H ($H-2^k$), CBA ($H-2^k$) and A ($H-2^a$) spleen cells. Little or
no stimulation was caused by DBA/1 ($H-2^q$), C57BL/6 ($H-2^b$),
ASW ($H-2^s$) or BALB/c ($H-2^d$) stimulator cells (3). Strong
cytotoxic activity specific for $H-2^k$ spleen blast cells or
tumor cells was also seen at that time (3). The cell line
was maintained a further two years in culture and then
assayed again for its functional specificity.

Cytotoxic Activity of C·C3·11·75. Cytotoxic effector
function assayed on $H-2^k$ target cells revealed that while C3H
spleen cells are lysed (Table 1) Rl(TL$^+$) tumor cells which
express both the K end private specificity H-2.23 and the D
end private specificity H-2.32 (6) are not. Syngeneic BALB/c
splenic blast cells are only lysed in the presence of phytohemagglutinin (Table 1). The failure of C·C3·11·75 to lyse
Rl(TL$^+$) suggests that this killer cell line does not recognize the K or D region coded antigens. In support of this,
Table 1 shows that not only C3H, but also B10A, B10A(4R) and
ATL, spleen blast cells are lysed. In contrast, C3H OL and
BALB/c blast cells are not lysed. Since Rl(TL$^+$) is not lysed,
this would suggest that the determinants recognized by this
cell line are encoded by genes to the right of the K region,
i.e., in the IA subregion.

TABLE 1
CYTOLYTIC ACTIVITY OF C·C3·11·75

Target	H-2	a/t	PHA (5µg/ml)	% Cytotoxicity
				5 hr
C3H blasts	kkkkkkk	30:1	-	37 ± 3
C3H blasts	kkkkkkk	10:1	-	19 ± 1
Rl(TL$^+$)	k.....k	30:1	-	<1
Rl(TL$^+$)	k.....k	10:1	-	<1
				3 hr
BALB/c blasts	ddddddd	50:1	-	<1
BALB/c blasts	ddddddd	15:1	-	<1
C3H blasts	kkkkkkk	50:1	+	43 ± 0.5
C3H blasts	kkkkkkk	15:1	+	37 ± 0.9
BALB/c blasts	ddddddd	50:1	+	45 ± 0.2
BALB/c blasts	ddddddd	15:1	+	36 ± 0.9
				3 hr
C3H blasts	kkkkkkk	50:1	-	40 ± 2.5
B10A blast	kkkdddd	50:1	-	43 ± 1.1
B10A (4R) blasts	kk**bbbbb**	50:1	-	42 ± 0.8
ATL blasts	skkkkkd	50:1	-	39 ± 1.1
C3H OL blasts	ddddkkk	50:1	-	4 ± 2.7
BALB/c blasts	ddddddd	50:1	-	<1

The cytotoxic activity of C·C3·11·75 reaches plateau
values at attacker to target cell ratios lower than 10:1 (4).
This supports the contention that this line is a rather homogeneous T killer cell population. Maximal cytolysis is always
found to be low (in the range of 30-45%) and may be due to
possible heterogeneity in the target population or
inhibition of the effector cells by soluble antigen.

Proliferative Specificity of C·C3·11·75. Since genes in
the I region are responsible for T cell proliferation it was
tested whether the spleen cells which are susceptible to lysis
by C·C3·11·75 are able to stimulate cell proliferation. In
Table 2 it is seen that C3H OL does not stimulate cell proliferation, while BALB/c consistently shows significant stimulation. It is not clear at present what the basis of this
syngeneic stimulation might be. Aside from the stimulation
by BALB/c, much higher stimulation is seen with C3H, B10A and
ATL spleen cells, which are good targets in the cytotoxic

TABLE 2

PROLIFERATIVE ACTIVITY OF C·C3·11·75

Responder[1]	Stimulator[2]	H-2	c.p.m. day[3] 2 - 3
5 x 10^4 C·C3·11·75	BALB/c	ddddddd	1,590 ± 192
5 x 10^4 C·C3·11·75	C3H OL	ddddkkk	168 ± 16
5 x 10^4 C·C3·11·75	C3H	kkkkkkk	12,138 ± 2,057
5 x 10^4 C·C3·11·75	B10A	kkkdddd	8,514 ± 723
5 x 10^4 C·C3·11·75	ATL	skkkkkd	5,802 ± 118
5 x 10^4 C·C3·11·75	Con A SN[4]	-	137 ± 22

[1] 5 x 10^4 C·C3·11·75 were cultured with 5 x 10^6 per ml 1000 r irradiated stimulator spleen cells.

[2] Background incorporation of ^{3}H TdR was between 70 and 115 cpm.

[3] Cultures were labeled with 0.5 μl ^{3}H thymidine on day 2 and harvested on day 3 (Ref. 2).

[4] Con A supernatant was prepared by culturing mouse spleen cells with concanavalin A for two days. The supernatant was harvested, filtered and tested as described in Ref. 8 and 9.

reaction. It therefore appears that the original population of killer cells was heterogeneous, consisting of cells which recognize more than one specificity expressed on both tumor cell lines and spleen blast cells. Prolonged selection of this cell line by periodic stimulation with C3H spleen cells has resulted in a population which is only stimulated by and only kills targets expressing antigens coded by the IA sub-region genes (4).

Specificity of Helper Activity of C·C3·11·75.
C·C3·11·75 lymphocytes and normal BALB/c T lymphocytes (both groups mitomycin/C treated) were added in varying numbers to B lymphocytes from B10.Br (H-2^k), B10 (H-2^b), and B10.D2 (H-2^d) mice. It can be seen from Figure 1A that both the BALB/c (H-2^d) and the C·C3·11·75 (H-2^d) T lymphocytes induced a positive allogeneic effect with the B10.Br B lymphocytes. The individual titration curves, however, differed between the two T cell preparations. The C·C3·11·75 cells displayed an 81 fold enrichment of helper function. Significant suppression was seen with cell numbers that, using BALB/c T cells, elicit optimal allohelp. When both groups of T cells

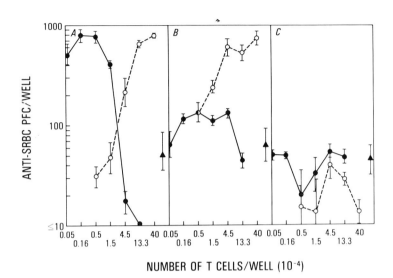

FIGURE 1. Nylon-wool column passed T cells from BALB/c
(o - - - o) and the C·C3·11·75 cell line (● —— ●), were
added to wells containing SRBC and 5 x 10^5 B cells from:
A. B10.Br mice; B. B10 mice; and C. B10.D2 mice. PFC responses were determined on day 4. Background responses of B
cells alone are indicated (▲).

were tested on B10 H-2^b) B lymphocytes the C·C3·11·75 cells
failed to give significant allohelp, demonstrating the
specificity of the cell line for the alloantigenic determinants used in their selection. In Figure 1C no positive
allogeneic effect can be seen when both groups of T cells
were tested on B cells expressing the syngeneic H-2^d haplotype.
Intra H-2 mapping of the genes coding for antigens required
in the induction of the positive allogeneic effect is shown
in Figure 2. C·C3·11·75 cells reproducibly showed a 27 fold
enrichment of effector function when compared with the response of BALB/c T cells. The number of plaque forming B
lymphocytes from the different intra-H-2 recombinant strains
was compared at the peak point. The C·C3·11·75 T cells
activated significant antibody synthesis in B10.Br, B10.A,
B10.AQR, and B10.A(4R) B cells, the B10.A(4R) giving as high
a response as B10.Br. B10.A(5R) B cells, expressing IJ^k and

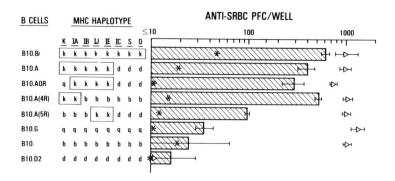

FIGURE 2.   T cells from BALB/c and C·C3·11·75 were added
to wells containing SRBC and B cells from the listed recombinant inbred mice.   The results represent the geometric mean
of PFC activated by 1.5 x 10^4 C·C3·11·75 T lymphocytes (peak
antibody response) (▨).   Background responses of B cells
alone are indicated (*).   Normal BALB/c T lymphocytes
routinely activated all the B cells listed except B10.D2 as
would be expected (Δ).   However, the peak response occurred
at a 27-fold higher concentration using these cells.

1E^k region homology with the stimulating haplotype exhibit a
significantly lower level of antibody synthesis.   Finally,
B10.G, B10, and B10.D2 B cells display no response, again
verifying the specificity of the C·C3·11·75 cell line for
H-2^k.   These results suggest that the IA subregion codes for
the alloantigens recognized in the induction of allohelp.

Specificity of an Allogeneic Effect Factor Derived from
C·C3·11·75.   It was tested whether an allogeneic effect
factor is secreted by confrontation of this cell line with
mitomycin/c treated B10.Br B lymphocytes and, if so, whether
this factor exhibits strain specific helper activity in the
primary humoral response to sheep erythrocytes.   Figure 3
demonstrates that a helper factor is released from C·C3·11·75
upon stimulation with B10.Br but not by stimulation with
B10.D2 B cells.   It can also be seen that the factor non-
selectively activates B lymphocytes from B10.A(4R), B10, and
B10.D2 mice and therefore can be considered non-specific.

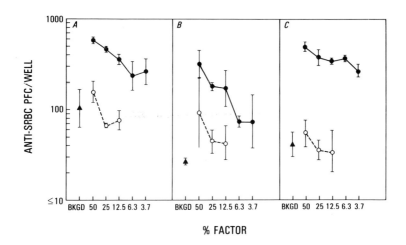

FIGURE 3. Varying concentrations of allogeneic effect
factor, derived from admixed C·C3·11·75 cells and either
10⁷ B10.D2 (o - - - o) or B10.Br (●——●) B lymphocytes
were added to wells containing SRBC and 5 x 10⁵ B lymphocytes
from: A. B10.A(4R); B. B10; and C. B10.D2.   PFC responses
were determined on day 4.   Background responses of B cells
alone are indicated (▲).

DISCUSSION

The cell line C·C3·11·75 propagated in tissue culture for
three years by repeated allostimulation is shown here to
exhibit specific cytotoxic and proliferative activity.   The
stimulating determinants and target cell antigens for lympholysis both appear to be coded by genes located in the IA
subregion of the mouse H-2 histocompatibility complex.   Therefore selection of this line resulted in loss of killer cells
specific for H-2K and D coded antigens while killer cells
specific for IA region coded antigens remained.   It is therefore possible that in this particular instance IAᵏ antigens
provide the stimulus for killing and cell proliferation to
the same cell, which could explain the relative advantage
these cells have in culture.   If this were correct one could
hypothesize that proliferation of K and D region specific
killer cells requires cooperation with I region gene product
specific helper T cells via soluble products.   It may be

relevant in this regard that this cell line appears to be
refractory to stimulation by lymphokines secreted by mitogen
activated T cells (Table 2). The cell line C·C3·11·75
displays another interesting function. If these cells are
mixed in small numbers with B cells and SRBC they are able
to cause a positive allogeneic effect under certain experimental conditions. The allogeneic effect is specific in
that the B cells activated had to share H-2 antigens with
the strain used for selection of the cell line. Intra H-2
mapping showed that genes in the IA subregion appeared to be
important for induction of the positive allogeneic effect.
Thus, the induction of help is due to recognition of the
H-2 subregion that is also responsible for proliferation and
cytotoxicity. A supernatant factor(s) secreted by this cell
line could substitute for the T cells in activation of the
in vitro humoral response. Although this factor(s) exhibited
no strain specificity in its action, its secretion was
dependent on allorecognition. It appears that the specificity seen in the positive allogeneic effect is a consequence
of the alloantigenic recognition receptors intrinsic to the
cell line, and not to any biologically restricting properties
of the allogeneic effect factor itself.

Demonstration of helper activity in a selected T cell
line contradicts an earlier finding failing to show similar
helper activity (7). The discrepancy, however, can be
explained by differences in the experimental system used:
C·C3·11·75 was not tested previously and the cell lines used
were tested three days after stimulation rather than six days.
This is important since at the earlier time C·C3·11·75 was
also suppressive.

Our findings raise certain questions regarding the homo-
geneity of the cell line. It is possible that more than one
subset of T lymphocyte has been selected for. Conversely,
one would have to assume that the cells of the allospecific
cell line are capable of performing more than one function.
Experiments utilizing anti-Ly sera, limiting dilution analysis,
and cloning of C·C3·11·75 are in progress to distinguish
between these possibilities.

ACKNOWLEDGMENT

We would like to acknowledge the technical assistance of
Ms. E. Waterfield, Ms. Sara Albanil, Mr. J. Kouba and
Mr. C. Crowley. We would also like to thank our colleagues
Drs. S. L. Swain and R. W. Dutton for valuable discussions
in parts of this study.

REFERENCES

1. Andersson, L. C., and Hayry, P. (1975). Transplant. Rev. 25, 121.
2. Dennert, G., and De Rose, M. (1976). J Immunol.116,1601.
3. Dennert, G., and Raschke, M. (1977). Eur. J. Immunol. 7, 352.
4. Dennert, G. (1979). Nature 277,476.
5. Fathman, C. G., and Hengartner, H. (1978). Nature 272,617.
6. Hyman, R., and Stallings, V. (1976).Immunogenetics 3, 75.
7. Dennert, G., De Rose, M., and Allen, R. (1977). Eur. J. Immun. 7, 487.
8. Gillis, S., and Smith, K. A. (1977). Nature 268, 154.
9. Nabholz, M., Engers, H. D., Collavo, D., and North, M. (1978). Current Topics in Microbiology and Immunology. 81,176

THE ESTABLISHMENT OF T CELL HYBRIDOMAS WITH
SPECIFIC SUPPRESSIVE FUNCTION

Masaru Taniguchi,[1] Takashi Saito,[1] Izumi Takei,[1]
and Tomio Tada[1,2]

Laboratories for Immunology, School of Medicine,
Chiba University, Chiba[1] and Department of Immunology,
Faculty of Medicine, University of Tokyo, Tokyo, Japan[2]

ABSTRACT Hybridomas continuously producing antigen-
specific suppressor molecules were established by the
fusion of an AKR thymoma cell line, BW5147, with keyhole
limpet hemocyanin (KLH)-specific enriched suppressor T
cells from C57BL/6 mice. They were positive for H-2^k,
H-2^b, I-J^b, Thy 1.1 and Thy 1.2 but lacked I-J^k alloantigens and surface immunoglobulins, and were trans-
plantable to (C57BL/6 x AKR)F$_1$ and (C57BL/6 x C3H)F$_1$
mice but not to either parental strains. By assaying
the activities of extracts or secreted materials, these
hybridomas were divided into three functional groups:
1. with antigen-specific suppressive activity, 2. with
antigen-nonspecific suppressive activity, and 3. without
detectable suppressive activity. The antigen-specific
suppressor molecule derived from group 1 cell lines
was invariably adsorbable to immunoadsorbents composed
of KLH, anti-H-2^b, and anti-I-J^b, but not to those of
unrelated antigen, anti-mouse Fab and anti-mouse immunoglobulins. The molecular size of the active factor was
found to be between 42,000 and 68,000 daltons. The
factor derived from group 1 suppressed the responses of
spleen cells from syngeneic or semisyngeneic mice,
C57BL/6 and (C57BL/6 x C3H)F$_1$ against dinitrophenylated
(DNP)-KLH, but not that from C3H mice. The factor from
group 2 hybrid cell lines with nonspecific activity
suppressed the response of any strains of mice.

INTRODUCTION

Previous studies demonstrated that antigen-stimulated
suppressor T cells and factors derived from them possessed
antigen-binding specificity. The suppressor molecule was
shown to have no known immunoglobulin isogeneic determinants,
and the molecular weight was estimated to be around 50,000.

The molecule has a determinant controlled by a gene or genes mapped in *I-J* subregion of the major histocompatibility complex (*H-2*) (1-9). The chemistry and the mode of action of the molecule have only been poorly analyzed because of paucity of the recovery of the molecule from antigen-specific suppressor T cells. The establishment of T cell hybridoma with specific suppressor function would provide a useful tool to chemically characterize the antigen-specific *I-J* bearing suppressor factor.

We have been successful in establishing a number of *I-J* positive hybrid cell lines by the fusion of T lymphoma cells with specifically enriched suppressor T cells. Some of the cell lines are continuously secreting molecules having antigen-specific suppressor function. The present communication describes some of the properties of suppressor molecules derived from hybridoma cell lines.

MATERIALS AND METHODS

The hybrids were made by the fusion of a hypoxanthine guanine phosphribosyl transferase negative AKR thymoma cell line, BW5147 (a gift of Dr. Takeshi Watanabe, Osaka University, Osaka, Japan) with enriched C57BL/6 suppressor T cells specific for keyhole limpet hemocyanin (KLH). The enrichment of the suppressor T cells was performed by adsorption to and elution from antigen-coated Petri dishes as described previously (7). The methods for cell fusion used in this paper have already been described in the previous paper (10,11). A mixture of 1-5 x 10^6 enriched suppressor T cells and equal to ten times excess of BW5147 thymoma cells in Dulbecco's modefied Eagle's mimimum essential medium (DMEM) was centrifuged at 400 g. To the pellet was added 2 ml of 42% (w/v) polyethylene glycol (PEG: mw 2,000) dimethylsulfoxide (DMSO) solution. This was gently mixed with a broadened pipette. Soon after this step, the mixture was transferred into 2 ml of 50% (w/v) PEG solution and mixed well. The suspension was gradually diluted by adding 16 ml of serum free DMEM, and further diluted with 180 ml of DMEM containing 13% fetal bovine serum (FBS). The mixtrue was then incubated at 37°C in 5% CO_2. Two to three hour after the incubation cells were washed 4 times with the medium, and were cultured at least for a week in HAT medium. Cells grown in HAT medium were stained by an anti-*I-J^b* antiserum (B10.A(5R) anti-B10.A (3R)) and fluorescein-conjugated rabbit anti-mouse Fab. The *I-J^b* positive hybrid cells were separated by fluorescence activated cell sorter, FACS-II (Becton-Dickinson Electronics Laboratory, Mountain View, California), and cloned in multi-well microplates (Falcon #3040) by limiting dilution or single cell manipulation. The established cell lines were charac-

terized for their surface markers, transplantability and their
suppressive activities. The materials extracted and secreted
from *I-J* positive hybrids were used to characterize suppressor
molecule. Cell-free extracts of cell lines were prepared by
freezing and thawing as described elsewhere (11). The secreted material was obtained as an ascites in (C57BL/6 x AKR)F$_1$
mice transplanted intraperitoneally with hybridomas. To
characterize hybridoma-derived suppressor factors, extracted
or secreted materials was absorbed with immunoadsorbents of
KLH, *Ascaris suum* extract, anti-mouse Fab, anti-mouse Igs,
anti-*H-2* and anti-I-J antisera. The suppressive activity was
tested in an *in vitro* secondary anti-DNP antibody response of
spleen cells from mice primed with DNP-KLH or DNP-EA. Generally, the extract equivalent to 3 x 10^5 hybridoma cells was
added to the culture. The anti-DNP plaque-forming cells (PFC)
was measured by the method of Cunningham and Szenberg 5 days
after the cultivation (2).

RESULTS AND DISCUSSION

Separation of *I-J* Positive Hybrids by Fluorescence Acti-
vated Cell Sorter (FACS). After the hybridization of BW5147
(*H-2*^{k}) with enriched KLH-specific C57BL/6 (*H-2*^{b}) suppressor
T cells, cells were allowed to grow in HAT medium for 7 days.
The cells were then reacted with anti-*I-J*^{b} antiserum or normal
C57BL/6 serum and stained with fluorescein-conjugated rabbit
anti-mouse Fab, which had been extensively absorbed with
BW5147 to avoid nonspecific staining. The fluorescence
profile by the FACS analysis is shown in Fig. 1. About 50%
of the total population was specifically stained. No staining
was observed with cells exposed to normal C57BL/6 serum. The
fluorescence positive (*I-J*^{b} positive) cells were separated and
cloned by limiting dilution and single cell manipulation.

Phenotypic Expressions on Established Cell Lines. The
cytotoxicity of hybrids with various alloantisera was assayed
by a conventional dye exclusion cytotoxic test using 1 x 10^4
cell in 10 μ*l* in the V bottomed microplate with rabbit complement. Fig. 2 shows that one of the established cell line,
9F18la, expresses *H-2* antigens of BW5147 (*H-2*^{k}) and C57BL/6
(*H-2*^{b}) parental haplotypes. The cell line possessed both
Thy 1.1 and Thy 1.2 antigens 4-6 week after the cell fusion
but lost Thy 1.2 expression 6 month after the cell hybridization. All the hybrid cell lines so far tested failed to react
with polyvarent rabbit anti-mouse Igs by the membrane fluorescence technique, being in agreement with those reported by
other investigators (12,13). They were also killed by anti-
I-J^b but not by anti-*I-J*^{k} antiserum.

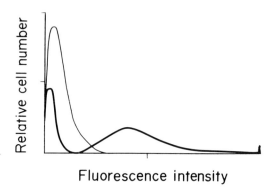

FIGURE 1.   Fluorescence profile of *I-J^b* positive hybrid cells. Cells reacted with anti-*I-J^b* antiserum (B10.A(5R) anti-B10.A(3R)) (———), and with normal C57BL/6 serum (———), respectively. Gain 1. Cell number analyzed: 1 x 10^4 cells.

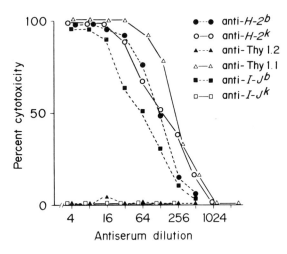

FIGURE 2.   Cytotoxic curves of the hybridoma 9F181a with various alloantisera. Cells were reacted with anti-*H-2^b* (B10.BR anti-B10), anti-*H-2^k* (B10 anti-B10.BR), anti-Thy 1.2 (AKR anti-C3H), anti-Thy 1.1 (C3H anti-AKR), anti-*I-J^b* (B10.A(5R) anti-B10.A(3R)) and anti-*I-J^k* (B10.A(3R) anti-B10.A(5R)), respectively.

It is well known that mouse alloantisera often contain antiviral activity. Therefore, T cell hybridomas are quite likely to carry viral products on their surface. In order to exclude this possibility, 25 μl anti-I-J^b antiserum, B10.A(5R) anti-B10.A(3R), extensively preabsorbed with BW5147 cells was absorbed 4 times with 1×10^8 spleen cells of various mouse strains at a dilution of 1:10 at 4°C for 45 min. The cytotoxic activity of absorbed anti-I-J^b antiserum was then tested by the conventional dye exclusion cytotoxic assay on the T cell hybridomas. Table 1 shows the some of the results. All of the established cell lines tested were killed by anti-I-J^b antiserum not being absorbed with spleen cells. Absorption of anti-I-J^b antisera with C57BL/6 spleen cells, however, lost their cytotoxic activity, whereas that with C3H spleen cells did not. Moreover, absorption with B10.A(3R) spleen cells, but not with B10.A(5R) spleen cells removed the activity against the hybrid cell lines. As the difference of H-2 haplotype between B10.A(3R) and B10.A(5R) is only I-J subregion, the products coded for by genes mapped in I-J subregion on the lymphoid cell surface can absorb the activity of anti-I-J^b antiserum. These results suggest that the cytotoxic activity of anti-I-J^b antiserum on the T cell hybridomas is not due to the contamination of antiviral antibodies, but due to the specific activity for the I-J determinants on the T cell hybridomas. Even 14 month after cell hybridization cell lines expressed H-2 antigens of both parental cells, together with I-J^b determinants introduced from C57BL/6 suppressor T cells.

TABLE I

SELECTIVE EXPRESSION OF I-J SUBREGION GENE PRODUCTS
ON T CELL HYBRIDOMAS

Anti-I-J^b absorbed with	I-J haplotype	% cytotoxicity		
		34S-18	34S-15	34S-281
None	——	90	89	100
C57BL/6	b	2	N.D.	20
C3H	k	79	N.D.	74
B10.A(3R)	b	0	13	15
B10.A(5R)	k	75	76	80

Transplantability of Hybrid Cells. The transplantability
of *I-J* positive hybridomas was studied by inoculating 2 x 10^6
cells in 0.1 m*l* intracutaneously into the shaved back of
C57BL/6 ($H-2^b$), C3H ($H-2^k$), AKR ($H-2^k$) and their F_1 hybrid
mice ($H-2^{b/k}$), (C57BL/6 x C3H)F_1 and (C57BL/6 x AKR)F_1, respectively. Fig. 3 shows the tumor growth curve of one of
the hybrid cell line 9F181a in C57BL/6, C3H and (C57BL/6 x
C3H)F_1 mice. The growth of the tumor as a solid form was
observed in (C57BL/6 x C3H)F_1 mice but neither in C3H nor in
C57BL/6 mice. The hybrids were also found to be transplant-
able into (C57BL/6 x AKR)F_1 but not into AKR mice (data not
shown). If the cells were transplanted intraperitoneally
into F_1 mice, a large quantity of ascites was produced.

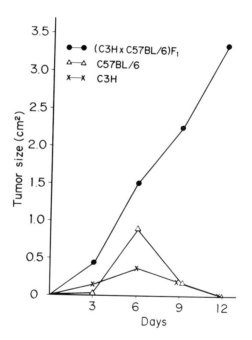

FIGURE 3.   The tumor growth curves of the
hybridoma 9F181a, in C57BL/6, C3H and (C3H x
C57BL/6)F_1 mice.

Effect of Hybridoma-Derived Factors on the *In Vitro* Secondary Antibody Response. Previous studies have established that the sonicated extract from KLH-specific, *I-J* positive suppressor T cells can specifically suppress the *in vivo* primary and *in vitro* secondary antibody responses against DNP-KLH (1,2). It was, therefore, of interest to study whether or not the ascites as well as the extract obtained from *I-J* positive hybridoma have suppressive activity. The established cell lines carrying *I-J* determinants were frozen in dry ice and thawed with warm water at 37°C for ten times. The cell free extract was obtained by ultracentrifugation at 20,000 g for 1 hr. The extracted or secreted materials were tested for their suppressive activity in an *in vitro* secondary anti-DNP PFC response. The dose of extracted materials corresponding to 3×10^5 hybrid cells was added to the culture of 4×10^6 spleen cells from C57BL/6 mice primed with 100 μg DNP-KLH or 100 μg DNP-EA plus pertussis vaccine. The number of anti-DNP IgG PFC was measured on day 5. Table II summarizes results obtained with extracts of some hybridoma cell

TABLE II

EFFECT OF HYBRIDOMA-DERIVED FACTORS ON THE *IN VITRO*
SECONDARY ANTIBODY RESPONSE

Suppressor factor	$I-J^b$ determinant on cells	Anti-DNP IgG PFC response to		Suppression
		DNP-EA	DNP-KLH	
——	——	1,460	1,566	——
BW5147	-	1,278	1,407	No
10L-11	-	1,407	1,480	No
9F-18	+	1,684	99	Specific
9F-181a	+	1,430	104	Specific
34S-11	+	2,025	491	Specific
34S-18	+	1,694	384	Specific
34S-70	+	1,332	149	Specific
9F-8	+	181	289	Nonspecific
8C-23	+	437	128	Nonspecific
34S-15	+	170	192	Nonspecific
34S-44	+	607	309	Nonspecific
34S-281	+	1,581	1,407	No
8C-19	+	2,153	1,407	No

lines in comparison with those of parental thymoma and *I-J* negative hybrid cell line (10L-11) expressing *H-2*^{b} and *H-2*^{k} antigens. Some of the *I-J*$^+$ hybridomas displayed suppressive activity in the *in vitro* secondary antibody responses either in antigen-specific and nonspecific fashion. Some other *I-J* positive hybridomas had no activities. The similar results were obtained in the previous report (10). This indicates that these hybridomas have different functional properties regardless their common expression of *I-J* determinants. Such functional differences may reflect the heterogeneity of *I-J* subregion gene products which are expressed on different sub-set of T cells (14).

The ascites from F$_1$ mice bearing the hybrid cell line 9F181a was also found to contain a strong antigen-specific suppressive activity. The results in Table III show that the addition of 1-50 µl of ascites to the cultured spleen cells suppressed anti-DNP IgG antibody response to DNP-KLH but not to DNP-EA.

Even 10 µl of ascites showed a maximal suppressive effect. The effect was comparable to that of extracted materials which corresponded to 3 x 10^5 hybrid cells. The same dose of extract from BW5147 had no effect on the responses against both antigens.

TABLE III

ANTIGEN-SPECIFIC SUPPRESSIVE EFFECT OF SECRETED OR EXTRACTED MATERIALS FROM THE *I-J*^{b} POSITIVE HYBRIDOMA

Suppressor factor	Dose	Anti-DNP IgG PFC	
		DNP-EA	DNP-KLH
Exp. A			
Not added	——	1,733	6,295
BW5147 extract	3 x 10^5	1,762	5,371
9F181a extract	3 x 10^5	1,697	417
Exp. B			
Not added	——	1,520	1,492
9F181a ascites	50 µl	1,521	213
	10 µl	1,307	149
	1 µl	1,379	625
	0.1 µl	1,648	1,762

Immunochemical Properties of Hybridoma-Derived Suppressor Factors. The suppressive extract as well as ascites was absorbed with immunoadsorbents composed of specific antigen (KLH), unrelated antigen (Ascaris extract), anti-*H-2*, anti-*I-J* antisera, polyvalent rabbit anti-MIgs and anti-mouse Fab antibodies. As shown in Table IV, the suppressive activity of both ascites and extract was completely removed by a passage through the immunoadsorbents of KLH, anti-*H-2b* and anti-*I-Jb*, but not by those of Asc, anti-MIgs, anti-mouse Fab and anti-*I-Jk* antibodies. These results indicate that the suppressor molecules both secreted and extracted from 9F181a possess antigen-binding site and *I-J* determinant. Most recently, we have shown the hybridoma-derived antigen-specific suppressor factor was removed by the immunoadsorbent of anti-V_H, but not that of anti-V_L antibodies. Thus it seems probably that the suppressor molecule contains at least two major components; *I-J* subregion gene products and immunoglobulin V_H gene product which is responsible for antigen-binding capacity. The molecular entity is as yet unknown. The molecular size of the hybridoma-derived suppressor factor was found to be between 42,000 and 68,000 daltons as determined by gel filtration, being similar to that of the previously reported suppressor factor from primed suppressor T cells (2).

TABLE IV

ABSORPTION OF SUPPRESSOR FACTOR ON ANTIGEN
OR ANTIBODY IMMUNOADSORBENT COLUMNS

Suppressive factor absorbed with	Anti-DNP IgG PFC/culture	
	Ascites	Extract
Not added	1,023	1,169
Unabsorbed	86	12
KLH	1,492	1,251
Asc	32	35
Anti-mouse Igs	96	47
Anti-mouse Fab	149	59
Anti-*H-2b*	1,204	1,180
Anti-*I-Jb*	1,364	947
Anti-*I-Jk*	149	24

    Effect of Hybridoma-Derived Suppressor Factors on the
Responses of Syngeneic and Allogeneic Spleen Cells. We have
previously demonstrated that the antigen-specific suppressor
factor from KLH-primed mice was able to suppress the response
of only *H-2* histocompatible strains. Thus, we attempted to
examine whether such a genetic restriction would exist in the
suppression mediated by the putatively homogenous factors
derived from hybrid cell lines having *I-J* determinants. Since
hybrids were made by the fusion of BW5147 ($H-2^k$) with C57BL/6
($H-2^b$) suppressor T cells, the factors secreted and/or extracted from hybrid cell lines were tested for their suppressive activity in the responses of spleen cells of parental
haplotype, C3H ($H-2^k$), C57BL/6 ($H-2^b$), and their F_1 hybrids
($H-2^{k/b}$). As shown in Table V, it was found that the factors
from the cell lines, 9F181a and 34S-18 having antigen-specific
activity, were able to suppress the responses of C57BL/6($H-2^b$)
and (C57BL/6 x C3H)F_1 ($H-2^{b/k}$), but not that of C3H ($H-2^k$)
spleen cells. The results are in agreement with our previous
findings that certain processes of suppressive cell interaction require the compatibility in *I-J* subregion genes between
the suppressor factor and the target cells (15). On the other
hand, the extract obtained from a cell line, 34S-44 with
antigen-nonspecific activity, suppressed the response of C3H
spleen cells in addition to those of C57BL/6 and (C57BL/6 x

TABLE V

EFFECT OF HYBRIDOMA-DERIVED FACTORS ON THE RESPONSES OF
C57BL/6, C3H AND THEIR F1 HYBRIDS

Suppressive factor	Antigen-specificity for KLH	Anti-DNP IgG PFC/culture		
		C57BL/6	BC3F1	C3H
Exp. A				
Not added	——	1,854	3,424	6,160
BW5147 extract	−	2,054	3,192	5,025
9F181a extract	+	134	586	5,382
9F181a ascites	+	682	1,008	6,545
Exp. B				
Not added	——	3,035	9,186	1,450
BW5147 extract	−	3,368	8,568	1,183
NG-38 extract	−	2,963	9,090	1,716
34S-18 extract	+	469	1,993	2,014
34S-44 extract	−	224	1,940	203

C3H)F_1. There were some other cell lines whose extracts had no suppressive activity. These results suggest that $I-J$ determinants are expressed on hybridomas with different functional properties. We are now exploring whether such a functional heterogeneity of $I-J$ bearing hybridomas is due to the structural and genetic differences of $I-J$ molecules. It is also suggested that the association of V_H gene product with $I-J$ subregion gene product would be attributed to the antigen-specificity of the suppressor molecule. In any events, the establishment of T cell hybridomas continuously producing antigen-specific suppressor molecules would provide a useful means to study on the chemical properties of the antigen-binding receptor on T cells.

ACKNOWLEDGEMENTS

We are grateful to Drs. M. Igarashi, K. Hiramatsu, Y. Hirai, K. Imai and H. Ra for their collaboration and criticism.

REFERENCES

1. Takemori, T., and Tada, T. (1975). J. Exp. Med. 142, 1241.
2. Taniguchi, M., Hayakawa, K., and Tada, T. (1976). J. Immunol. 116, 542.
3. Taniguchi, M., and Miller, J.F.A.P. (1978). J. Immunol. 120, 21.
4. Théze, J., Kapp, J.A., and Benacerraf, B. (1977). J. Exp. Med. 145, 839.
5. Kontiainen, S., and Feldmann, M. (1977). Eur. J. Immunol. 7, 310.
6. Tada, T., Taniguchi, M., and David, C.S. (1976). J. Exp. Med. 144, 713.
7. Taniguchi, M., and Miller, J.F.A.P. (1978). J. Exp. Med. 146, 1450.
8. Théze, J., Waltenbaugh, C., Dofr, M.E., and Benacerraf, B. (1977). J. Exp. Med. 146, 287.
9. Murphy, D.B., Herzenberg, L.A., Okumura, K., Herzenberg, L.A., and McDevitt, H.O. (1976). J. Exp. Med. 144, 699.
10. Taniguchi, M., and Miller, J.F.A.P. (1978). J. Exp. Med. 148, 373.
11. Taniguchi, M., Saito, T., and Tada, T. Nature in press.
12. Kohler, G., Lefkovits, I., Elliott, B., and Coutinho, A. (1977). Eur. J. Immunol. 7, 758.
13. Goldsby, R.A., Osborne, B.A., and Herzenberg, L.A. (1977). Nature 267, 707.
14. Tada, T., Nonaka, M., Okumura, K., Taniguchi, M., and Tokuhisa, T. Leukocyte Culture Conference, in press.
15. Taniguchi, M., Tada, T., and Tokuhisa, T. (1976). J. Exp. Med. 144, 20.

MURINE CYTOLYTIC T-CELL LINES : STABILITY OF FUNCTIONAL
PHENOTYPE AND EXPRESSION OF CELL SURFACE MARKERS[1]

Markus Nabholz,[2] Marcel North,[2] Howard Engers,[3] Dino
Collavo,[2,4] Harald von Boehmer,[5] Werner Haas,[5] Hans Hengartner[5]
and Ian F.C. McKenzie[6]

Genetics Unit[2] and Dept. of Immunology[3], Swiss Institute for
Experimental Cancer Research, CH-1066 Epalinges s/Lausanne,
Laboratory of Experimental Oncology, Institute of Pathological
Anatomy, University of Padua[4], Basel Institute of Immunology[5],
Department of Medicine, University of Melbourne[6].

ABSTRACT   The stability of the lytic activity of two
cloned murine cytolytic T-cell lines was investigated
by analysis of subclones. In one line a large degree of
interclonal variation persisted even after repeated subcloning. Variation among subclones of the other line was
lower. The frequency of totally inactive variants does
not exceed a few percent in subclones of either line
several months after derivation. These lines express
Thy-1 and Ly-2 antigens but not Ly-1. Initial expression
of Ly-3 was lost in one line.

INTRODUCTION

Establishment of clonable cell-lines which stably express
T-lymphocyte functions would greatly expand the possible
approaches to the study of the mechanisms involved. It would,
in particular, provide us with a source material for an analysis of these functions by means of somatic cell genetics.
Attempts to derive cytolytically active T-cell lines by transformation with oncogenic DNA- or RNA-viruses, or by somatic
cell hybridization with tumor derived cell lines have, so far,
been unsuccessful. Recently, however, several groups have
reported that when murine spleen cells are first stimulated
with antigen and then transfered to medium containing supernatant from concanavalin A (Con A) stimulated mouse or rat
spleen cells (Con A supernatant = CS) long term proliferation

[1]This work was supported by grants from the
Fonds National Suisse de la Recherche Scientifique.

of cytolytic T-lymphocytes can be obtained. Such cell populations have been established from cells immunized first in vivo
and then restimulated in vitro with allogeneic tumor cells (1),
from female cells primed similarly with syngeneic male cells
(2), or from cultures of naive spleen cells repeatedly stimulated with allogeneic leukocytes (3).

They grow, apparently, indefinitely and maintain, in the
majority of cases, their cytolytic activity. Cloned lines can
be established from them by plating them in soft agar or by
limiting dilution in liquid cultures (2,3,4). We have derived
a number of such lines and maintained them for up to 500 days
after transfer to CS-medium. As our principal aim is to use
such cells as source material for an analysis of T-cell functions by means of somatic cell genetics we have sought to
determine whether such an approach is feasible by obtaining
information on (1) the stability of phenotypic expression of
the T-cell functions investigated, i.e. in our case, specific
determinant recognition and cytolytic activity and (2) the
expression of cell surface markers which may possibly be related to the cytolytic phenotype of these cells.

MATERIALS AND METHODS

Cytolytic Cell Lines and Culture Methods. The origin and
methods of derivation of the cell populations and cell lines
used in the experiments described here have been reported in
earlier publications. DA-7 is a cloned line derived from
(AKR x DBA/2)Fl cells originally stimulated with C57Bl/6 (B6)
cells (3). The B6.1 clone stems from a culture of female B6
cells immunized in vivo and restimulated in vitro with syngeneic male cells (2). These lines and their subclones depend
on CS (20%) for growth. Cell lines were cloned in semi-solid
agar, cells, or by limiting dilution, in wells of flat-bottom
micro-titer plates. In both cases feeder layers of irradiated
peritoneal exudate cells were used. The number of wells with
growth when different cell concentrations are plated follows
Poisson statistics. Details have been reported elsewhere (2,3).

Assay for Cytolytic Activity. Cytolytic activity of the
cell lines was measured as previously described (5) in a ^{51}Cr
release assay (6) against 10^4 targets (tumor cell lines or
LPS-blasts (7)).

To assay the cytolytic activity of large numbers of individual clones the cytolytic cell lines were plated as for
cloning at a concentration of 1 cell/well. After 10 to 15 days

cells from individual wells were transferred to round bottom
micro-titer plates, and their activity assayed against 10^4
^{51}Cr-labelled targets for 5 hrs.

Antisera and Monoclonal Antibodies. The following alloantisera were used : C3H anti-CE (Ly-1.2), C57BR anti-CE
(Ly-2.1), (C3H x BDP)F1 anti-B10.BR (Ly-2.2), (CBA x SJL)F1
anti-C58 (Ly-3.1) and C58 anti-CE (Ly-3.2). The production
and properties of these reagents are described elsewhere (8,9)
Origin and specificity of the monoclonal antibodies used is
given in table 4.

Micro-Absorption and Micro-Cytotoxicity Assays (Complement mediated lysis). In 50 μl of antiserum diluted to the
lowest concentration giving maximal killing on the test cells
were absorbed essentially as described previously (10). The
activity of absorbed antisera and monoclonal antibodies was
tested in a microcytotoxicity test essentially as described
by Amos et al. (11). Unabsorbed and agarose absorbed rabbit
serum was used as complement   with the cytolytic cell lines
and normal cells, respectively.

RESULTS

Functional Stability of the Cytolytic T-Cell Lines.

Quantitative Variation of Cytolytic Activity among
Subclones of DA-7 and B6.1. Three generations of subclones
were derived from DA-7. The first and second subcloning were
carried out in soft agar and the plating efficiency was .5
and 2% respectively with 500 or 1000 cells/30mm dish. The
third subcloning by limiting dilution gave a plating efficiency of approximately 80%. The cytolytic activity of a number
of clones derived from each cloning step was tested on the
C57B1/6 derived thymoma EL-4. The results (Fig.1) clearly demonstrate that a large degree of quantitative variation in
the cytolytic activity was regenerated relatively rapidly
within each subclone. The activity of most subclones remained
quite stable over one to several months, but some quantitative
fluctuations in the relative strengh of the different clones
were observed. One subclone, DA-7.8, displayed high levels of
activity for the first three months after isolation. Its lytic
potential then rapidly declined and was undetectable 2 months
later, even in the presence of the lectins PHA or Con A, which

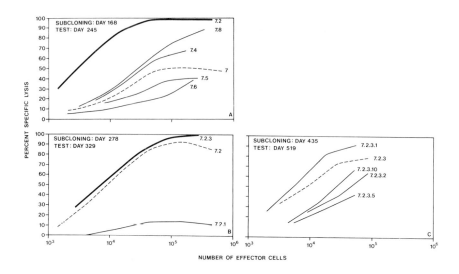

FIGURE 1. Quantitative variation of lytic activity in three generations of subclones of DA-7. In each panel the activity of the parental clone (---) is compared to that of the subclones derived from it, including the clone (heavy lines) from which the next generation of subclones was derived.

were added to circumvent the requirement for specific antigen recognition (unpublished results).

Seven subclones were derived from line B6.1. Comparison of their activity on LPS-induced blasts from various strains showed that the line and its active subclones kill specifically both male target cells from strains carrying the H-2D^b allele or cells of either sex from strains carrying the H-2D^d allele (2). Repeated tests on the BALB/c - (H-2^d) myeloma S194 showed that 5 of the subclones had identical lytic capacity, while B6.1.1 gave about 10 fold less activity and B6.1.3 almost none (Fig. 2). Thus, this line appears to be more stable than DA-7 with regard to quantitative variation in lytic capacity when its activity against targets expressing the appropriate determinants is measured. On EL-4, an H-2^b target which does not express H-Y determinants, most of the B6.1 subclones show some albeit much lower activity and the variation among the clones is much greater than with S194 (Fig. 2). We also found substantial variation in the growth rates of the group of B6.1-subclones with identical activity (unpublished results).

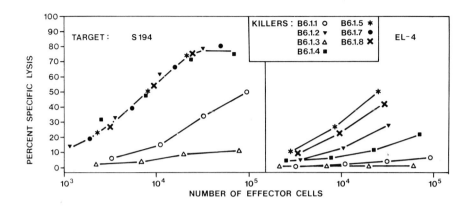

FIGURE 2. Lytic activities of subclones of B6.1.

Apparent Loss of Specificity of Line DA-7.2.3. The specificity of line DA-7 and its subclones was assessed by comparing their activity against a number of tumor targets. DA-7 gave good activity against a number of C57Bl/6-derived tumors but was at least 200 fold less active on P815 (H-2^d), LSTRA (H-2^d), BW5147 (H-2^k) and AKR-A (H-2^k). In further experiments P815 and BW5147 were used as negative control targets. When testing line DA-7.2.3 initially no killing against P815 or BW5147 was observed but at later times the same line became increasingly more active against P815 and S194 (H-2^d), and it lyses P815 now only 2 to 4 times less efficiently than EL-4. It still shows essentially no activity against BW5147. Strong lysis against the latter is, however, seen in the presence of Con A. When the activity of DA-7.2.3 against different LPS-blast targets was measured we found that the line lysed with equal efficiency all targets tested, including C57Bl/6 and (AKR x DBA/2)F$_1$ cells (results not shown).

Qualitative Assessment of the Stability of the Cytolytic Phenotype by screening Large Numbers of Subclones. In the experiments described above one totally inactive line was discovered among a total of 13 subclones of DA-7 and none among 7 subclones of B6.1.

In order to obtain more accurate information on the frequency of such totally inactive variants we set up experiments allowing a qualitative screening of larger numbers of clones. To this end, cells were plated at an average concentration of 1 cell/well. Colony growth was scored by eye and the activity

of the cells in the individual wells was tested 10 to 15 days
after plating. Although the plating efficiency varies from experiment to experiment the frequency of wells with growth at
different cell concentrations follows Poisson statistics (2).
Fig. 3 shows the data obtained from one such experiment.

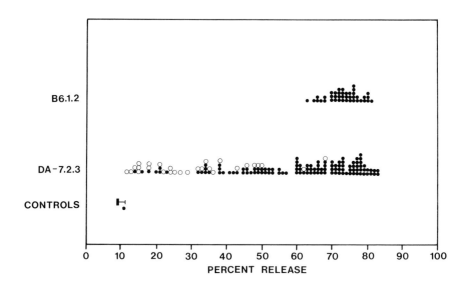

FIGURE 3. Lytic activities of single colonies derived
from DA-7.2.3 and B6.1.2 against S194. Empty symbols indicate
wells with barely discernible growth. Controls : Mean + 4SD
and maximal release of 68 empty wells.

The results obtained so far are summarized in Table 1. The
fact that almost all subclones of B6.1.3, a line with very low
activity (Fig. 2), showed some activity above background demonstrates the relative sensitivity of the method. While some
of the variation in the activity of the DA-7.2.3 derived
colonies is expected from the results described above, it is
confounded in these experiments with the effects of the large
variability in colony size. Although larger numbers of subclones have yet to be scored our results demonstrate that in
spite of the large quantitative variation between subclones
of some lines the frequency of totally inactive variants does
not exceed a few percent and may be much lower.

TABLE I
CYTOLYTIC ACTIVITY OF SINGLE COLONIES

Subline	Age[1] (Days)	Plating[2] Efficiency (%)	Wells with growth	Clones[3] tested	Inactive wells
DA-7.2.3	197	90	39	24	0
	263	34	147	122	0
B6.1.2	80	5	30	30	0
	129	12	42	37	0
B6.1.3	80	33	126	108	5
B6.1.7	64	33	31	18	0

[1] Days of culture after derivation of subline.
[2] Estimated from proportion of wells without growth.
[3] Expected number of wells containing a single colony.

Expression of Lymphocyte Specific Alloantigens on
Cytolytic Cell lines. We have tested the lines described here
for the expression Thy-1 and Ly-1,2,3,4,6 and 7 antigens using
conventional alloantisera in microabsorption assays or monoclonal antibodies with direct complement mediated cytotoxicity.
(The use of conventional alloantisera in direct cytotoxicity
assays on the cell lines gives completely unreliable results).
The data obtained in individual experiments are shown in figure 4, and table 2 gives a summary of the results obtained with
the conventional anti-Ly-1,2 and 3 reagents. DA-7 and B6.1 can
completely absorb appropriate anti-Ly-2 and anti-Ly-3 sera,
but do not remove any anti-Ly-1.2 activity. DA-7.2.3 appears
to express a greatly reduced amount of Ly-3.1 compared to
DA-7. Neither DA-7.2.3 nor the non-cytolytic subline DA-7.8
react with a monoclonal anti-Ly-3.1 antibody, but both give
strong reactions with monoclonal anti-Thy-1.2 and anti-Thy-1.1
antibodies, while B6.1.2 is lysed only by the former reagent
(Table 3). DA-7 can also completely absorb anti-Ly-4.2, 6.2
and 7.2 activity (unpublished results).

DISCUSSION

After transfer to CS-medium the cytolytic cell populations gradually adapt to in vitro culture conditions : They
become easier to manipulate, their growth rate, saturation density and cloning efficiency tends to increase. We have reported earlier a case of an uncloned population which was over-

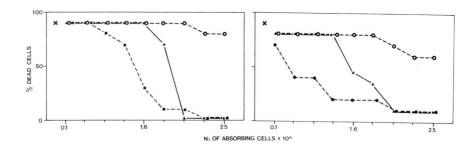

FIGURE 4. Absorption of anti-Ly sera with DA-7. A:anti-
Ly-3.1, target cells:B6.Ly-2.1, 3.1 thymocytes, B:anti-Ly-2.1,
target cells:B6.Ly-2.1 thymocytes. Absorbing cells:B6 (O),
B6.Ly-2.1 (●), B6.Ly-2.1,3.1 (■), DA-7 (▲).

TABLE II
ABSORPTION OF ANTI-Ly ANTISERA[1]

Antiserum	Control[2]	DA-7	DA-7.2.3	B6.1
Ly-1.2	0.8-1.6	>25	ND	>25
Ly-2.1	0.1-0.4	1.25	1.6	ND
Ly-2.2	ND	ND	ND	0.4
Ly-3.1	1.6-6.5	3.0	>25	ND
Ly-3.2	3.5	ND	ND	0.8

[1]Results are expressed as number of cells (x 10^6) required to reduce antiserum activity on thymocytes from
appropriate C57Bl/6 congenic strains by 50 %.
[2]For positive and negative controls sera were absorbed
with thymocytes from appropriate C57Bl/6-congenic strains.
Figures refer to absorption by positive control cells.

grown by one clone carrying a marker chromosome (3) and we believe that within most populations there is strong selection
for variants particularly well adapted to the culture conditions. After some months most populations are easily distinguishable from each other on the basis of their morphology and
growth pattern. Cloned cell lines tend to regenerate a certain degree of variation within the line, affecting lytic activity, growth rate and morphology.

TABLE III

REACTION OF CYTOLYTIC CELL LINES WITH MONOCLONAL ANTIBODIES[1]

Antibody	Origin[2]	Specificity	Thymocytes		Cell Lines		
			AKR	DBA/2	DA-7.2.3	DA-7.8	B6.1
AT83A	a	Thy-1.2	< 1	7	4	4	4
22-1	b	Thy-1.1	7	< 1	4	4	< 1
F-9	b	Ly-3.1	7	< 1	< 1	< 1	< 1

[1]Titres as Log_{10} of highest dilution still giving maximum killing (> 90 % for all positive reactions).
[2]a: F.W. Fitch, Dept. of Pathology, University of Chicago, b: M.L. Gefter, Dept. of Biology, MIT.

Our data concerning the variability in lytic activity among subclones seem to be in contrast with the findings reported by Baker et al. (4). Possibly the cell line that they have studied is more stable in this respect but their published data do not rule out some amount of inter-subclonal variation.

Our experience leads us to interpret any results concerning specificity obtained with tumor target cells with great caution : The lytic efficiency of a cell line on different target cells may vary because it "sticks" better to some due to non-specific surface properties rather than because of differing affinity of its determinant specific receptors.

In spite of the quantitative variation among subclones the frequency of variants without detectable activity appears not to exceed a few percent in sublines several months after cloning. Thus the frequency by which such variants arise may be very low, in particular as they may have a selective advantage over active cells. This is suggested by our observations that clones with low or undetectable activity tend to grow faster and to higher densities than those with high lytic efficiency. Overgrowth by a negative variant may have occurred in the case of subline DA-7.8. In any case it appears from our results that the frequency of variants with a complete loss of functional activity may not exceed that of chain loss variants in some myeloma lines (12,13).

Our preliminary results on the expression of lymphocyte differentiation markers confirm the T-cell origin of the cytolytic cell lines. Expression of Ly-2 and Ly-3 by DA-7 and absence of Ly-1 corresponds to the phenotype expected from the distribution of these antigens on normal alloreactive T-cells.

Line B6.1, derived from an anti-syngeneic male killer cell population expresses the same Ly antigens.

The fact that DA-7.2.3 still is able to absorb anti-Ly-
2.1 but not anti-Ly-3.1 and that this line as well as DA-7.8
do not react with a monoclonal anti-Ly-3.1 antibody may indicate that loss of expression of this antigen occurs commonly
in long term cytolytic cell lines. But we cannot yet draw any
implications concerning the role of this antigen in the cytolytic function as we have not tested these cell lines for the
expression of the Ly-3.2 allele contributed by the DBA/2
parent.

ACKNOWLEDGMENTS

We thank Drs F.W. Fitch and M.L. Gefter for generous
gifts of monoclonal antibodies and hybridomas. Rats were
a gift of Sandoz Co, Basel. Catherine Dysli and Josiane Duc
typed the manuscript and P. Dubied prepared the figures.

REFERENCES

1. Gillis, S., and Smith, K.A. (1977). Nature 268, 154.
2. v. Boehmer, H., Hengartner, H., Nabholz, M., Lenhardt, W.,
    Schreier, M.H., Haas, W. (1979). Eur. J.Immunol., in press.
3. Nabholz, M., Engers, H.D., Collavo, D., North, M. (1978).
    Current topics in Microbiology and Immunology 81, 176.
4. Baker, P.E., Gillis, S., and Smith, K.A. (1979)
    J. Exp. Med. 149, 273.
5. Nabholz, M., Vives, J., Young, H.M., Meo, T., Miggiano, V.,
    Rijnbeck, A.M., Schreffler, D.C. (1974).Eur.J.Immunol.4,378.
6. Cerottini, J.-C., and Brunner, K.T. (1971). In "In vitro
    Methods in Cell-Mediated Immunity". (Bloom, B.R. and Glade,
    P.R. eds.)Academic Press, New York, pp. 369-373.
7. Nabholz, M., Young, H., Rijnbeck, A., Boccardo, R., David,
    C.S., Meo, T., Miggiano, V., and Shreffler, D.C. (1975)
    Eur. J. Immunol.5, 594.
8. Shen, F., Boyse, E.A., Cantor,H.(1975).Immunogenetics 2,591.
9. McKenzie, I.F.C., and Potter, T. (1979).Adv. Immunol., in press.
10. McKenzie, I.F.C., Morgan, G.M., Melvold, R.W., Kohn, H.I. (1976).
    Immunogenetics 3, 241.
11. Amos, D.B., Bashir, H., Boyle, W., MacQueen, M.,
    Tilikainen, A. (1969). Transplantation 7, 220.
12. Coffino, P., and Scharff, M.D. (1971). Proc. Nat. Acad. Sci. 68, 219.
13. Cotton, R.G.H., Secher, D.S., Milstein, C.(1973).Eur.J.Imm.3,135.

INDUCTION OF CONTINUOUS CYTOTOXIC T
CELL LINES TO SYNGENEIC PLASMACYTOMA ANTIGENS[1]

Janis V. Giorgi and Noel L. Warner

Departments of Pathology and Medicine
University of New Mexico School of Medicine
Albuquerque, New Mexico 87131

ABSTRACT: A variety of tumor associated antigens have
been detected on plasma cell tumors (PCTs). In an
attempt to obtain homogeneous populations of cytotoxic
T cells which are specific for individual PCT antigens,
several continuous cytotoxic T lymphocyte lines (CTLLs)
have been generated. These lines show a substantial
enrichment of cytotoxic activity against the tumor cell
line against which they were generated as compared to
cytotoxic T cells generated in a primary in vitro
induction. In addition, these lines show different
patterns of reactivity from one another when tested
against a range of tumor cell targets which are known
to share antigens in common with the stimulating PCT.
These CTL lines may be of considerable value in further
studies on major histocompatibility restriction of
cytotoxic T cell responses to individual PCT antigens.

INTRODUCTION

A variety of tumor associated antigens (TAAs) have been
detected on murine plasma cell tumors (PCTs) by in vivo
transplantation and humoral immunity studies (1,2,3,4,5,6).
Analysis of the cytotoxic T cell (Tc) responses to PCT antigens and the detailed target specificities against which
these responses are directed has progressed largely as a
result of in vitro methods for generating and detecting Tc
responses against TAAs (6,7).
The antigens which have been recognized on PCTs include
unique TAAs found on individual PCTs (8), oncofetal antigens
(9), PCT specific antigens which are shared by PCTs derived
from several different mouse strains (10), antigens shared by
several PCTs and T lymphomas (11), and PCT specific antigens
which are shared by several PCTs from one mouse strain, but

[1]This work was supported by USPH Research Grants CA22268
and F32 CA0591.

are not expressed on PCTs derived from other strains (12).
The definition of these various PCT antigens has been made
by analysis of the specificity of Tc populations which have
been generated and then tested for cytolytic activity
against various tumor targets. These studies have, in general indicated that each population of responding T cells is
heterogeneous, thereby rendering further dissection of any
specific anti-tumor response relatively difficult, unless
a selective enrichment or cloning of the individual populations could be achieved.

Such an approach has recently been developed for alloreactive Tc populations (13,14), employing repeated antigenic
stimulation followed by continued growth stimulation using
supernatants from Conconavalin A (Con A) activated lymphocytes. This procedure has also been used in allogeneic
stimulations with tumor cells to develop tumor specific
cytotoxic T cell lines (14,15). In these present studies,
we now describe the development of cytotoxic T lymphocyte
lines (CTLLs or CTL lines) against TAAs of PCTs which have
been developed from syngeneic in vitro immunizations. Our
preliminary results indicate that cloned CTL lines would
provide a useful and effective approach to defining and
characterizing TAAs.

MATERIALS AND METHODS

The tumors used in these studies were maintained as
established tissue culture lines in Dulbecco's Modified
Eagles Medium supplemented with 10% fetal bovine serum
(DMEF). The tumor lines which were used (with strain of
origin) were: plasmacytomas: MPC-11, MOPC-315 (BALB/c),
and Cl.18 (C3H); T lymphomas: WEHI-7 and WEHI-22 (BALB/c).
All tumor lines were cultured as previously described (16),
and were used during log phase of growth.

The production of CTLLs was initiated by exposing
spleen cells from BALB/c or (BALB/c x C57BL/6)F1 (CB6F1)
mice to irradiated MPC-11 tumor cells using the conditions
which have been described for induction of primary Tc
responses in vitro to PCT antigens (17). Briefly, these
conditions were to culture 15×10^6 spleen cells with $1.5 \times
10^5$ MPC-11 cells in the wells of Sterilin culture plates.
Each culture contained 4 ml of medium (DMEF supplemented
with 10^{-4} M 2-mercaptoethanol); 40 culture wells were set
up initially. At day 5 after the initiation of the induction, and again at day 10, 3 ml of the medium in these
cultures was replaced without disrupting the cells.

At day 14 of culture, the remaining cells were spun
down and were exposed to fresh irradiated MPC-11 tumor

cells. For this second stimulation, 8×10^6 viable spleen
cells and 1.6×10^5 MPC-11 tumor cells were placed in each
4 ml well of Sterilin trays. The cells were incubated for
9 to 10 more days and 3 ml of the medium was replaced with
fresh medium once during this second culture period.

At the end of the second in vitro stimulation period,
the remaining cells were spun down and continuous growth
in culture was initiated by placing 1 to 5×10^5 viable cells
in 5 ml of TCGF 50. TCGF 50 is DMEF which contains 50% TCGF
(see below), 10^{-4} M 2-mercaptoethanol and non-essential
amino acids. The cells were fed or split every two to five
days in order to maintain their growth using TCGF 50.

T cell growth factor (TCGF) was prepared using spleen
cells from rats and Con A at 5 μg/ml (14). After 46 hours
of incubation, the rat cells were spun out by centrifugation
(1200g, 20 min) and the supernatant was used as TCGF without
further purification.

Cell-mediated cytotoxicity assays were performed using
the CTLL cells as effectors. These assays were performed
essentially as described previously (17). Assays which were
performed to evaluate the cytotoxic activity of cells from
primary in vitro inductions were performed after 5 days of
incubation of the responder and stimulator cells followed by
one day of incubation in fresh medium.

Visual immunofluorescence of the cells was carried out
using the monoclonal anti-Thy-1.2 (H-12) kindly provided by
Drs. J. Ledbetter and L.A. Herzenberg of Stanford University,
using FITC-goat-anti-rat Ig as the second step reagent.
Further cell surface and cell volume analyses were carried
out using the Los Alamos Scientific Laboratories multiparameter cell sorter (18) in order to compare the profile of
the population of cells which was obtained after a primary
induction to the profile of the CTLL populations. Methanol
fixed, Giemsa stained smears of these two populations were
also prepared.

RESULTS

Growth of CTLLs. Three separate CTL lines have been
initiated. CTLL-1 was initiated from a BALB/c anti-MPC-11
induction and was only maintained for two weeks in TCGF.
CTLL-2 was also initiated from a BALB/c anti-MPC-11
induction, and has been maintained at present for 75 days
in TCGF. CTLL-3, initiated from a CB6F1 anti-MPC-11 induction, has been in TCGF dependent culture for 70 days.

After about 11 days of relatively rapid proliferation,
with a doubling time of 32 to 38 hours, CTLL-2 and -3 went
through periods during which proliferation was interupted

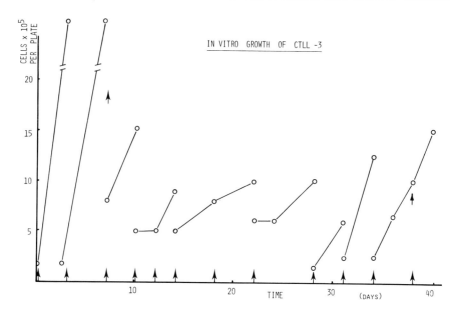

FIGURE 1.   Growth of CTLL-3 in TCGF.   Arrows indicate when the culture was fed or split.

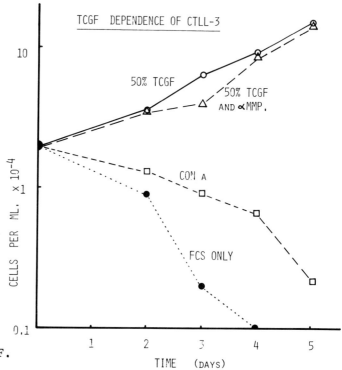

FIGURE 2.
Dependence of
CTLL-3 on TCGF.

and no overall increase in cell number occurred in the
population. The growth of these lines has now stabilized
with an average doubling time of about 28 hours in TCGF 50.
An example of the growth pattern during the first 40 days
of TCGF dependent culture for one line (CTLL-3) is shown in
FIGURE 1. Cultures which grow to a maximum of 3×10^5 cells
per ml and are fed or split every three days exhibit the
greatest population expansion.

The dependence of CTLL-3 on TCGF for growth was demonstrated by plating the cells in different media after 40 days
of growth in TCGF 50 (FIGURE 2). CTLL-3 grew in the presence
of TCGF 50 but did not grow in medium supplemented with FCS
(DMEF) in the absence of TCGF. Furthermore, that the active
factor that supports the growth of these CTL lines is not Con
A itself was demonstrated in that CTLL-3 did not grow when
Con A (2.5 μg/ml) was added to DMEF, and 2-methyl mannoside
(60 mM) did not inhibit the growth promoting effect of TCGF.

Cytotoxic Activity of CTLLs. FIGURE 3 shows a comparison of the lysis of MPC-11 mediated by the CTL lines
after about 2 weeks of TCGF dependent culture and the lysis
mediated by Tc populations generated in primary in vitro
inductions of BALB/c or CB6F1 against MPC-11. All three
CTL lines had more lytic activity than the corresponding
primary Tc populations.

As shown in FIGURE 3-left, 20% specific lysis of MPC-11
occurred at a 20:1 ratio of primary BALB/c anti-MPC-11 Tc
to MPC-11 target cells. In contrast, 20% specific lysis of
MPC-11 occurred at a 5:1 ratio of CTLL-1 to MPC-11 target
cells and at a 3:1 ratio of CTLL-2 to MPC-11 target cells.
CTLL-1 was tested after 11 days of TCGF dependent culture
and CTLL-2 was tested after 12 days. This observation
suggests that these CTL lines have from 4 to 7 times as
many cytotoxic cells as the primary Tc population. In data
not shown, after 32 days of TCGF dependent culture, CTLL-2
retained a strikingly similar lytic activity against MPC-11
with 20% lysis still occurring at a 20:1 ratio of CTLL to
MPC-11 target cells.

FIGURE 3-right shows that an even greater increase in
the proportion of cytotoxic cells occurred in the generation
of CTLL-3. Here, 50% specific lysis of MPC-11 occurred with
a CTLL to MPC-11 target cell ratio of less than 1:1. In
contrast, 50% specific lysis of MPC-11 required a primary Tc
to MPC-11 ratio of 20:1. When CTLL-3 was tested after 36
days of TCGF dependent culture (data not shown), similar
lytic activity against MPC-11 was present.

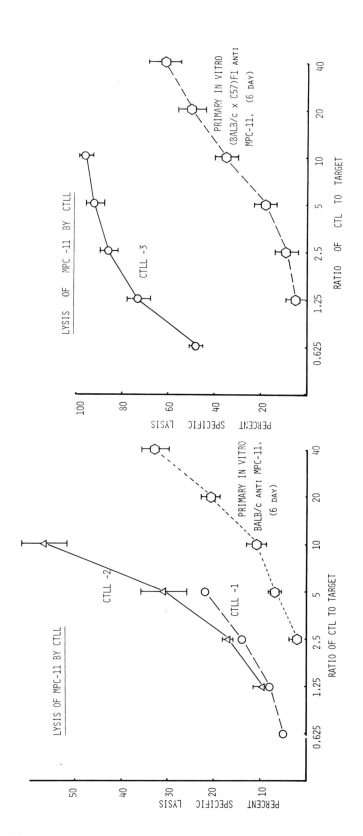

FIGURE 3. Lysis of MPC-11 by CTLL-1, CTLL-2 and primary BALB/c anti-MPC-11 Tc populations (left), and by primary CB6F1 anti-MPC-11 Tc populations and CTLL-3 (right).

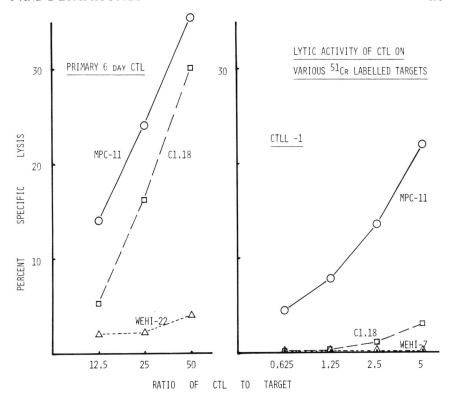

FIGURE 4. Specificity of lytic activity of a primary
BALB/c anti-MPC-11 Tc population (left), and CTLL-1 (right).

Specificity of the Cytotoxic Activity of CTLLs. The
three CTLLs which were generated displayed quite different
patterns of cross-reactivity when tested against a range of
target cells bearing several types of TAAs which have been
previously described on PCTs. FIGURE 4-left shows the lytic
activity of a primary Tc population on MPC-11, Cl.18, and
WEHI-22; FIGURE 4-right shows the activity of CTLL-1 on
MPC-11, Cl.18, and WEHI-7. Whereas the primary BALB/c anti-
MPC-11 Tc population killed both MPC-11 and Cl.18 (a C3H
PCT), suggesting that this population was reacting with at
least one PCT antigen which is shared by MPC-11 and Cl.18,
CTLL-1 killed only MPC-11, and thus appeared to be a population which was reacting either against a unique MPC-11 PCT
antigen, or against an H-2^d restricted PCT antigen. No lytic
activity against the T lymphomas was observed in either the
primary Tc population or in the CTLL-1 population.

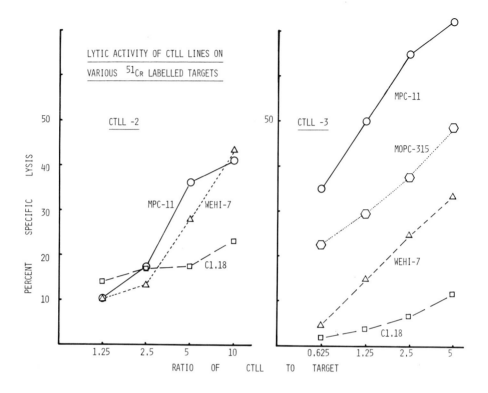

FIGURE 5. Specificity of lytic activity of CTLL-2
(left) and CTLL-3 (right).

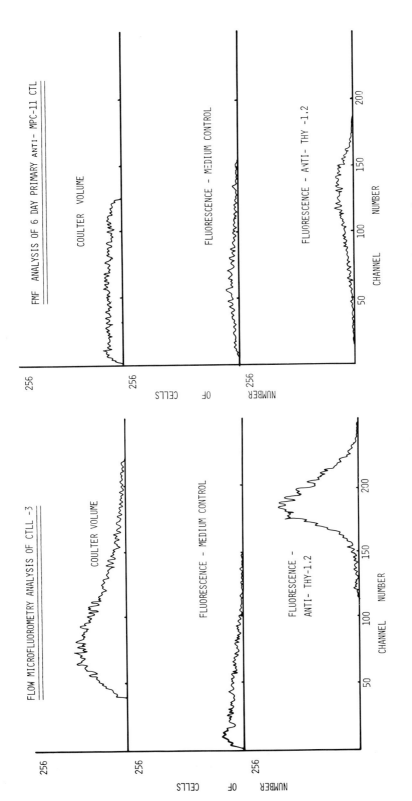

FIGURE 6. Flow microfluoremetry analysis of CTLL-3 (left) and primary anti-MPC-11 Tc population.

As shown in FIGURE 5-left, the lytic activity of CTLL-2 against MPC-11, Cl.18, and WEHI-7 after 32 days of TCGF dependent culture suggests that autoreactivity or a broad tumor specific reactivity may predominate in this population. There was still marked cross-reactivity in this population when it was tested after 71 days of TCGF dependent culture (data not shown).

The lytic activity of CTLL-3 against MPC-11, MOPC-315, Cl.18, and WEHI-7 was tested after 36 days in TCGF and the results are shown in FIGURE 5-right. These results suggest that CTLL-3 may contain a mixed population of cytotoxic cells. Although it is difficult to interpret directly from direct specific lysis data due to the fact that the degree to which these target cells can be lysed varies, the results are compatible with the presence in this population of cells reactive against a BALB/c specific PCT antigen (MPC-11 and MOPC-315), and cells reactive with a TAA which is shared by T lymphomas and PCTs. This latter type of antigen has previously been shown to be recognized by CB6F1 mice (11).

General Characteristics of CTLLs Induced against Syngeneic PCTs. Giemsa stained preparations of characteristic cells from the CTLL-3 population at day 42 of TCGF dependent culture showed a most atypical appearance for T cells. The CTLL cells were relatively large, vacuolated, and contained certain granular structures. In contrast, the cells from a primary in vitro induction after 5 or 6 days of culture with MPC-11 are typically small to medium lymphocytes.

The coulter profile of CTLL after 44 days in TCGF is shown in FIGURE 6-left(top). This profile indicates that the cells in CTLL-3 are relatively homogeneous, are quite large, and have a size distribution which is characteristic of a rapidly dividing population. The immunofluorescence profile of these cells in the presence of a monoclonal hybridoma to Thy-1.2 followed by FITC-goat-anti-rat Ig is shown in FIGURE 6-left(bottom) and indicates that this population is virtually entirely composed of T cells with a moderate Thy-1.2 density.

The coulter profile of cells after primary in vitro induction is shown in FIGURE 6-right(top). These cells are a heterogeneous population of cells which are smaller than the CTLL cells. Although most of the cells in this population are T cells, the average fluorescence of the population with anti-Thy-1.2, shown in FIGURE 6-right(bottom), is only approximately 1/10 that of CTLL-3.

CONCLUSIONS

Experiments described in this report indicate that it
is possible to generate cytotoxic T cell lines against TAAs
of PCTs. The lines described here were developed from
syngeneic in vitro immunizations of normal spleen cells
against irradiated tumor cells, and were stimulated to grow
continuously in culture for at least 75 days in TCGF.

The cell lines which were generated by these procedures
show a considerable enrichment of cytotoxic activity against
the stimulating tumor as compared to the primary in vitro
response from which they were initiated. These results
suggest that many of the cells which survive in TCGF dependent culture are specific cytotoxic T cells that have been
stimulated by antigens during the primary and secondary in
vitro exposures to the PCT cells. Other types of T cells,
such as PCT specific suppressor or helper cells, as well as
a population of nonspecific T cells might also be present
in the proliferating CTLL populations, and further tests to
elucidate the composition of the CTLL populations are
currently underway.

Tests to evaluate the specificity of the three CTL lines
that have been generated indicate that they have different
and restricted anti-tumor specificities. The antigens which
are recognized by these lines are apparently identical to the
TAAs of PCTs which have been described previously (8,10,11).
It must be stressed that at this time, the CTL lines have
not been cloned, and therefore, probably contain several
distinct Tc populations against several of these PCT antigens.
By cloning these lines, we may obtain restricted populations
of Tc against individual antigenic specificities. These
clones would be of considerable value since they would allow
analysis of a number of issues which have been difficult to
approach due to the heterogeneous nature of the Tc populations obtained by conventional in vitro sensitization techniques. These issues include analysis of MHC restriction
(or not) in tumor specific lysis, and definition of tumor
specific antigens that can be recognized by individual
populations of cytotoxic T cells

ACKOWLEDGEMENTS

We are most appreciative of the excellent technical
assistance of Mrs. Eva Barry. We also wish to acknowledge
the participation of Mr. Scott McLaughlin (Los Alamos
Scientific Laboratories) in the multiparameter cell sorter
analyses.

REFERENCES

1. Lynch, R.G., Graff, R.J., Sirisinha, S., Simms, E.S., and Eisen, H.N. (1972). Proc. Nat. Acad. Sci. 69, 1540.
2. Rollinghoff, M., Rouse, B.T., and Warner, N.L. (1973). J. Natl. Cancer Inst. 50, 159.
3. Kolb, J.P., Poupon, M.F., and Lespinats, G. (1974). J. Natl. Cancer Inst. 52, 723.
4. McCoy, J.L., Dean, J.H., Law, L.W., Williams, J., McCoy, N.T., and Holiman, B.J. (1974). Int. J. Cancer 14, 264.
5. Boyer, P.J., and Fahey, J.L. (1976). J. Immunol. 116, 202.
6. Burton, R.C., Chism, S.E., and Warner, N.L. (1978). In Contemp. Top. Immunobiol. 8, (N.L. Warner and M.D. Cooper, eds.), pp. 69-106. Plenum Press, New York.
7. Warner, N.L., Giorgi, J.V., and Daley, M.J. (1979). In Immunobiology and Immunotherapy of Cancer, (W.D. Terry and Y. Yamamura, eds.). Elsevier, North Holland.
8. MacKenzie, M.R., Burton, R.C., and Warner, N.L. (1978). Intl. J. Cancer 21, 789.
9. Chism, S.E., Burton, R.C., and Warner, N.L. (1976). J. Natl. Cancer Inst. 57, 377.
10. Burton, R.C., and Warner, N.L. (1977). J. Natl. Cancer Inst. 58, 301.
11. Burton, R.C., and Warner, N.L. (1978). Austr. J. Exp. Biol. 56, 587.
12. Burton, R.C., and Warner, N.L. (1978). Fed. Proc. 37, 1569.
13. Gillis, S., and Smith, K.A. (1977). Nature 268, 155.
14. Nabholz, M., Engers, H.D., Collavo, D., and North, M. (1978). In Current Topics in Microbiology and Immunology 81: Lymphocyte Hybridomas, (F. Melchers, M. Potter and N. Warner, eds.), pp. 176-187. Springer-Verlag, Berlin.
15. Baker, P.E., Gillis, S., and Smith, K.A. (1979). J. Exp. Med. 149, 273.
16. Harris, A.W., and Horibata, K. (1970). Exp. Cell Res. 60, 61.
17. Burton, R.C., Thompson, J., and Warner, N.L. (1975). J. Immunol. Methods 8, 133.
18. Steinkamp, J.A., Fulweiler, M.J., Coulter, J.R., Hiebert, R.D., Horney, J.L., and Mullaney, P.F. (1973). Rev. Sci. Inst. 44, 1301.

WORKSHOP #15: T and B Cell Hybrids-I. T Cell Hybrids
Elizabeth Simpson and Vernon T. Oi, Department of Genetics,
Stanford Univ Schl Med, Stanford, CA 94305

T cell hybrids with biological function were considered
under the headings: 1) suppression; 2) help; 3) cytotoxicity;
4) other functions.

Suppressor hybrids were described by three participants-
Taniguchi, Kontiainen and Liew. In each case hybridization
was performed with BW5147 as the tumor parent, and the normal
parental lymphocytes were selected as populations of primed
spleen cells with high levels of the desired antigen specific
activity. Taniguchi and Kontiainen both used KLH as antigen;
Taniguchi selected I-J$^+$ cells from primed spleens, fused with
BW, selected hybrids in HAT and subsequently with the FACS for
I-J$^+$ hybrids. Kontiainen fused in vitro KLH induced supressors
with BW, and selected in HAT. Both reported high incidence
of hybrids with suppressor function, some antigen specific,
some not antigen specific, plus the occasional production
of hybrids which enhanced responses. Taniguchi tested hybrid
cell extracts or serum from mice bearing hybrid tumors.
Kontiainen tested hybrid supernatants. Such suppressor factors
from each lab bore I-J determinants, bound KLH but not other
antigens, or immunoglobulin. Taniguchi's factors were V$_H$
positive, Kontiainen's bore both "constant" and "variable"
determinants detected by sera raised against "conventional"
KLH specific suppressor factors. The activity of Taniguchi's
factors were genetically restricted in the in vitro assay.
This contrasted with the lack of genetic restriction shown by
Kontiainen's conventional suppressor factor. Taniguchi had
tested his hybrid lines for cell surface Ia determinants, and
found them positive using cytotoxic anti-I-J sera, following
absorption of such sera with appropriate recombinant mouse
strain spleen cells, and with BW, to remove anti-viral activity.
The hybrid lines also bound radio-iodinated KLH; such binding
could be inhibited by cold KLH. Kontiainen briefly discussed
both helper and suppressor hybrids to NP. Activities of some
supernatants were heteroclytic.

Liew's suppressor lines were developed by fusing BW with
spleen cells from CBA mice immunized with SRBC in such a way as
to induce suppressor cells to the induction of DTH in vivo
against SRBC. The supernatants or serum from mice bearing
hybrid tumors suppressed either expression of DTH (7 hybrids,
6/7 antigen specific) or induction of DTH (3 hybrids, 1/3
antigen specific). The suppressor factor had a MW between 30-
50 K, bore I-J determinants, was not genetically restricted in
its expression, but was very unstable, even in liquid nitrogen.
This instability contrasted with the stability of Taniguchi's
and Kontiainen's suppressor factors.

Discussion of suppressor factors focused on their possible mode of action, since they were specific for multi-determinant antigens. It was agreed that anti-idiotype activity was thus unlikely, and that they were more likely to work via antigen.

Also discussed were the use of other tumor lines as hybrid parents. EL-4 had been used by several people, and found to be relatively unsatisfactory. The failure of everyone to obtain hybrids with cytotoxic function was underlined by Nabholz's finding that even a female B6 α-male cytotoxic T cell clone lost its activity after fusion with BW, although such hybrids had H-2^b markers.

Kurnich discussed experiments in which human allo-killers or antigen specific T cells (from PPD or Tetanus Toxin sensitized donors) were maintained in vitro, stimulated with antigen plus syngeneic irradiated lymphocytes. Such cells could be cloned by limiting dilution on feeder layers and the necessary interaction between cultured cell and feeder cells was HL-D restricted.

Nancy Ruddle reported SRBC and ABA-SRBC binding hybrids made between BW and mouse spleen cells. It was not known whether binding was via a hybrid produced receptor but a molecule could be isolated from rosetting cells which bound to SRBC.

Howard reported CSF producing hybrids between BW and PWM activated mouse spleen cells. Such hybrids produced fewer species of CSF than whole spleen, and the hybrids could be grown in serum free medium in which inclusion of LPS increases production of factors.

WORKSHOP #15: T and B Cell Hybrids-II. B Cell Hybrids
Vernon T. Oi, Department of Genetics, Stanford University
School of Medicine, Stanford, CA, 94305

The original protocol described by Köhler and Milstein
four years ago to generate antibody-producing hybrid cell
lines with desired reactivities by somatic cell hybridization,
has now been modified by many different laboratories to meet
their individual requirements. The initial focus of work done
with hybridoma cell lines was on reporting new hybridoma antibody reactivities, but this approach to generating specific
antibody probes has now been well established and such reports
no longer have merit in and of themselves. The focus of the
workshop was in three areas: (1) improved technologies to increase relevant somatic cell fusion events and to decrease the
time in generating monoclonal antibody-producing hybrid cell
lines; (2) the nature of hybridoma antibody serology; and (3)
uses of somatic cell genetics in other areas of immunology.

The most straightforward improvement in hybridoma technology is the use of non-producing myeloma parental cell lines.
This eliminates the problem of producing mixed molecules in
hybrid cell lines generated from tumor parents synthesizing
irrelevant immunoglobulin chains. Two such non-producing cell
lines are (1) SP2/0 (M. Shulman et al., 1978, Nature 276:339),
and (2) P3X63 Ag2653 (from J. Kearney, G. Hämmerling and K.
Rajewsky). A rat myeloma cell line suitable for somatic cell
hybridization has also been described in the literature
(G. Galfrè et al., 1979, Nature 227:131).

Pre-fusion enrichment of spleen cells reactive with the
ARS-hapten was used by S.M. Robertson, J.D. Capra, and J.R.
Kettman in generating anti-ARS hybridoma cell lines. They
reported increased, relevant fusion events when spleen cells
used for hybridization were enriched for ARS-reactive cells by
in vitro stimulation with dextran sulfate, LPS, and antigen
prior to fusion with the MPC-11 cell line. Post-fusion enrichment for relevant antibody-producing cells was also described.
Specific antigen-binding hybridoma cells, 16 days after fusion
and HAT selection were sorted and directly cloned by the fluorescence-activated cell sorter (FACS) (D.R. Parks et al., 1979,
PNAS, 76: in press). Antigen-binding was visualized with
antigen covalently coupled to fluorescent, latex microspheres.
With electronic modifications, the FACS directly sorted and
deposited single antigen-binding hybrid cells into individual
microculture wells. Other selection systems were also
discussed.

From the beginning, when hybridoma antibodies were first
described, we expected that homogeneous antibodies would provide unique probes of antigenic determinants. J. Howard des-

cribed a rat Ag-B antigenic determinant, which on appropriate
rat red cells is accessible to a cytotoxic hybridoma antibody,
but is masked on appropriate rat lymphocytes. On rat lymphocytes from a recombinant rat strain, which is a recombinant
derived from strains positive and negative for this antigenic
marker on red cells, the lymphocyte determinant is unmasked
and accessible to the cytotoxicity of the hybridoma antibody.
The nature and location of this determinant on the Ag-B molecule has not yet been resolved, but clearly an additional
level of complexity of the nature of cell surface antigens
has been unraveled by this hybridoma antibody reactivity.

In another study of hybridoma antibodies four and probably
five allotypic determinants on mouse γ_{2a} Ig heavy chains were
localized to the hinge region, and the C_H2 and C_H3 domains,
indicating that the gene segments coding for these structures
are polymorphic. Genetic mapping with these antibody probes
reactive with the b allotype of mouse γ_{2a} Ig was done and no
recombination within this genetic cistron was found in the
inbred mice tested.

Finally, W. Raschke described his initial experience with
somatic cell hybridization using B-lymphomas with membrane Ig
as parental cell lines. Generally, it is known that these
lymphomas can be induced to secrete Ig by fusion with a secreting cell line; however, Raschke's initial results show that
fusion of these lymphomas with normal spleen cells does not
give rise to new membrane Ig chains (derived from spleen cell
parents) in the hybrid cells. The ability to extend somatic
cell genetics techniques to generate hybridoma membrane-bound
antibody cell lines with desired reactivities then, awaits
further development, but the approach has exciting possibilities.

All of the abstracts received for this workshop merited
formal presentation, but this was a difficult task to accomplish as the topic around which this workshop was organized was
basically a technique. The questions addressed by the investigations presented involved a number of diverse research
interests and coordinating these diverse interests in a single
workshop was not possible. The technique and approach of
using somatic cell gentics in understanding immunological
problems has been well established; therefore, I believe this
should be the last workshop specifically held on hybridomas.
Like any technique, somatic cell genetic techniques are only
as good as the problems posed by the investigator using the
technique. Most of the abstracts discussed in the workshop
addressed specific problems that would have been better discussed in other workshops.

INDEX

Numbers refer to the chapters in which the entries are discussed.

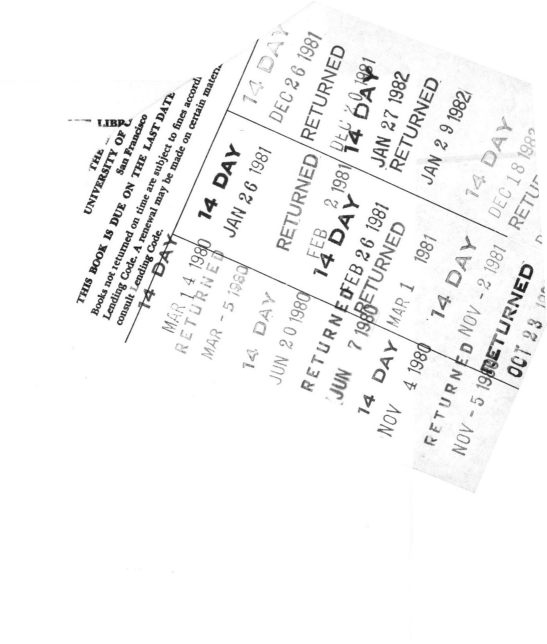